Care of Adults with Chronic Childhood Conditions

Mariecel Pilapil · David E. DeLaet
Alice A. Kuo · Cynthia Peacock
Niraj Sharma
Editors

Care of Adults with Chronic Childhood Conditions

A Practical Guide

SGIM
Society of General Internal Medicine
Creating Value for Patients

Springer

Editors
Mariecel Pilapil, MD, MPH
Assistant Professor, Department of Medicine and Pediatrics
Hofstra Northwell School of Medicine
Hempstead, NY, USA

David E. DeLaet, MD, MPH
Associate Professor, Department of Medicine and Pediatrics
Icahn School of Medicine at Mount Sinai
New York, NY, USA

Alice A. Kuo, MD, PhD
Professor and Chief, Medicine-Pediatrics Health Care Transitions Research Network UCLA
Los Angeles, CA, USA

Cynthia Peacock, MD
Associate Professor, Department of Medicine and Pediatrics
Baylor College of Medicine
Houston, TX, USA

Niraj Sharma, MD, MPH
Assistant Professor of Medicine and Pediatrics, Harvard Medical School
Brigham and Women's Hospital
Boston Children's Hospital
Boston, MA, USA

ISBN 978-3-319-43825-2 ISBN 978-3-319-43827-6 (eBook)
DOI 10.1007/978-3-319-43827-6

Library of Congress Control Number: 2016947511

Printed on acid-free paper

This Springer imprint is published by Springer Nature
The registered company is Springer International Publishing AG Switzerland

The editors would like to dedicate this book to all of our colleagues who spent time away from family and friends to write chapters in this book and to the young adults we care for daily.

In Memoriam

To Brendan Kelly, MD and Alexander Djuricich, MD, two tireless Med-Peds educators and advocates who touched the lives of hundreds of Med-Peds students and residents with their kind hearts, wit, and dedication to their friends, colleagues, and learners. They will be missed.

Preface

Who Are Adults with Chronic Childhood Conditions?

Adults with chronic childhood-onset conditions are a special population with unique needs. As children, they are often termed children or youth with "special health care needs" (CYSHCN). CYSHCN are defined by the U.S. Health Resources and Services Administration (HRSA)'s Maternal and Child Health Bureau (MCHB) as "children who have or are at increased risk for a chronic physical, developmental, behavioral, or emotional condition and who also require more than routine health and related services" [1]. Each year nearly half a million children with chronic conditions become adults [2]. Moreover, roughly 20 % of young adults have a chronic childhood-onset condition [1].

A Note on Terminology

Many terms have been used to describe the population we are covering in this book. Variations to the MCHB term CYSHCN exist, such as "adolescents and young adults with special health care needs (AYASHCN)" or "young adults with special health care needs (YASHCN)." Some prefer to refer to "chronic conditions" or "chronic medical conditions." Also, the terms "youth", "emerging adults" and "young adults" often overlap.

Because of the collaborative nature of this book and the contributions of dozens of authors, we chose to respect the individual author's preferences for terminology. We have tried to streamline and stay consistent in places where it did not seem to matter as much. For the most part, "adolescents" refer to individuals age 14–18 years, "emerging adults" to individuals age 19–25 years, and "young adults" to individuals age 26–30 years.

Audience

This book is for the practicing adult healthcare provider—either generalist or specialist. For primary care physicians, this book provides a new framework for thinking about care of young adults and identifying opportunities to impact patient health outcomes over a life trajectory. For others, this book serves as a reference with approaches for caring for young adults with specific conditions acquired in childhood. While we understand that we have not presented every chronic childhood condition, we chose the most common conditions based on data on CYSHCN from the U.S. Department of Health and Human Services needs or conditions that are illustrative of broader approaches.

This book also discusses the challenges facing this special population of patients as they transition from the pediatric healthcare system to the adult health care system and highlights why this period is often associated with poor outcomes. Ultimately, we provide some strategies to improve health outcomes for CYSHCN and assist adult health providers in better understanding the challenges they face.

In a recent publication, the following questions were articulated regarding healthcare transitions: "Who most needs a deliberate transition plan, at what age should transition planning begin, how should the transfer of medical care occur, what preparation is required, and in what manner should the actual transfer of care take place?" Also, one of the most basic questions remains: What are the effective strategies to engage the adult healthcare system in the care of these young people? Targeting this book to adult healthcare providers will hopefully help bridge the gap that exists between the pediatric and adult healthcare systems.

Understanding and Responding to Emerging Adulthood

This book is grounded in several guiding principles: patients live in the context of their families and communities, social determinants of health influence health outcomes and quality of life, and preventive measures and interventions applied in young adulthood can have a tremendous impact on an individual's life trajectory. The practice of internal medicine has been to date very medically focused, particularly in approaching chronic diseases of middle age and geriatrics. In order to take advantage of the opportunities to change the health trajectories of adults, both without and with chronic childhood conditions, the practice of internal medicine needs to shift towards a preventive paradigm in which the primary care physician provides anticipatory guidance to help patients change health behaviors that could be detrimental.

In this book, we present a model of primary and secondary prevention for emerging adulthood—primary prevention in which all young adults are screened for high-risk behaviors and health needs and secondary prevention in which young adults with chronic childhood conditions are optimized through coordinated care, connections to community resources, and social/family support. The second part of this book details the new developmental period of emerging adulthood and the opportunities for primary care physicians to optimize health during this time.

Transition from Pediatric to Adult Health Care as a Major Determinant of Adult Health Outcomes

Although the importance of transitional care and excellent health care for this population is widely recognized, research regarding the effectiveness of such programs is lacking. A 2012 review of transition program research found no randomized controlled trials or similar strong study designs. It found that introduction to adult care providers or the use of care coordinators may be effective, but the level of evidence was weak [3]. Some have said there is an urgent need for research to evaluate current transitional care practices for youth with SHCN. In general, the needs of young adults and the challenges they face do not receive widespread attention in research or in policy making, although many are starting to pay attention as this is a generation of individuals who may have the worst health outcomes to date.

A recent publication showed some promise, finding that practices that implemented the Center for Health Care Transition's Six Core Elements and utilized their resources were able to conduct transition readiness assessments for more than 70 % of patients [4]. Still, comprehensive transition plans were developed for only about 30 % of patients, demonstrating that much work remains to be done. Therefore, we hope more adult healthcare practices are able to adopt these steps and achieve the triple aim of better healthcare individual outcomes, better population health, and reduced costs [5].

In order to implement these steps for the excellent care of adults with childhood-onset chronic conditions, there is also the requirement that physicians and other healthcare professionals develop the knowledge and skills required to provide high quality, developmentally appropriate health care to this population. Young adults with childhood-onset chronic conditions are very different than typical adult patients, and therefore adult providers may need specialized training to care for them [3]. Adult providers have cited concerns about their ability to provide needed care coordination and social supports (e.g., social workers) that are thought to be more available in pediatric settings and about financial constraints from payers that may prevent them from spending sufficient time with newly transitioned youth. Training and education, as well as structural reforms, may be needed to overcome this problem. There are several health professional education resources on the "Got Transition?" program website, including links to CME courses, webinars, and online course modules that we encourage all health care professionals working with this population to investigate (www.gottransition.org).

Structure of This Book

This book is organized in five parts. Part I provides a detailed overview of the healthcare transition from pediatrics to adult medicine from both a policy and practice perspective. We review the literature on healthcare transition and describe the efforts of the Maternal and Child Health Bureau (MCHB)-funded Center for Health Care Transition Improvement (Got Transition). In the second part, we introduce the concept of emerging adulthood as a developmental period and provide strategies to the adult primary care provider for providing improved comprehensive care for this age group. Part III is divided into condition-specific chapters, each of which details a specific chronic childhood condition, starting with a clinical case and ending with summary reports that can be used as a quick guide. The fourth part ties very closely to the third and reviews additional clinical considerations that are not necessarily condition-specific, but are highly relevant to the care of many young adults with chronic childhood conditions. Finally, Part V describes certain socio-legal issues adult providers should be aware of when caring for this population.

There are several simple steps that adult primary care providers and their practices can implement immediately [6]:

(1) Meet with colleagues, ideally in their practice and in practices from which patients often transition, to create a healthcare policy statement that can be distributed to young adults and their families.
(2) Use a transition readiness assessment tool to track readiness for adult health care for young adults entering their practice, especially those with childhood-onset chronic conditions.
(3) Ensure direct contact with the childhood primary care provider and other childhood providers prior to or at the beginning of the transfer of care, and obtain all relevant medical records.
(4) Start every relationship with a transitioning young adult patient, in particular those with childhood-onset chronic conditions, with goal-setting and the creation of a comprehensive written healthcare plan.

Most of what is recommended in this book is based on pediatric literature and the care of children or youth who have the disease. Much of the information is derived from consensus statements among experts who have cared for young adults but not from randomized treatment control trials or blinded studies for this specific population of patients. Some inroads are being made to identify the appropriate care for young adults surviving with childhood conditions, but much more needs to be done.

Much more discussion needs to take place on how we care for a generation of individuals who are just recently having their healthcare needs recognized as a national issue. For more information and to use as a resource, we recommend *Investing in the Health and Well-Being of Young Adults*, authored by the Committee on Improving the Health, Safety and Well-Being of Young Adults; Board on Children, Youth, and Families with the Institute of Medicine and the National Research Council [7]. Arguably, this is a population in whom the U.S. healthcare system needs to invest as the returns to this nation could be not only a healthy workforce but also a much healthier economy.

Hempstead, NY, USA Mariecel Pilapil
New York, NY, USA David E. DeLaet
Los Angeles, CA, USA Alice A. Kuo
Houston, TX, USA Cynthia Peacock
Boston, MA, USA Niraj Sharma

References

1. Newacheck PW, Strickland B, Shonkoff JP, Perrin JM, McPherson M, McManus M, Lauver C, Fox H, Arango P. An epidemiology profile of children with special health care needs. Pediatrics 1998;102:117–23.
2. American Academy of Pediatrics, American Academy of Family Physicians, and American College of Physicians, Transitions Clinical Report Authoring Group. Pediatrics 2011;128:82.
3. Bloom SR, Kulthau K, Van Cleave J, Knapp AA, Newacheck P, Perrin JM. Health care transition for youth with special health care needs. J Adolesc Health 2012;51:213–19.
4. McManus M, White P, Barbour A, Downing B, Hawkins K, Quion N, Tuchman L, Cooley WC, McAllister JW. Pediatric to adult transition care: a quality improvement model for primary care. J Adolesc Health 2015;56:73–8.
5. Berwick DM, Nolan TW, Whittington J. The triple aim: care, health, and cost. Health Aff (Millwood) 2008;27:759–69.
6. Institute of Medicine and National Research Council. Investing in the health and well-being of young adults. Washington, DC: The National Academies Press; 2015.

Acknowledgments

The development of this book was supported by the Society of General Internal Medicine. We wish to acknowledge the members and staff of the SGIM Adults with Chronic Conditions Originating in Childhood (ACCOC) Task Force. We also acknowledge the support of the federal Maternal and Child Health Bureau's Health Care Transitions Research Network and Center for Health Care Transitions Improvement in the development of this book.

I am so thankful that we have had the opportunity to put this book together. This book was—as Alice put it—truly a "labor of love." First and foremost, I want to acknowledge my co-editors Dave, Alice, Cynthia, and Niraj who have been a joy to work with. I am a witness to how truly passionate they are in caring for this population and I have learned tremendously from each of them during the development of this book.

I would like to thank my mentors, both past and present. A special thank you to David DeLaet, who first motivated me to go into med-peds and has been an unfailing source of guidance throughout residency and beyond. My love for med-peds, in no small way, has also been encouraged by the mentorship of Eva Waite and Joseph Truglio. Thank you to my division chiefs Joseph Conigliaro and Minu George whose support and enthusiasm enable me to love my job on a daily basis. I am also grateful to work with Daniel Coletti and Cindy Rabey on our transition program—the care and empathy they provide our young adult patients is inspiring.

A heartfelt thank you to my family: my parents, Lillian and Alfredo, for their selflessness and love; my brother Brian, whose kindness and intellect never cease to amaze me; my husband and best friend Matt, who makes each day better than the last; and to our son James—you bring us pure joy.

Finally, I want to acknowledge my young adult patients and their families who inspire me with their strength and courage, and remind me of how much there is to be thankful for.

Mariecel Pilapil

I want to begin by thanking my adolescent and young adult patients. The relationships that I have developed with them over the years have inspired me to advocate on their behalf.

I also want to recognize my mentors and colleagues who have helped to guide me in my journey. As a medical student, I chose to pursue training in internal medicine-pediatrics in no small part because of the example set by stellar residents such as Chad Brands and Tom Webb. As a resident and junior faculty member at the University of Cincinnati, Joe Barrocas, Phuong Le, Frank Biro, and Caroline Mueller were mentors upon whom I could always rely for sound advice. I will forever be grateful to Eva Waite for giving me an opportunity to join the med-peds faculty at Mount Sinai and for her endless support and friendship.

I further want to acknowledge my co-editors. Alice, Cynthia, Niraj, and Mariecel. It has been such a pleasure working with each of them in the development of this book. Their passion and creativity during this project only further demonstrated to me the dedication and enthusiasm each of them have for the care of their patients. I especially want to note how proud I am of the leadership role Mariecel took in assuring this book was delivered on time; it does not seem so long ago that I had the opportunity to first work with her during her second year of medical school.

Lastly, I want to thank my family: my late father Jack and my mother Sandra, for their guidance and support over the years; my wife, Rebecca, who amazes me daily in her ability to so adeptly balance family and work, and my children Jack (age 14) and Allison (age 13), who patiently allowed me the time to contribute to this book. I can finally answer, "Now," to their oft repeated question, "When are you going to be done with the book?"

David E. DeLaet

I have been extremely fortunate in my career to work with outstanding trainees and colleagues at UCLA. My med-peds residents and graduates are a constant source of pride and joy for me and give me optimism that our future is in good hands. Our Medicine-Pediatrics division at UCLA is the result of support from Jan Tillisch and Alan Fogelman, two amazing leaders with a spirit of innovation that I admire and try to emulate. I am also indebted to Eric Curcio, the Medical Director of the Medicine-Pediatrics Comprehensive Care Center, and all my faculty for taking multiple leaps of faith with me when we try innovative models of care delivery. Our med-peds group is truly my academic family.

I must also thank my Maternal and Child Health colleagues, from Michael Lu and his staff at the federal Maternal and Child Health Bureau to my own MCH colleagues at UCLA: Faye Holmes, Bobby Verdugo, Lynette Lau, Mischka Garel, and Tara Crapnell. I am also indebted to Neal Halfon, a visionary leader and change agent of systems of care for children in this country.

Paul Shattuck and his Life Course Outcomes team at the AJ Drexel Autism Institute are great research collaborators and have furthered my thinking on neurodiversity, disability rights, and social justice. When Paul and I started the Health Care Transitions Research Network in 2014, we embarked on a journey to raise awareness in the research community and general public of the challenges faced by families of young adults on the autism spectrum and to encourage new ideas and models of care to bridge the transition from childhood to adulthood.

At home, I could not work on projects such as these without the unwavering support of my husband John, and my two sons, Matthew (age 8) and Noah (age 4). Our own experiences with special education and those of their friends have helped shaped my practice and views on caring for children with special needs.

Finally, I am grateful for the opportunity to care for my patients, both neurotypical and with disabilities. The stories of their triumphs and challenges as they navigate the world of developmental and social services inspire me to continue working to improve the problem of pediatric to adult transition.

Alice A. Kuo

In 2005 I started a clinic to care for young adults with chronic childhood conditions. The medicine and pediatric departments at Baylor College of Medicine in collaboration with Texas Children's Hospital (TCH) recognized this patient population needed assistance establishing an adult medical home. I am encouraged and honored that they have supported my work of raising awareness about young adults aging out of the pediatric healthcare system and their unique ongoing healthcare needs. I am indebted to Dr. Ralph Feigin, who at the time was the pediatric chair at Baylor College of Medicine and the President of Texas Children's Hospital, for it was he who saw that I had the talent to build not only a clinic but a program that would address transition healthcare issues. There are so many who support and passionately believe in the clinic's mission that it would take pages to list them. Advocates, interest groups, local and state agencies, colleagues, patients and families whose efforts helped create TCH-Baylor Transition Medicine Clinic. The clinic's success and national recognition is in part due to them. My daily inspiration comes from patients and their families for who I care for and who continue to challenge me to learn and to teach a new generation of healthcare providers an innovative model of health care. Over 30 years ago, Surgeon General C. Everett Koop brought to the nation's attention that young adults with chronic childhood conditions need assistance transitioning into the adult healthcare system. My colleagues who worked hard on this book realize we still have miles to go to solve this healthcare problem; my hope is this book will spark an interest for other healthcare providers to follow and join us in the effort.

Cynthia Peacock

I would to like to begin by thanking my co-editors. Having the opportunity to work with Mariecel, David, Alice, and Cynthia has been an absolute honor. I have learned so much from each of you.

I must acknowledge all the patients who have motivated me over the years to be a better physician and to work towards improving transition care.

I have been honored to serve as a residency training director for over 16 years. The residents and medical students I have taught during this time are constantly inspiring me to be a better teacher and doctor. In particular, I would like to thank Colleen Monaghan, MD, Kitty O'Hare, MD, and

Ahmet Uluer, DO who are amazing colleagues and leaders in Boston in medical education and transition care. I must include all of my colleagues in the Medicine-Pediatrics Program Directors Association for their friendship over the years.

There are three leaders in particular who have been meaningful in my career. Charles Christianson, MD, was my mentor in medical school who taught me what it means to be an ideal primary care physician. Charles Pegelow, MD, served as my residency Program Director and inspired me to pursue a career in medical education. Gwendolyn Scott, MD, first taught me about the transition of youth born with HIV and motivated me to research ways to improve their care.

I would like to thank my parents, Dr. Dharmendra and Santosh Sharma for their love and for raising me to be the man I am today. Most importantly, I would like to thank my wife, Tanvi Sharma, MD, MPH and our two brilliant daughters, Amari and Aesha, who truly give me inspiration, love, energy, and happiness on a daily basis.

Niraj Sharma

Contents

Editors and Contributors

About the Editors

Mariecel Pilapil, MD, MPH is Assistant Professor of Internal Medicine and Pediatrics at Hofstra Northwell School of Medicine. She is a clinician-educator providing primary care to both children and adults and is developing a multidisciplinary primary care transition program at Northwell Health. She has presented nationally on transition and care of young adults with chronic childhood conditions and is a recipient of the David E. Rogers Junior Faculty award for her workshop on preventive screening on young adults with special healthcare needs. She holds regional leadership positions in the Society of General Internal Medicine (SGIM) and is an active member of the SGIM Task Force on Adults with Chronic Conditions Originating in Childhood.

David E. DeLaet, MD, MPH is Associate Professor of Internal Medicine, Pediatrics, and Medical Education at the Icahn school of Medicine at Mount Sinai. He is a national leader in scholarly activities pertaining to young adults with special healthcare needs and the transition of this population from pediatric-oriented to adult-oriented healthcare systems. He has multiple publications in peer-reviewed journals and has contributed several invited publications on this topic. Additionally, he has been an invited speaker at numerous regional medical institutions on the topic of care of the young adult with special healthcare needs and has developed and presented workshops at both the regional and national level regarding this unique and rapidly growing patient population. He is an active member of the Society of General Internal Medicine Task Force on Adults with Chronic Conditions Originating in Childhood.

Alice A. Kuo, MD, PhD is Professor of Internal Medicine and Pediatrics at the David Geffen School of Medicine at UCLA, and of Health Policy and Management at the UCLA Fielding School of Public Health. She is a national expert on child health policy and healthcare transitions for children with special healthcare needs, currently serving as Director of the Maternal and Child Health Bureau's Health Care Transitions Research Network. She is also the Director of the Transition Committee of the Medicine-Pediatrics

Program Directors Association and has served on the Steering Committee on Pediatric to Adult Care Transition Initiative of the American College of Physicians, the Task Force on Adults with Chronic Conditions Originating in Childhood of the Society for General Internal Medicine, and the Health Care Transitions writing group for the Society for Adolescent Health and Medicine. She is also the founding medicine-pediatrics residency program director and medicine-pediatrics division chief at UCLA.

Cynthia Peacock, MD is Associate Professor of Internal Medicine at Baylor College of Medicine. She is the medical director of the Texas Children's Hospital -Baylor Transition Medicine Clinic for young adults and adults with chronic conditions of childhood that has been nationally recognized as an academic model of care for a population of medically complex patients aging out of a pediatric healthcare system. She also is the director of the Center for Transition Medicine at Baylor College of Medicine. She is recognized nationally as an expert on the care of adults with chronic conditions of childhood and the use of the medical home model in the delivery of transition healthcare needs. She has served on numerous committees in regard to transition health care and currently serves on the Task Force on Adults with Chronic Conditions Originating in Childhood of the Society for General Internal Medicine. Additionally she is Associate Program Director for the Baylor Medicine Residency Program and the former Medicine-Pediatrics Residency Program Director.

Niraj Sharma, MD, MPH is Assistant Professor of Internal Medicine and Pediatrics at Harvard Medical School. He is the Director of the Medicine-Pediatrics Unit in the Brigham and Women's Hospital (BWH) Department of Internal Medicine, Division of General Medicine and is the Associate Director of the Weitzman Family Bridges Adult Transition Program at Boston Children's Hospital (BCH). He also serves as the Director of the Internal Medicine-Pediatrics Residency Training Program at BWH/BCH. He is a national leader in the field of transition medicine with numerous peer-reviewed publications, presentations, and grants in the field. He has built clinical programs to improve the transition process at BWH, BCH, and Partners Healthcare. He has also held a number of national positions, including former Co-Site Director and Cabinet Member of the Got Transition National Learning Collaborative and Director of the Medicine-Pediatrics Program Directors Association Transition Committee. He is currently a member of the American College of Physicians Committee on Pediatric to Adult Care Transition Initiative and the Society for General Internal Medicine Task Force on Adults with Chronic Conditions Originating in Childhood.

Contributors

William J. Barbaresi Division of Developmental Medicine, Department of Medicine, Boston Children's Hospital, Harvard Medical School, Boston, MA, USA

Tara Lynn Barto Division of Pulmonary, Sleep and Critical Care Medicine, Baylor College of Medicine, Houston, TX, USA

Kimberly Carter Bates Internal Medicine Residency, Department of Graduate Medical Education, Gwinnett Medical Center, Lawrenceville, GA, USA

Paul Bixenstine Combined Internal Medicine and Pediatrics Residency Program, University of California, Los Angeles, CA, USA

Peter D. Bulova Department of Internal Medicine, General Internal Medicine, Montefiore Hospital, University of Pittsburgh Medical Center, Pittsburgh, PA, USA

Elizabeth O. Buschur Department of Internal Medicine, Division of Endocrinology, Diabetes, and Metabolism, The Ohio State University Wexner Medical Center, Columbus, OH, USA

Jennifer H. Chuang Craig-Dalsimer Division of Adolescent Medicine, Children's Hospital of Philadelphia, Philadelphia, PA, USA

Daniel J. Coletti Department of General Internal Medicine, Hofstra Northwell School of Medicine, Great Neck, NY, USA

Kamala Gullapalli Cotts Department of Internal Medicine, University of Chicago Medicine, Lagrange, IL, USA

Tara Crapnell MCHB Health Care Transitions Research Network (HCT-RN), Los Angeles, CA, USA

David E. DeLaet Departments of Medicine and Pediatrics, Icahn School of Medicine at Mount Sinai, New York, NY, USA

Tiffiny Diers Department of Internal Medicine, University of Cincinnati Medical Center, Cincinnati, OH, USA

Miguel X. Escalon Department of Rehabilitation Medicine, Icahn School of Medicine at Mount Sinai, New York, NY, USA

Ellen Fremion Department of Internal Medicine and Pediatrics, Baylor College of Medicine, Houston, TX, USA

Elba Y. Gerena Maldonado Montana Providence Health and Services, Montana Spine and Pain Center, Missoula, MT, USA

Christopher D. Hanks Department of Internal Medicine, The Center for Autism Services and Transition, The Ohio State University Wexner Medical Center, Hilliard, OH, USA

Elizabeth B. Harstad Division of Developmental Medicine, Department of Medicine, Boston Children's Hospital, Harvard Medical School, Boston, MA, USA

Kathryn Hassell Division of Internal Medicine/Hematology, University of Colorado School of Medicine, Aurora, CO, USA

Susan Hunt Departments of General Internal Medicine and Pediatric Medicine, University of Washington Medical Center and Seattle Children's Hospital, Seattle, WA, USA

Jill Ann Jarrell Section of Palliative Care and Academic General Pediatrics, Texas Children's Hospital, Clinical Care Center, Baylor College of Medicine, Houston, TX, USA

Kristin M. Jensen Departments of Pediatrics and Internal Medicine, Adult and Child Consortium for Outcomes Research and Delivery Science, University of Colorado School of Medicine, Aurora, CO, USA

Naomi S. Kane Clinical Psychology Health Emphasis Program, Ferkauf Graduate School of Psychology, Yeshiva University, Bronx, NY, USA

Daniel Karlin Combined Internal Medicine and Pediatrics Residency Program, University of California, Los Angeles, CA, USA

Jane Subak Kennedy Department of Social Work and Family Services, Children's Hospital of Philadelphia, Philadelphia, PA, USA

Rose Khavari Department of Urology and Restorative Pelvic Medicine, Department of Internal Medicine, Houston Methodist Hospital, Houston, TX, USA

Ross C. Klingsberg Department of Medicine, Tulane/Southeast Louisiana Veteran's Healthcare System, New Orleans, LA, USA

Alice A. Kuo Departments of Medicine and Pediatrics, Health Care Transitions Research Network, University of California, Los Angeles, CA, USA

Michael Landry Department of Internal Medicine, Southeast Louisiana Veterans Healthcare System and Tulane University School of Medicine, New Orleans, LA, USA

Lynette Lau MCHB Health Care Transitions Research Network (HCT-RN), University of California, Los Angeles, CA, USA

Stephanie Lawrence Department of Internal Medicine, The Ohio State University Wexner Medical Center, Grandview Heights, OH, USA

Jennifer M. LeComte Transition Care and Pediatric Practices, Christiana Care Health System, Wilmington, DE, USA

Jenny M. Lieberman Department of Rehabilitation Medicine, The Mount Sinai Hospital, New York, NY, USA; New York, NY, USA

Barry Love Department of Pediatrics, Icahn School of Medicine at Mount Sinai, New York, NY, USA

Elana Maser Division of Gastroenterology, Mt. Sinai Hospital, New York, NY, USA

Margaret McManus The National Alliance to Advance Adolescent Health, Washington, DC, USA

Deonna Monnahan Department of Nutrition, Seattle Children's Hospital, Seattle, WA, USA

Larissa Nekhlyudov Harvard Medical School, Brigham and Women's Hospital, Boston, MA, USA

Christina Nicolaidis School of Social Work, Portland State University, Portland, USA; Schools of Medicine and Public Health, Oregon Health and Science University, Portland, OR, USA

Cory Ellen Nourie Division of Transition of Care, Nemours Alfred I. duPont Hospital for Children, Wilmington, DE, USA

Linda S. Overholser Department of General Internal Medicine, University of Colorado Denver/University of Colorado Health, Aurora, CO, USA; Division of General Internal Medicine, University of Colorado School of Medicine, Aurora, CO, USA

Kitty O'Hare Department of Medicine, Boston Children's Hospital, Boston, MA, USA; Department of Medicine, Brigham and Women's Hospital, Boston, MA, USA; Harvard Medical School, Boston, MA, USA

James Passamano Sufian & Passamano, LLC, Houston, TX, USA

Anish Patel Department of Gastroenterology/Hepatology, Carl R. Darnall Army Medical Center, Fort Hood, TX, USA

Cynthia Peacock Department of Internal Medicine and Pediatrics, Baylor College of Medicine, Houston, TX, USA

Nirupa Jaya Raghunathan Department of Medicine, Memorial Sloan Kettering Cancer Center, New York City, NY, USA

Tova Ronis Department of Pediatrics, Division of Rheumatology, Children's National Health System, Washington, DC, USA

Faysal Saab Combined Internal Medicine and Pediatrics Residency Program, University of California, Los Angeles, CA, USA

Gregory S. Sawicki Division of Respiratory Diseases, Boston Children's Hospital, Harvard Medical School, Boston, MA, USA

Linnaea Schuttner Combined Internal Medicine and Pediatrics Residency Program, University of California, Los Angeles, CA, USA

Amy Sopchak Sufian & Passamano, LLC, Houston, TX, USA

David S. Stein Division of Developmental Medicine, Department of Medicine, Boston Children's Hospital, Harvard Medical School, Boston, MA, USA

Heather Stewart Division of Pediatric Nephrology and Hypertension, Department of Pediatrics, University of South Carolina School of Medicine - Palmetto Richland Children's Hospital, Columbia, SC, USA; New York, NY, USA

Julie N. Stewart Department of Urology and Restorative Pelvic Medicine, Department of Internal Medicine, Houston Methodist Hospital, Houston, TX, USA

Beth Sufian Sufian & Passamano, LLC, Houston, TX, USA

Gregg Talente Department of Internal Medicine, University of South Carolina School of Medicine, Columbia, SC, USA

Jonathan Tolentino Department of Pediatrics, Stony Brook University, Stony Brook, NY, USA

Joseph Truglio Departments of Internal Medicine, Pediatrics and Medical Education, Icahn School of Medicine at Mount Sinai, New York, NY, USA

Devesh Upadhya Department of Internal Medicine and Pediatrics, Baylor College of Medicine, Houston, TX, USA

Eva Waite Departments of Internal Medicine and Pediatrics, Mount Sinai Medical Center, New York, NY, USA

Stacey Weinstein Medicine-Pediatrics Transition Care Program, Departments of Medicine and Pediatrics, University of California, Los Angeles, CA, USA

Patience H. White Department of Medicine and Pediatrics, George Washington University School of Medicine and Health Sciences, Washington, DC, USA; The National Alliance to Advance Adolescent Health, Washington, DC, USA; Got Transition: the Center for Health Care Transition Improvement, Department of Medicine and Pediatrics, George Washington University School of Medicine and Health Sciences, Washington, DC, USA

Angelica Zen Combined Internal Medicine and Pediatrics Residency Program, University of California, Los Angeles, CA, USA

Part I

Facilitating the Transition from Pediatric-Oriented to Adult-Oriented Primary Care

1 Facilitating the Transition from Pediatric-Oriented to Adult-Oriented Primary Care

Patience H. White and Margaret McManus

Defining Pediatric to Adult Transition

"Transition is the purposeful, planned movement of adolescents and young adults with chronic physical and medical conditions from child-centered to adult-oriented health care systems" [1]. It represents not only the passage from one developmental stage to another (dependence to independence), but also represents the passage from one type of care (pediatric/family-centered care to adult/patient-centered care) and often the change to a different health care setting. Although all youth transit to adult-focused care, usually between the ages of 18 and 21, youth with special health care needs (YSHCN) typically require an expanded process of transition planning to address the exchange of more complex health information, competencies for self-care, transfer of specialty care, and issues related to public program eligibility, decision-making supports, and coordination with community services.

Transition from pediatric to adult health care refers to a set of actions designed to ensure continuity of care between pediatric and adult health care settings and improve health literacy so that youth and young adults understand and manage their own health needs and navigate the health care system. Transition takes place over time, beginning in early adolescence in pediatric settings and continuing into young adulthood in adult settings. It is a predictable life-course change that affects all youth, especially those with chronic conditions. Even if a youth remains with the same provider into adulthood, preparation for adult-focused care is necessary. Because of the mobility of youth and young adults, the likelihood that they will change providers is almost certain, and thus the need to establish a systematic transition process.

Transition Landscape

United States: National Transition Context

Affordable Care Act

The Patient Protection and Affordable Care Act (ACA), passed in 2010, has accelerated interest in transitional care in general. The Centers for Medicare & Medicaid Services (CMS) has

P.H. White (✉)
Department of Medicine and Pediatrics, George Washington University School of Medicine and Health Sciences, 1615 M Street, NW, Suite 290, Washington, DC 20036, USA
e-mail: PWhite@thenationalalliance.org

P.H. White · M. McManus
The National Alliance to Advance Adolescent Health, 1615 M Street NW, Suite 290, Washington, DC 20036, USA
e-mail: mmcmanus@thenationalalliance.org

M. Pilapil et al. (eds.), *Care of Adults with Chronic Childhood Conditions*,
DOI 10.1007/978-3-319-43827-6_1

supported numerous payment and service delivery innovations to improve hospital-to-home transitions. It also established the Community-based Care Transitions Program for Medicare beneficiaries at high risk of hospital readmission [2]. Further, CMS implemented a new health home-state Medicaid plan amendment to improve transitional care for children and adults with chronic conditions, and 19 states and the District of Columbia had implemented this option at the end of 2015 [3]. Additional transition-related efforts in the ACA include support for accountable care organizations, advanced primary care initiatives, and insurance expansions. These have all contributed to the growing national interest in transition, including pediatric to adult transition.

Healthy People 2020 and Title V National Performance Goals

National goals articulated in Healthy People 2020 and the federal Maternal and Child Health Title V Block Grant call for improving transition support to youth with and without special health care needs. As many as 32 state Title V programs across the country have selected transition from pediatric to adult health care as their priority and are in the process of developing 5-year statewide action plans [4]. Although these programs have historically served only children, many of them are beginning to reach out to adult clinical leaders and their professional organizations. They are also starting to establish quality improvement, consumer education, and training efforts that are aligned with the American Academy of Pediatrics/American Academy of Family Physicians/American College of Physicians (AAP/AAFP/ACP) clinical report on transition [5] and the Six Core Elements of Health Care Transition [6] (described in detail later).

Medical Home Certification Standards and Electronic Health Records Meaningful Use Standards

Other national efforts influencing national attention on transition include the 2014 National Committee on Quality Assurance's medical home standards [7], which calls for the practice to collaborate with the patient/family to develop and implement a written care plan for patients transitioning from pediatric to adult health care. The CMS Meaningful Use Measures call for the use of certified electronic health records (EHR) technology in ways that can be measured to improve quality and safety, including the electronic sharing of a summary of care record for patients moving from one setting of care or provider to another [8].

Youth in Transition

Who Are They?

More than 30 million youth are between the ages of 18 and 24 in the United States [9]. According to the 2011/12 US National Survey of Children's Health, 25 % of the adolescent population, ages 12–17, has a special health care need [10]. Although comparable special needs prevalence estimates are not available for the young adult population, ages 18–24, related literature reveals that at least 30 % of young adults have 1 or more chronic conditions [11], and about 5 % of young adults report having a disability that affects their daily functioning [12]. In sum, there are estimated 9 million young adults in the US with a chronic condition, including 1.5 million with a disability, who are transitioning to adult-centered care.

According to the Institute of Medicine, "young adults are surprisingly unhealthy," as evidenced by the peaking of many risky behaviors in the age group, the onset of serious mental health conditions, unintentional injury, substance abuse, and sexually transmitted infections [13]. Despite these health risks, young adults' utilization of health services is significantly lower than adolescents and adults over the age of 25, and, unfortunately, their emergency room use is higher [14]. In 2014, 25 % of young adults in the US were without a usual source of medical care [14]. Despite improvements in insurance access among this age group as a result of the ACA, their connection to health care is tenuous at best.

What is Their Experience?

Several US national studies have examined the experience of youth and young adults transitioning to adult-focused care. According to the 2009/2010 National Survey of Children with Special Health Care Needs, 60 % of youth with special health care needs are not receiving from their health care providers the necessary preparation to transition from pediatric to adult health care [15]. Those least likely to receive transition support are male; Hispanic; Black; low to moderate income; with emotional, behavioral, or developmental conditions; without a medical home; and publicly insured or uninsured.

Published studies both internationally and in the US consistently show that youth/young adults often feel lost, unclear about the distinctions between pediatric and adult care, confused about the logistics for accessing adult health care, and unprepared about assuming self-care and self-advocacy responsibilities [16–19]. Also, from the youth/young adult perspective, certain adult provider characteristics negatively affect satisfaction with their transition experience, including decision-making opportunities, time alone without parents, and providers' social skills (talking, listening, showing understanding, and honesty) [20].

Without transition support, YSHCN transitioning to adult health are not only at risk of dissatisfaction and unnecessary worry, but also at increased risk for poor health outcomes [21]. The literature shows that youth and young adults are often unable to name their own health condition, relevant medical history, prescriptions, and insurance. Their adherence to care is lower, and medical complications are increased. In addition, many reports having difficulty finding an adult provider willing and interested in accepting them as a new patient, particularly those with developmental disabilities, mental health conditions, and complex medical conditions.

Provider Transition Barriers

Both pediatric and adult providers within the US and internationally identify many obstacles to offering transition services. The most common barriers are the lack of communication, infrastructure to support care coordination, time and reimbursement, guidelines, and protocols between the two systems [20, 22–24]. In addition, both provider groups report issues with youth/young adult's non-compliance with treatment—lack of disease knowledge, self-care skills, and independence—and challenges addressing psychosocial issues affecting transition-aged youth and young adults [25, 26]. Both groups acknowledge the difficulty that pediatric providers have in breaking the bond with adolescents who have long been in their practice and the difficulty that parents have in ceding decision-making authority to their youth when they are with adult providers [20, 23]. Conversely, adult providers acknowledge that for young adults with more complex chronic conditions, the lack of parental involvement after transfer to adult care is a barrier to transition [20]. Both the provider groups acknowledge that young adults and parents often have unrealistic expectations of adult providers especially around time and attention [20, 27].

There are also barriers specific to each provider group. Pediatric providers consistently cite concerns about adult health care, including lack of confidence in adult care especially around the comparability and organization of care that youth/young adults with special health care needs receive in the adult system [22, 24]. In addition, pediatric providers frequently report difficulty in finding adult providers [24] and, in particular, those with specialized knowledge about young adults with pediatric-onset chronic diseases, including intellectual/developmental and mental health conditions [20, 28].

For adult providers, research studies point to several transition impediments, including the lack of medical records and follow-up recommendations from their new patients' past pediatric providers [29, 30]. Adult providers cite concerns about their limited knowledge and training in pediatric-onset diseases, adolescent development and behavior, and available community resources [22, 31]. In addition, they are concerned that there are not enough adult subspecialty or mental health providers to care for the young adults they accept into their practices [28].

Transition Models/Approaches and Professional Recommendations

Transition Models/Approaches

Transition models are variable in their structure and provider roles, but they align across broad categories of actions needed to improve transition for youth with and without special needs. They usually offer a common set of services: a designated transition coordinator, patient education and activation, a transition plan of care, and assistance with transfer and follow-up. Models often vary in terms of the timing and duration of the transition intervention, the scope of transition planning (e.g., health care primarily or health/education/employment/independent living), and the patient population involved (typically youth with specific chronic conditions or with complex conditions). Oftentimes transition models are established as separate clinics, typically based on hospital ambulatory settings, located in either the pediatric or adult medical settings where youth at a certain age will obtain the necessary preparation and assistance in moving from one system to the next and can involve being seen jointly by both the pediatric and adult provider.

The action steps within these models fall into the broad categories of preparation, transfer, and post-transfer/integration into adult approach to care. Based on an examination of US and international transition recommendations and systematic reviews, the following summarizes common elements of each of these three action steps:

1. *Preparation/Planning:*
   - Practice policy/approach that is shared with the youth/family
   - Assessment of transition readiness that addresses knowledge of disease and health systems, self-management, and advocacy
   - Plan of care that often includes overarching goals in education, independent living, employment along with supporting health goals
   - Care coordination across many domains
   - Support for independence (e.g., visits alone with health care provider and honoring adult approach to care at age 18), self-management, and self-advocacy through education and sometimes peer support
   - Medical summary and emergency care plan
   - List/assistance with selecting adult provider, arranging initial visit, and sometimes joint pediatric/adult visits
   - Tracking mechanism to assure planning support received
   - Designated member of practice who coordinates transition process in pediatric/adult setting
2. *Transfer:*
   - Transfer package
   - Communication between pediatric and adult provider, including clarification of residual pediatric responsibilities before initial adult visit
3. *Post-Transfer/Integration into Adult Approach to Care*
   - Information/orientation for new patient about adult practice, sometimes including policy, welcome letter, frequently asked questions (FAQs), pre-visit call, and identification of preferred communication methods
   - Follow-up with new young adult patient after transfer
   - Feedback from youth/young adult/family about transition experience

United Kingdom and American Professional Organizations Recommendations

National Institute for Health and Care Excellence (NICE) Guideline, "Transition from

Children's to Adults' Services for Young People Using Health or Social Care Services"

NICE develops national clinical guidelines to offer consistent high-quality, evidence-based care for patients using the National Health Service in the United Kingdom. In 2016, NICE published transition recommendations that offer guidance for practitioners in children's and adult health, mental health and social care services, and education and employment [32]. Their overarching principles call for involvement of youth and their caregivers and the provision of a developmentally appropriate, strength-based and person-centered approach. They also recommend children's and adult's service managers work together to develop [32]:

1. Joint vision and shared transition protocols
2. Early transition planning (ages 13 and 14) with a transition plan
3. A designated "worker" to coordinate transition support
4. Involvement of young people to build independence with parents and caregivers
5. Transfer support and information about the youth's health condition, emergency care, strengths, and future goals
6. Support after transfer to ensure engagement with adult care and services
7. Senior leadership support, and
8. Ongoing feedback, planning and education for all involved.

American Academy of Pediatrics/American Academy of Family Physicians/American College of Physicians Clinical Report on Transition to Adulthood in the Medical Home

In 2011, the American Academy of Pediatrics (AAP), the American Academy of Family Physicians (AAFP), and the American College of Physicians (ACP) published a joint statement describing a recommended clinical approach for transition to adulthood for all youth, not just for youth with special needs [5]. According to this consensus statement, transition planning, "should be a standard part of providing care for all youth and young adults" and "should involve the engagement and participation of the medical home team, the family and other caregivers, and the individual youth should be collaborating in a positive and mutually respectful relationship." Starting early in adolescence and continuing into young adulthood, Step 1 of this practice algorithm begins with a discussion of the office transition policy with youth and families and an assessment of transition readiness. Step 2 continues with a transition readiness assessment and transition plan of care, and Step 3 involves implementing and updating the plan of care to prepare for adult care. Step 4, beginning at age 18, calls for an adult model of care and assistance in preparing for transfer to an adult provider. Step 5 consists of identifying an adult practice prepared to accept the new patient and coordinating the transfer, and Step 6 is documenting transfer completion. In 2016, the AAP reaffirmed their commitment for the principles in the 2011 Clinical Report and, in 2017, the AAP/ACP/AAFP plan to update the original Clinical Report.

To promote implementation of the Clinical Report, Got Transition, the Center for Health Care Transition Improvement, developed a structured approach in 2011, called the "Six Core Elements of Health Care Transition" with sample tools and transition measurement options [6] (described below). From 2011 to 2013, 5 US transition learning collaboratives piloted this approach and sample tools and demonstrated that the Six Core Elements approach and tools were feasible and adaptable for use in a variety of primary and specialty clinical settings and resulted in measurable improvements in the health care transition process [33]. In 2014, the original Six Core Elements were updated based on the learnings from the national quality improvement projects, the literature, and reviews from more than 100 provider and consumer experts [6].

The Six Core Elements define the basic components of health care transition support. Providers can choose to implement all or only a few core elements according to their patients' needs and available practice resources. They can also choose to customize the sample tools to align with practice policy, disease-specific interests, and other patient population needs.

For *adult practices,* the Six Core Elements include: (1) a transition and young adult care policy, (2) tracking and monitoring, (3) orientation to adult practice, (4) integration into adult approach to care, (5) initial visit, and (6) ongoing care.

For *pediatric practices*, the Six Core Elements are slightly different and consist of: (1) a transition policy, (2) a method for tracking and monitoring, (3) a transition readiness assessment, (4) transition planning, (5) transfer of care, and (6) transfer completion (see Fig. 1.1).

For providers who care for youth throughout the lifespan, such as family practitioners and med-peds-trained providers, the Six Core Elements offer ways to transition to an adult approach to care at age 18 and, if needed in the future, preparation for a new adult provider.

Specifically, for adult providers who are accepting a young adult, consider the following ways to implement the six core elements (examples of the tools mentioned can be found at www.gottransition.org): Create a transition policy that will inform the young adult what to expect when coming to your practice, especially around confidentiality and consent, and share with all new young adults with chronic conditions of childhood (YACCC) patients. Create a welcome letter with office FAQs and share with pediatric practices who could offer it to their patients as they are planning to transfer to your practice, or give the welcome letter and FAQs along with the transition policy to the YACCC at the initial visit and discuss any questions they might have with regard to interfacing with you and your practice. As YACCC often do not follow-up consistently and are tech savvy, discuss with YACCC ways that your office can contact them for appointments such as texting them reminders and connecting them to your online chart information if available. If the YACCC does not come with a readiness assessment done by the pediatric office, consider giving a self-care assessment to the YACCC at the first or second visit to learn what aspects of their health and adult health care they do not know. A plan for gaining the knowledge needed from the self-care assessment can be added to their plan of care. This self-care assessment can be repeated during the first year the YACCC is in the practice to be sure they are prepared to take better care of their health. To further engage YACCC in their care, consider giving a follow-up survey asking YACCC how the integration into your practice went so they understand that your practice is interested in their opinion about how to improve the transition process in your practice.

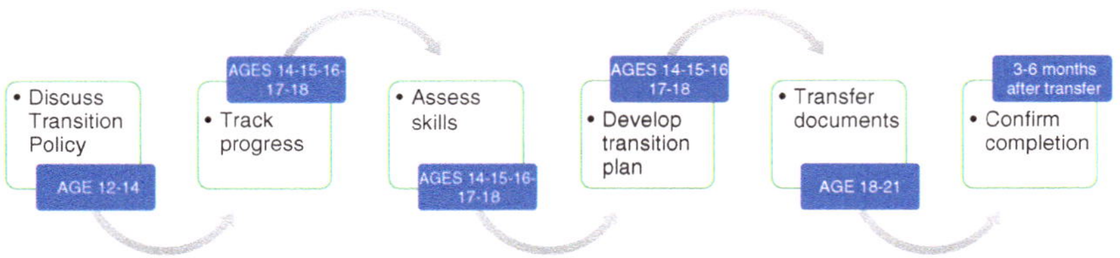

Practice/ Provider	#1 Transition policy	#2 Tracking and Monitoring	#3 Transition readiness/ Orientation to adult practice	#4 Transition planning/ Integration	#5 Transfer of care/Initial visit	#6 Transition Completion/ Ongoing care
Pediatric	Create and discuss with youth/family	Track progress of youth/family readiness for transition	Transition readiness assessment (RA)	Develop transition plan including needed RA skills	Transfer of care with information and communication	Obtain feedback on the transition process
Adult	Create and discuss with young adult (YA)/ guardian, if needed	Track progress to increase YA's knowledge of health and adult health care system	Share/discuss Welcome and FAQs letter with YA/guardian, if needed	Update transition plan with additional skills required	Self care assessment	Ongoing care with selfcare skill building

Fig. 1.1 Summary of six core elements of transition approach and timeline for pediatric and adult practices

Starting a Transition Improvement Process and Measuring Impacts

To transition patients more effectively, a team-based approach is needed where both the pediatric and adult provider teams are engaged with the process. Quality improvement strategies have been shown to improve health care processes and can be used by pediatric and adult provider teams to improve transition care for YACCC.

Starting a Transition Improvement Process

Much has been written about implementing practice improvements, particularly related to the US medical home model [34]. Many of these same steps apply to transition whether in primary or specialty practices or within different insurance schemes such as a US health plan or accountable care organization. There are several guiding principles that serve as a foundation for all transition efforts: they should involve youth and parent consumers; they should be person-centered, and culturally and developmentally appropriate; they require collaborations between pediatric and adult providers/systems; and they should be part of routine care and linked to insurance coverage and other community-based transition supports.

Got Transition: Center for Health Care Transition Improvement has a practice resource on starting a quality improvement transition process [35]. This resource describes four steps: (1) securing senior leadership support, (2) forming a transition improvement team, (3) defining transition processes for improvement, and (4) dedicating time to implement transition improvements. Other key lessons learned from implementing transition quality improvements with pediatric and adult sites and health plans confirm the significance of customizing the tools that will be used for transition planning, transfer, and integration. This process ensures buy-in and enables sites to ensure that their patient population needs are addressed and that practice and state-specific information is incorporated, as needed. Another critical lesson is that starting a transition process may involve distinct patient populations—those who are 18 and older and need to transfer relatively quickly, those who are new young adult patients and who have received no orientation to adult care, and those who are ages 12–14 with whom clinicians have the time to plan for a smooth transfer and integration into adult care. More lessons have been summarized in recent quality improvement efforts directed by Got Transition [33, 36].

Measurement Options for Assessing Quality, Experience, and Costs

A 2014 systematic review of transition measures identified the range of "Triple Aim" measures used in published studies with a rigorous evaluation design [21]. This study concluded, however, that "transition programs are inconsistently evaluated in terms of their impact on population health, patient and provider experience, and cost [21]". Despite the nascent field of pediatric to adult transition evaluation, there are several options for measuring transition performance among individual providers, practices, and networks/systems. With respect to *transition process measurement*, the Six Core Elements include two options for measuring implementation of the Six Core Elements: (1) the "Current Assessment of Health Care Transition Activities" is a qualitative self-assessment method for determining the level of health care transition support currently available and (2) the "Health Care Transition Process Measurement Tool" is an objective scoring method for assessing implementation of the Six Core Elements. Either one of these tools can be used in transition quality improvement initiatives as a baseline measure and then repeated periodically to assess progress.

With respect to *transition measures related to population health*, there are several that could be considered, including self-care skills, adherence to care, and continuity of care (including medications). Other population health measures, such as disease-specific measures, quality of life, and mortality have been used to evaluate transition performance. However, the extent to which transition interventions should be held accountable for potentially influencing these outcomes is a subject of debate. Certainly, these measures are important to assess in terms of the provision of care in general.

With respect to *transition consumer experience measures*, the Six Core Elements includes a "Health Care Transition Feedback Survey" that can be used in full or part to elicit youth, young adult, and/or parent experience regarding transition preparation, transfer, and integration into adult care. Another consumer experience instrument, the "Mind the Gap Scale," has been used in transition studies for youth with arthritis [37]. There is a dearth of measures/instruments for eliciting provider experience in implementing specific transition approaches. One study, using a structured interview format, obtained provider feedback on implementing the Six Core Elements [33]. Specifically, clinicians were asked about the quality improvement process, implementation of each core element, major challenges, and potential for spread of transition. For the most part, published literature is limited to describing common barriers impeding the provision of transition services.

With respect to measures for utilization and costs, there are several options to consider, including changes in the use of ambulatory care, emergency rooms, and hospitalizations. What is intended for transition is that more youth and young adults have a usual source of sick and preventive care; more make an annual preventive/primary care visit; the time between the last pediatric visit and the initial adult visit is reduced; and the no-show rate among young adults is lowered. All of these intended effects are measurable, including their associated costs.

United States Training Competencies Related to Transition

Adult providers, as described previously, are interested in training in the specific diseases they had little exposure to during training [22, 30]. They also welcome consultative support from their pediatric colleagues. An important transition educational effort is being conducted by the American College of Physicians (ACP) Council on Subspecialty Societies (CSS). They partnered with Got Transition and formed specialty society work groups to customize the Six Core Elements for particular condition groups to strengthen internists' ability to care for young adults with congenital or childhood-onset conditions. The specialty societies' subgroups customized at least three tools from the six Core Elements: (1) a transition readiness assessment (for use in pediatric care), (2) a self-care assessment (for use in adult care), and (3) a medical summary/transfer record containing the essential information needed for communication between pediatric and adult clinicians for practices. These new condition-specific transition tools are now available and were developed for use in general and specialty practices caring for transitioning patients [38].

Professional societies have made available modules and curriculum for residents both in pediatrics and internal medicine. The American Academy of Pediatrics offers a series of five case-based educational modules designed to be incorporated into existing curriculum by pediatric residency program directors and faculty. The modules focus on educating residents about characteristics and benefits of the patient- and family-centered medical home, care coordination, care planning, transition to adult care, and team-based care [39]. In addition, the Association of American Medical Colleges has a transition case scenario called *But Tommy Likes It Here: Moving to Adult Medicine* available on their Website [40]. This case discusses the process for a transition for a youth with a chronic illness covering barrier and resistance issues that may be encountered and how a physician could handle the issue. The case suggests areas of discussion such as age-appropriate care, handling of intrusive parents, feelings of the patient and provider, and problem-solving skills. The Medicine-Pediatrics Program Directors Association, through a Health Resources and Services Administration-funded effort in 2013–2015, developed a transition curriculum for primary care residents that incorporate training around the needs of YSHCN and the transition process and shows where the learning objectives demonstrate components of the Six Core Elements (publication forthcoming).

There are examples of training approaches within adult medicine residency programs that can address training in childhood-onset diseases. Studies have been conducted with internal medicine residents about their exposure and preferences around transition from pediatric to adult health care. They have shown that internal medicine residents receive little exposure to transition issues or young adult patients in their training [31, 41], and they prefer to receive their education mainly through clinical exposure and case discussions. Several academic medical centers have started joint pediatric and adult residency training sessions addressing transition and caring for young adults with congenital or childhood-onset conditions, such as Brigham and Women's Hospital and Boston Children's Hospital (The WISHES project) [41] and the George Washington University Medical Center and Children's National Medical Center in Washington, DC. Other training approaches include exposing internal medicine residents to young adult patients in continuity clinics so that they can gain experience in caring for this distinctive age group or offering electives in college/university health clinics so residents can learn if they have a special interest in caring for this population.

Payment for Transition Services Within the United States Health Care System

Payment for the added time, training, and infrastructure necessary to ensure effective transition to adult care is typically cited as one of the most important concerns affecting adult and pediatric providers in the US. Costs associated with transition quality improvements, electronic medical records (EMR) modifications, consumer outreach, and health professional training related to transition and to the care of young adults with childhood-onset conditions are seldom covered, except through grant mechanisms. Non face-to-face services, including care coordination, identification of adult specialists, and care plan development are seldom compensated. To overcome these payment barriers, multiple strategies need to be considered.

Improvements in Coding and Reimbursement

Several important options are currently available for adult physicians to code and are described in a Got Transition Practice Resource [42]. To assess a new patient's self-care skills, adult practices can bill under CPT 99420 so long as they are using a standardized scorable tool, such as Got Transition's Self-Care Assessment Tool [43] or the Patient Activation Measure. To develop or update a plan of care that incorporates transition, adult practices can use either the CPT code for care plan oversight services (CPT 99339-40) or for complex chronic care managements services (CPT 99487-90). To educate new patients about self-care skills, several codes are available, including CPT codes for office visits (CPT99211-15), prolonged services (993544-55), or education and training services for patient self-management (CPT 99860-62). To provide hospital-to-home transition support, there is a relatively new transitional care management services code (CPT 99495-96) that covers a bundled set of face-to-face and non face-to-face services. Other codes that may be part of transition support include interprofessional telephone and Internet consultations (CPT 99446-49), online medical evaluation (CPT 99444), telephone services (CPT 99441-43), and medical team conference (CPT 99366). Coding for services does not equate with reimbursement. However, without accurate coding, reimbursement will never be possible. Practice contract negotiations and affiliation with state ACP, AAFP, and AAP chapters are critical in order to address transition payment gaps.

Because of the tremendous workforce shortages among adult primary care providers, payers and plans may be receptive to alternative payment strategies to expand the availability of adult providers willing to care for young adults with complex medical conditions, intellectual/developmental disabilities, and/or mental health conditions. The set of payment options are described in detail elsewhere [42]. For example, payers may want to experiment with bonuses for adult practices willing to accept a certain volume of new young adult patients with chronic conditions tied with care coordination support and pediatric consultation support. Recognizing the added complexity of serving young adults with high no-show rates, payers may want to consider monthly care management fees to ensure that this vulnerable population is adequately oriented, with active outreach and follow-up. Another payment innovation that payers could consider is a pay-for-performance strategy linked to improvements made in the use of the Six Core Elements or to evidence of shared accountability between pediatric and adult providers for transfer and integration into adult health care.

Infrastructure Funding

Aligning with the increased interest in transition, opportunities for infrastructure investments may be possible by linking with hospital-to-home transition efforts, accountable care organizations, medical or health home efforts, Medicaid performance improvement efforts, state innovation models, care coordination programs, and state Title V programs for children with special needs, many of whom are reaching out to partner with adult providers and state medical professional organizations and training programs.

Conclusion

Many transition improvements are being introduced into clinical practice and training programs to address the inherent challenges in moving from pediatric to adult health care. These improvements—directed at transition preparation, transfer, and integration into adult care/post-transfer—are based on professional consensus recommendations, the new tested quality improvement approach ("Six Core Elements"), and a broad set of US and international transition interventions. Progress in measuring and paying for pediatric to adult care transitions is still in its infancy, however.

References

1. Rosen DS, Blum RW, Britto M, Sawyer SM, Siegel DM. Transition to adult health care for adolescents and young adults with chronic conditions: position paper of the Society for Adolescent Medicine. J Adolesc Health. 2003;33:309–11.
2. Centers for Medicare & Medicaid Services (CMS). Community-based care transitions program. https://innovations.cms.gov/initiatives. Accessed 23 March 2016.
3. Medicaid. Approved health home state plan amendments. https://www.medicaid.gov/State-Resource-Center/Medicaid-State-Technical-Assistance/Health-Homes-Technical-Assistance/Approved-Health-Home-State-Plan-Amendments.html. Accessed 23 March 2016.
4. McManus M, Beck D, White P. State title V health care transition performance objectives and strategies: current snapshot and suggestions. Washington, DC: Got Transition; 2016.
5. American Academy of Pediatrics, American Academy of Family Physicians, American College of Physicians, Transitions Clinical Report Authoring Group. Clinical Report—Supporting the health care transition from adolescence to adulthood in the medical home. Pediatrics. 2011;128:182–200.
6. Got Transition. Six core elements of health care transition 2.0. http://gottransition.org/resourceGet.cfm?id=206. Accessed 23 March 2016.
7. National Committee on Quality Assurance (NCQA). Patient-centered medical home (PCMH) certification standards 2014. www.ncqa.org. Accessed 23 March 2016.
8. Centers for Medicare & Medicaid Services (CMS). Electronic health records (HER) incentive programs. https://www.cms.gov/Regulations-and-Guidance/Legislation/EHRIncentivePrograms/index.html?redirect=/ehrincentiveprograms/ Accessed 23 March 2016.
9. United States Census Bureau. Age and sex composition: 2010. 2010 Census Briefs. http://www.census.gov/prod/cen2010/briefs/c2010br-03.pdf. Accessed 23 March 2016.
10. 12 National Survey of Children's Health. Child and Adolescent Health Measurement Initiative (CAHMI), "2011–2012 NSCH: Child Health Indicator and

Subgroups SAS Codebook, Version 1.0" 2013, Data Resource Center for Child and Adolescent Health, sponsored by the Maternal and Child Health Bureau. http://childhealthdata.org/docs/nsch-docs/sas-codebook_-2011–2012-nsch-v1_05-10-13.pdf. Accessed 23 March 2016.
11. The National Alliance to Advance Adolescent Health. From prevalence data from the National Health Interview Survey and the Substance Abuse and Mental Health Services Administration. http://www.thenationalalliance.org/.
12. Brown B, Moore K, Bzostek S. A portrait of well-being in early adulthood. Washington, DC: Child Trends; 2003.
13. Committee on Improving the Health, Safety and Well-Being of Young Adults. Investing in the health and well-being of young adults. Washington, DC: The National Academies Press; 2014.
14. National Health Interview Survey estimates prepared by the State Health Access Data Assistance Center for The National Alliance to Advance Adolescent Health, 2016.
15. McManus MA, Pollack LR, Cooley WC, McAllister JW, Lotstein D, Strickland B, Mann MI. Current status of transition preparation among youth with special needs in the United States. Pediatrics. 2013;131:1090–7.
16. Plevinsky JM, Gumidyala AP, Fishman LN. Transition experience of young adults with inflammatory bowel diseases (IBD): a mixed methods study. Child Care Health Dev. 2014;41:755–61.
17. Rutishauser C, Akre C, Suris JC. Transition from pediatric to adult health care: expectations of adolescents with chronic disorders and their parents. Eur J Pediatr. 2011;170:865–71.
18. Van Staa AL, Jedeloo S, van Meeteren J, Latour JM. Crossing the transition chasm: experiences and recommendations for improving transitional care of young adults, parents and providers. Child Care Health Dev. 2011;37:821–32.
19. Wong LHL, Chan FWK, Wonk FYY, Wong ELY, Huen KF, Yeoh E, Fok T. Transition care for adolescents and families with chronic illnesses. J Adolesc Health. 2010;6:540–546.
20. Sonneveld HM, Strating MMH, van Staa AL, Nieboer AP. Gaps in transitional care: what are the perceptions of adolescents, parents and providers? Child Care Health Dev. 2012;39:69–80.
21. Prior M, McManus M, White P, Davidson L. Measuring the "Triple Aim" in transition care: a systematic review. Pediatrics. 2014;134:e1648–61.
22. Okumura MJ, Kerr EA, Cabana MD, Davis MM, Demonner S, Heisler M. Physician views on barriers to primary care for young adults with childhood-onset chronic disease. Pediatrics. 2010;125(4):e748–54.
23. Davidson LF, Chhabra R, Cohen HW, Lechuga C, Diax P, Racine R. Pediatricians transitioning practices, youth with special health care needs in New York State. Clin Pediatr (Phila). 2015;11:1051–8.
24. Reale L, Frassica S, Gollner A, Bonati M. Transition to adult mental health services for young people with attention deficit hyperactivity disorder in Italy: parents' and clinicians experiences. Postgrad Med. 2015;127(7):671–6.
25. Heldman MR, Sohn MW, Gordon EJ, Butt Z, Mohammed S, Alonso EM, et al. National survey of adult transplant hepatologists on the pediatric-to-adult care transition after liver transplantation. Liver Transpl. 2015;21(2):213–23.
26. Sebastian S, Jenkins H, Mccartney S, Ahmad T, Arnott I, Croft N, et al. The requirements and barriers to successful transition of adolescents with inflammatory bowel disease: differing perceptions from a survey of adult and paediatric gastroenterologists. J Crohns Colitis. 2012;6(8):830–44.
27. Wright EK, Williams J, Andrews JM, Day AS, Gearry RB, Bampton P, et al. Perspectives of paediatric and adult gastroenterologists on transfer and transition care of adolescents with inflammatory bowel disease. Intern Med J. 2014;44:490–6.
28. McLaren S, Belling R, Paul M, Ford T, Kramer T, Weaver T, et al. 'Talking a different language': an exploration of the influence of organizational cultures and working practices on transition from child to adult mental health services. BMC Health Serv Res. 2013;13:254–64.
29. Hunt S, Sharma N. Pediatric to adult-care transitions in childhood-onset chronic disease: hospitalist perspectives. J Hosp Med. 2013;8(11):627–30.
30. Suh E, Daugherty CK, Wroblewski K, Lee H, Kigin ML, Rasinski KA, et al. General internists' preferences and knowledge about the care of adult survivors of childhood cancer: a cross-sectional survey. Ann Intern Med. 2014;160(1):11–7.
31. Mennito S. Resident preferences for a curriculum in healthcare transitions for young adults. South Med J. 2012;105(9):462–6.
32. National Institute for Health and Care Excellence (NICE). Transition from children's to adults' services for young people using health or social care services. February 2016. nice.org.uk/guidance/ng43. Accessed 23 March 2016.
33. McManus M, White P, Barbour A, Downing B, Hawkins K, Quion N, Tuchman L, Cooley WC, McAllister JW. Pediatric to adult transition: a quality improvement model for primary care. J Adolesc Health. 2015;1:73–78.
34. Wagner EH, Coleman K, Reid RJ, Phillips K, Sugarman JR. Guiding transformation: how medical practices can become patient-centered medical homes. New York, NY: Commonwealth Fund; 2012.
35. White P, Cooley WC, McAllister J. Starting a transition improvement process using the six core elements of health care transition. Washington, DC: Got Transition; 2015.
36. McManus M, White P, Pirtle R, Hancock C, Ablan M, Corona-Parra R. Incorporating the six core elements of health care transition into a medicaid

managed care plan: lessons learned from a pilot project. J Pediatr Nurs. 2015;30:700–13.
37. Shaw KL, Southwood TR. British Society of Paediatric and Adolescent Rheumatology. Development and preliminary validation of the 'Mind the Gap' scale to assess satisfaction with transitional health care among adolescents with juvenile idiopathic arthritis. Child Care Health Dev. 2007;33:380–8.
38. American College of Physicians. Pediatric to adult care transitions initiative. https://www.acponline.org/clinical-information/high-value-care/resources-for-clinicians/pediatric-to-adult-care-transitions-initiative. Accessed 23 March 2016.
39. American Academy of Pediatrics. Module 4: facilitating the transition from pediatric to adult care. 2015. https://www.aap.org/en-us/Documents/clinicalsupport_module_4_medical_home_modules_pediatric_residency_education.pdf. Accessed 23 March 2016.
40. Association of American Medical Colleges. But Tommy Likes it here: moving to adult medicine. July 3, 2012. https://www.mededportal.org/publication/9190. Accessed 23 March 2016.
41. Patel MS, O'Hare K. Residency training in transition of youth with childhood-onset chronic disease. Pediatrics. 2010;126(Suppl 3):S190–3.
42. McManus M, Molteni R. Coding and reimbursement tip sheet for transition from pediatric to adult health care. Washington, DC: Got Transition; 2016.
43. Got Transition. Sample transition readiness assessment for youth/young adults. http://www.gottransition.org/resourceGet.cfm?id=239. Accessed 23 March 2016.

Part II

Care of the Emerging Adult

2 Care of the Emerging Adult

Stacey Weinstein, Paul Bixenstine, Daniel Karlin, Faysal Saab, Linnaea Schuttner, Angelica Zen and Alice A. Kuo

Introduction

When was the last time you saw a 22-year-old male in your clinic? How long was the visit and what issues were addressed? It is possible that certain assumptions were made regarding that individual—about where they lived, their level of education, their personal life, and their health.

For most internists, visits with young adults are often brief and "easy visits." After seeing multiple middle-aged or elderly patients with multiple chronic medical conditions, internists often find that there is not much to discuss in their visits with young adults, and may even view these visits as opportunities to catch up or even get ahead in their schedule. Most young adults are healthy, and these patients are sent on their way after a brief exam and a few routine labs. In fact, browsing through the United States Preventive Services Task Force (USPSTF) guidelines for a 22-year-old male, the guidelines can be summarized in a few words: check blood pressure and screen for tobacco use and sexually transmitted infections (STIs).

But why then, does this 22-year-old male become a 50-year-old obese male who develops diabetes, hypertension, and cardiovascular disease, who ends up on dialysis because of diabetic nephropathy and needs a 3-vessel coronary artery bypass graft (CABG) from severe coronary artery disease (CAD)? What was missed during those routine "easy" visits with him when he was younger and healthy? Was there anything that could have been prevented?

As it turns out, the answer is yes. During the young adult years, there are many opportunities

S. Weinstein
Medicine-Pediatrics Transition Care Program, Departments of Medicine and Pediatrics, University of California, Los Angeles, CA, USA
e-mail: sweinstein@mednet.ucla.edu

P. Bixenstine · D. Karlin · F. Saab · L. Schuttner · A. Zen
Combined Internal Medicine and Pediatrics Residency Program, University of California, Los Angeles, CA, USA
e-mail: pbixenstine@mednet.ucla.edu

D. Karlin
e-mail: dkarlin@mednet.ucla.edu

F. Saab
e-mail: fsaab@mednet.ucla.edu

L. Schuttner
e-mail: l.schuttner@gmail.com; lschuttner@mednet.ucla.edu

A. Zen
e-mail: azen@mednet.ucla.edu

A.A. Kuo (✉)
Departments of Medicine and Pediatrics, Health Care Transitions Research Network, University of California, Los Angeles, CA, USA
e-mail: AKuo@mednet.ucla.edu

M. Pilapil et al. (eds.), *Care of Adults with Chronic Childhood Conditions*,
DOI 10.1007/978-3-319-43827-6_2

for early intervention that can alter the patient's life course. This might not be so apparent to internists, who primarily see older adult patients who have already developed fixed habits and lifestyles and already suffer from several chronic medical conditions. In fact, many adult health conditions originate in childhood and adolescence during critical periods of development [1]. Combined internal medicine and pediatric (med-peds) physicians and family physicians are more familiar with these childhood and adolescent antecedents to chronic medical conditions, as they often witness firsthand the evolution of these conditions as their patients grow older and transition into adulthood. All primary care providers have an obligation to help minimize risk factors that can cause cardiovascular disease, cancer, and other adult chronic conditions, and to help maximize health-promoting protective factors that can facilitate development along optimal health trajectories.

Emerging Adulthood

The period of transition to adulthood, between 18 and 25 years, now commonly referred to as "emerging adulthood" is a distinct phase in life that was first described originally by Arnett [2], and is a unique period involving a transition to independence. This phase is wrought with its challenges and changes that can impact the health of a person for years to come. As described by Arnett, emerging adulthood can be defined as an age of identity exploration, instability, self-focus, feeling in between, and possibilities [3]. It is a state of flux and transition, and one in which medical providers can take part to help navigate young adults toward their future paths.

Unlike other age groups, emerging adulthood is characterized by demographic heterogeneity. For example, most 30-year olds live independently, are in long-term relationships, and have clear career paths ahead of them. Similarly, most 16-year olds live with their parents, have just entered the dating scene, and attend high school. However, those in the 18–25 age group do not fit such generalizations—40 % of them are not enrolled in college while 60 % entered college immediately after graduating high school, 33 % are unmarried but 67 % of them live with their partner, and only 40 % have full-time jobs [4–7]. Such statistics speak to the wide demographic variety of this patient population, and affirm the importance of clarifying such issues with the patient to better understand their life circumstances, many of which may be important determinants of their adult health.

However, there are many issues that are unique to emerging adulthood. It is well known that young adulthood is the time during which people have the most weight gain and increased risk for being overweight in the future [8]. This has been accentuated in recent decades by the development of cheap, processed food high in processed sugars and saturated fats that individuals are more likely to buy due to price and convenience, as they become more responsible for food planning and preparation [9, 10]. In fact, rates of obesity at age 25 have increased by 30 % in recent cohorts [11].

Another major issue in young adulthood that can predict future behaviors is substance use. This often commences with exploratory behaviors in adolescence, but peaks during young adulthood and can predict future behavior. For example, regular alcohol consumption at a younger age is associated with increased problem drinking in adolescence and alcohol use disorder in adulthood [12, 13].

Sexual risk behavior should also be addressed during regular visits in the emerging adulthood period. Although people aged 15–24 years represent only 25 % of the overall population, they account for nearly half of all the new cases of STIs each year [14]. Moreover, it is important for providers to be aware of how new technology may be impacting sexual behaviors. People who seek partners online have reported higher risk sexual behaviors including more unprotected sex, more sexual partners, and more STIs [15–18].

How HEADDSS Impacts Prevention

Much of these behaviors can be uncovered by performing a thorough HEADDSS (home, education/employment, activities, drugs, diet, sexuality, suicide) assessment (Table 2.1) [8, 12, 13, 19–28]. Although commonly taught in medical schools to be used primarily for adolescents, this tool can be instrumental in identifying key patient demographic features, which can reveal potential risk behaviors that would benefit from intervention. For example, such an assessment can facilitate questions about drug addiction, sexual promiscuity, and symptoms of depression, all of which are important issues that if intervened on at the right time, can impact future health. As stated earlier, a routine health visit with a young adult would be incomplete if a provider simply referenced the age-specific USPSTF guidelines; completing a HEADDSS assessment is equally critical during these visits. The HEADDSS assessment delves into topics not touched upon by the USPSTF, but which have clear evidence supporting their discussion in a primary care setting.

The following cases will highlight crucial topics that, if addressed at opportune times, can redirect an at-risk emerging adult and prevent unhealthy habits and lifestyles from becoming into irreversible chronic medical conditions.

Preconception Counseling and the Emerging Adult

Lisette is a 24-year-old woman coming to see you to establish care. When you first meet her, she is a pleasant, well-groomed female. Her vital signs are notable for a body mass index (BMI) of 30, but are otherwise within normal limits. You start to flip through her chart, asking the occasional clarification question about her past medical history, which seems relatively benign, and she does not seem to have any alcohol or substance use problems. She does tell you, when you ask about sexual history, that she is monogamous with her boyfriend, and gives you a little smile, admitting she met him on Tinder. You collect the rest of the history without much standing out, and you move on to the physical exam, which is within normal limits except for her weight. You also do her Pap smear, as she is due, and collect a sample for STIs while doing her pelvic exam. You finish your exam and finalize your electronic charting, and are pleased to note that you are running 5 min ahead on your 30-min new patient exam slot time. As you stand up to leave, Lisette asks, somewhat shyly, if she can have a prescription for "birth control." You've already asked her sexual history, and she tells you she uses condoms, but she and her boyfriend want to start having unprotected sex and she also heard that the pill can help her cycles, which are annoying her with their irregularity. When you ask her about her condom use, she blushes and reveals that her boyfriend only starts using protection halfway through the intercourse act. She shrugs when you ask what her thoughts are if she should become pregnant. You agree condoms might not be a good choice for her, and explain to her a little about the options of birth control. You end up writing her a prescription for some standard-dose oral contraceptives based on her answers. You remind her about using a backup method, answer her last questions, and move on to your next patient.

Lisette's case provides an illustration of many of the routine women's health issues faced by the internist. While obese, she is generally healthy, but is dealing with a multitude of topics that have serious implications for her future health and quality of life, specifically, her choice and pattern of contraception, her obesity and its impact on her future fertility, her attitude about pregnancy, the vague signs and symptoms that could be consistent with polycystic ovarian syndrome (PCOS), and her use of a social media application for dating. Each of these offers a thread that if followed, leading to highly relevant health topics that are frequently overlooked by the busy provider.

First and foremost, Lisette's choice of and pattern of condom use should be explored, as it foreshadows a risk of unintended pregnancy. According to data from the 2006 to 2010 National Survey of Family Growth conducted by the Centers for Disease Control and Prevention (CDC), 37 % of pregnancies were unintended (either unwanted or mistimed) among women who had ever been married. For women like Lisette, between 15 and 24 years old and not married or cohabitating, a full 79 % of live births were unintended. Even when looking at married women ages 25–44 years, almost one in five

Table 2.1 Adapting the HEADDSS for use with emerging adults [8, 12, 13, 19–28]

H Home/Family/Community environment	Important social determinant of health and education	A positive family environment during adolescence (low family conflict, high family warmth, effective child management) predicted higher levels of educational attainment in early adulthood [19] Maltreatment in the home environment "is associated with adverse outcomes in physical health, brain development, cognitive and language skills, and social–emotional functioning [20]"
E Education plans, employment goals	Promotes financial security	Higher level of education directly correlates with lower unemployment rate and higher median weekly earnings
A Activities, hobbies, exercise	Key factors that contribute to health outcomes	The ability to access safe environments for recreational activities may influence exercise activity [21] Physical activity during adolescence predicted change in body mass index (BMI) during young adulthood. Sedentary behaviors during adolescence predicts type 2 diabetes mellitus (DM) during young adulthood [22]
D Diet	Decreases obesity epidemic	Most weight gain occurs during young adulthood and increases risk of being overweight in the future [8]
D Drugs	Prevents addiction behaviors	Initiating alcohol use earlier and heavier alcohol use during adolescence and young adulthood predict a higher likelihood of lifetime substance and alcohol abuse [12, 13, 23]
S Sex, contraception, relationships, reproductive planning, and preconception care	Prevents unwanted pregnancies, STDs	Rates of unintended pregnancy are highest among women aged 18–24 [24] "The pregnancy rate among women attending the trained clinics for pregnancy prevention was about 8 pregnancies per 100 women per year, compared to about 15 pregnancies per 100 women per year among those at the untrained clinics" [25]
S Suicide, mental health	Identifies thoughts and/or behaviors before they have permanent consequences	"Up to 45 % of individuals who die by suicide have visited their primary care physician within a month of their death" [26] Training healthcare providers in suicide prevention can decrease rates of suicide [27] Screening for major depression using Patient Health Questionnaire-2 (PHQ-2) in a primary care setting had 86 % sensitivity and 78 % specificity with a score of 2 or higher; for the PHQ-9, they were 74 and 91 %, respectively, with a score of 10 or higher [28]

The original HEADSS assessment was developed by Dr. Henry Berman in 1972 for use with adolescents

births were unintended during this time period [29]. When considering the factors leading up to unintended pregnancy, Lisette is not unique in her sporadic condom use. Sixty-one percent of all women using condoms do so inconsistently, a number related to a woman's prior experience with unintended pregnancy (she is 40 % more likely to use them consistently if she has been through this experience) and with feeling that avoiding pregnancy is a little or not important (these women are 2.6 times less likely to report consistent use than a woman who believes this is very important) [30]. If Lisette does want to avoid pregnancy, finding a contraceptive method that she likes and will use is important; 95 % of unintended pregnancies occur among women who use contraception incorrectly or inconsistently [31]. At minimum, discussing with Lisette her options of long-acting contraception may be in order, as both oral contraceptives and condoms have high failure rates with typical use at 9 and 18 %, respectively, over the course of 1 year [32]. If Lisette's approach to pregnancy changes or if she continues to have sporadic use of contraception, it may be beneficial to suggest she begin taking a prenatal vitamin on a routine basis.

Another aspect of Lisette's visit that should be addressed is her obesity. Given that you were trying to cover a broad range of her health history and focus on her contraceptive needs, her weight and its implications on her current and future fertility were not a significant topic of your discussion. While she may feel ambivalent toward pregnancy now, she may have a harder time getting pregnant when she does desire pregnancy, with 3 times higher rates of ovulatory infertility for overweight females (BMI $\geq$ 27 kg/m^2) [33]. Once she is pregnant, obese women (BMI $\geq$ 30 kg/m^2) are at higher risk of adverse outcomes, including gestational hypertension and diabetes, pre- and post-term birth, fetal growth and congenital anomalies, cesarean delivery, and postpartum hemorrhage. In one review, the relative risk of fetal death increased 1.21 (95 % CI 1.09–1.35) for every 5-unit increase in maternal BMI, for stillbirth 1.24 (1.18–1.30) and for perinatal death 1.16 (1.00–1.35) [34]. Weight loss prior to pregnancy reduces many of these risks, although the data are less clear on the effect on mortality. Having a chance to speak with Lisette about her weight and other aspects of prenatal care before she becomes pregnant is a opportunity that few providers utilize—only 18 % of women 18–44 years old who delivered a live infant in 2009 reported receiving preconception counseling, although 66 % of women 18–44 years overall had an annual routine check-up [35].

Reproductive planning in general is a crucial topic for women in their 20s and 30s, and Lisette's cavalier attitude is unfortunately common. This age is a time of relentless career pursuit or higher education for some, and fertility is either purposefully delayed or something not even considered for many. Unfortunately, as is well known to many doctors, but less commonly known to patients, biology is rarely forgiving. Using data from the CDC's 2012 report on Assisted Reproductive Technology (ART), women are less likely to become pregnant and then to carry that pregnancy to term as they age, with a drop off that occurs in the mid- to late-30s. While about 40 % of ART cycles for women at age 30 will result in a live birth, this number is closer to 30 % by age 36, and reaches 12 % by age 41. Carrying a pregnancy to term becomes a single-digit feat by the time a woman is age 42 [36]. For those who successfully deliver, the risk of birth defects increases with age. Comparing women 25–29 years to those 40 years and older, babies born to older women had a higher risk of cardiac defects (adjusted odds ratio [aOR] 2.2–2.9), esophageal atresia (aOR 2.9), hypospadias (aOR 2.0), and craniosynostosis (aOR 1.6) [37]. The risk of her 16-week-old fetus having Down syndrome, the most common genetic abnormality, is 1:733 for a 30-year-old woman, 1:265 for a 35-year-old, and 1:60 for a 40-year-old. Bringing up these statistics with a young woman can help her to plan her future.

Lisette's fertility may be additionally impacted by your suspicion of polycystic ovarian syndrome (PCOS). Many young patients may have additional signs and symptoms of PCOS not readily apparent to the provider. Women often depilate unsightly hair, so asking about the patient's grooming habits can be a key part of the history. PCOS is not a trivial disorder. Patients who have PCOS are at increased risk for endometrial hyperplasia and future infertility given their chronic anovulatory cycles, and also can have hirsutism, insulin resistance, and dyslipidemia. Weight loss is a first-line intervention for the underlying hormonal and metabolic dysregulation. Those not pursuing pregnancy benefit from oral contraceptives to regulate menses, and other adjunctive medication for the hirsutism, such as spironolactone, anti-androgens, or topical hair removal agents.

Finally, Lisette's brief mention of the social media application Tinder requires the modern internist to at least have a rudimentary grasp of the habits and knowledge of this demographic. While the technology is rapidly evolving, social media has become a primary means to meet new romantic partners discretely and quickly, and is a mainstay of the generation. In 2013, one in five adults of 25–34 years old and one in ten of all adults of 18 and older were dating online, either through cell phone applications or online dating websites [38]. While some smartphone or Internet applications have respectable reputations, others can be a synonym for a quick way to meet a partner for a one-night stand. Knowing which means which can help tailor your line of questions to screen for high-risk sexual behaviors accordingly. A brief primer to show the diversity and range of choices is listed in Table 2.2, although the technology is rapidly evolving.

Mental Health and Substance Use in the Emerging Adult

Joe is a 25-year-old male presenting to your urgent care clinic with a complaint of palpitations. He is wearing a T-shirt, shorts, and sandals, and sports a few days' worth of stubble. His heart rate is 92, and he appears to be in no acute distress in your office. As you begin your questioning, he describes

Table 2.2 Common social network Internet sites or applications used for dating

Website or application	Type	Description
Facebook	Online website with cell phone application	Networking with all levels of casual friends and acquaintances. Potential for connecting romantically via private messaging or "friending" someone, but generally used platonically
Coffee Meets Bagel and Hinge	Cell phone applications	Daily potential matches sent to your phone, selected from mutual Facebook connections. If both users accept, a private chat opens. Considered friendly, mostly young adult-based dating applications
Tinder	Cell phone application	"Swipe" to search through potential matches. A mutual match between users opens a message. Initially a "hook-up" app, now becoming respectably mainstream for longer term dating
Grindr	Cell phone application	Successful application geared toward gay or bisexual men, with "hook ups" as predominant goal
Match.com	Online website with cell phone application	Longstanding subscription dating website and newer cell phone application with almost 35 million users (2015), for those looking for long-term relationships. Considered more sincere, likely due to the cost associated with signing up
Jdate	Online website with cell phone application	Specific for Jewish singles looking to meet for long-term relationships
OkCupid	Online website with cell phone application	One of the most popular free dating websites, uses extensive data to match profiles of users looking for relationships
Meetup	Online website with cell phone application	Geared toward connecting people with similar interests, not technically a dating website

occasional moments where he feels his heart racing and a sensation of his heartbeat against his chest. Flushing of the face and a wave of nausea overtakes him and he feels the need to remove himself from whatever social situation he is in. After a cursory and benign cardiac exam, you obtain an electrocardiogram (EKG), which demonstrates a normal sinus rhythm with no evidence of hypertrophy. Reassured, you diagnose him with panic disorder and prescribe an as-needed short-acting benzodiazepine. As you are about to leave, he asks if it is all right to continue smoking marijuana when he takes the benzodiazepine. Inquiring further, he reveals that he has been smoking marijuana nightly and occasionally using edibles to help "calm his nerves," especially after he has arguments with his parents.

Joe clearly wants to discuss his family situation further, and you get the sense that this is the first time he has spoken to anyone about this. He says that he was laid off from his first job after college just 6 months ago, and recently had to move back in with his parents. His mother has a long history of bipolar disorder that has recently become more difficult to manage, and he often gets into heated arguments with her. He feels defeated about his work prospects and is having difficulty adjusting to his recent change in environment. You tell Joe that you will put in a referral for a therapist.

Joe's case features many themes that pervade medical care for emerging adults. Mental health disorders, potentially related to a prior family history of such disorders, often present as mild physical complaints and may be self-treated with illicit substances. Moreover, depression and anxiety may represent difficulty adjusting to new degrees of independence or lack thereof, as many emerging adults are moving back home due to poor job prospects.

Mental health disorders frequently present in early adulthood, *with 74 % of all mental health disorders presenting before age 25* and 46 % of all college-age adults reporting a psychiatric diagnosis within the past year [39]. These may be preceded by a family history of mental health disorders, as well as earlier childhood events that contribute to later presentations; for example, about 20 % of college students report a diagnosis of a personality disorder, which typically are present prior to age 18 [39]. Joe's family history of bipolar disorder places him at a 20–30 % risk of developing a major affective disorder in his lifetime; if both parents are affected with bipolar disorder, the risk jumps to 50–75 % of any affective disorder [40]. Similarly, marijuana use prior to age 18 increases the risk of schizophrenia [41].

Joe's complaint of palpitations is not an unusual presentation for an underlying psychiatric disorder. Across all age ranges, somatic complaints of mood disorders are often the primary concern of patients presenting for medical treatment. As many as 45–95 % of patients with depression report only somatic complaints, with a twofold risk of a somatic presentation in patients who do not have a definite ongoing relationship with a set primary care provider [42]. Substance use may often serve as a means of self-medication, as evidenced by frequent presentations of "dual diagnoses." Alcohol is reported as a means of tempering the symptomatology of the extremes of mania or depression, just as marijuana is often used for anti-anxiety purposes.

The legalization of marijuana in Colorado by Amendment 64 in 2012, and its subsequent enactment in January 2014, is emblematic of a growing shift in the use of drugs once heavily controlled or considered taboo. Young adults, similar to the overall population and yet to a greater intensity, have had shifting definitions as to what constitutes "problematic use" of a particular drug. Joe's use of marijuana is not atypical for marijuana users of his age group. A shift from purely recreational use to "instrumental use" (the goal of use being to achieve a desired effect rather than for pure recreation) has led to a greater trend of daily use, especially in young adults who seek out marijuana's anti-anxiety properties [43]. Though overall use has decreased in the past 5 years, the proportion of teenagers who perceive great risk from daily marijuana use has dropped to 36 % from 52 % in 2009 [44]. Even in cases of cannabis hyperemesis syndrome, where chronic daily use is linked to persistent cycles of vomiting, young adults have difficulty linking their usage with ill effects, as they cite marijuana's anti-emetic properties as a reason to continue using it. As such, problematic marijuana use is increasingly difficult to categorize, yet negative effects of chronic heavy usage have been defined, as evidenced by a decrease in IQ by 8 points among daily marijuana users from prior to age 18 [45]. Exposure to marijuana in the critical neuroplasticity period of young adulthood is a risk factor for the presentation of schizophrenia, with earlier use leading to a greater risk of schizophrenia than later use [41].

Changing usage patterns for other drugs are given as examples in Table 2.3 [46]. While problematic drug use was often understood within the framework of addiction, tolerance, and withdrawal, many newer drugs (or newer usage patterns of common drugs) do not have the typical physical manifestation of tolerance or withdrawal, or are used in specific contexts, and thus many young adults do not see their usage as characterized by addiction, and therefore, not problematic. While Joe may not characterize his marijuana use as a problem, he is still certainly at risk for long-term deleterious effects of its use. In addition, although Joe reports using marijuana, he should still be screened for tobacco and alcohol, as these substances are still widely used in this age group.

Underlying many of the psychological stressors is the shifting landscape of employment opportunities for emerging adults. In the years following the economic recession of the late 2000s, the proportion of 18- to 29-year olds holding full-time jobs has dropped to the low 40s [47, 48] which according to the Bureau of Labor Statistics is the lowest proportion since the bureau first started collecting data in the 1940s. Faced with poor economic opportunities in the post-college environment, the emerging adults returning to live with their parents have earned the label of "boomerang children" (Pew Social Trends). In this critical period of identity formation and establishment of autonomy and independence from one's parents, young adults are caught in a difficult situation, where many economic forces are pushing them to rely on their parents for support.

With the advent of the Affordable Care Act, young adults can remain on their parents' insurance plans until age 26. Thereafter, young adults may not often consider a need for health insurance, or may opt for high-deductible catastrophic insurance. Qualitative work [49] demonstrates a perceived lack of value of health insurance for young adults, especially in those who were previously covered under their parents' insurance. Responders frequently stated that they were at a lower risk for health problems and thus the financial burden of paying for insurance was felt to be low value for the actual cost. Lower health literacy among young adults is widespread, with less than a third aware of health insurance marketplaces and less than a quarter aware of the

Table 2.3 Changes in usage pattern of recreational drugs

Drug	Change in usage pattern
Marijuana	Daily usage for anti-anxiety properties. Increasing diversity in routes of administration, e.g., concentrated resin ("dabs"), edibles, lozenges, vaporizers
Stimulants (cocaine, methamphetamine)	Use in work-related contexts for increased feeling of energy and focus
Heroin	Transition from abused prescription opioids to heroin as a cheaper alternative
Synthetic Marijuana (K2)	Increasing usage in areas where marijuana is difficult to obtain. A cheaper alternative with greater potency but also greater proportion of adverse effects
Party Drugs (MDMA, ketamine)	Frequent use in certain social contexts is not seen as problematic, as it is only limited to that context, in spite of significant risk of harm during usage and long-term neurologic changes associated with repeated use [46]

MDMA 3,4-Methylenedioxymethamphetamine

Table 2.4 Paradigm shift for the primary care of emerging adults

Old paradigm	New paradigm
Prescribe birth control and do Pap smear	Explore healthy relationships and reproductive planning
Thinking medically (i.e., ordering Holter on someone with palpitations)	Thinking biopsychosocially (i.e., exploring anxiety sources for palpitations)
Ask about substance use to document them	Actively engage in motivational interviewing and other resources to decrease substance use (recognizing it may be easier to get someone to quit if they have only been using for 4 years as opposed to 40 years)

Medicaid expansion [50]. Though coverage for preventive health visits is mandatory within the Affordable Care Act, emerging adults are less likely to request health maintenance visits. When Joe turns 26 and is faced with difficulty obtaining employer-based health insurance due to poor employment prospects, he is less likely to obtain a sufficient coverage plan and will probably opt for a high-deductible plan, which will be unlikely to include sufficient coverage for mental health services. Fewer opportunities to interact with emerging adults in a healthcare setting, as well as a predilection for urgent care presentations, ultimately translate to an increased importance of discussing underlying health and social issues with each point of contact with a young adult patient.

A Paradigm Shift for Approaching the Emerging Adult/Young Adult Preventive Visit

Primary care providers should recognize these predominant health issues of the emerging adult (18–25 years) and young adult (26–35 years) populations and the potential to optimize the health trajectory over the entire adult life span. At a minimum, mental health issues should be screened for and addressed, given the potential morbidity and mortality from these in quality of life and suicide risk, both now and later on in adulthood. Substance use should be examined as well, and motivational interviewing skills applied with vigor, recognizing that it can be easier to work with a patient to reduce or quit substance use earlier than after decades of use. Finally, unlike in the adolescent period when pregnancy is virtually never desired, contraceptive care should be tailored to anticipate potential pregnancy within 1–3 years; and preconception care should be practiced to not only anticipate a potential pregnancy but also to optimize a woman's health prior to conception to ensure a healthy pregnancy and decrease the risk of birth defects and/or birth complications. Table 2.4 demonstrates the shift that we propose for adult primary care providers in their care of emerging adults.

Emerging Adults with Chronic Childhood-Onset Conditions

Emerging adults with chronic childhood-onset conditions have increased medical and psychosocial needs, and without additional support may experience worse outcomes, compared with other young adults. Emerging adults with complex medical conditions in general have lower educational achievement and incomes, and more limited work experience than their peers [51]. Emerging adults with chronic conditions are also at higher risk for developmental difficulties, unnecessary dependency, and psychosocial delay [52]. However, a successful transition to adult health care may help prevent this inequality in outcomes by increasing a sense of personal responsibility, enhancing autonomy, and facilitating self-reliance [52].

Despite the benefit of excellent transition care for these emerging adults, studies have shown that their transition to adult health care is often poor. In one study only about 20 % of young adults were found to have made a successful transition to adult health care. In another, less than 25 % of young adults reported that they had received appropriate transition counseling [53]. Rates of these discussions may be even lower among minorities. In general, racial/ethnic minorities and those with problems with access to care or gaps in health insurance may have poorer transition outcomes.

Patient-Centered Medical Home

The patient-centered medical home (PCMH) has been promoted as a promising model for care delivery for all patients, in particular adults with chronic childhood-onset conditions. The first Maternal and Child Health Bureau (MCHB) core outcome explicitly specifies that children with special health care needs (SHCN) should "receive coordinated ongoing comprehensive care within a medical home" [54]. The PCMH is a model of primary care transformation that seeks to meet the health care needs of patients and to improve patient and staff experiences, outcomes, safety, and system efficiency—in other words, to achieve the "Triple Aim" [55].

The National Committee for Quality Assurance (NCQA), which offers PCMH accreditation, requires six standards for certified PCMHs: (1) patient-centered access, (2) team-based care, (3) population health management, (4) care management and support, (5) care coordination and care transitions, and (6) performance measurement and quality improvement. According to the 2011 American Academy of Pediatrics (AAP), American Academy of Family Physicians (AAFP) and American College of Physicians (ACP) Transitions Clinical Report Authoring Group, "planned care, as the product of a partnership among health care professionals, youth, and families, has become an essential characteristic of the primary care medical home" [56].

Chronic Care Model and Other Models of Chronic Disease Care

The chronic care model was developed in Seattle by the Improving Chronic Illness Care program, sponsored by the Robert Wood Johnson Foundation. It is one of the most popular models for comprehensive care of chronic illnesses. It uses a systematic approach to restructure medical care to create partnerships between health systems and communities with the goal of improving interactions between providers and patients, and in turn, health care outcomes. There are six areas of emphasis: (1) organization of health care (e.g., removing barriers to care and mobilizing sufficient care resources); (2) community linkages (e.g., creating partnerships with community-based resources and public health agencies); (3) self-management support (e.g., facilitating patient empowerment and skill-based learning); (4) delivery system design (e.g., coordinating and streamlining care processes and workflows); (5) decision support (e.g., providing guidance for providers through the electronic medical records (EMR) and other means to provide evidence- and value-based care); and (6) clinical information systems (e.g., tracking meaningful outcomes and providing feedback to both patients and providers) [57].

Other models have broadened the definition of comprehensive care for chronic conditions. These include the innovative care for chronic conditions (ICCC) model published by the World Health Organization (WHO) [58] and the expanded chronic care model proposed by Barr et al. [59]. These models also incorporate prevention efforts, social determinants of health, and enhanced community participation as core components of chronic disease care [57]. The ICCC also has a larger focus on supporting "positive policy environments" (e.g., partnerships, legislative frameworks, human resource allocation, leadership, and financing) in community and health care organizations [58].

Steps for Caring for Adults with Chronic Childhood-Onset Conditions

We here present our interpretation of the ten essential steps for adult primary care physicians (PCPs) accepting care for young adults with chronic childhood-onset conditions to provide them with the excellent, comprehensive care they deserve ("Appendix"). We assume care takes place in the context of a PCMH that embraces comprehensive chronic disease management as defined by the chronic care model and other models. These steps have been adapted for adult practices from steps for children's practices that serve children with SHCN, such as those created by the national "Got Transition?" campaign.

Step 1: Health Care Policy Statement

The first step for a practice that will be caring for adults with a chronic childhood-onset condition is developing a written health care policy statement for the transition and future care of the young adult. Attention to care transitions is an explicit part of the National Committee for Quality Assurance (NCQA) PCMH designation. This health care policy should be developed with input from young adults transitioning to adulthood. Ideally, it may also be developed jointly with children's practices from which the adult practice often accepts transitioning patients. The policy should explicitly state the practice's expectations of the young transitioning adults and their families, and describe the practice's transition and future care process.

After the policy is developed, all practice staff should be educated and trained with regard to its implementation, including the specific roles of the patient, the family, and the health care team members. The policy should be prominently displayed and readily available to patients and their families.

Step 2: Tracking and Monitoring: Utilizing Clinical Information Systems

As specified in the chronic care model, practices should use clinical information systems to improve their practice [57]. Performance measurement and quality improvement is also part of NCQA PCMH accreditation. All transitioning young adults should be entered into a registry with tracking of data related to achievement of successful transition. Each adult practice should develop its own measures to define success, such as completion of each step of the transition process and improvement in relevant patient disease outcomes. It should also include measures addressing social determinants of the patient's health (see Step 8).

For each patient, the registry should be used to track the young adults' progress and health status. If possible this registry data should be incorporated into the electronic health records (EHR). This registry will enable "empanelment" of patients. This means linking each patient to a care team and PCP [60]. In turn this enables each physician and team to later engage in population health management (see Step 10).

Step 3: Transition Readiness Assessment and Goal-Setting

A transition readiness assessment should be conducted before the young adult transitions from the children's practice to the adult practice. Ideally, these assessments would have been performed at least yearly beginning no later than age 14 (www.gottransition.org), but this may not be within the adult practice's control. The assessment should include evaluation of competencies for self-care; insurance status with regard to eligibility for adult services; entitlements and guardianship; cultural and religious preferences; and young adult's ability to perform self-care management tasks such as manage medications, keep appointments, track health issues, discuss their care with providers, manage their lifestyle choices, and perform other transition-related activities. There are several validated transition tools available, such as the Transition Readiness Assessment Questionnaire (TRAQ).

Perhaps the most important part of the transition process is the development of goals for successful health care. These goals should be developed collaboratively between the health care team, young adult, and family. These goals again will ideally be created by the young adult's pediatric practice, but regardless will need to be (re-)addressed by the accepting adult practice. These goals should be individualized based upon factors identified during the readiness assessment, such as the young adult's medical status, intellectual ability, independence and future functioning goals, and guardianship status [56]. Goals should be set with regard to future functional status, employment, romantic relationships, and end-of-life care [56].

This time is also an opportunity to encourage the young adult to begin to assume more responsibility for his/her health care, if he or she has not already [61]. The physician should attempt to ensure that the young adult understands his/her condition and medications, and, if parents are still closely involved, work with them to gradually release responsibility to their young adult. If the young adult is with his or her parents at the initial visit, physicians should also meet privately with the young adult, with the goal of encouraging their independence, if developmentally appropriate.

Step 4: Written Health Care Plan

For each young adult transitioning to adult care, a written health care plan should be developed. The basic structure and elements of this plan should be standardized by each practice. However, every plan should be customized and adapted to each patient's unique needs [56]. Like the readiness assessment, this plan should ideally be completed by the pediatric practice no later than age 14 [62]; however, it again will need to be (re-)addressed and customized by the adult practice. Once transition goals have been created (see Step 3), the written plan should contain a list of prioritized actions to achieve these goals. Each action should have a process and time deadline for completion. Actions will need to be taken in many areas, including, but not limited to the following.

Creation of Health Care Team

Team-based care in an essential element of the PCMH (see Step 6). Health care team members need to be explicitly identified, including, most importantly, a point person for the young adult's care. The ideal point person is located in the accepting adult PCP's practice and can work closely with this physician. This person should act as an advocate and primary contact for the young adult and his/her family in navigating the transition process [52].

The point person and the physician cannot care for the patient alone. Advance PCMH practices involve many others, particularly in the care of complex patients such as young adults with chronic childhood-onset conditions. These might include nutritionist/dieticians, pharmacists, behavioral health workers or psychiatrists, social workers, care managers, even peer health coaches. Each care team will need to be customized to the needs of the patient and the environment and resources of the primary care practice.

Adult specialty physicians will also likely need to be identified and plans made to coordinate with these physicians and their practices (see Step 7). A plan should be made as well for where to receive emergency care and any inpatient tertiary care. It may also be worthwhile to review which medical situations merit emergency room visitation versus clinic phone calls or appointments.

Insurance

The patient's insurance status should be scrutinized to ensure that care with all planned adult providers as well as any emergency care will be covered. If not, new providers may need to be selected or new insurance obtained. Patients and their families may need assistance in this process from a social worker or other community resources. Ideally, this insurance would also reimburse the new adult providers for transition planning and care coordination [62].

Guardianship

For families of young adults with intellectual disabilities, it is important to plan early to address guardianship issues. The legal age of majority in most states is 18 years. The Health Insurance Portability and Accountability Act (HIPAA) dictates that a physician cannot release information about a patient over 18 without the patient's consent, regardless of the intellectual level or communication abilities of the patient [61]. Therefore, parents should be informed that if and when their young adult becomes 18 they will not be able to be given health information about their adult child without his or her consent or legal guardianship. There are less restrictive forms of guardianship that can provide specific decision-making support while not completely denying the young adult's participation in that decision. Families will need assistance deciding which form of guardianship best meets their needs and then pursing this. For more details, please see Chap. 30 of this book.

Culturally and Religiously Appropriate

Great care should be taken to ensure that the health care goals and corresponding actions are sensitive to cultural and religious practices and beliefs. For example, the emergency care plan may need to specify certain measures that are not to be taken, e.g., blood transfusions. Patient or family's beliefs or preferences, such as preferred degree of involvement in decision-making and method and frequency of contact, and characteristics such as their health care literacy and level of understanding of the child's chronic condition(s) should be taken into account and accommodations written into the health care plan.

Update Process

With each interaction, and no less than yearly, the young adults' primary care provider and rest of his/her health care team should reevaluate the health care plan. In light of potential changes in the child's medical and social status the plan should be updated as appropriate [62]. Any patient or family concerns may also warrant revision of the health care plan.

Step 5: Transfer of Care

Transition to adult care should occur when appropriate based upon a young adult's developmental level, medical status, and relevant policy/licensing requirements, e.g., age of transition from pediatric practices. Whenever possible patients should only be transferred when medically stable, the adult primary care provider should confirm acceptance of care of the young adult with the childhood primary care provider's team. A pre-transfer visit to the adult practice may also be advised in the year before the transfer of care [56].

The accepting adult practice should ensure they have all relevant previous medical information to assume care of the young adult. This should include the child's complete medical records, which may require obtaining a release of medical information, as well as hopefully an updated medical summary prepared by the childhood provider's health care team. This medical summary should include all information relevant to the patient's present medical care and social situation. A copy should also be given to the family. There should also be a direct handoff of care between the childhood primary care provider and the accepting adult PCP, either in person or by phone [56]. A similar handoff between present and future point persons, if not the PCPs, should also occur.

The adult practice should ensure there is an emergency care plan, and if needed a condition fact sheet and appropriate legal documents, such as those detailing guardianship. The adult primary care provider should share this information with any adult specialists as well. Examples of a transition action plan, portable medical summary, and emergency care plan are available at www.gottransition.org.

Someone from the accepting adult primary care practice health care team should contact the childhood primary care provider within 3 months of the transition to confirm that the transition of care has been successful. Feedback should be also elicited from this children's practice on the transfer process, so as to improve and streamline this transition process for subsequent patients.

Ideally, ongoing collaborative partnerships may be forged between childhood and adult providers. Practices should also ask patients and their families for feedback on their experience with the transfer process. The health care team should be sure all relevant data from the transition is entered in the registry so that this may be used for iterative future improvement.

Step 6: Team-Based Care

Once the health care team has been created and the transition of care made, great attention should be paid to provide excellent, organized team-based care going forward. Clear roles for team members should be established. Ideally, roles should be constructed such that each individual is practicing "at the top of his/her license." All team members should be able to coordinate with each other. Optimally, this will involve frequent communication, both in person and via the EHR. Huddles—that is quick in-person meetings at the beginning/end of the day or even before/after individual patient visits—are one common excellent practice to make sure all team members are on the same page. All members should also be empowered to do their jobs individually. This may include standing orders from physicians to enable non-physician staff to complete tasks such as ordering labs or changing medications [60]. There will need to be frequent reflection to ensure workflows are optimized among team members. This is a key part of delivery system design under the chronic care model [57].

Step 7: Care Coordination

In particular for young adults with a chronic childhood-onset conditions, attention should be paid to the process of continued seamless coordination with specialists, who may also be transitioning from child to adult providers. Care plans or patient data registries may need to be developed to share among these providers and there may need to be planning for coordinated visits with multiple specialists and other activities of "chronic condition management" [56]. For patients with multiple adult providers, the medical summary may be shared digitally among them to aid in the coordination of care [62]. A shared document in the EHR may be the ideal mechanism for this, if all providers have access. Otherwise, more traditional means such as faxing records and phone calls will be needed to coordinate care.

The PCP and his/her health care team should put forethought into what situations necessitate consultation or referral to specialty providers. Ideally, the PCP should obtain relevant diagnostic studies before referral, preventing the need for unnecessary repeat specialty visits. E-consults, or other consultation with specialists that does not involve in-person visits, may also save time and expense. Similar thought should be put into referral to tertiary or emergency care. If such care is necessary, the adult practice should be sure to provide extra support upon discharge to prevent readmission. There may be a case manager in the practice whose sole function is managing this care coordination.

Step 8: Address the Social Determinants of Health

The social determinants of health are everything that affects a person's health besides their actual disease process, i.e., where he/she lives, works, eats, and plays. These social determinants may have up to a five times greater impact on health outcomes than medical care alone.

To address the social determinants of health, practices need to assess patient's needs with regard to income, housing, education, access to food, etc. Then, when issues are identified, patients need to be connected to resources to address these issues. Just as important as connection to resources within the health care system is connection to resources in the community. Recall, the foundation of the chronic care model is partnership between health systems and communities [57]. As more recent models for comprehensive management of chronic disease, such as the ICCC, have noted, community participation is essential to address the social determinants of health.

Each practice will need to identify relevant community resources in their community. These may include such varied resources as job training programs, food kitchens, Goodwill stores, etc. A social worker may be a good person to start with to help patients connect to these resources; however, all members of the health care team should see it as their job to address these issues. This may involve a substantial culture shift within the PCP's practice.

Step 9: Self-Management Support

Young adult patients should be empowered to become managers of their own health. To do so requires support and education in self-care. Diabetes is an excellent example. Research has shown that diabetes self-management education (DSME) that teaches patients how to manage their diabetes can dramatically improve diabetes control. There are now national standards for DSME, including skill-based education on using medications safely and effectively; preventing, detecting, and treating acute and chronic complications; physical activity and nutrition; and personal strategies to address psychosocial issues. While there may not be national standards for all chronic childhood-onset conditions, the same principles should be expanded to help aging young adults to successfully manage their own health. This may take many forms, including group classes, online modules or videos, or one-on-one tutorials.

Step 10: Population Health Management & Continuous Improvement

The final step of successful care for adults with childhood-onset chronic conditions is population health management. This is again an essential element of the PCMH, as well as a core element of the Triple Aim. Population health was initially defined by Kindig and Stoddart [63] as "the health outcomes of a group of individuals, including the distribution of such outcomes within the group." Now, though, it has come to mean much more, including (1) addressing not only health but social determinants of health, (2) focusing not just on treatment but on prevention, and (3) assuming shared responsibility as a health care team for patient outcomes [64]. Population health management is enabled by clinical information systems (See Step 3).

Using the patient data established in Step 3, the health care team should periodically and continually reflect on performance for all of their patients, regardless of whether or not these patients have scheduled visits upcoming. As mentioned, data should include disease measures as well as measures of social determinants of health. Data should be relevant to both providers and patients and therefore include both process and outcome measures. Practices should reflect on their performance and seek to improve it. This improvement should happen continuously using quality improvement methodology such as plan–do–study–act cycles. Quality improvement is the final necessary element of a PCMH. To improve performance, practices will need to work on improving all aspects of their practice, such as steps 6–9.

Conclusion

Young adults with childhood-onset chronic conditions are at increased risk for poor developmental and health outcomes, and therefore ensuring they receive excellent transition services and then excellent adult care is even more important than for other young adults. Excellent care for such patients requires (1) developing a health care policy statement; (2) utilizing clinical information systems to track and monitor patient outcomes; (3) conducting transition readiness assessments and goal-setting; (4) written, comprehensive health care planning; (5) transferring of care; (6) team-based care; (7) care coordination; (8) addressing social determinants of health; (9) self-management support; and (10) population health management and quality improvement. By implementing these steps, adult providers can achieve better, more equitable outcomes for young adults with childhood-onset chronic conditions.

Appendix

10 Steps for caring for adults with chronic childhood-onset conditions

1. Health Care Policy Statement
   - written, posted and readily available
   - developed with input of young adults and their families
   - educate and train all health care staff
   - discuss with all entering young adults
2. Tracking & Monitoring
   - data on all patients, including detailed status of each individual
   - measures of disease status and social determinants
   - use for iterative improvement
   - ideally integrate into the EHR
3. Readiness Assessment/Goal-Setting
   - use a validated questionnaire
   - address: self-care, insurance, guardianship, culture/religion, self-management, etc.
   - develop goals for functional status, employment, romantic relationships, end of life care
4. Written Health Care Plan includes:
   - creation of health care team
   - insurance
   - guardianship
   - cultural/religious beliefs
   - update process
5. Transfer of Care
   - time when appropriate
   - obtain all relevant medical info
   - obtain direct handoff
6. Team-Based Care
   - clear roles, top of license
   - empowered
   - frequent communication and reflection
7. Care Coordination
   - criteria for referral and escalation or care
   - communication, especially via EHR
   - consider case manager
8. Address Social Determinants of Health
   - screen for income, food, housing, etc.
   - connect with internal and community-based resources
9. Self-Management Support
   - Educate patients for self-care
10. Population Health Management & Quality Improvement
    - monitor performance measures on all patients
    - use quality improvement strategies to continually improve

References

1. Kuo AA. Life course health development. In: Kuo AA, Coller RJ, Stewart-Brown S, Blair M (eds). Child health. Oxford: Oxford University Press; 2015. p. 111–32. Available from: http://www.oxfordmedicine.com/view/10.1093/med/9780199309375.001.0001/med-9780199309375-chapter-6 Accessed 8 June 2016.
2. Arnett JJ. Emerging adulthood: A theory of development from the late teens through the twenties. Am Psychol. 2000;55(5):469.
3. Munsey C. Emerging adults: the in-between age. Monit Psychol. 2006;37(6):68.
4. U.S. Census Bureau. American Community Survey: 2005. 2005.
5. Goldscheider F, Goldscheider C. Leaving and returning home in 20th century America. Washington, DC: Population Reference Bureau. Popul Bull. 1994;48 (4):1–35.
6. Michael RT, Gagnon JH, Laumann EO, Kolata G. Sex in America: a definitive survey. Boston, MA: Little, Brown; 1994.
7. Bianchi SM, Spain D. Women, work, and family in America. Population Bulletin. 1996;51(3):1–48.
8. Dummer TJ, Kirk SF, Penney TL, Dodds L, Parker L. Targeting policy for obesity prevention: identifying the critical age for weight gain in women. J Obes. 2012;2012:934895.
9. Hebden L, Chan H, Louie J, Rangan A, Allman-Farinelli M. You are what you choose to eat: factors influencing young adults' food selection behaviour. J Hum Nutr Diet. 2015;28(4): 401–8.
10. Laska MN, Graham DJ, Moe SG, Van Riper D. Young adult eating and food-purchasing patterns: food store location and residential proximity. Am J Prev Med. 2010;39(5):464–7.
11. Reither EN, Hauser RM, Yang Y. Do birth cohorts matter? Age-period-cohort analyses of the obesity epidemic in the United States. Soc Sci Med. 2009;69 (10):1439–48.
12. Hingson RW, Heeren T, Winter MR. Age at drinking onset and alcohol dependence: age at onset, duration, and severity. Arch Pediatr Adolesc Med. 2006;160 (7):739–46.
13. Pitkänen T, Lyyra A, Pulkkinen L. Age of onset of drinking and the use of alcohol in adulthood: a follow-up study from age 8–42 for females and males. Addiction. 2005;100(5):652–61.
14. Centers for Disease Control and Prevention (CDC). Sexual risk behaviors: HIV, STD, & Teen Pregnancy Prevention. Last updated April 15, 2016. http://www.cdc.gov/healthyyouth/sexualbehaviors/ Accessed 15 June 2016.
15. Bull SS, McFarlane M. Soliciting sex on the Internet: what are the risks for sexually transmitted diseases and HIV? Sex Transm Dis. 2000;27(9):545–50.
16. Grov C, DeBusk JA, Bimbi DS, Golub SA, Nanin JE, Parsons JT. Barebacking, the Internet, and harm reduction: an intercept survey with gay and bisexual men in Los Angeles and New York City. AIDS Behav. 2007;11(4):527–36.
17. McFarlane M, Bull SS, Rietmeijer CA. The Internet as a newly emerging risk environment for sexually transmitted diseases. JAMA. 2000;284(4):443–6.
18. McFarlane M, Bull SS, Rietmeijer CA. Young adults on the Internet: risk behaviors for sexually transmitted diseases and HIV. J Adolesc Health. 2002;31(1):11–6.
19. Martin MJ, Conger RD, Sitnick SL, Masarik AS, Forbes EE, Shaw DS. Reducing risk for substance use by economically disadvantaged young men: positive family environments and pathways to educational attainment. Child Dev. 2015;86(6):1719–37.
20. Harden BJ. Safety and stability for foster children: a developmental perspective. Future Child. 2004;14 (1):31–47.
21. Eriksson U, Arvidsson D, Sundquist K. Availability of exercise facilities and physical activity in 2,037 adults: cross-sectional results from the Swedish neighborhood and physical activity (SNAP) study. BMC Public Health. 2012;12(1):1.
22. Lee PH. Association between adolescents' physical activity and sedentary behaviors with change in BMI and risk of type 2 diabetes. PLoS ONE. 2014;9(10): e110732.
23. Zucker RA. Alcohol use and the alcohol use disorders: a developmental-biopsychosocial systems formulation covering the life course. In: Cicchetti D, Cohen DJ, editors. Developmental psychopathology, volume 3: risk, disorder, and adaptation. 2nd ed. Hoboken, NJ: Wiley; 2006. p. 620–56.
24. Finer LB, Henshaw SK. Disparities in rates of unintended pregnancy in the United States, 1994 and 2001. Perspect Sex Reprod Health. 2006;38 (2):90–6.
25. Harper CC, Rocca CH, Thompson KM, Morfesis J, Goodman S, Darney PD, et al. Reductions in pregnancy rates in the USA with long-acting reversible contraception: a cluster randomised trial. The Lancet. 2015;386(9993):562–8.
26. Reed J. Primary Care: A Crucial Setting for Suicide Prevention [Internet]. SAMHSA-HRSA/Suicide Prevention in Primary Care. http://www.integration.samhsa.gov/about-us/esolutions-newsletter/suicide-prevention-in-primary-care Accessed 8 June 2016.
27. Washington State Department of Health. Report to the Legislature: Suicide Education Study. December 2013. http://www.doh.wa.gov/portals/1/documents/pubs/631049.pdf Accessed 8 June 2016.
28. Arroll B, Goodyear-Smith F, Crengle S, Gunn J, Kerse N, Fishman T, et al. Validation of PHQ-2 and PHQ-9 to screen for major depression in the primary care population. Ann Fam Med. 2010;8(4):348–53.
29. Mosher WD, Jones J, Abma JC. National Center for Health Statistics (US). Intended and unintended births

in the United States: 1982–2010. National Health Statistics Reports, Number 55, July 24, 2012. http://www.cdc.gov/nchs/data/nhsr/nhsr055.pdf Accessed 15 June 2016.
30. Frost JJ, Darroch JE. Factors associated with contraceptive choice and inconsistent method use, United States, 2004. Perspect Sex Reprod Health. 2008;40 (2):94–104.
31. Gold RB, Sonfield A, Richards CL, Frost JJ. Next steps for America's family planning program: leveraging the potential of Medicaid and Title X in an evolving health care system. Guttmacher Institute; 2009. https://www.guttmacher.org/sites/default/files/pdfs/pubs/summaries/NextStepsExec.pdf Accessed 15 June 2016.
32. Trussell J. Contraceptive failure in the United States. Contraception. 2011;83(5):397–404.
33. Grodstein F, Goldman MB, Cramer DW. Body mass index and ovulatory infertility. Epidemiology. 1994;5:247–50.
34. Aune D, Saugstad OD, Henriksen T, Tonstad S. Maternal body mass index and the risk of fetal death, stillbirth, and infant death: a systematic review and meta-analysis. JAMA. 2014;311(15):1536–46.
35. Robbins CL, Zapata LB, Farr SL, Kroelinger CD, Morrow B, Ahluwalia I, et al. Core state preconception health indicators-pregnancy risk assessment monitoring system and behavioral risk factor surveillance system, 2009. Morb Mortal Wkly Rep. 2014;63 (3):1–62.
36. Centers for Disease Control and Prevention, American Society for Reproductive Medicine, Society for Assisted Reproductive Technology. 2012 Assisted Reproductive Technology National Summary Report. Atlanta, GA: US Department of Health and Human Services; 2014. https://www.cdc.gov/art/pdf/2012-report/national-summary/art_2012_national_summary_report.pdf Accessed 15 June 2016.
37. Gill SK, Broussard C, Devine O, Green RF, Rasmussen SA, Reefhuis J, et al. Association between maternal age and birth defects of unknown etiology: United States, 1997–2007. Birt Defects Res A Clin Mol Teratol. 2012;94(12):1010–8.
38. Smith A, Duggan M. Online dating & relationships. Washington, DC: Pew Research Center's Internet and American Life Project; 2013 Oct. Available from: http://www.pewinternet.org/files/old-media//Files/Reports/2013/PIP_Online%20Dating%202013.pdf Accessed 9 June 2016.
39. Blanco C, Okuda M, Wright C, Hasin DS, Grant BF, Liu S-M, et al. Mental health of college students and their non-college-attending peers: results from the National Epidemiologic Study on Alcohol and Related Conditions. Arch Gen Psychiatry. 2008;65 (12):1429–37.
40. National Coalition for Health Professional Education in Genetics. Empiric risk data. http://www.nchpeg.org/index.php?option=com_content&view=article&id=120&Itemid=118 Accessed 10 June 2016.
41. Arseneault L, Cannon M, Poulton R, Murray R, Caspi A, Moffitt TE. Cannabis use in adolescence and risk for adult psychosis: longitudinal prospective study. BMJ. 2002;325(7374):1212–3.
42. Simon GE, VonKorff M, Piccinelli M, Fullerton C, Ormel J. An international study of the relation between somatic symptoms and depression. N Engl J Med. 1999;341(18):1329–35.
43. Boys A, Marsden J, Strang J. Understanding reasons for drug use amongst young people: a functional perspective. Health Educ Res. 2001;16(4):457–69.
44. Substance Abuse and Mental Health Services Administration,(SAMHSA). Results from the 2012 national survey on drug use and health: Summary of national findings. Rockville, MD: Substance Abuse and Mental Health Services Administration; 2013. (NSDUH Series H-46). Report No.: HHS Publication No. (SMA) 13-4795.
45. Meier MH, Caspi A, Ambler A, Harrington H, Houts R, Keefe RS, et al. Persistent cannabis users show neuropsychological decline from childhood to midlife. Proc Natl Acad Sci. 2012;109(40):E2657–64.
46. Obrocki J, Buchert R, Thomasius R, Beyer W, Schiemann T. Ecstasy-long-term effects on the human central nervous system revealed by positron emission tomography. Br J Psychiatry. 1999;175(2):186–8.
47. Wang W, Morin R. Home for the Holidays… and Every Other Day. Pew Research Center's Social & Demographic Trends Project. 2009. http://www.pewsocialtrends.org/2009/11/24/home-for-the-holidays-and-every-other-day/ Accessed 10 June 2016.
48. Gallup Inc. In U.S., Fewer Young Adults Holding Full-Time Jobs in 2013. Gallup.com. http://www.gallup.com/poll/163727/fewer-young-adults-holding-full-time-jobs-2013.aspx Accessed 10 June 2016.
49. Dauner KN, Thompson J. Young adult's perspectives on being uninsured and implications for health reform. Qual Rep. 2014;19(4):1.
50. Long SK, Kenney GM, Zuckerman S, Goin DE, Wissoker D, Blavin F, et al. The Health Reform Monitoring Survey: addressing data gaps to provide timely insights into the Affordable Care Act. Health Aff (Millwood). 2014;33(1):161–7.
51. Bloom SR, Kuhlthau K, Van Cleave J, Knapp AA, Newacheck P, Perrin JM. Health care transition for youth with special health care needs. J Adolesc Health. 2012;51(3):213–9.
52. Rosen DS, Blum RW, Britto M, Sawyer SM, Siegel DM. Transition to adult health care for adolescents and young adults with chronic conditions: position paper of the Society for Adolescent Medicine. J Adolesc Health. 2003;33(4):309–11.
53. Sawicki GS, Lukens-Bull K, Yin X, Demars N, Huang I-C, Livingood W, et al. Measuring the transition readiness of youth with special healthcare needs: validation of the TRAQ—Transition Readiness Assessment Questionnaire. J Pediatr Psychol. 2011;36(2):160–71.

54. U.S. Department of Health and Human Services, Health Resources and Services Administration, Maternal and Child Health Bureau. National Survey of Children with Special Health Care Needs 2005–2006: Core Outcomes Introduction. Rockville, MD: U.S. Department of Health and Human Services; 2008. http://mchb.hrsa.gov/cshcn05/mco/intro.htm Accessed 10 June 2016.
55. Jackson GL, Powers BJ, Chatterjee R, Bettger JP, Kemper AR, Hasselblad V, et al. The patient-centered medical home: a systematic review. Ann Intern Med. 2013;158(3):169–78.
56. Cooley WC, Sagerman PJ. Supporting the health care transition from adolescence to adulthood in the medical home. Pediatrics. 2011;128(1):182–200.
57. Stellefson M, Dipnarine K, Stopka C. The chronic care model and diabetes management in US primary care settings: a systematic review. Prev Chronic Dis. 2013;10:E26.
58. World Health Organization. Innovative care for chronic conditions: Building blocks for actions: global report. 2002. http://www.who.int/chp/knowledge/publications/icccglobalreport.pdf Accessed 15 June 2016.
59. Barr VJ, Robinson S, Marin-Link B, Underhill L, Dotts A, Ravensdale D, et al. The expanded chronic care model: an integration of concepts and strategies from population health promotion and the Chronic Care Model. Healthc Q. 2003;7(1):73–82.
60. Bodenheimer T, Ghorob A, Willard-Grace R, Grumbach K. The 10 building blocks of high-performing primary care. Ann Fam Med. 2014;12(2):166–71.
61. Lemly DC, Weitzman ER, O'Hare K. Advancing healthcare transitions in the medical home: tools for providers, families and adolescents with special healthcare needs. Curr Opin Pediatr. 2013;25(4):439–46.
62. American Academy of Pediatrics. American Academy of Family Physicians, American College of Physicians-American Society of Internal Medicine. A consensus statement on health care transitions for young adults with special health care needs. Pediatrics. 2002;110(Suppl 3):1304–6.
63. Kindig D, Stoddart G. What is population health? Am J Public Health. 2003;93(3):380–3.
64. Stoto MA. Population health in the Affordable Care Act era, vol. 1. Washington, DC: Academy Health; 2013.

Part III

Case-Based Examples of Management of the Young Adult with a Chronic Childhood Condition

Attention-Deficit/Hyperactivity Disorder (ADHD)

3

David S. Stein, Elizabeth B. Harstad and William J. Barbaresi

Case Presentation

Mr. S is a 24-year-old man who presents for an initial visit with concerns about attention-deficit/hyperactivity disorder (ADHD). In the second grade, he had difficulty with schoolwork, was frequently sent out of class for distracting other students, and was formally diagnosed with ADHD, combined type (currently referred to as "ADHD of the Combined Presentation") [1]. Neuropsychological testing at that time revealed high average cognitive ability, especially in verbal skills. Between the third and eighth grades, he tried several stimulant medications with suboptimal improvement in his ADHD symptoms, eventually responding well to dexmethylphenidate XR daily on weekdays and dexmethylphenidate after school as needed for homework. During high school, Mr. S was in several minor traffic accidents. Between ages 10 and 20, he required emergency room care on 4 occasions due to lacerations (twice) and fractures of his arm and leg. He began to use marijuana on a daily basis and has continued to use intermittently since. During his senior year in high school, he was diagnosed with mild depression, and was treated with fluoxetine for 1 year, in addition to dexmethylphenidate. His teachers recommended him to go to vocational school, but he chose to attend a traditional 4-year high school and then attended a community college, but failed to graduate. During college, he discontinued treatment with stimulant medication.

Mr. S received special educational services throughout late elementary, middle, and high school, primarily due to difficulty in organizing and completing his work in a timely fashion. He held several jobs during high school and while attending community college. He has been fired several times in the past 2 years due to tardiness and making frequent, careless errors on the job. He is currently working as an administrative assistant in a car dealership. Mr. S regularly drinks alcohol but denies symptoms of dependence. He intermittently uses marijuana. He recently had another car accident, requiring an emergency room visit for treatment of bruised ribs. Mr. S attends this visit along with his live-in girlfriend, with whom he has had a turbulent and inconsistent relationship, and who is currently pregnant.

Mr. S informs you that he was previously diagnosed with ADHD as a child and that he would like to resume treatment, because he believes that he continues to have significant

D.S. Stein (✉) · E.B. Harstad · W.J. Barbaresi
Division of Developmental Medicine, Department of Medicine, Boston Children's Hospital, Harvard Medical School, Fegan 10, 300 Longwood Avenue, Boston, MA 02115, USA
e-mail: David.Stein@childrens.harvard.edu

E.B. Harstad
e-mail: Elizabeth.Harstad@childrens.harvard.edu

W.J. Barbaresi
e-mail: William.Barbaresi@childrens.harvard.edu

M. Pilapil et al. (eds.), *Care of Adults with Chronic Childhood Conditions*,
DOI 10.1007/978-3-319-43827-6_3

problems at work and at home due to his tendency to be distracted, disorganized, and impulsive.

Case Discussion

The case of Mr. S highlights many of the common challenges seen among adults with ADHD. Adults with ADHD typically have increased rates of medical problems, specifically in physical health, mental health, and substance abuse. Adults with ADHD exhibit poor habits related to smoking and limited exercise [2, 3] and engage in more risky behaviors. Health care costs throughout childhood are double for subjects with ADHD compared to their non-ADHD peers in a 9-year study of median annual health care costs [4]. Mr. S is not currently noted to exhibit substantial physical health challenges. However, his challenges with organization, holding a job, history of depression, and intermittent substance abuse may predict poorer habits and resultant physical health problems as he ages. In addition, Mr. S has experienced several car accidents, and ADHD is associated with impairment with driving. This association appears to be related to increased distractibility, risk-taking, and impulsive behaviors while driving for those with ADHD relative to controls, who also engage in more defensive driving practices [5]. Mr. S was involved in a recent accident and subsequent emergency room visit as an adult, suggesting that his driving impairment persists.

Mr. S exhibited struggles with mental health issues, including depression diagnosed in late adolescence. Adults with persistent ADHD, as seems to be the case for Mr. S, are far more likely to experience other psychiatric disorders, at a rate of 81 versus 35 % of non-ADHD controls in one large cohort study [6]. The risk of death from suicide in those with ADHD versus controls is also substantially elevated [6], and Mr. S's struggles with depression and substance abuse likely place him at higher risk for suicidality. Mr. S uses alcohol and marijuana, consistent with the increased rates of substance abuse in adults with ADHD. Individuals seeking substance abuse treatment have far higher rates of ADHD [7] and adults with a history of childhood ADHD exhibit higher rates of drug dependence in adulthood, including new onset dependence [8]. Thus, Mr. S's use of marijuana and alcohol may be an indicator of risk for further substance use problems, including dependence, in adulthood. However, the fact that Mr. S is seeking treatment may be a positive prognostic indicator for his risk for substance abuse and dependence. Male adolescents with ADHD who were treated with stimulant medication showed reduced rates of substance use disorders relative to those who were untreated [9], and recent studies suggest that adults with ADHD who are medically treated also have reduced risk for substance abuse [10].

Mr. S chose a common route for secondary and postsecondary education by attending a typical high school and then community college. However, Mr. S did not graduate community college, a common outcome among persons with ADHD. Individuals with ADHD typically struggle in school, with higher rates of learning disabilities [11, 12], absenteeism, and grade retention, coupled with lower academic achievement scores and rates of high school graduation [13]. While we do not have specific information about Mr. S's academic achievement, his failure to complete community college in the context of high average verbal cognition certainly suggests suboptimal academic achievement. Notably, treatment with stimulant medication in childhood and adolescence moderates negative school outcomes. Children and adolescents treated with medication exhibit reduced absenteeism and grade retention, as well as modest increases in achievement scores for reading [13]. It is possible, then, that Mr. S's completion of high school was aided, in part, by his previous treatment. It is also possible that Mr. S's lack of treatment during college contributed to difficulty completing this experience. While the moderating effects of medication treatment in adulthood on vocational outcomes are not well understood, several studies have demonstrated the efficacy of medication treatment in treating core symptoms of ADHD in adults [14]. Further, the childhood and adolescent data, as well as Mr. S's history and trajectory (i.e., that he graduated high school while being treated, and did not complete community college without treatment), suggest that resumption of medical treatment would be beneficial for him. Stimulant treatment has also been shown to improve driving in adults with ADHD [15].

In the social domain, Mr. S is exhibiting many typical challenges for adults with ADHD. While Mr. S is cohabitating with his girlfriend, the relationship has been inconsistent and the couple is expecting a child. Adults with ADHD are noted to have more difficulties with adult relationships and often become parents at an early age [2]. This may also predict financial challenges for Mr. S and the couple. Mr. S has struggled to hold a job consistently due to apparent difficulties with executive function, particularly organization. Adults with ADHD are more likely to struggle to meet job requirements, to be perceived negatively by employers, and to be fired from jobs [16]. The added stress of child-rearing for a couple with a tumultuous relationship may only worsen Mr. S's emotional status and further limit his job performance, particularly without treatment. As will be discussed further, Mr. S would likely benefit from working with a rehabilitation agency and/or an executive function coach to learn both the skills to manage his adult life, as well as to build his self-advocacy skills.

Treatment approaches for childhood ADHD are well established. The American Academy of Pediatrics [17] has issued a guideline for the diagnosis and treatment of ADHD in children and adolescents. In preschool-age children, behavior therapy focused on parent training is the first-line intervention, and this can be followed by combined treatment with stimulant medication if behavioral treatment is insufficient. In school-aged children, the guidelines recommend combined treatment that includes medication, behavioral therapies, and school-based accommodations. When combined, these treatments are the most effective in addressing core symptoms; associated social, emotional, and academic issues; and allow for maintenance on lower doses of stimulant medication. These treatment recommendations are based on the Multimodal Treatment of ADHD Study, [18] which represents the largest and most rigorous comparative trial of ADHD treatments in children and adolescents.

In adults with ADHD, medication treatment is effective in symptom management and is well tolerated [14]. Medication is the primary mode of intervention and leads to improved functioning, though long-term functional outcomes have not been sufficiently studied to date. As noted previously, Mr. S would likely benefit from medication treatment. In addition to medical intervention, however, there is evidence that psychotherapy, and specifically targeted cognitive behavioral therapy (CBT), has a role in the treatment of adults with ADHD [19, 20]. CBT may address skill deficits such as issues with executive function—likely at least in part due to improved understanding and enhanced self-awareness—and may also help to manage comorbid psychiatric conditions that have a major impact upon functioning. For Mr. S, who struggles with executive function and has a history of depression, CBT would likely be an effective adjunct to medication treatment. It is also important to note that skill deficits and their impact upon employment may be somewhat moderated by working with a rehabilitation agency. State rehabilitation agencies work with adults who have any impairing condition, including ADHD, and who would benefit from vocational assessments, job training, or job placement assistance. Information about rehabilitation agencies in each state in the United States is available at www.rehabnetwork.org.

Mr. S would likely derive great benefit from working with a rehabilitation agency that could help him to find suitable employment and also advocate for supports to help him perform in the workplace.

Definition

ADHD is a neurobehavioral condition characterized by significant inattention and/or hyperactivity/impulsivity across at least 2 different settings, such as home and work. Symptoms must be present from early childhood, by age 12 years according to the Diagnostic and Statistical Manual of Mental Disorders (DSM)-5 [1], although it is possible for symptoms to only become apparent with increasing attentional and organizational demands of late childhood, or even adulthood. Individuals can be diagnosed with ADHD of the predominantly inattentive presentation, ADHD of the predominantly hyperactive/impulsive presentation, or ADHD of the combined presentation. For adults, 5 out of 9 of the inattentive and/or 5 out of 9 of the hyperactive/impulsive symptoms are the minimum criteria necessary to fulfill diagnostic criteria, whereas for children the threshold is higher, with 6 symptoms of either required (see Box 3.1) [1]. Some research suggests that only 4 symptoms either of inattention or hyperactive/impulsivity should be sufficient to meet diagnostic criteria for adults and that requiring 5 symptoms may be too restrictive [6].

The predominant features of ADHD may differ in children versus adults, with adults showing more inattention and relatively less hyperactivity. Common manifestations of ADHD in adulthood include difficulties with organizing activities, prioritizing tasks, and meeting deadlines, as well as quitting jobs without any alternatives, reckless driving, and terminating valued relationships [21]. Many adults with ADHD experience mood lability, irritability, and low frustration tolerance, which can result in the inability to manage uncomfortable emotions and the tendency to become overwhelmed [22, 23].

Box 3.1 DSM-5 Diagnostic Criteria for ADHD [1]

Inattention
- Fails to give close attention to detail or makes careless mistakes in schoolwork, at work, or with other activities
- Has trouble holding attention on tasks or play activities
- Does not seem to listen when spoken to directly
- Does not follow through on instructions and fails to finish schoolwork, chores, or duties in the workplace (e.g., loses focus, side-tracked)
- Has trouble organizing tasks and activities
- Avoids, dislikes, or is reluctant to do tasks that require mental effort over a long period of time (such as schoolwork or homework)
- Loses things necessary for tasks and activities (e.g., school materials, pencils, books, tools, wallets, keys, paperwork, eyeglasses, mobile telephones)
- Often easily distracted
- Often forgetful in daily activities

Hyperactivity and Impulsivity
- Fidgets with or taps hands or feet, or squirms in seat
- Leaves seat in situations when remaining seat is expected
- Runs about or climbs in situations where it is not appropriate (adolescents or adults may be limited to feeling restless)
- Unable to play or take part in leisure activities quietly
- Is often "on the go," acting as if "driven by a motor"
- Often talks excessively
- Blurts out an answer before a question has been completed
- Has trouble in waiting his/her turn
- Often interrupts or intrudes on others (e.g., butts into conversations or games)

Epidemiology

The prevalence of ADHD among US adults ages 18–44-years old is reported to be 4.4 % [24]. However, this prevalence estimate may vary depending on which methods (such as simple reporting of symptoms versus use of structured diagnostic interview) are used to assess for an ADHD diagnosis in adults [25]. ADHD may be underdiagnosed in lower income or minority racial/ethnic groups [26, 27]. Increased availability of specialists in underserved areas and culturally competent approaches to assessing ADHD in African-Americans may help to decrease this disparity [27, 28]. ADHD is more common in males than females, with pediatric studies reporting that males are 2–3 times more likely to have ADHD [29, 30].

Factors to Consider in Making a Diagnosis in Adults

The Diagnostic and Statistical Manual of Mental Disorders (DSM-5) criteria for ADHD were developed to diagnose ADHD in children, and thus it may be difficult to directly apply these criteria to adults. According to the DSM-5, signs and symptoms of ADHD must be present prior to age 12 years—although this criterion can pose a challenge when adults seek treatment for ADHD, since there are conflicting findings on the accuracy of adult recall of childhood ADHD symptoms [31, 32]. A recent prospective outcome study demonstrated that adults were able to accurately report their childhood ADHD symptoms when they were asked about specific symptoms as part of a structured diagnostic interview [25]. If possible, review of childhood medical records or school report cards/progress notes could help to determine if childhood symptoms were present.

Another challenge with making the diagnosis of ADHD in adults is that symptoms must cause impairment in 2 or more settings [1]. While a childhood diagnosis relies on use of rating scales completed by teachers and parents, it may not be possible to obtain ADHD rating scales from informants such as employers and spouses in adulthood, given concerns about patient confidentiality. Self-report of impairment may not be accurate since respondents often rate themselves overly positively [33]. The use of a brief, structured, diagnostic interview of ADHD symptoms, and related impairments may more accurately identify adult ADHD [25]. The Mini International Neuropsychiatric Interview (M.I.N.I. ADHD) [34] is an example of a structured diagnostic interview that can be administered by clinicians to help determine whether or not an adult presenting with ADHD concerns meets diagnostic criteria for ADHD.

It is also important to assess for other medical conditions that can cause inattention and/or hyperactivity/impulsivity, such as depression, anxiety, mood disorders, substance use, thyroid disease, or sleep disorders. These conditions must be considered as they may cause ADHD-like symptoms and/or they may co-occur with ADHD. Additionally, the potential for malingering for an adult presenting with new onset ADHD symptoms should be considered, as an ADHD diagnosis could be sought for secondary gain (such as to obtain stimulant medications, which have a high rate of abuse and diversion). However, it is important to emphasize that there is no evidence that adults with ADHD themselves abuse stimulant medications; rather, they have increased rates of substance use disorders involving alcohol, marijuana and, less commonly, other drugs of abuse [8]. While brain imaging and electroencephalographic studies are used in research settings to better understand brain function in ADHD, they are not currently recommended for clinical diagnosis or management, in the absence of other neurological concerns.

Risk Factors

The etiology of ADHD is not fully understood, although genetics and environmental factors may both play a role in the development of ADHD. Familial and twin studies show that the risk of ADHD in parents and siblings of children with ADHD is increased 2–8 times, [35] and heritability has been estimated at 76 % [36]. A number of genes involved in dopamine and serotonin pathways may underlie the symptoms of ADHD [36]. Additionally, 1 case–control study showed that children with ADHD had a higher rate of copy number variants than controls (15.6 vs. 7.5 %) thus supporting the genetic contribution to ADHD [37].

While genetics clearly play a role in the development of ADHD, findings from studies evaluating the association between environmental factors and ADHD are less definitive. In utero environmental exposures including prenatal exposure to tobacco, alcohol, or illicit substances may increase risk for ADHD [38]. Elevated blood lead levels are associated with increased risk for ADHD [38, 39]. One US population-based cross-sectional study found that children with higher levels of urinary metabolites of organophosphate pesticides were more likely to meet diagnostic criteria for ADHD, although prospective studies are needed to establish whether this association is causal [40]. Dietary influences on development of ADHD have also been studied, although at this time there is no conclusive research to recommend dietary modifications as a means to prevent or treat ADHD, outside of the standard medical recommendations to maintain a healthy, well balanced diet [41]. Recent studies have suggested a link between electronic media exposure and ADHD symptoms, although the direction of the association is unclear [42]. It may be that individuals with ADHD choose to engage in more electronic media use, rather than that electronic media use causes ADHD symptoms.

Pathophysiology

Brain imaging studies indicate that there is dysfunction of the fronto-subcortical and parietal circuits in adults with ADHD, with the most prominent abnormalities in the prefrontal cortex and its projections to subcortical structures [43, 44]. Pediatric studies have shown reduced global activation and reduced local activation in the area of the basal ganglia and the anterior frontal lobe [45]. Neuroimaging studies also show that ADHD is associated with a delay in cortical maturation [46]. Animal studies suggest that an imbalance between the norepinephrine and dopamine systems in the prefrontal cortex (decrease in dopaminergic activity and increase in norepinephrine activity) contributes to the development of ADHD [47]. In a small human study, patients with ADHD were reported to have an increase in dopamine transporter density compared to controls, meaning that the dopamine was cleared from the synapse too quickly and there was relatively less available dopamine [48].

Associated Conditions

ADHD in adults is associated with a high rate of comorbid conditions. ADHD is associated with higher rates of obesity, which in turn can cause various medical problems, such as hypertension and hyperlipidemia, although ADHD itself is not reported to be directly linked to these conditions or to higher rates of cancer [49]. Some of the most commonly reported comorbid conditions for adults with ADHD are substance use disorders, antisocial personality disorders, mood disorders, anxiety, and depression [6, 50]. With increasing age, psychiatric comorbidities may become more evident and problematic. Therefore, it is imperative to routinely screen for, and treat if present, any comorbid conditions for adults with ADHD.

Adults with ADHD may experience a range of adverse psychosocial outcomes and ADHD should be seen as a significant chronic health condition that confers increased risk for early death related to suicide. One longitudinal, population-based study confirmed that childhood ADHD is associated with significantly increased risk for early death from suicide, with highest risk for those with comorbid substance use disorders or other comorbid psychiatric disorders [6]. Other problems associated with adult ADHD include reduced educational achievement, unemployment, increased risk of traffic and other accidents, and criminality [6, 51, 52].

Special Issues in Transition to Adulthood

Given the adverse impact of both core ADHD symptoms, and commonly occurring comorbidities, youth with ADHD must be followed closely during their transition to adulthood.

Treatment, Monitoring, and Side Effects

Treatment of both ADHD symptoms and comorbidities should be optimized. Medication treatment for ADHD usually involves stimulant medications, such as methylphenidate or amphetamine preparations, both of whose suspected mechanism of action is to increase the amount of available dopamine [53]. While stimulant medications have a higher likelihood of reducing ADHD symptoms of inattention, impulsivity, and hyperactivity compared to other medications [17], atomoxetine has US Food and Drug Administration (FDA) approval for treatment of ADHD in adults, and alpha-agonists and antidepressants also have some evidence suggesting they may reduce ADHD symptoms in adults [53]. Table 3.1 provides a list of commonly prescribed medications to treat adult ADHD. When medication is used to treat ADHD, it is started at a relatively low dose and the dose is titrated upward until ADHD symptoms are appropriately controlled, side effects become intolerable, or the maximum dosage of medication is reached. In children and adolescents, use of standardized ADHD rating scales at baseline and after dose changes (which usually occur 1 week to 1 month apart) can help to determine if the core symptoms of ADHD have diminished with medication treatment. For the reasons noted earlier in this chapter, it can be more difficult to obtain valid information about ADHD symptoms in adults. There are self-report questionnaires available, primarily based on the DSM-IV TR diagnostic criteria for ADHD [54]. However, the symptoms of ADHD in DSM-IV TR, versus the recently published DSM-5 criteria, differ primarily in the number of symptoms required for a diagnosis [1], so DSM-IV TR-based questionnaires are still clinically useful, and newer versions will undoubtedly become available. Examples include the Adult ADHD Self-Report Scale-V1.1 (ASRS-V1.1) [55] and the Conners' Adult ADHD Rating Scales [56]. Perhaps more importantly, assessment of treatment response should include a review of aspects of function that are impacted by the patient's ADHD symptoms, such as task-completion at work, interactions with peers and significant others, and driving. Specific targets of treatment will vary, and assessment of treatment should be guided by an understanding of the areas of function that were determined to be most significantly impacted by ADHD symptoms at baseline, prior to the initiation of treatment.

Common side effects of stimulant medications include diminished appetite, delayed sleep onset,

Table 3.1 Commonly prescribed medications to treat adult ADHD

Class	Trade name	Generic name	Side effects	Dosing considerations
Stimulants				
Methylphenidate	Ritalin; Ritalin LA; Ritalin SR	Methylphenidate	Common: Diminished appetite, delayed sleep onset, headaches, and irritability Rare: Psychosis, priapism	Initial dose: 20 mg/day Adjust in weekly 20 mg increments
	Metadate CD	Methylphenidate		Initial dose: 20 mg/day Adjust in weekly 10–20 mg increments
	Focalin; Focalin XR	Dexmethylphenidate		Dexmethylphenidate: Initial dose: 5 mg/day Adjust in weekly 2.5 mg increments Dexmethylphenidate extended release: Initial dose: 5 mg/day Adjust in weekly 5 mg increments
	Concerta	Methylphenidate		Initial dose: 18–36 mg/day Adjust in weekly 18 mg increments
Amphetamine	Adderall; Adderall XR	Mixed amphetamine salts		Mixed amphetamine salts: Initial dose: 5 mg/day or BID Adjust in weekly 2.5 mg increments Mixed amphetamine salts, extended release: Initial dose: 10 mg/day Adjust in 5–10 mg weekly increments
	Vyvanse	lisdexamfetamine		Initial dose: 30 mg/day adjust in 20 mg weekly increments
Nonstimulants				
Selective norepinephrine reuptake inhibitor	Strattera	Atomoxetine	Gastrointestinal distress, headache, sedation, suicidal ideation, transient growth effects, elevated blood pressure or heart rate Rare: Hepatotoxicity, priapism	Initial dose: 40 mg/day, increase to 80 mg/day after 3 days Increase after 2–4 weeks if optimal response not achieved
Alpha agonists	Kapvay	Clonidine	Gastrointestinal distress, headache, decreased blood pressure or heart rate, sedation	Initial dose: 0.1 mg/day Adjust in 0.1 mg increments weekly
	Intuniv	Guanfacine		Initial dose: 1 mg/day Adjust in increments of no more than 1 mg weekly

headaches, and irritability. Rare, but more serious side effects, include psychosis (more common in those with underlying mood disorder already associated with psychosis) and priapism. Monitoring of heart rate and blood pressure is warranted at clinical visits (initially monthly while making dosage changes and then every 3–4 months) because stimulant medications are associated with a slight increase in systolic and diastolic blood pressure (3–5 mmHg) and heart rate (5 beats per minute) [57]. Recent data on cardiovascular risks of stimulant medications suggests no increased risk of a serious cardiac event from stimulant medications for those with an otherwise healthy heart [58, 59]. Consultation with a cardiologist should be considered for patients with underlying cardiac defects, arrhythmias, or cardiac complaints while on stimulant medications. Stimulant medications are considered pregnancy class C; thus, prescribing during pregnancy should be done after careful risk/benefit consideration for each patient. While primary care providers may manage many patients with ADHD, consultation with a neurologist or psychiatrist should be considered for complicated cases, such as in patients with severe comorbid mental health disorders or substance abuse. Whether used as an adjunct to medication treatment or alone, there is accumulating research suggesting that participation in cognitive behavioral therapy can help reduce ADHD symptoms for adults [60]. Therefore, both medication and psychotherapy should be considered as potential treatment options for adults with ADHD.

Workplace Accommodations

In addition to medication and therapy, workplace accommodations may benefit adults with ADHD. ADHD is associated with higher levels of unemployment compared to control groups [61]. In one study involving a workplace simulation laboratory, adults with ADHD reported internal restlessness, intolerance of boredom, and difficulty maintaining vigilance, which are likely to adversely impact workplace performance [62]. Adults with ADHD may benefit from accommodations in the workplace, such as frequent breaks.

Conclusion

Additional Considerations

Screening for substance use disorders, anxiety, and depression should be part of routine clinical care for adolescents and adults with ADHD, given the high risk for these comorbidities to occur and the benefits that early detection and intervention can provide (Appendix). Anticipatory guidance around safe stimulant prescribing practices is also recommended, given the high rate of misuse and diversion of stimulant medications [63]. Counseling should include directions to keep stimulant medication in a secure location and information about the risks of stimulant abuse and diversion. Caregivers should provide oversight at the time that the adolescent or young adult assumes responsibility for medication administration. Using a weekly pillbox can allow the individual with ADHD autonomy over self-administration and also enable a visual check-in from a caregiver or significant other to ensure that the medication is taken each day.

Given the chronic nature of ADHD, and its association with adverse employment, relationship, and overall health outcomes, regular clinic visits with an adult provider are necessary to monitor treatment, assess for comorbidities, and ensure optimal outcomes.

Appendix

Attention-deficit/hyperactivity disorder (ADHD) condition fact sheet

Definition	Attention-deficit/hyperactivity disorder (ADHD) is a chronic neurodevelopmental disorder that often affects individuals throughout the lifespan. ADHD is characterized by impairing symptoms of inattention and/or hyperactivity/impulsivity across at least 2 different settings, such as home and work • Associated deficits in executive function (organization, planning) are common
Epidemiology	• The prevalence of ADHD among US adults ages 18–44-years old is reported to be 4.4 % • ADHD is more common in males than females, with pediatric studies reporting that males are 2–3 times more likely to have ADHD, while the male to female ratio is lower among affected adults • Rates of diagnosed ADHD are lower among minority populations, potentially due to under identification • ADHD is significantly more common among first-degree relatives of affected individuals, reflecting the high heritability of ADHD
Special considerations	**Individuals with ADHD have high rates of comorbid mental health and other chronic conditions, including:** • Depression/Mood disorders • Suicidality • Anxiety disorders • Substance use disorders • Learning disorders • Antisocial personality disorder • Obesity **Individuals often have impairment in multiple domains including:** • Employment and occupational functioning • Relationships • Driving

Suggested Reading List

- Barkley RA, Murphy KR, Fischer M. ADHD in Adults: What the Science Says. New York, NY: The Guilford Press. 2008.
- Barkley RA. Taking Charge of Adult ADHD. New York, NY: The Guilford Press. 2010.

Patient/Caregiver Resources

- Barkley RA. Taking Charge of Adult ADHD. New York, NY: The Guilford Press. 2010.
- Children and Adults with Attention Deficit Disorder (www.chadd.org)

References

1. American Psychiatric Association. Diagnostic and Statistical Manual of Mental Disorders. 5th ed. Washington: American Psychiatric Association; 2013.
2. Barkley R, Murphy KFM. ADHD in adults: What the science says. New York, NY: Guilford Press; 2008.
3. Kollins SH, McClernon J, Fuemmeler BF. Association between smoking and Attention Deficit/ Hyperactivity Disorder symptoms in a population-based sample of young adults. Arch Gen Psychiatry. 2005;62(10):1142–7.
4. Leibson C, Katusic SK, Barbaresi WJ, Ransom J, Brien PCO. Use and Costs of Medical Care For Children Attention-Deficit/Hyperactivity Disorder. JAMA. 2001;285(1):60–6.

5. Merkel RL, Nichols JQ, Fellers JC, Hidalgo P, Martinez LA, Putziger I, et al. Comparison of on-road driving between young adults with and without ADHD. J Atten Disord [Internet]. 2013;1087054712473832. Available from: http://jad.sagepub.com/content/early/2013/02/08/1087054712473832.abstract.
6. Barbaresi WJ, Colligan RC, Weaver AL, Voigt RG, Killian JM, Katusic SK. Mortality, ADHD, and psychosocial adversity in adults with childhood ADHD: a prospective study. Pediatrics [Internet]. 2013;131(4):637–44. Available from: http://pediatrics.aappublications.org.ezp-prod1.hul.harvard.edu/content/131/4/637.
7. Schubiner HI, Tzelepis A, Milberger S, Lockhart N, Kruger M, Kelley BJSE. Prevalence of attention-deficit/hyperactivity disorder and conduct disorder among substance abusers. J Clin Psychiatry. 2000;61(4):244–51.
8. Levy S, Katusic SK, Colligan RC, Weaver AL, Killian JM, Voigt RG, et al. Childhood ADHD and risk for substance dependence in adulthood: a longitudinal, population-based study. PLoS One [Internet]. 2014;9(8):e105640. Available from: http://www.pubmedcentral.nih.gov/articlerender.fcgi?artid=4146503&tool=pmcentrez&rendertype=abstract.
9. Katusic SK, Barbaresi WJ, Colligan RC, Weaver AL, Leibson CL, Jacobsen SJ. Psychostimulant treatment and risk for substance abuse among young adults with a history of attention-deficit/hyperactivity disorder: a population-based, birth cohort study. J Child Adolesc Psychopharmacol. 2005;15(5):764–76.
10. Wilens T. Impact of ADHD and its treatment on substance abuse in adults. J Clin Psychiatry. 2004;65 (Suppl 3):38–45.
11. Yoshimasu K, Barbaresi WJ, Colligan RC, Killian JM, Voigt RG, Weaver AL, et al. Gender, ADHD, and reading disability in a population-based birth cohort. Pediatrics. 2010;126(4):e788–95.
12. Yoshimasu K, Barbaresi WJ, Colligan RC, Killian JM, Voigt RG, Weaver AL, et al. Written-language disorder among children with and without ADHD in a population-based birth cohort. Pediatrics. 2011;128(3):e605–12.
13. Barbaresi WJ, Katusic SK, Colligan RC, Weaver AL, Jacobsen SJ. Modifiers of long-term school outcomes for children with attention-deficit/ hyperactivity disorder: does treatment with stimulant medication make a difference ? Results from a population-based study. J Dev Behav Pediatr [Internet]. 2007;28:274–87. Available from: http://www.ncbi.nlm.nih.gov/pubmed/17700079.
14. Kolar D, Keller A, Golfinopoulos M, Cumyn L, Syer C, Hechtman L. Treatment of adults with attention-deficit/hyperactivity disorder. Neuropsychiatr Dis Treat. 2008;4(2):389–403.
15. Barkley R, Murphy KR, O'Connell T, Connor DF. Effects of two doses of methylphenidate on simulator driving performance in adults with attention deficit hyperactivity disorder. J Saf Res. 2005;36(2):121–31.
16. Barkley R, Fischer M, Smallish L, Fletcher K. Young adult outcome of hyperactive children: adaptive functioning in major life activities. J Am Acad Child Adolesc Psychiatry. Am Acad Child. Adolesc Psychiatry [Internet]. 2006;45(2):192–202. doi:10.1097/01.chi.0000189134.97436.e2.
17. American Academy of Pediatrics. ADHD: Clinical practice guideline for the diagnosis, evaluation, and treatment of attention-deficit/hyperactivity disorder in children and adolescents. Pediatrics [Internet]. 2011;128(5):1007–22. Available from: http://pediatrics.aappublications.org/cgi/doi/10.1542/peds.2011-2654.
18. MTA Cooperative Group. A 14-month randomized clinical trial of treatment strategies for attention-deficit/hyperactivity disorder. Arch Gen Psychiatry. 1999;56(12):1073–86.
19. Safren SA, Otto MW, Sprich S, Winett CL, Wilens TE, Biederman J. Cognitive-behavioral therapy for ADHD in medication-treated adults with continued symptoms. Behav Res Therapy [Internet]. 2005;43(7):831–42. Available from: http://linkinghub.elsevier.com/retrieve/pii/S0005796704001366.
20. Rostain AL, Ramsay JR. A combined treatment approach for adults with ADHD—results of an open study of 43 patients. J Atten Disord [Internet]. 2006;10(2):150–9. Available from: http://www.ncbi.nlm.nih.gov/pubmed/17085625.
21. Haavik J, Halmoy A, Lundervold AJFO. Clinical assessment and diagnosis of adults with attention-deficit/hyperactivity disorder. Expert Rev Neurother. 2010;10:1569–80.
22. TE Barkley RAB. Unrecognized attention-deficit/hyperactivity disorder in adults presenting with other psychiatric disorders. CNS Spectr. 2008;13:977.
23. Rapport LJ, Friedman SL, Tzelepis A, Van Voorhis A. Experienced emotion and affect recognition in adult attention-deficit hyperactivity disorder. Neuropsychology [Internet]. 2002;16(1):102–10. Available from: http://doi.apa.org/getdoi.cfm?doi=10.1037/0894-4105.16.1.102.
24. Kessler RC, Adler L, Barkley RA, Biederman J, Conners CK, Demler O, et al. The prevalence and correlates of adult ADHD in the United States: results from the National Comorbidity Survey Replication. Am J Psychiatry. 2006;163(4):716–23.
25. Barbaresi WJ, Weaver AL, Voigt RG, Killian JM, Katusic SK. Comparing methods to determine persistence of child hood ADHD into adulthood: a population-based study. J Atten Disord. 2015 Dec 22. pii: 1087054715618791. [Epub ahead of print]. PMID: 26700793.
26. Fayyad J, DeGraaf R, Kessler R, Tenaere KD, Girolamo GDE, Haro JM, Kar EG. Cross-national prevalence and correlates of adult attention-deficit hyperactivity disorder. Br J Psychiatry. 2007;190:402.
27. Ramsay JR. Health care systems issues and disparities in ADHD care for African American adults. J Clin Psychiatry. 2014;75(12):e32.

28. Waite R. Culturally competent approaches to assessing ADHD in African American adults and overcoming cultural issues with patients and families. J Clin Psychiatry. 2015;76(3):e7.
29. Visser SN, Danielson ML, Bitsko RH, Holbrook JR, Kogan MD, Ghandour RM, Perou R, Blumber S. Trends in the parent-report of health care provider-diagnosed and medicated ADHD: United States, 2003–2011. J Am Acad Child Adolesc Psychiatry. 2014;53(1):34–46.
30. Froehlich TE, Lanphear BP, Epstein JN, Barbaresi WJ, Katusic SK, Kahn RS. Prevalence, recognition, and treatment of attention-deficit/hyperactivity disorder in a national sample of US children. Arch Pediatr Adolesc Med. 2007;161(9):857–64.
31. Barkley RA, Fischer M, Smallish L, Fletcher K. The persistence of attention-deficit/hyperactivity disorder into young adulthood as a function of reporting source and definition of disorder. J Abnorm Psychol. 2002;111(2):279–89.
32. Dias G, Mattos P, Coutinho G, Segenreich D, Saboya E, Ayrão V. Agreement rates between parent and self-report on past ADHD symptoms in an adult clinical sample. J Atten Disord [Internet]. 2008;12(1):70–5. Available from: http://www.ncbi.nlm.nih.gov/pubmed/18192619.
33. Faraone SV, Antsel K. Diagnosing and treating ADHD in adults. World Psychiatry. 2008;7(3):131–6.
34. Sheehan DV, Lecrubier Y, Sheehan KH. The Mini-International Neuropsychiatric Interview (M.I.N.I.): the development and validation of a structured diagnostic psychiatric interfiew for DSM-IV and ICD-10. J Clin Psychiatry. 1998;59(Suppl 20):22–33.
35. Smith AK, Mick E, Faraone SV. Advances in genetic studies of attention-deficit/hyperactivity disorder. Curr Psychiatry Rep. 2009;11(2):143–8.
36. Faraone SV, Mick E. Molecular genetics of attention deficit hyperactivity disorder. Psychiatr Clin North Am [Internet]. 2011;33(1):1–20. Available from: http://www.pubmedcentral.nih.gov/articlerender.fcgi?artid=2847260&tool=pmcentrez&rendertype=abstract.
37. Williams NM, Zaharieva I, Martin A, Langley K, Mantripragada K, Fossdal R, et al. Rare chromosomal deletions and duplications in attention-deficit hyperactivity disorder: a genome-wide analysis. Lancet [Internet]. Elsevier Ltd; 2010;376(9750):1401–8. Available from: http://linkinghub.elsevier.com/retrieve/pii/S0140673610611099.
38. Froehlich TE, Anixt JS, Loe IM, Chirdkiatgumchai V, Kuan L, Gilman RC. Update on environmental risk factors for attention-deficit/hyperactivity disorder. Curr Psychiatry Rep [Internet]. 2011;13(5):333–44. Available from: http://www.pubmedcentral.nih.gov/articlerender.fcgi?artid=3277258&tool=pmcentrez&rendertype=abstract.
39. Kim S, Arora M, Fernandez C, Landero J, Caruso J, Chen A. Lead, mercury, and cadmium exposure and attention deficit hyperactivity disorder in children. Environ Res [Internet]. Elsevier; 2013;126:105–10. Available from: http://www.pubmedcentral.nih.gov/articlerender.fcgi?artid=3847899&tool=pmcentrez&rendertype=abstract.
40. Bouchard MF, Bellinger DC, Wright RO, Weisskopf MG. Attention-deficit/hyperactivity disorder and urinary metabolites of organophosphate pesticides. Pediatrics [Internet]. 2010;125(6):e1270–7. Available from: http://pediatrics.aappublications.org/cgi/doi/10.1542/peds.2009-3058.
41. Millichap JG. Etiologic classification of attention deficit/hyperactivity disorder. Pediatrics [Internet]. 2008;121(2):358–65. Available from: http://pediatrics.aappublications.org/content/121/2/e358.full.html.
42. Weiss MD, Baer S, Allan BA, Saran K, Schibuk H. The screens culture: impact on ADHD. Atten Defic Hyperact Disord [Internet]. 2011;3(4):327–34. Available from: http://www.pubmedcentral.nih.gov/articlerender.fcgi?artid=3220824&tool=pmcentrez&rendertype=abstract.
43. Cortese S, Kelly C, Chabernaud C, Proal E, Di Martino A, Milham MP, et al. Toward systems neuroscience of ADHD: a meta-analysis of 55 fMRI studies. Am J Psychiatry [Internet]. 2012;169:1038–55. Available from: http://www.ncbi.nlm.nih.gov/pmc/articles/PMC3879048/pdf/nihms535797.pdf.
44. Kasparek T, Theiner P, Filova A. Neurobiology of ADHD from childhood to adulthood: findings of imaging methods. J Atten Disord [Internet]. 2013; Available from: http://www.ncbi.nlm.nih.gov/pubmed/24097847.
45. Rubia K, Smith A, Brammer M, Toone B, Taylor E. Abnormal brain activation during inhibition and error detection in medication-naive adolescents with ADHD. Am J Psychiatry [Internet]. 2005;162(6):1067–75. Available from: http://www.ncbi.nlm.nih.gov/pubmed/15930054.
46. Shaw P, Eckstrand K, Sharp W, Blumenthal J, Lerch JP, Greenstein D, et al. Attention-deficit/hyperactivity disorder is characterized by a delay in cortical maturation. Proc Natl Acad Sci U S A [Internet]. 2007;104(49):19649–54. Available from: /pmc/articles/PMC2148343/?report=abstract.
47. Russell V, Allie S, Wiggins T. Increased noradrenergic activity in prefrontal cortex slices of an animal model for attention-deficit hyperactivity disorder—the spontaneously hypertensive rat. Behav Brain Res. 2000;117:69.
48. Dougherty DD, Bonab AA, Spencer TJ, Rauch SL, Madras BK, Fischman AJ. Dopamine transporter density in patients with attention deficit hyperactivity disorder. The phantom of progressive dementia in epilepsy. Lancet [Internet]. 1999;354:2132–3. doi:10.1016/S0140-6736(99)04030-1.
49. Aguirre Castaneda RL, Kumar S, Voigt RG, Leibson CL, Barbaresi WJ, Weaver AL, et al. Childhood attention-deficit/hyperactivity disorder, sex, and obesity: a longitudinal population-based study. Mayo Clin Proc. 2016;91(3):352–61.
50. Biederman J, Mick E, Faraone SV. Age-dependent decline of symptoms of attention deficit hyperactivity

disorder: impact of remission definition and symptom type. Am J Psychiatry. 2000;157(5):816–8.
51. Ebejer JL, Medland SE, van der Werf J, Gondro C, Henders AK, Lynskey M, et al. Attention deficit hyperactivity disorder in Australian Adults: prevalence, persistence, conduct problems and disadvantage. PLoS One. 2012;7(10):1–10.
52. Chang Z, Lichtenstein P, D'Onofrio BM, Sjolander ALH. Serious transport accidents in adults with ADHD and the effect of medication: a population-based study. JAMA Psychiatry. 2014;71 (3):319–3235.
53. Wilens TE, Morrison NR, Prince J. An update on the pharmacotherapy of ADHD in adults. Expert Rev Neurother. 2011;11:1443.
54. American Psychiatric Association. Diagnostic and Statistical Manual of Mental Disorders, Fourth Edition, Text Revision [Internet]. Text. 2000. 943p. Available from: http://scholar.google.com/scholar?hl=en&btnG=Search&q=intitle:Diagnostic+and+statistical+manual+of+mental+disorders#3.
55. Hines JL, King TS, Curry WJ. The adult ADHD self-report scale for screening for adult attention deficit-hyperactivity disorder (ADHD). J Am Board Fam Med [Internet]. 2012;25(6):847–53. Available from: http://www.ncbi.nlm.nih.gov/pubmed/23136325.
56. Conners CK, Erhardt D, Epstein JN, Parker JDA, Sitarenios G, Sparrow E. Self-ratings of ADHD symptoms in adults I: Factor structure and normative data. J Atten Disord [Internet]. 1999;3(3):141–51. Available from: http://jad.sagepub.com/content/3/3/141.abstract.
57. Wilens TE, Hammerness PG, Biederman J, Kwon A, Spencer TJ, Clark S, et al. Blood pressure changes associated with medication treatment of adults with attention-deficit/hyperactivity disorder. J Clin Psychiatry. 2005;66(2):253–9.
58. Habel LA, Cooper WO, Sox CM, Chan KA, Fireman BH, Arbogast PG, et al. ADHD medications and risk of serious cardiovascular events in young and middle-aged adults. JAMA [Internet]. 2011;306 (24):2673–83. Available from: http://www.pubmedcentral.nih.gov/articlerender.fcgi?artid=3350308&tool=pmcentrez&rendertype=abstract.
59. Schelleman H, Bilker WB, Kimmel SE, Daniel GW, Newcomb C, Guevara JP, et al. Methylphenidate and risk of serious cardiovascular events in adults. Am J Psychiatry. 2012;169(2):178–85.
60. Knouse L, Safren S. Current status of cognitive behavioral therapy for adult attention-deficit hyperactivity disorder. Psychiatr Clin North Am [Internet]. 2010;33(3):497–509. Available from: http://europepmc.org/articles/PMC2909688.
61. Biederman J, Mick E, Faraone SV. Normalized functioning in youths with persistent attention-deficit/hyperactivity disorder. J Pediatr. 1998;133(4):544–51.
62. Fried R, Surman C, Hammerness P, Petty C, Faraone S, Hyder L, et al. A controlled study of a simulated workplace laboratory for adults with attention deficit hyperactivity disorder. Psychiatry Res [Internet]. Elsevier; 2012;200(2–3):949–56. Available from: http://www.pubmedcentral.nih.gov/articlerender.fcgi?artid=3426653&tool=pmcentrez&rendertype=abstract.
63. Harstad E, Levy S. Attention-deficit/hyperactivity disorder and substance abuse. Pediatrics [Internet]. 2014;134(1):e293–301. Available from: http://pediatrics.aappublications.org/cgi/doi/10.1542/peds.2014-0992.

4 Autism

Tara Crapnell, Lynette Lau, Christopher D. Hanks, Christina Nicolaidis and Alice A. Kuo

Case Presentation

Allen is a 21-year-old male with autism spectrum disorder (ASD) and mild intellectual disability who presents to establish care. He is accompanied by his mother who says he refused to return to his previous Internal Medicine physician because the physician "did not know what to do with him." One year ago, his pediatrician had suggested that they find an adult doctor but they have had difficulty finding the right physician. Allen graduated from high school with a diploma and spent some time in a vocational training program. After completing that, he struggled to find work and spent about 1 year at home with no regular daily activities. He recently obtained some support through his local Board of Developmental Disabilities and he is now working part-time at a local grocery store bagging groceries and retrieving shopping carts with a job coach for support. They feel he is capable of more than this but have not been able to find the right fit for him.

Allen appears well-groomed, quiet, and avoids eye contact. He answers questions with short responses and at times takes longer than expected to answer. He is unable to answer some of the questions about his medical history. His mother at times needs to reword the questions asked so that he can understand them. His mother

T. Crapnell · L. Lau · A.A. Kuo
MCHB Health Care Transitions Research Network (HCT-RN), University of California, 10960 Wilshire Blvd, Suite 960, Los Angeles, CA 90024, USA
e-mail: Crapnellt@outlook.com

L. Lau
e-mail: lynette@ucla.edu

C.D. Hanks
Department of Internal Medicine, The Center for Autism Services and Transition, The Ohio State University Wexner Medical Center, 3691 Ridge Mill Dr, Hilliard, OH 43026, USA
e-mail: christopher.hanks@osumc.edu

C. Nicolaidis
School of Social Work, Portland State University, 1600 SW 4th Avenue, Portland, USA
e-mail: nicol22@pdx.edu; christina.nicolaidis@pdx.edu

C. Nicolaidis
Schools of Medicine and Public Health, Oregon Health and Science University, Portland, OR 97201, USA

A.A. Kuo (✉)
Departments of Medicine and Pediatrics, Health Care Transitions Research Network, University of California, Los Angeles, 757 Westwood Plaza, Suite 7501, Los Angeles, CA 90095, USA
e-mail: AKuo@mednet.ucla.edu

M. Pilapil et al. (eds.), *Care of Adults with Chronic Childhood Conditions*,
DOI 10.1007/978-3-319-43827-6_4

reports he had attention-deficient/hyperactivity disorder (ADHD) and was on a stimulant through high school, but he has not taken it for several years. He is also on an atypical antipsychotic, which was started 8 years ago due to explosive outbursts. He has not had any outbursts for years and they are not sure if he should continue this medication or not. They also wonder if restarting his stimulant would help him focus at work. He exhibits some intermittent rocking in his chair and several episodes of hand-flapping that become more prominent as the visit progresses. Exam is only remarkable for being overweight, ticklish during the abdominal exam, and refusal of the genital exam.

Allen reports that when he is not at work he spends most of his day playing video games or watching videos online. His mother expresses concern about his weight, which has been steadily increasing since he graduated from high school. Additionally, he resists brushing his teeth and bathing himself because he does not like how the toothpaste and soap feel. She also notes that he is struggling to develop relationships with friends and has seemed more withdrawn recently. When asked about these things, he is reluctant to discuss it.

Case Discussion

This case illustrates some of the challenges that both individuals on the autism spectrum and their parents face when they reach adulthood. Many people with ASD struggle to maintain close relationships with others once they leave the structured environment of high school. Youth with ASD can be "disconnected" in the years after aging out of school, meaning that they are not in any employment or postsecondary education setting. Additionally, parents of young adults on the autism spectrum struggle to find the balance of allowing autonomy and independence while ensuring safety and support for their children.

In Allen's case, he is struggling to express himself and communicate with his physician. This can occur due to several causes, including anxiety, challenges with communicating feelings and needs, or sensory processing difficulties that may inhibit him from performing at his highest level of ability. His physician should explore how he best communicates and seek accommodations to help him remain engaged in the encounter. The provider should try to use precise, literal language to help improve the effectiveness of his or her communication. Encouraging him to come prepared with questions that are preplanned or written down may be beneficial. Additionally, Allen is demonstrating challenges that could benefit from services such as occupational therapy (OT) to improve his self-care skills and address possible sensory processing challenges associated with bathing and brushing his teeth. This would help improve his level of independence as well as functional and meaningful participation in other activities of interest.

Since Allen is on the autism spectrum and has an intellectual disability, you should consider referring him for genetic testing because the genes that have been linked to autism can also be associated with cancers, leading to a need to adjust the cancer-screening timeline. Genetics programs at major academic centers will often have a cancer-screening clinic for individuals who are at risk for early cancers.

Allen's mother coached and supported him through this encounter, which allowed Allen to stay more involved in the discussion. However, many parents or caregivers struggle to find the right balance in supporting independence while also ensuring essential information is conveyed. Providers may need to coach parents to allow the individual to interact with the provider at their highest potential. Parents and caregivers can perform important roles in helping patients learn their medical needs and learn to self-advocate. Depending on patient preference, effort should be made to allow the patient some time with the physician without a parent or caregiver present to allow development of comfort with the medical provider as well as allow discussion of topics that may be difficult to discuss with parents present.

Several important medical and social issues were raised in this case. Obesity is common in adults with ASD. His "disconnectedness" over the past several years may be contributing to this, as he has limited opportunity to get out of the home, be active, interact with others, and develop friendships. Assisting Allen and his parents in identifying opportunities for work that fit his strengths, interests, and needs will be important for him to maintain a healthy lifestyle. While helping patients in this dilemma is beyond the purview of a typical primary care office, making recommendations to parents to connect with the Department of Vocational Rehabilitation, a local Family Resource Center, or the public Department of Developmental Services in the area is a good place to help them get started.

Finally, many individuals on the autism spectrum are treated with medication for behavioral issues. Commonly used medications include selective serotonin reuptake inhibitors (SSRIs), antipsychotics, and stimulants, as well as antiepileptic medications. Many of these medications have significant adverse effects and need monitoring with labs or other clinical assessments. Additionally, polypharmacy concerns are common in patients on multiple psychotropic medications. In this case, the provider should consider a trial discontinuation of the atypical antipsychotic, as the risks associated with antipsychotics may outweigh the benefit in this patient who has not had an aggressive outburst in many years. In many cases, primary care providers may not feel comfortable managing these medications, and patients should be referred to a psychiatrist or neurologist who has more experience managing these medications with people on the autism spectrum.

Medical Model Versus Social Model of Disability

Of relevance to this case study and discussion is the concept of the medical model versus the social model of disability. For several decades, approaches and interventions for individuals on the autism spectrum have largely focused on the individual, their impairment, and remediation of skills so that individuals can progress along the typical developmental pathway of their peers. The medical model has defined how we see and describe individuals on the autism spectrum, the interventions that have been developed over the past several decades, and the treatments to which we often refer individuals and families. While it is known that individuals on the autism spectrum experience significant challenges in areas such as social and communication skills and sensory processing, and various interventions have proven to be effective in improving these areas, we should also have an understanding of ASD through the lens of the social model. The social model views disability as a result of societal and environmental barriers. As physicians, we should consider the individual within their context, and the social and environmental factors that may be influencing our interactions with individuals and exacerbating their symptoms during office visits or in their day-to-day life. Examples of this include our own personal biases and assumptions, as well environmental factors, such as lights or sounds in the waiting room. Many of the tips provided in this chapter focus on low-cost accommodations that could be implemented in practice. These accommodations can help create a more supportive environment and increase the chances of a successful checkup or office visit for those on the autism spectrum.

While it is important to understand the individual challenges experienced by those on the autism spectrum and the impact of social and environmental factors, it is also important to acknowledge the individual strengths of our patients. Examples of strengths unique to individuals with ASD include detailed thinking, good long-term memory, and the ability to analyze information [1]. Identifying and focusing on the strengths of your patients with ASD can assist individuals in seeing their own strengths. While this can positively affect the attitudes and beliefs of the individuals and parents, it can also help providers identify and make proper referrals to services and community programs, and can assist individuals and families to realize the different opportunities one could pursue in adulthood with the proper supports in place.

The following sections provide information on the phenomenology and etiology of ASD, comorbidities and risk factors associated with

ASD, and special issues arising during the transition to adulthood that may be important for primary care providers to be aware of, as well as brief descriptions of the interventions and treatments that individuals on the autism spectrum may receive or benefit from and practical tips for facilitating health care.

Background

Definition

Autism spectrum disorder is a complex, lifelong neurodevelopmental condition that is marked by deficits in social communication and interaction, and repetitive or restrictive patterns of behavior, interests, or activities [2]. Signs and symptoms are present in early childhood, but may not become obvious until later childhood or adulthood, when demands increase [2]. Individuals on the autism spectrum may also experience a lack of coordination, motor planning, and atypical sensory processing, such as oversensitivity to auditory, tactile, and visual input [3, 4]. Furthermore, an intellectual disability may or may not be present [5]. Symptoms and behaviors associated with autism often result in decreased social participation, occupational and other areas of functional participation, and may change over time with development and life stages [2, 6, 7].

Prevalence

Over the past several years, the prevalence of ASD has increased 123 % from 2002 to 2008 [5]. The reasons for the increasing prevalence of ASD remains unclear, however, it is suspected that it is related to factors such as increased awareness and diagnostic practices [8, 9]. The current estimated prevalence of ASD in the United States is 14.7 per 1000 (1 in 68) children aged 8 years [5]. In addition, it has been found that prevalence does not change with age [10]. While ASD is reported to occur in all racial/ethnic and socioeconomic groups, prevalence estimates vary between these groups, as there are reported gender [11, 12], ethnic, and racial disparities in the identification of ASD [13, 14].

Etiology and Risk Factors

The etiology of ASD is not fully understood, however, several studies have identified various risk factors associated with ASD. Genetic factors have long been thought to influence autism and are one of the most extensively studied factors in epidemiologic research. Studies have found a 40 to 90 % heritability rate [15, 16] and associations with fragile X syndrome, 15q11-13 duplications, genetic variants, and de novo mutations [17, 18]. More than 100 mutated genes have been found to be associated with ASD [19]. Gene mutations in ASD are believed to be a result of spontaneous mutations, suggesting gene–gene interaction [20], gene–environment [21], and epigenetic programming early in life [22–25], as well as windows of vulnerability that may influence ASD [26] during fetal development and in early childhood. While studies indicate there is a neurogenetic component to ASD, some studies suggest there are associations between ASD and prenatal exposures and perinatal factors [27–32]. However, it should be noted that there are limitations associated with these studies.

Associated Morbidity

Autism spectrum disorders have been commonly researched within the disciplines of psychiatry and neurology. However, evidence has shown that individuals on the autism spectrum experience high rates of co-occurring mental and physical conditions, shifting the focus from solely neurodevelopmental and behavioral to a more complex process. Research indicates that specific medical conditions are more prevalent in individuals with autism compared to the neurotypical population. Medical conditions that are reported to occur at higher rates in people on the autism spectrum include: eczema, allergies, asthma, ear and respiratory infections, gastrointestinal problems, severe headaches and migraines, sleep disorders, and epilepsy [33]. People on the autism spectrum are also at heightened risk for chronic health conditions in adulthood, such as diabetes, coronary heart disease, cancer [34], and mental health conditions [33, 35, 36]. These co-occurring conditions have been found to negatively impact functional ability of individuals on the autism spectrum within the areas of behavior, communication, cognition, and sensory processing.

Genetics and Cancer Screening

Recent studies have suggested that ASD has a strong genetic component with potential links to cancer [37–40]. Findings have indicated associations between ASD and up regulation of the PI3K (phosphatidylinositol 3-kinase)–Akt–mTOR (mammalian target of rapamycin) growth-signaling pathway [41–45], which has been associated with the development of cancers [46, 47]. Individuals with autism have been found to have similar mutations in the gene, PTEN, as seen in various forms of cancer [39]. PTEN is a tumor suppressor gene that helps prevent cells from becoming cancerous and is a negative regulator of PI3K–Akt–mTOR signaling. Mutations in PTEN have been associated with cognitive impairments and abnormalities in brain structure and various forms of cancer, including cancers of the breasts, kidney, prostate, and brain. In addition, the neurofibromatosis gene NF1, which is also a tumor suppressor and negative regulator of the PI3K–Akt–mTOR pathway, has been associated with ASD [48]. Because recent evidence suggests individuals with ASD are at heightened risk for cancer, a referral for genetic testing and cancer screening is recommended (see Box 4.1).

Box 4.1 Genetics and cancer screening

- The American Academy of Neurology and the Child Neurology Society recommend referring individuals with ASD for high-resolution chromosome studies (karyotype) and DNA analysis for Fragile X, particularly if
  - intellectual disability is present (or cannot be excluded)
  - there is a family history of Fragile X or undiagnosed intellectual disability
  - dysmorphic features are present

  Note, however, there is little likelihood of positive karyotype or Fragile X testing in the presence of autism without intellectual disability
- Genetic counseling for individuals with ASD (and their families) should always accompany genetic evaluation
- Routinely include age-appropriate cancer-screening procedures during health maintenance visits

Seizure Disorder

Individuals on the autism spectrum are reported to experience higher rates of epilepsy than the general population, with a prevalence rate of 12.5 % in children with ASD, which increases to 26 % by adolescence [49, 50]. Seizure disorder has been associated with increased age, lower intellectual functioning, and decreased adaptive behavior. Epilepsy can be easily misdiagnosed in individuals with intellectual disabilities as a result of misinterpretation of behavioral, physiological, and psychological events [51]. Undiagnosed or misdiagnosis can potentially have fatal implications. Therefore, further evaluation, such as electroencephalogram (EEG), and/or referral to a specialist should be considered when patients present with changes in behavior that could be related to seizures [52].

Gastrointestinal Disorder

Individuals on the autism spectrum are reported to experience higher rates of gastrointestinal problems, including diarrhea, constipation, vomiting, and abdominal pain. These symptoms can have negative implications on behavior. Evaluation and management of gastrointestinal problems in individuals on the autism spectrum is not yet fully understood [53], however, it is recommended that individuals should receive the same thoroughness and standard of care as patients without ASD.

Furthermore, gastrointestinal workup should be considered with change in behavior.

Sleep Disturbances

Sleep disturbances are commonly reported in individuals on the autism spectrum across the lifespan [54–57]. Sleep disturbances can negatively impact daily functioning and quality of life [58, 59]. Sleep problems may be a result of obstructive sleep apnea and gastrointestinal reflux, and have been associated with emotional and behavioral problems as well as psychiatric conditions [60]. Melatonin and other behavioral interventions have been found to be effective in improving sleep [54, 61].

Mental Health Conditions

Individuals on the autism spectrum are reported to experience high rates of mental health conditions [33, 35, 36], with anxiety and depression being the most commonly reported co-occurring conditions. In addition, reports suggest around 30 % of individuals on the autism spectrum meet the criteria for ADHD [62]. While anxiety is reported to occur in children with ASD, studies have indicated that anxiety often increases in adolescence and adulthood. Assessment and diagnosis of anxiety and depression can be challenging as individuals may have difficulties with communicating feelings and symptoms. While various interventions including using components of cognitive behavioral therapy (CBT) have been proven to be effective in improving anxiety symptoms in ASD [63, 64], there is often a lack of mental health providers trained to serve adults with ASD. Effort should be made to identify mental health providers with experience treating those with ASD, if possible.

Special Issues that Arise in the Transition to Adulthood

It is estimated that approximately 500,000 individuals on the autism spectrum will transition into young adulthood each year in the United States. Youth on the autism spectrum are especially vulnerable during the transition to adulthood due to the inherent characteristics of ASD, such as challenges with communication and social interaction, [2], comorbid physical and mental health problems [36], and societal biases and discrimination [65]. These pervasive challenges often result in complex service needs that cut across sectors and require high levels of care coordination, further complicating this transitional period [66–69].

Based on Part B of the Individuals Disability Education Act (IDEA), children and youth are eligible to receive special education-related services from 3 to 22 years of age [70]. The IDEA ensures that while children are in school and of eligible age (3–22 years of age), they are entitled to services that will help them function within their current educational setting and prepare them for adulthood within the areas of education, employment, and independent living [70]. However, upon reaching their 22nd birthday, individuals essentially experience a "services cliff" where they go from receiving several hours of services to no services, despite the need for continued supports and services to assist them during and after the transition to community-based settings.

Although this is a time of much needed support, the gap between service needs and receipt increases as many individuals on the spectrum exit the special education system and attempt to access adult systems of care. Evidence has shown less optimal outcomes for young adults on the autism spectrum with high rates of disconnectedness upon leaving high school [71, 72]. It is reported that one-third of young adults are disconnected after high school (never had a job or continued education after high school) and approximately 26 % receive no services that would help them become employed, continue their education, or live more independently [72]. In addition, only 36 % ever attend postsecondary education and 58 % work for pay outside of the home between high school and their early 20s [72].

Evidence suggests that many individuals on the autism spectrum continue to lack skills, such as self-care and daily living skills that are foundational and necessary for achieving functional and meaningful participation in adulthood [73–75]. In addition, marked social deficits may become increasingly problematic in adolescence when social expectation demands increase and social network heightens [76]. Symptoms of autism do not disappear when an individual becomes an adult [77] and many could benefit from continued support and services throughout life [75, 78]. Educating and assisting individuals on the autism spectrum and their families to connect to services within their community—such as the Department of Vocational Rehabilitation, Department of Developmental Services, and community centers—can help reduce disconnectedness and improve outcomes in adulthood for those on the autism spectrum.

Interventions and Treatment

There is a wide range in severity of symptoms in autism. Families may pursue treatments including behavioral, psychological, educational, and alternative treatments. Interventions are generally targeted at improving social communication and interaction, increasing and maintaining adaptive behaviors, functional skills, and increasing meaningful participation. Below are common interventions provided to individuals on the autism spectrum.

Applied Behavioral Analysis

Applied behavioral analysis (ABA) is an evidence-based intervention for children on the autism spectrum that uses principles of learning theory to try to bring about meaningful and positive change in behavior. The goal of ABA is to increase and maintain functional and adaptive behaviors, decrease maladaptive behaviors, teach new skills, and generalize skills to other environments. Functional behavioral assessments include identifying antecedents, behaviors, and consequences of behavior, and developing individualized treatment plans that will increase the frequency of a targeted behavior and adaptive behavior. It is important to note that although ABA is commonly used in children on the autism spectrum, autistic rights advocates have raised significant concerns about ABA [79] and there is very limited evidence to support this intervention for adults on the autism spectrum.

Cognitive Behavioral Therapy

Cognitive behavioral therapy (CBT) is used to help individuals on the autism spectrum improve behaviors and self-regulation. Cognitive behavioral therapy is an approach that aims to change perceptions of thoughts. It is an approach that has been proven to help reduce anxiety and depressive symptoms. While CBT can help reduce symptoms and challenging behaviors, such as obsessive thoughts, it teaches individuals how to cope, manage, and reduce unwanted feelings.

Speech and Language Therapy

Speech and language therapy aims to improve social communication and interaction, self-advocacy, and other language impairments in individuals on the autism spectrum. Intervention includes a variety of modalities to help support and improve social interaction and verbal and nonverbal communication, including activity schedules/visual supports and/or augmentative and alternative communication (AAC). Augmentative and alternative communication includes supplementing or replacing natural speech with aided or unaided symbols. Examples of these devices, include, but are not limited to Picture Exchange Communication System (PECS), speech generative devices, and manual signs or gestures. These approaches have been proven to be effective in improving communication skills, social skills and interactions, and self-advocacy and self-determination in individuals on the autism spectrum.

Occupational Therapy

Occupational therapy (OT) is a client-centered profession that assists individuals to achieve the highest degree of independence. Occupational therapy aims to improve performance and participation in daily occupations, such as self-care routines, leisure activities, and school- or work-related tasks. Occupational therapy works on developing and maintaining individual skills and modifying the environment to create a person–environment fit. Occupational therapy also uses sensory integration (SI) alone or as part of therapy. The goal of SI is to remediate processing and integration of sensory information to allow the individual to adapt and interact with their environment.

Practical Tips to Facilitate Health Care

Limited communication and social interactions as well as sensory processing challenges experienced by individuals on the autism spectrum can make it challenging for medical providers to identify health complications in individuals on the autism spectrum. Adults on the autism spectrum report greater unmet healthcare needs, lower use of preventive services, and greater use of the emergency department than adults without ASD [80], placing them at risk for less optimal health outcomes. A recent qualitative study indicated that poor provider and patient level interactions contribute to negative healthcare experiences. Individuals on the autism spectrum have a significant need for services and supports to help increase quality of life and function and to treat co-occurring medical conditions. Timely, accurate information with care coordination can help improve outcomes in adulthood.

The following sections provide practical tips from the Academic Autistic Spectrum Partnership in Research and Education (AASPIRE) for healthcare providers when managing and providing care of individuals with ASD. The complete list of helpful tips can be found on their Website at: www.autismandhealth.org.

Communication and Interaction

Individuals on the autism spectrum are reported to have various strengths and challenges in verbal and nonverbal communication, receptive and expressive skills, and ability to process information. In addition, individuals on the autism spectrum commonly take language literally and require information to be provided to them in a way that is precise, concrete, and specific (Box 4.2). Understanding a patient's communication needs is very important to providing quality care.

Box 4.2 Tips on communication and interaction

- Do not assume that a patient cannot understand healthcare information or communicate when he/she does not speak fluently. In addition, do not assume that a patient who speaks fluently does not have significant communication challenges
- Obtain individualized information on communication needs and preferences
- Be precise, concrete, and specific
- Do not assume a patient is distracted or inattentive because he/she is fidgeting, making repetitive movements, or avoiding eye contact
- Give adequate time for individuals to process information they need to see, hear, or feel before they respond

Sensory Challenges

Individuals on the autism spectrum commonly have atypical sensory processing. Individuals may be hyper-responsive or hypo-responsive to sounds, lights, smells, touch, or taste. As a result, some environments can be over stimulating for some individuals. Environments that are not sensitive to their sensory need can have a negative impact on their healthcare experience and social interactions. In addition, individuals may have difficulties with body awareness, making it difficult for them to discriminate between different tactile inputs and location of symptoms. Therefore understanding these sensory challenges and creating a sensory-friendly environment can create more positive experiences for the patient on the spectrum (Box 4.3).

Box 4.3 Tips on sensory challenges

- Use natural light or make the lighting dim
- See the patient in a quiet room
- Avoid unnecessarily touching the patient and warn him/her if you will use touch for a physical examination
- Suggest that the patient bring manipulatives or other physical supports to help reduce or increase sensory stimuli

Planning and Organizing

Some individuals on the autism spectrum experience difficulties with executive functioning within the areas of planning, organizing, and sequencing information. Individuals on the autism spectrum also commonly have difficulties adapting to new environments and situations, creating a need for routine and consistency. See Box 4.4 for tips on the types of supports that can assist individuals in making decisions, following through with information, and decreasing the stress of attending a healthcare appointment.

Box 4.4 Tips on planning and organizing

- Identify patient needs and necessary accommodations prior to the visit by having patients complete a pre-visit assessment or complete a Personalized Accommodations Report by going to www.autismhealth.org/AHAT
- Let the patient and/or his/her supporter know what will occur at the appointment
- Provide visual supports to help the patient through the healthcare routine
- Write up step-by-step instructions
- Have staff assist the patient in scheduling follow-up visits, referrals, or tests
- Contact and follow-up with the patient and/or supporter after the visit

Exams and Procedures

Tolerating examinations, tests, and procedures may be challenging for individuals on the autism spectrum due to reasons mentioned previously. See Box 4.5 for tips to help people on the autism spectrum better tolerate these medical procedures.

Box 4.5 Tips on exams and procedures

- Explain to the patient what is going to be done before doing it
- Slowly expose individuals to different equipment and perform a "trial run" if possible
- Give patients extra time to process information he/she sees, hears, or feels before they respond
- Order blood tests only when absolutely necessary
- Have staff assist the patient in scheduling follow-up visits, referrals, or tests
- Use a numbing spray, cream, or provide the patient with anti-anxiety medication, if necessary, before a blood draw

Conclusion

Understanding the challenges that individuals on the autism spectrum experience, and how social and environmental factors affect them can allow for better provider–patient interactions, successful checkups, and can assist providers in making proper referrals to services and community resources (Appendix) [33, 34, 36, 37]. Utilizing the tips discussed earlier and creating a supportive environment can help improve your practice and delivery of care to adults on the autism spectrum and their families.

Appendix

Autism Spectrum Disorders (ASD) Condition Fact Sheet

Definition	**Autism spectrum disorders (ASD) is a lifelong neurodevelopmental condition characterized by** • Deficits in social communication and interaction • Repetitive or restrictive patterns of behavior, interests, or activities • Additional deficits include lack of coordination, motor planning, and abnormalities in sensory processing • Individuals may or may not have co-occurring intellectual deficits
Epidemiology	• In the United States, 14.7 per 1000 (1 in 68) children aged 8 years have an ASD • ASD is 5 times more common in males (1 in 42) than females • Prevalence of ASD in white non-Hispanic children is 15.7 per 1000, 12.1 per 1000 black non-Hispanic children, and 10.8 per 1000 in Hispanic children • Identical twins are at increased risk for ASD and will occur 36–95 % of the time and 0–31 % of the time in non-identical twins • Parents with 1 child with autism have a 2–18 % chance of having a second child with an ASD
Special considerations	**Individuals on the autism spectrum disorder have high rates of comorbid physical and mental health conditions, including:** [33, 34, 36, 37] • Eczema • Allergies • Asthma • Ear and respiratory infections • Gastrointestinal problems • Severe headaches and migraines • Sleep disorders • Epilepsy • ADHD • Anxiety and depression **Individuals are at heightened risk for chronic conditions, including** • Diabetes • Coronary heart disease • Cancer
Recommended screening	**All individuals with a diagnosis of an autism spectrum disorder should have genetic screening, particularly** • Females • Co-existing intellectual disability • Known sibling with an autism spectrum disorder

References

1. Robertson SM. Neurodiversity, quality of life, and autistic adults: shifting research and professional focuses onto real-life challenges. Disabil Stud Q. 2009;30(1). http://dsq-sds.org/article/view/1069. Accessed 12 Aug 2016.
2. American Psychiatric Association. Diagnostic and statistical manual of mental disorders. 5th ed. Arlington: American Psychiatric Association; 2013.
3. Kern JK, Trivedi MH, Garver CR, Grannemann BD, Andrews AA, Savla JS, et al. The pattern of sensory processing abnormalities in autism. Autism. 2006;10(5):480–94.
4. Fournier KA, Hass CJ, Naik SK, Lodha N, Cauraugh JH. Motor coordination in autism spectrum disorders: a synthesis and meta-analysis. J Autism Dev Disord. 2010;40(10):1227–40.
5. Investigators DDMNSYP, (CDC) CfDCaP. Prevalence of autism spectrum disorder among children aged 8 years—autism and developmental disabilities monitoring network, 11 sites, United States, 2010. MMWR Surveill Summ. 2014;63(2):1–21.
6. Sukhodolsky DG, Scahill L, Gadow KD, Arnold LE, Aman MG, McDougle CJ, et al. Parent-rated anxiety symptoms in children with pervasive developmental disorders: frequency and association with core autism symptoms and cognitive functioning. J Abnorm Child Psychol. 2008;36(1):117–28.
7. Cheely CA, Carpenter LA, Letourneau EJ, Nicholas JS, Charles J, King LB. The prevalence of youth with autism spectrum disorders in the criminal justice system. J Autism Dev Disord. 2012;42(9):1856–62.
8. Blumberg SJ, Bramlett MD, Kogan MD, Schieve LA, Jones JR, Lu MC. Changes in prevalence of parent-reported autism spectrum disorder in school-aged U.S. Children: 2007 to 2011–2012. Natl Health Stat Rep. 2013;65:1–11.
9. Schieve LA, Rice C, Devine O, Maenner MJ, Lee L-C, Fitzgerald R, et al. Have secular changes in perinatal risk factors contributed to the recent autism prevalence increase? Development and application of a mathematical assessment model. Ann Epidemiol. 2011;21(12):930–45.
10. Brugha TS, McManus S, Bankart J, Scott F, Purdon S, Smith J, et al. Epidemiology of autism spectrum disorders in adults in the community in England. Arch Gen Psychiatry. 2011;68(5):459–65.
11. Giarelli E, Wiggins LD, Rice CE, Levy SE, Kirby RS, Pinto-Martin J, et al. Sex differences in the evaluation and diagnosis of autism spectrum disorders among children. Disabil Health J. 2010;3(2):107–16.
12. Rivet TT, Matson JL. Review of gender differences in core symptomatology in autism spectrum disorders. Res Autism Spectr Disord. 2011;5(3):957–76.

13. Mandell DS, Wiggins LD, Carpenter LA, Daniels J, DiGuiseppi C, Durkin MS, et al. Racial/ethnic disparities in the identification of children with autism spectrum disorders. Am J Public Health. 2009;99(3):493–8.
14. Jo H, Schieve LA, Rice CE, Yeargin-Allsopp M, Tian LH, Blumberg SJ, et al. Age at autism spectrum disorder (ASD) diagnosis by race, ethnicity, and primary household language among children with special health care needs, United States, 2009–2010. Matern Child Health J. 2015;19(8):1687–97.
15. Folstein SE, Rosen-Sheidley B. Genetics of austim: complex aetiology for a heterogeneous disorder. Nat Rev Genet. 2001;2(12):943–55.
16. Bailey A, Lecouteur A, Gottesman I, Bolton P, Simonoff E, Yuzda E, et al. Autism as a strongly genetic disorder—evidence from a british twin study. Psychol Med. 1995;25(1):63–77.
17. O'Roak BJ, Vives L, Fu W, Egertson JD, Stanaway IB, Phelps IG, et al. Multiplex targeted sequencing identifies recurrently mutated genes in autism spectrum disorders. Science. 2012;338(6114):1619–22.
18. O'Roak BJ, State MW. Autism genetics: strategies, challenges, and opportunities. Autism Res. 2008;1(1):4–17.
19. De Rubeis S, He X, Goldberg AP, Poultney CS, Samocha K, Cicek AE, et al. Synaptic, transcriptional and chromatin genes disrupted in autism. Nature. 2014;515(7526):209–15.
20. Hallmayer J, Cleveland S, Torres A, Phillips J, Cohen B, Torigoe T, et al. Genetic heritability and shared environmental factors among twin pairs with autism. Arch Gen Psychiatry. 2011;68(11):1095–102.
21. Grafodatskaya D, Chung B, Szatmari P, Weksberg R. Autism spectrum disorders and epigenetics. J Am Acad Child Adolesc Psychiatry. 2010;49(8):794–809.
22. Taylor SE, Way BM, Welch WT, Hilmert CJ, Lehman BJ, Eisenberger NI. Early family environment, current adversity, the serotonin transporter promoter polymorphism, and depressive symptomatology. Biol Psychiatry. 2006;60(7):671–6.
23. Wadhwa PD, Buss C, Entringer S, Swanson JM, editors. Developmental origins of health and disease: brief history of the approach and current focus on epigenetic mechanisms. Seminars in reproductive medicine; 2009: NIH Public Access.
24. Kuzawa CW, Thayer ZM. Timescales of human adaptation: the role of epigenetic processes. Epigenomics. 2011;3(2):221–34.
25. Borghol N, Suderman M, McArdle W, Racine A, Hallett M, Pembrey M, et al. Associations with early-life socio-economic position in adult DNA methylation. Int J Epidemiol. 2012;41(1):62–74.
26. Dietert RR, Dietert JM. Potential for early-life immune insult including developmental immunotoxicity in autism and autism spectrum disorders: focus on critical windows of immune vulnerability. J Toxicol Environ Health B Crit Rev. 2008;11(8):660–80.
27. Gardener H, Spiegelman D, Buka SL. Prenatal risk factors for autism: comprehensive meta-analysis. Br J Psychiatry. 2009;195(1):7–14.
28. Suren P, Roth C, Bresnahan M, Haugen M, Hornig M, Hirtz D, et al. Association between maternal use of folic acid supplements and risk of autism spectrum disorders in children. J Am Med Assoc. 2013;309(6):570–7.
29. Rogers EJ. Has enhanced folate status during pregnancy altered natural selection and possibly autism prevalence? A closer look at a possible link. Med Hypotheses. 2008;71(3):406–10.
30. Lyall K, Schmidt RJ, Hertz-Picciotto I. Maternal lifestyle and environmental risk factors for autism spectrum disorders. Int J Epidemiol. 2014;43(2):443–64.
31. Leeming R, Lucock M. Autism: Is there a folate connection? J Inherit Metab Dis. 2009;32(3):400–2.
32. Gardener H, Spiegelman D, Buka SL. Perinatal and neonatal risk factors for autism: a comprehensive meta-analysis. Pediatrics. 2011;128(2):344–55.
33. Kohane IS, McMurry A, Weber G, MacFadden D, Rappaport L, Kunkel L, et al. The co-morbidity burden of children and young adults with autism spectrum disorders. PLoS One. 2012;7(4):e33224.
34. Tyler CV, Schramm SC, Karafa M, Tang AS, Jain AK. Chronic disease risks in young adults with autism spectrum disorder: forewarned is forearmed. Am J Intellect. 2011;116(5):371–80.
35. Levy SE, Giarelli E, Lee LC, Schieve LA, Kirby RS, Cunniff C, et al. Autism spectrum disorder and co-occurring developmental, psychiatric, and medical conditions among children in multiple populations of the United States. J Dev Behav Pediatr. 2010;31(4):267–75.
36. Joshi G, Petty C, Wozniak J, Henin A, Fried R, Galdo M, et al. The heavy burden of psychiatric comorbidity in youth with autism spectrum disorders: a large comparative study of a psychiatrically referred population. J Autism Dev Disord. 2010;40(11):1361–70.
37. Kao HT, Buka SL, Kelsey KT, Gruber DF, Porton B. The correlation between rates of cancer and autism: an exploratory ecological investigation. PLoS One. 2010;5(2):e9372.
38. Chiang HL, Liu CJ, Hu YW, Chen SC, Hu LY, Shen CC, et al. Risk of cancer in children, adolescents, and young adults with autistic disorder. J Pediatr. 2015;166(2):418–23.
39. Frazier TW, Embacher R, Tilot AK, Koenig K, Mester J, Eng C. Molecular and phenotypic abnormalities in individuals with germline heterozygous PTEN mutations and autism. Mol Psychiatry. 2015;20(9):1132–8.
40. McBride KL, Varga EA, Pastore MT, Prior TW, Manickam K, Atkin JF, et al. Confirmation study of PTEN mutations among individuals with autism or developmental delays/mental retardation and macrocephaly. Autism Res. 2010;3(3):137–41.

41. Belmonte MK, Bourgeron T. Fragile × syndrome and autism at the intersection of genetic and neural networks. Nat Neurosci. 2006;9(10):1221–5.
42. Kwon CH, Luikart BW, Powell CM, Zhou J, Matheny SA, Zhang W, et al. Pten regulates neuronal arborization and social interaction in mice. Neuron. 2006;50(3):377–88.
43. Neves-Pereira M, Muller B, Massie D, Williams JH, O'Brien PC, Hughes A, et al. Deregulation of eif4e: a novel mechanism for autism. J Med Genet. 2009;46 (11):759–65.
44. Serajee FJ, Zhong H, Nabi R, Huq AHMM. The metabotropic glutamate receptor 8 gene at 7q31: partial duplication and possible association with autism. J Med Genet. 2003;40(4):e42.
45. Hoeffer CA, Klann E. Mtor signaling: at the crossroads of plasticity, memory and disease. Trends Neurosci. 2010;33(2):67–75.
46. Bunney TD, Katan M. Phosphoinositide signalling in cancer: beyond PI3K and PTEN. Nat Rev Cancer. 2010;10(5):342–52.
47. Ciuffreda L, Di Sanza C, Incani UC, Milella M. The mtor pathway: a new target in cancer therapy. Curr Cancer Drug Targets. 2010;10(5):484–95.
48. Marui T, Hashimoto O, Nanba E, Kato C, Tochigi M, Umekage T, et al. Association between the neurofibromatosis-1 (NF1) locus and autism in the japanese population. Am J Med Genet Part B Neuropsychiatric Genet. 2004;131(1):43–7.
49. Woolfenden S, Sarkozy V, Ridley G, Coory M, Williams K. A systematic review of two outcomes in autism spectrum disorder—epilepsy and mortality. Dev Med Child Neurol. 2012;54(4):306–12.
50. Viscidi EW, Triche EW, Pescosolido MF, McLean RL, Joseph RM, Spence SJ, et al. Clinical characteristics of children with autism spectrum disorder and co-occurring epilepsy. PLoS One. 2013;8(7):e67797.
51. Chapman M, Iddon P, Atkinson K, Brodie C, Mitchell D, Parvin G, et al. The misdiagnosis of epilepsy in people with intellectual disabilities: a systematic review. Seizure. 2011;20(2):101–6.
52. Stokes T, Shaw E, Juarez-Garcia A, Camosso-Stefinovic J, Baker R. Clinical guidelines and evidence review for the epilepsies: diagnosis and management in adults and children in primary and secondary care. London: Royal College of General Practitioners; 2004. p. 397.
53. Buie T, Campbell DB, Fuchs GJ IIIrd, Furuta GT, Levy J, Vandewater J, et al. Evaluation, diagnosis, and treatment of gastrointestinal disorders in individuals with ASDS: a consensus report. Pediatrics. 2010;125(Suppl 1):S1–18.
54. Malow BA. Sleep disorders, epilepsy, and autism. Ment Retard Dev Disabil Res Rev. 2004;10(2):122–5.
55. Øyane NM, Bjorvatn B. Sleep disturbances in adolescents and young adults with autism and asperger syndrome. Autism. 2005;9(1):83–94.
56. Polimeni MA, Richdale AL, Francis AJ. A survey of sleep problems in autism, Asperger's disorder and typically developing children. J Intellect Disabil Res. 2005;49(Pt 4):260–8.
57. Matson JL, Ancona MN, Wilkins J. Sleep disturbances in adults with autism spectrum disorders and severe intellectual impairments. J Ment Health Res Intellect Disabil. 2008;1(3):129–39.
58. Patzold LM, Richdale AL, Tonge BJ. An investigation into sleep characteristics of children with autism and Asperger's disorder. J Paediatr Child Health. 1998;34(6):528–33.
59. Schreck KA, Mulick JA, Smith AF. Sleep problems as possible predictors of intensified symptoms of autism. Res Dev Disabil. 2004;25(1):57–66.
60. Sivertsen B, Posserud MB, Gillberg C, Lundervold AJ, Hysing M. Sleep problems in children with autism spectrum problems: a longitudinal population-based study. Autism. 2012;16(2):139–50.
61. Meltzer LJ, Mindell JA. Nonpharmacologic treatments for pediatric sleeplessness. Pediatr Clin North Am. 2004;51(1):135–51.
62. Leyfer OT, Folstein SE, Bacalman S, Davis NO, Dinh E, Morgan J, et al. Comorbid psychiatric disorders in children with autism: interview development and rates of disorders. J Autism Dev Disord. 2006;36(7):849–61.
63. White SW, Schry AR, Miyazaki Y, Ollendick TH, Scahill L. Effects of verbal ability and severity of autism on anxiety in adolescents with asd: one-year follow-up after cognitive behavioral therapy. J Clin Child Adolesc Psychol. 2015;44(5):839–45.
64. Spain D, Sin J, Chalder T, Murphy D, Happe F. Cognitive behaviour therapy for adults with autism spectrum disorders and psychiatric co-morbidity: a review. Res Autism Spectr Dis. 2015;9:151–62.
65. Billawala A, Wolbring G. Analyzing the discourse surrounding autism in the New York times using an Ableism lens. Disabil Stud Q. 2014;34(1). http://dx.doi.org/10.18061/dsq.v34i1.3348. Accessed 12 Aug 2016.
66. Brookman-Frazee LI, Taylor R, Garland AF. Characterizing community-based mental health services for children with autism spectrum disorders and disruptive behavior problems. J Autism Dev Disord. 2010;40(10):1188–201.
67. Garland AF, Hough RL, Landsverk JA, Brown SA. Multi-sector complexity of systems of care for youth with mental health needs. Child Serv Soc Policy Res Pract. 2001;4(3):123–40.
68. Burns BJ, Costello EJ, Angold A, Tweed D, Stangl D, Farmer E, et al. Children's mental health service use across service sectors. Health Aff. 1995;14(3):147–59.
69. Farmer TW, Farmer EM. Developmental science, systems of care, and prevention of emotional and behavioral problems in youth. Am J Orthopsychiatry. 2001;71(2):171–81.
70. Committee on Health E, Labor, and Pensions. Senate report 108–185—individuals with disabilities education act. Washington, DC: U.S. Government Publishing Office; 2003.

71. Wei X, Wagner M, Hudson L, Jennifer WY, Shattuck P. Transition to adulthood employment, education, and disengagement in individuals with autism spectrum disorders. Emerg Adulthood. 2014:2167696814534417.
72. Roux AM, Shattuck PT, Rast JE, Rava JA, Anderson KA. National autism indicators report: transition into young adulthood. Philadelphia, PA: Life Course Outcomes Research Program, A.J. Drexel Autism Institute, Drexel University; 2015.
73. Matthews NL, Smith CJ, Pollard E, Ober-Reynolds S, Kirwan J, Malligo A. Adaptive functioning in autism spectrum disorder during the transition to adulthood. J Autism Dev Disord. 2015;45(8):2349–60.
74. Smith LE, Maenner MJ, Seltzer MM. Developmental trajectories in adolescents and adults with autism: the case of daily living skills. J Am Acad Child Adolesc Psychiatry. 2012;51(6):622–31.
75. Bal VH, Kim SH, Cheong D, Lord C. Daily living skills in individuals with autism spectrum disorder from 2 to 21 years of age. Autism. 2015;19(7):774–84.
76. Mitchel K, Regehr K, Reaume J, Feldman M. Group social skills training for adolescents with Asperger syndrome or high functioning autism. J Dev Disabil. 2010.
77. Seltzer MM, Shattuck P, Abbeduto L, Greenberg JS. Trajectory of development in adolescents and adults with autism. Ment Retard Dev Disabil Res Rev. 2004;10(4):234–47.
78. Taylor JL, Seltzer MM. Changes in the autism behavioral phenotype during the transition to adulthood. J Autism Dev Disord. 2010;40(12):1431–46.
79. Jones J, Lerman DC, Lechago S. Assessing stimulus control and promoting generalization via video modeling when teaching social responses to children with autism. J Appl Behav Anal. 2014;47(1):37–50.
80. Nicolaidis C, Raymaker D, McDonald K, Dern S, Boisclair WC, Ashkenazy E, et al. Comparison of healthcare experiences in autistic and non-autistic adults: a cross-sectional online survey facilitated by an academic-community partnership. J Gen Intern Med. 2013;28(6):761–9.

Cerebral Palsy

5

Jonathan Tolentino and Gregg Talente

Case Presentation

Ann is a 20-year-old young woman with cerebral palsy (CP) presenting to the primary care office to establish care. She is accompanied by her mother at this visit. She was last seen by her primary care pediatrician 2 years ago before moving away to college. She has recently left school and moved back home after a 2-week hospitalization for pneumonia that forced her to withdraw from her coursework. The hospital physician instructed her to find a primary care physician for follow-up.

Ann appears as a well-groomed young woman sitting in one of the wheelchairs from the office. She expresses that her main goal for the visit is to get well enough to return to school for the next semester. Since her hospitalization she has had increased difficulty with ambulation and routine daily activities requiring more assistance from her parents than normal. She has also lost 12 lb.

Ann's medical history is significant for premature birth at 32 weeks gestation. She was diagnosed with cerebral palsy in infancy. Her cognitive development was normal. Speech early on was impacted by mild dysarthria, which improved with speech therapy as a child. She had significant gross and fine motor delay and spasticity predominantly in her left arm and leg. She has had difficulty swallowing and with weight gain throughout her life and has a gastrostomy tube in place, although she has not used this in the last few years. In addition to her recent hospitalization she has been hospitalized a few other times for pneumonia as a child. Her only current medication is ibuprofen, which she uses as needed but somewhat frequently for hip and back pains.

On review of systems, Ann reports fatigue, back and left hip pain, the weight loss previously mentioned, and some recent difficulty swallowing certain foods since her discharge. She also reports issues with constipation. She reports that typically she can ambulate independently using a cane for balance but that since her hospitalization she has needed additional assistance and because of this has limited her activities considerably compared to when she was in school. She states that the nurses had her use the office wheelchair to make it easier for her to get back to the exam room.

On exam her vital signs are normal. Her body mass index (BMI) is 18 kg/m^2. She is a thin but well-appearing young woman. She has some

J. Tolentino (✉)
Department of Pediatrics, Stony Brook University, HSC Level 11, Room 040, 101 Nicolls Road, Stony Brook, NY 11794-8111, USA
e-mail: Jonathan.Tolentino@stonybrookmedicine.edu

G. Talente
Department of Internal Medicine, University of South Carolina School of Medicine, 2 Medical Park, Suite 502, Columbia, SC 29203, USA
e-mail: Gregg.Talente@uscmed.sc.edu

M. Pilapil et al. (eds.), *Care of Adults with Chronic Childhood Conditions*,
DOI 10.1007/978-3-319-43827-6_5

difficulty getting on the exam table. Her musculoskeletal exam is significant for some mild scoliosis, hypertonicity particularly in the left arm and leg, with a mild reduction of extension of the left knee. She has tenderness over the lumbar region of the back and the left hip on palpation and apparent discomfort on movement of the left hip on exam.

Case Discussion

This case illustrates many of the problems adults with cerebral palsy face and provides an example that highlights the most important aspect of managing adults with cerebral palsy. What is most important is exactly what Ann states as her goals: wellness, functioning, and participation in normal aspects of adult life such as higher education and her social connections with friends. The case fails, though, to fully capture what it means to be an adult with cerebral palsy because cerebral palsy is an extremely variable condition. Even though there are many commonalities, each person's experiences, problems, and needs are unique.

The primary symptoms of cerebral palsy are spasticity, joint contractures, motor control difficulties, and musculoskeletal deformities. These lead to issues with mobility, fine motor dexterity and, in some cases, communication and learning. These problems can result in decreased overall health, less independence, and less participation, all of which are illustrated in Ann's case. Her pneumonia was likely more serious because of her cerebral palsy, and she has had a decrease in her motor function due to the prolonged hospitalization that has forced her to leave school.

While the underlying insult in cerebral palsy is not progressive, individuals can have deterioration in the severity of their symptoms that can cause progressive loss of function as they age. Contractures can worsen over time and strength can deteriorate. Inactivity is the most common risk factor for worsening contractures, so it is not surprising that Ann's hospitalization has led to decreased functioning. In caring for cerebral palsy patients, constant surveillance and early intervention to preserve strength and function are important. Collaboration with a physical and occupational therapist to develop a plan to assist Ann in regaining the mobility she had prior to hospitalization would be the recommended approach.

Pain control is another important component of managing adults with cerebral palsy. Many have chronic pain that can be from the inherent spasticity of the condition or a number of other sources. Chronic pain can also have a significant impact on function. It is clear from the history that Ann is dealing with pain even though this is not her main complaint. Assessment of her pain severity and its impact on her function would be a critical component of her care. Simple interventions such as anti-inflammatory medications and physical therapy are effective, but in some patients, more aggressive interventions are needed. If her pain is related to uncontrolled spasticity and it is difficult to control, assistance from a physiatrist and consideration of interventions such as botulinum A toxin injection or intrathecal baclofen are necessary.

Cerebral palsy is associated with a number of other conditions, some of which are demonstrated in this case. She reports difficulties with swallowing, weight loss with her low BMI suggesting that her nutritional status may be less than ideal, and issues with constipation. An important aspect of managing patients with cerebral palsy is to have familiarity with the many issues they may face, to do a thorough review of systems, and to manage these issues as they are discovered. In Ann's case it might be beneficial to refer her to a nutritionist and, based on the recommendations, consider supplementing her diet possibly by use of her gastrostomy tube. A bowel regimen consisting of increased fiber in the diet, increased hydration, and the initiation of an osmotic laxative would help with her constipation.

The key to managing Ann as a patient begins with listening to her stated goals. Cerebral palsy cannot be fixed or cured. What is important is helping Ann to live with cerebral palsy in the way that she wants. The main goal is to help her regain enough strength and mobility to restart school. This may be done with simple exercise guided by a physical therapist, or it may require finding new solutions to increase her mobility and ability to participate at school. In addition, to best help her with her goals, a thorough evaluation with specific attention to possible problems related to her cerebral palsy should be undertaken. Finally, routine preventive health should be provided. At this time, Ann requires only sexually transmitted infection (STI) screening, but as she ages these preventive measures should not be neglected, though they frequently are in adults with cerebral palsy. She should also receive counseling on reproductive health issues.

Definition

Cerebral palsy is defined as a group of permanent disorders affecting development of movement and posture causing activity limitations and attributed to nonprogressive injury of the developing fetal or infant brain [1]. This encompasses a broad spectrum of conditions with diverse symptoms and presentations. Individuals with cerebral palsy are often further classified by the location of the brain lesion, the types of motor symptoms displayed, the extremities affected, and the severity of the symptoms.

Classification by brain lesion requires magnetic resonance imaging (MRI) and typically divides cases into cortical, pyramidal tract, extrapyramidal tract, and cerebellar groupings. Symptom classification usually divides patients based on the primary motor symptom: spasticity, dyskinesia, athetoid, or ataxic cerebral palsy. Another classification is by the affected extremities, dividing cerebral palsy into diplegic, hemiplegic, and quadriplegic groups [1]. Scales exist that are commonly used to classify cerebral palsy based on the severity of motor dysfunction. The Gross Motor Function Classification System (GMFCS) and the Minimal Ability Classification System (MACS) are two scales that are commonly used in the literature on cerebral palsy [2, 3].

While classification has its importance for research and transfer of knowledge, no system of classification can truly represent the needs of an individual patient and, practically, classification is less important than assessing each individual's functional needs, risks, and treatment goals. This focus on function is what led the International Classification of Functioning Disability and Health (ICF) sponsored by the World Health Organization (WHO) to promote a shift in how disability is discussed. Traditionally, conditions are considered using a linear model where disease leads to a damaged organ or organ system that, in turn, leads to disability. The WHO recommends instead an integrative model focusing on the condition and the contextual factors impacted and impacting the condition, promoting a focus on functional activity in the framework of the patient's condition [4]. Practically, the use of a classification system such as the GMFCS (described in detail later) can be a useful tool to assist in communication between providers sharing care of a young adult with cerebral palsy and in communication with the patient and family about prognosis.

Prevalence

Cerebral palsy occurs in 2–3 of 1000 children born [1]. The prevalence of cerebral palsy has been mostly stable over time. Risk factors for cerebral palsy include prematurity and low birth weight. Most infants born with cerebral palsy will live into adulthood. Studies suggest that 98 % of children with cerebral palsy not classified as severe reach age 20, and up to 85 % of children with severe cerebral palsy reach age 20. It is estimated that there are about half a million adults with cerebral palsy living in the US.

Life expectancy of adults with cerebral palsy is less than that of the general population, though a significant percentage of patients reach age 50 and older [1]. In patients with higher function, mortality is similar to that of the general population. However, those who have lost the ability to ambulate by age 60 are more likely to have poorer survival. Mortality in patients in the third and fourth decade of life is usually due to respiratory complications, while mortality in the fifth and sixth decade of life is usually due to cardiovascular or oncologic diseases [5–7]. Intellectual disability was found to be the greatest single predictor of mortality, while severe motor impairment increased the risk for early mortality [8].

Pathophysiology

Cerebral palsy is most commonly caused by interference in brain development in utero, though it has been attributed to injury occurring perinatally. Hypoxic injury or neonatal asphyxia was traditionally thought to be the cause of the brain injury, though currently asphyxia is believed to impact only 10–20 % of cases of cerebral palsy. Other causes of developmental injury leading to cerebral palsy include genetic causes, infection, and thromboembolic causes [1].

Clinical Presentation

Patients with cerebral palsy will often present to the general internist with abnormalities in motor function secondary to abnormal tone, weakness, difficulty with mobility and balance, and poor control of motor movement, with accompanying abnormalities in sensation, cognition, communication, and behavior [9]. While cerebral palsy is often considered a nonprogressive disorder, the motor abilities of adults with cerebral palsy often decline over time, affecting gross and fine motor function and ambulation [10].

A number of non-neuromuscular comorbidities are associated with cerebral palsy that should be co-managed between the general internist, neurologist, physiatrist, and other subspecialists (Table 5.1) [1, 9–11]. Most commonly seen disorders include musculoskeletal disorders, epilepsy, intellectual disability, speech disorders, obesity, dysphagia, bladder and gastrointestinal problems, and dental problems [5, 12, 13]. Patients with more severe functional impairment and higher GMFCS scores have increasing problems with age, including disorders associated with decreased movement such as osteopenia [5].

Quality of Life

Multiple studies have shown that the reported health and quality of life of patients with cerebral palsy is lower compared to non-disabled populations, particularly in the domains of motor and social functioning, but better compared to other diseases such as multiple sclerosis [14–17]. Adults report a deterioration of gross motor function and quality of life as they age, with the most decline occurring by the middle of the fifth decade rather than during the young adult transition period [14, 16, 18, 19]. Physical function has a greater effect in adolescent CP patients, while psychological and emotional aspects play a greater role in older patients [17, 20]. Other factors that influence quality of life include sports participation, chronic pain, chronic fatigue, deterioration of function, living alone, unemployment, and low sense of coherence [21, 22]. Many cerebral palsy patients separate physical health from overall health, and one study reported that the subjective well-being and general satisfaction of life in a cross section of adults with CP was not decreased [23].

Transition Issues

Most patients presenting to the general internist for continuity of care usually have come from a pediatric institution that provided care involving a multidisciplinary team, including physical therapists, occupational therapists, orthopedic surgeons, physiatrists, and neurologists to provide coordinated care [1, 9, 24–27]. In addition, many adult practitioners are unfamiliar with the unique needs of CP patients and struggle with dealing with the needs of cognitively limited patients with limited communication skills, leading to access issues [24, 28, 29]. The heterogeneity of the CP population is a challenge, ranging from autonomous patients with

Table 5.1 Common comorbidities associated with adults with cerebral palsy [1, 9–11]

Cerebral Palsy: common adulthood comorbidities	
HEENT:	**Gastrointestinal**
Saliva control	Gastroesophageal reflux disease (GERD)
Visual problems	Delayed gastric emptying
Strabismus	Constipation
Visual field defects	Bowel and bladder dysfunction
Myopia	Problems with feeding, swallowing
Hypermetropia	Bowel motility
Severe visual and hearing impairment	Poor nutrition and growth
Speech disorders	**Psych**
Poor dental health	Chronic pain
Neurological	Chronic fatigue
Epilepsy (severe CP)	**Bone Health**
Partial epilepsy (unilateral spastic CP)	Hip dislocation
Sensorineural deafness	Scoliosis
Infectious Disease	Cervical instability and spinal arthritis
High rates of infection	Osteopenia and osteoporosis
Cellulitis and decubitus ulcers	
Urinary tract infection (UTI)	

normal intelligence to those with severe cognitive deficit requiring coordinated specialty and supportive care [30]. New clinical and transition programs are being designed at some pediatric and adult centers targeting the adult cerebral palsy patient, but long-term outcomes for these programs remain limited [31–34].

Cerebral palsy patients find it difficult to transition because of child-centered providers, youth and parental reluctance to transition to adult care, and unease and lack of training among adult providers in cerebral palsy [35]. The lack of cooperation or communication between providers, the feeling of abandonment, and the lack of knowledge or support through the transition process further complicates this period of transition [36, 37]. The transition process also demonstrates a new focus in shift of care from normalization of function, which is a primary focus of therapy treatments in childhood, to the accommodation of function, which is increasingly becoming the focus of therapy across the lifespan [38]. Compared to their peers, patients with CP lagged behind in several milestones in achieving independence in transition, such as housing, employment, and relationships [39]. In addition, many patients will remain dependent on parents for both emotional and financial support, causing stress for both patient and parents [40, 41].

Medical Issues of CP Patients

Neuromuscular Function Issues

The general internist will co-manage many of the neuromuscular issues experienced by adults with cerebral palsy with physical therapists, occupational therapists, physiatrists, and possibly neurologists and orthopedic surgeons. The Gross Motor Function Classification System (GMFCS) is commonly used to describe function in cerebral palsy patients (see Box 5.1) [2].

Box 5.1: Expanded and revised Gross Motor Function Classification System (GMFCS) for children 12–18 years [2, 51]

GMFCS Level I: Youth walk at home, school, outdoors, and in the community. Youth are able to climb curbs and stairs without physical assistance or a railing. They perform gross motor skills such as running and jumping, but speed, balance, and coordination are limited

GMFCS Level II: Youth walk in most settings but environmental factors and personal choice influence mobility choices. At school or work they may require a handheld mobility device for safety and climb stairs holding onto a railing. Outdoors and in the community, youth may use wheeled mobility when traveling long distances

GMFCS Level III: Youth are capable of walking using a handheld mobility device. Youth may climb stairs holding onto a railing with supervision or assistance. At school they may self-propel a manual wheelchair or use powered mobility. Outdoors and in the community youth are transported in wheelchair or use powered mobility

GMFCS Level IV: Youth use wheeled mobility in most settings. Physical assistance of 1–2 people is required for transfers. Indoors, youth may walk short distances with physical assistance, use wheeled mobility or a body support walker when positioned. They may operate a powered chair, otherwise are transported in a manual wheelchair

GMFCS Level V: Youth are transported in a manual wheelchair in all settings. Youth are limited in their ability to maintain antigravity head and trunk postures and control leg and arm movements. Self-mobility is severely limited, even with the use of assistive technology

In patients with cerebral palsy, an estimated 21–43 % were hemiplegic, 29–35 % were diplegic, and 12–22 % were quadriplegic; approximately a fifth of adult patients had dyskinesia [3, 42, 43]. Between 28 and 77 % of adults with CP reported the use of a wheelchair, with up to 40 % of wheelchair users being ambulatory previously [3, 9, 10, 43, 44]. Some adults with CP have stopped ambulating as they aged by choice due to fatigue and pain leading to inactivity, deconditioning, and contractures. Decline in function may happen early in life, but up to a fourth of those with CP may show decline in gross neuromuscular function later into adult life, with declines occurring between the second and fourth decade [9, 16, 19, 45]. The decline may be a function of changes in muscle flexibility, increased spasticity, falls, fractures, pain, and fatigue [10].

The management of neuromuscular problems in patients with cerebral palsy requires the coordination between physical therapy, occupational therapy, and physiatry [25–27]. The primary medical therapies include muscle relaxants and anti-dystonic drugs (Tables 5.2, 5.3) [1, 46, 47]. Baclofen is most often used and has been very effective; however, sudden withdrawal can lead to rebound spasticity, seizures, and hallucinations [47]. Second-line agents, such as tizanidine and dantrolene, are effective in reducing spasticity, but their use is limited by their adverse effects. Physiatry will typically be able to assist with the use of other interventions, such as the use of botulinum toxin (e.g., Botox®) injections that have some efficacy in the pediatric population, with initial studies in the adult CP population also demonstrating some improvement in function [47, 48]. Botox effects usually peak within 4–6 weeks but wane after 12 weeks; patients will need repeated planned injections every 12 weeks [47]. Physical therapy will be able to assist in interventions for mobility, improvements in biomechanics, assistive technology, and movement dysfunction [27].

More invasive therapies include selective dorsal rhizotomy, which severs problematic nerve roots, and intrathecal baclofen pump placement. Selective dorsal rhizotomies are usually performed in ambulatory patients and improve body function and spasticity, but has no evidence of influence on long-term activity and participation [1, 49]. Intrathecal baclofen has been shown to be effective in reducing short-term spasticity, but its effect on gross motor function, improvement in comfort, ease of care, and quality of life is not as well established [50].

Orthopedic Issues

A number of orthopedic issues affect patients with cerebral palsy, many of which are the result of the long-standing contractures (see Box 5.2) [45]. Hip displacement is fairly common, affecting up

Table 5.2 Medical management of patients with dystonia [46]

Medical management of patients with dystonia		
Medication	Target population	Typical dose
Carbidopa–Levodopa	Early onset dystonia	Begin 1 mg/kg/day divided BID into TID. Increase by 1 mg/kg/week, up to 5 mg/kg/d for at least 4 weeks
Benzodiazepines	Early onset dystonia Late onset dystonia	Clonazepam: 0.5–10 mg QD Diazepam: 2–100 mg QD Lorazepam: 0.5–8 mg QD
Baclofen	Craniofacial dystonia Early onset dystonia	Begin 2.5–5 mg QHS Increase by 2.5 or 5 mg QD to total daily dose of 80 mg
Trihexyphenidyl	Early onset dystonia Late onset dystonia	Adults typically tolerate 8–12 mg QD
Tetrabenazine	Tardive dystonia	12.5–200 mg QD

Adapted with permission from Bragg et al. [46]

Table 5.3 Medical management of patients with spasticity [47]

Medication	Indication	Typical dose	Side effects
Baclofen	Preferred oral antispasticity drug	Starting dose 5 mg three times daily; titration 5–10 mg weekly; maximum dose 90–120 mg/day divided into three doses; lower doses in renal failure; taper by up to 15 mg/week	Weakness, drowsiness, dizziness, sexual dysfunction, and urinary incontinence. Sudden withdrawal may cause rebound spasticity, seizures, and hallucinations. Should be used with caution during pregnancy
Tizanidine	Second-line treatment if baclofen is not tolerated or not effective	Starting dose 2 mg at bedtime; titration, increased by 2 mg weekly; maximum dose 36 mg/day divided into 3 or 4 doses; taper by 4 mg/week	Dry mouth, gastrointestinal disturbance, hypotension, and acute hepatitis. Monitor liver enzymes
Dantrolene	Second-line treatment if baclofen is not tolerated or not effective	Starting dose 25 mg/day; titration, increase in steps of 25 mg/week; maximum dose 100 mg 3 or 4 times daily, taper by 25 mg/week	Hepatotoxicity, weakness, dizziness, and diarrhea. Monitor liver enzyme levels
Gabapentin	Spasticity associated with pain	300 mg once daily on day 1, then 300 mg twice daily on day 2, then 300 mg 3 times daily on day 3, then increased according to response in steps of 300 mg every 2 or 3 days, up to maximum of 3600 mg daily	Weight gain, gastrointestinal disturbance, confusion, depression, hostility, and sleep disturbances. Need electrocardiography to monitor for QT interval prolongation

Reprinted with permission from Nair and Marsden [47]

to a third of patients with cerebral palsy, especially the non-ambulatory [1, 51]. Hip dislocation most commonly occurs in patients with quadriplegia, with nearly half of these hips becoming painful and affecting function [45]. Asymptomatic hip dislocation can also be seen with severe spastic quadriplegia and severe hemiplegia, but the long-term impact is unknown [51, 52]. Neuromuscular scoliosis affects between 15 and 80 % of patients with CP, particularly the non-ambulatory and less functional patients [45, 51]. Corrective surgeries such as spinal fusion to the pelvis with rod insertions have good outcomes in more than 90 % of cases, with a significant improvement in comfort, health, and overall quality of life, but functional improvement was not as notable [53, 54]. Patella alta causes anterior knee pain and is more commonly seen in patients with spastic diplegia, leading to stress fractures, tendonitis, and subluxations/dislocations [45]. The most common foot deformities include equinus, planovalgus, and equinovarus/equinocavovarus, which can lead to functional issues with gait and pain [55]. Ankle deformities include valgus and hallux valgus [56].

Box 5.2: Secondary orthopedic conditions [45]

- Patella alta
- Hip displacement
- Spondylosis
- Cervical stenosis
- Scoliosis
- Foot deformities

Correction of musculoskeletal deformities should take into account the functional needs, pain, and the overall benefit of surgical correction. In patients with hip dislocations, surgical correction should be based upon the presence of pain or impact on function. Conservative nonsurgical management should be reserved for asymptomatic hip dislocation, especially in the non-ambulatory patient. Scoliosis should continue to be monitored into adulthood as curve angles may continue to progress even after skeletal maturity is achieved and the need for future corrective surgery may need to be entertained to avoid complications such as restrictive lung pathologies [51]. For patients with foot and ankle deformities, a combination of foot and ankle orthotics, physical therapy, spasticity reduction, and surgical correction are the mainstay of therapy [55]. Surgical correction is typically reserved for patients with significant deformity, pain, or inability to use orthotic and modified shoes [57, 58]. Due to chronic abnormal gait and movement, management of acquired degenerative changes of the knee and the hip must also be managed by the generalist [58]. Collaborative management between orthopedic surgery, physical therapy, and physiatry is necessary to assure management with the focus on improvement in function.

Osteopenia

Patients with cerebral palsy are at increased risk for a number of normal conditions associated with aging in the general population. These conditions need to be monitored for and treated, as they are associated with increased morbidity. One such condition that is common in cerebral palsy is poor bone health (osteopenia and osteoporosis) and the risk for fracture associated with low bone mineral density. Low bone mineral density is often found much earlier in cerebral palsy patients than the general population [59, 60]. Physicians caring for adults with cerebral palsy need to be aware of this and consider early screening and intervention.

Risk factors for developing low bone mineral density in patients with cerebral palsy include poor nutrition, greater severity of neurologic symptoms, non-ambulatory status, poor vitamin D and calcium intake, and periods of immobility [61]. Thus patients with more severe motor dysfunction, those who are non-ambulatory, and those with nutritional issues are probably the ones in whom early screening is most likely to be of benefit. Unfortunately, there is not enough data available to develop a standard recommendation for screening in the cerebral palsy population. Existing risk stratification tools used in the general adult population have not been studied in cerebral palsy. Physicians should use their judgment and knowledge of the risk factors and consider bone density testing even in high-risk young adults.

If screening is to be done, dual-energy X-ray absorptiometry (DEXA) scans would be the test of choice. One potential challenge for this is that many cerebral palsy patients are not capable of being positioned for all of the images typically obtained in this assessment. Cost and insurance coverage of this test should also be considered.

Treatment of low bone mineral density in cerebral palsy should involve three combined approaches. First, nutritional interventions are important. Both vitamin D and calcium supplementation and overall nutrition are important for promoting higher bone density, so in addition to advising supplements, ensuring adequate overall caloric intake should be done. Increased physical activity is also helpful in improving bone density. Exercise regimens under the guidance of a therapist should be considered for patients diagnosed with osteopenia [61]. Finally, studies in cerebral palsy patients suggest a benefit from the use of bisphosphonates [62–66]. Bisphosphonate therapy increases bone mineral density in children with cerebral palsy and osteopenia. Adult studies have not been done and no definitive guidelines exist, but treatment with bisphosphonates can be considered in adult cerebral palsy patients, although the consequences of long-term use of bisphosphonates are not understood. Co-management with an endocrinologist may be helpful.

Pain

Pain is a common and important problem in adults with cerebral palsy. Multiple studies suggest that up to two-thirds of patients with cerebral palsy suffer from pain in one or more sites of longer than 3 months duration [67]. Thus the majority of adult cerebral palsy patients meet the criteria for suffering from chronic pain. The incidence of chronic pain in cerebral palsy increases with increasing age [68]. Back pain is the most common site of pain with hip and leg pain being the next most common [69].

The source of pain is mostly from the underlying movement impairments of the condition, spasticity, and joint deformity. Other orthopedic causes include scoliosis, joint subluxation, joint dislocation, and degenerative arthritis. Low bone mineral density can lead to fracture. Dental pain is common as well since many patients have dental disease and lack access to dental care. Gastrointestinal causes of pain are common including gastrostomy tube site pain, constipation, and pain from gastroesophageal reflux. Pain from pressure sores and skin injury in less mobile patients and those with poor nutrition are common as well [67].

Evaluation and management of pain in cerebral palsy is best undertaken with a detailed history and examination to determine the cause of the pain. If feasible, specific interventions for the underlying cause, such as repair of dental issues and treatment of gastroesophageal reflux, should be undertaken. Otherwise, management of pain in cerebral palsy should be done according to the principles used to treat all chronic pain.

There is little specific data on what works to treat pain in cerebral palsy patients. Improved coping strategies such as task persistence and attention diversion and avoidance of catastrophic thinking seem to be associated with better pain control [70]. As in all chronic pain management, there is a role for counseling-based interventions. Exercise is also useful as an intervention for pain management [71, 72].

Use of medications in the management of pain in patients with cerebral palsy is best done by treating the underlying cause such as spasticity and dystonia, as described earlier. Nonsteroidal anti-inflammatory medications are also useful. Narcotic pain medications, as in any form of chronic non-cancer pain, should be used judiciously and as a last resort.

Gastrointestinal Issues

There are four common gastrointestinal issues associated with cerebral palsy: gastroesophageal reflux disease (GERD), swallowing concerns, nutrition, and bowel function. Their impact can range from mild to severe. They can be a source of pain, have an impact on function and participation, and impact risk for morbidity and mortality. Thus screening for and management of gastrointestinal issues in adult cerebral palsy patients is an important aspect of care.

Dysphagia and difficulty swallowing are common [73]. These issues are frequently diagnosed in childhood and often infancy, with common presenting symptoms including poor feeding, choking, and spitting. Assessment of swallowing is most commonly done by video-assisted swallowing testing sometimes combined with upper gastrointestinal imaging when esophageal reflux is also suspected [74, 75]. Speech therapy is the most common intervention. Placement of a gastrostomy tube is done when swallowing issues present too great a risk for aspiration, or inhibit adequate nutrition. While most often identified and treated in childhood, adults with CP sometimes will present with new or worsening complaints of dysphagia. Such complaints are often related to the underlying motor issues of CP exacerbated by factors that lead to decreased functioning such as acute illness or poor nutrition. They can be caused though by any typical adult illness associated with dysphagia. Adult providers should monitor their patients for swallowing issues.

Gastroesophageal reflux is very common in cerebral palsy. It can present at any age as simple heartburn, respiratory symptoms, or as anemia alone [75]. Because reflux is related to the central developmental brain injury and resulting motor dysfunction, it can be refractory to medical therapy. Despite this, the initial intervention is acid blockade with H_2 receptor blockers or proton pump inhibitors. In severe, refractory cases fundoplication should be considered, especially if comorbid complications develop such as recurrent aspiration pneumonitis or pneumonia [73].

Constipation is common in cerebral palsy. It results from delayed colonic transit and incoordination of the anal sphincter and pelvic floor musculature [76, 77]. It is often exacerbated by immobility and dietary factors. Treatment of constipation should include dietary fiber, hydration, and when needed the use of osmotic laxatives or stimulants [78].

Poor nutrition is also common in cerebral palsy patients. Typically, it is due to other gastrointestinal issues, particularly dysphagia. Due to impacted mobility and activity levels, particularly in more severe cases of cerebral palsy, estimating ideal metabolic needs can be challenging. Delivery of nutrition is also problematic. Many patients are entirely or partially fed using gastrostomy tubes. Assessment of nutritional status, tracking of weight with attention to periods of weight loss, and collaboration with a nutritionist are recommended in managing adults with cerebral palsy [73].

Immobility-Related Issues

Urinary Dysfunction and Urinary Tract Infections

An estimated 16–60 % of cerebral palsy patients have some degree of urinary incontinence [79–82]. Patients at highest risk include those who are obese, non-ambulatory, and have higher GMFCS scores [79, 82, 83]. Incontinence interfering with life is commonly seen in both men and women. While men often complain of urgency, women were more likely to leak with cough, exercise, or sneezing [82]. Conservative nonsurgical management of urinary dysfunction is successful in 75–91 % of CP patients, including toileting education, medications such as oxybutynin, padding and perineal hygiene and, when needed, clean intermittent catheterization for bladder management [80, 83].

Urinary tract infections are most often seen with poor perineal hygiene and the use of an external urinary collection device or an indwelling Foley catheter [79]. Management of acute urinary tract infections should be based upon established guidelines for urinary tract infections in the general population and local antibiotic resistance patterns and should be considered complex urinary tract infection in patients with CP [84]. Prevention of urinary tract infections should include good conservative management of urinary dysfunction and avoiding the use of indwelling Foley catheters for urologic management of incontinence.

Skin Breakdown and Infections

Cerebral palsy patients who are quadriplegic and have significant limitations in mobility are at risk for complications associated with skin breakdown. While literature in the ambulatory non-hospitalized cerebral palsy patient is limited, it is well established that patients with CP admitted to the hospital are at risk for skin-related complications [85]. Most commonly, post-surgical infections after spinal fusion were due to gram-negative bacilli [86]. About 21 % of paraplegic and 23 % of quadriplegic patients have pressure ulcers, commonly affecting the sacrum, ischium, and the heel [87, 88]. Management of pressure ulcers requires appropriate staging using the European Pressure Ulcer Advisory Panel (EPUAP) guidelines. Nonsurgical management by general internists should be in consultation with a wound care provider and often includes hydrocolloid and hydrogel dressings for stage I and stage II ulcers. Complex stage II ulcers and higher should be managed with a wound care provider, and recalcitrant ulcers typically will require co-management with a plastic surgeon [88, 89]. Suspicion for an infected ulcer should include workup for potential osteomyelitis, including evaluation of inflammatory markers, blood cultures, and appropriate imaging such as MRI (care should be taken for those who have prior rod placement).

Obesity and Cardiometabolic Risk

Compared to other disorders with cognitive and physical disabilities, patients with cerebral palsy generally have lower BMIs and rates of obesity [90, 91]. Estimated obesity rates range from 9.7 to 41.5 %, with prevalence rates increasing in many countries, most notably in the US (from 7.7 to 16.5 %) [91–95]. Obesity risk was seen more in female, hemiplegic, and ambulatory patients [93, 94]. Non-ambulators were more likely to be underweight [93]. Cerebral palsy patients may have a degree of muscle atrophy and decreased bone density, and despite a normal BMI, actually have excess body fat. Coupled with the relative sedentary lifestyle, CP patients may have increased cardiovascular mortality at "normal" weights [96]. New research suggests the need for lower BMIs to predict cardiometabolic risk for patients with limited mobility, such as BMI of 20 kg/m^2 for boys and 19 kg/m^2 for girls, and suggests that waist circumference (80 cm for women, 94 cm for men) and waist-to-hip ratios may be a better predictor for cardiometabolic risk for hypertension and dyslipidemia in adults [96–98]. Mortality due to cardiovascular diseases is the most common in the oldest age groups, but there is substantial excess mortality from ischemic heart disease and cerebrovascular diseases in those under 35 years [6]. An estimated 20 % of ambulatory adults and 28.6 % of non-ambulatory adults have metabolic syndrome.

Management of obesity in patients with neuromuscular disability is focused on lifestyle changes and improvement in function. Patients with spastic cerebral palsy, especially lower functioning patients, are sedentary and are less likely to participate in moderate to vigorous physical activity [92, 99]. Moderate physical activity has shown improvement in waist–height ratio, waist circumference, systolic and diastolic blood pressure, and is encouraged, especially for ambulators [92]. Activities such as interval training and strength and aerobic training have shown short-term improvement and positive trends [100]. Other medical weight management treatments, including the use of metformin, phentermine, and topiramate, have not been studied in the CP population. The role of bariatric surgery has not been established in these patients, but a small case series of patients with neuromuscular disability did show some short-term weight benefit [101]. Patients at risk for the development of metabolic syndrome or cardiovascular risks should be screened using evidence-based guidelines, such as guidelines published by the United States Preventive

Services Task Force, American Diabetes Association, and the American College of Cardiology, and managed appropriately.

Vision, Hearing, and Communication

Vision, hearing, and communication can all be affected in patients with cerebral palsy. Vision and hearing problems may develop later on in adulthood, whereas communication issues are more likely to be noted early in childhood [10]. Regardless, adult providers should screen for deficits in all three of these areas during routine health assessments. Vision and hearing testing should be ordered whenever any concern is noted.

Dysarthria is the most common cause of communication limitations in cerebral palsy patients. Dysarthria is caused by interference with the muscle function related to speech production [10]. It is worth noting that receptive communication issues can also occur in cerebral palsy patients with comorbid intellectual disability. Speech therapy is the first intervention for dysarthria. Studies have suggested that intrathecal baclofen can improve dysarthria. Finally, assistive technology should be considered in more severe cases. In line with the goal of focusing on function, addressing communication, vision and hearing deficits should be a priority of managing adults with cerebral palsy.

Psychosocial and Mental Health Issues

For young adults with CP, psychosocial well-being improves as patients age, although psychosocial well-being is not strongly associated with overall functional status [15, 102]. Participation by cerebral palsy patients of normal intelligence in daily activities and in social roles (i.e., leisure activities, community living, and employment) is more restricted, especially in those with lower motor function, advanced age, and lower education level [103]. Nearly, two-thirds reportedly have difficulty with mobility, recreation, and housing, and nearly half have difficulties with personal care and employment [104]. Loneliness in patients with cerebral palsy was noted to be higher than in the general population [105]. Patients with CP are more likely to participate in leisure activity if mobility is good and if the environment facilitated leisure (such as adaptive transport, services, and computer aides) [106].

Educational attainment is possible for many patients with cerebral palsy, with a good proportion completing high school and college with appropriate support systems and accommodations [43]. While many who are completing undergraduate courses have received helpful accommodations such as individualized educational plans (IEPs) and Section 504 plans, including access to speech and occupational therapy, young adults must discuss with colleges and higher education institutions continuation of their services including test accommodations [9]. Completion of community college or supplemental job training does improve the chances for employment opportunities. For patients with developmental disabilities who are unable to continue onto higher education, special education high schools end at age 21 years and can provide a useful bridge to additional adult educational enrichment programs in the community [9]. Employment for those with a college education is nearly twice more likely than in those with only a high school degree or less, and the rate of employment decreases as patients with disabilities age [107].

Employment rates remain low, with reported rates between 10 and 48 % [9, 42, 43, 106]. Patients with higher IQ, higher education, better mobility, supportive family, improved physical health, decreased pain, completion of regular high school, improved speech ability, and normal hearing and vision are more likely to have regular employment [9]. Nearly half of young adults with CP were employed by 20–24 years of age, which is still lower than the non-CP population. Patients with more severe GMCFS rates were less likely to be employed, and nearly 25 % experienced some sort of medical or physical limitation during employment [108]. Accommodations in the workplace for older CP patients are essential to reduce the early employment loss, and the need to develop vocational rehabilitation plans for employment needs throughout the lifespan is necessary [107].

For living arrangements, approximately 60–80 % of young adult CP patients live with their parents, while approximately 60 % of older CP patients in the 30–40 years of age range live independently [43]. Among the older CP adults, approximately 20–28 % are either married or live with a partner. However, at least 60 % report difficulties with mobility, recreation, and housing, and about a fourth reported issues with personal care and employment [104]. Patients with more severe forms of spastic cerebral palsy and with developmental disabilities can often reside in group homes and assisted living arrangements [9, 43].

Reproductive Health and Sexuality

As cerebral palsy patients mature through young adulthood, they actively participate in healthy relationships and are actively engage in sex. Between 52 and 76 % of young adults with CP report having been in a relationship, with a quarter reporting being in a current relationship [109–111]. A little over half of young adults with CP report being sexually active, but compared to non-disabled peers, rates of experiences are lower [110–112]. Social barriers to starting a relationship include lack of self-confidence, being treated differently, and physical disabilities; nearly half also felt that it was difficult to find a partner due to the disability itself [113]. Physical obstacles include spasticity, difficulty with spreading legs and pelvic tilt, increased stiffness of joints and muscles, and fatigue [112, 113]. Most CP young adults have received sexual education regarding reproduction, birth control, and sexually transmitted diseases, mostly through school, parents, pamphlets, radio/television, and peers, but often not by providers [112, 113]. Generalists should provide appropriate preventative care for CP adults, including education regarding sexuality, treatment, and evaluation of sexual difficulties and prevention of sexually transmitted diseases.

During pregnancy, women should be counseled regarding the complications associated with pregnancy, including falls, urinary tract and bladder problems, mobility issues associated with wheelchair use, worsening shortness of breath, increased spasticity, and bowel management difficulties [114]. Spasticity does worsen with pregnancy, and the teratogenic effects of the medications are not well established. Many of the antispasmodic medications are secreted in the breast milk, and should be used cautiously in breastfeeding mothers [47]. For CP patients during delivery, a paucity of evidence is available regarding the use of spinal anesthesia, although a few case reports have demonstrated its safe use without complications [115].

Conclusion

Overview and Recommendations for Practice

1. The goal of therapy for adults with CP should be to maximize function even if accomplished through the use of assistive technology so that these individuals can achieve their life goals.
2. Internists should familiarize themselves with the treatments for the neuromuscular complications of CP, be comfortable medically managing dystonia and spasticity with oral medications, and identify referral sources for more invasive treatments if required ("Appendix").
3. Management of adults with CP should include surveillance for the common complications associated with cerebral palsy as listed in Table 5.1.
4. Adults with CP should receive all the normal counseling and preventive health measures appropriate for their age.
5. Important partners in managing adults with CP should include a physical therapist, a physiatrist, and orthopedist, and other specialists as needed based on the individual's unique problems.

Appendix

Cerebral palsy (CP) condition fact sheet

Definition	**Cerebral palsy** is defined as a group of permanent disorders affecting development of movement and posture causing activity limitations and attributed to nonprogressive injury of the developing fetal or infant brain • This encompasses a broad spectrum of conditions with diverse symptoms and presentations • Symptom classification usually divides patients based on the primary motor symptom: spasticity, dyskinesia, athetoid, or ataxic cerebral palsy • Another classification is by the affected extremities, dividing cerebral palsy into diplegic, hemiplegic, and quadriplegic groups • Individuals may or may not have co-occurring intellectual deficits
Epidemiology	• Cerebral palsy occurs in 2–3 of 1000 children born • The prevalence of cerebral palsy has been mostly stable over time • Risk factors for cerebral palsy include prematurity and low birth weight • Most infants born with cerebral palsy will live into adulthood • It is estimated that there are about half a million adults with cerebral palsy living in the US • Life expectancy of adults with cerebral palsy is less than that of the general population though a significant percentage of patients reach age 50 and older
Special considerations	Individuals with cerebral palsy have high rates of comorbid physical and mental health conditions, including the following: • Speech disorders • Bladder dysfunction • Poor dental health • Constipation • Epilepsy • Chronic Pain • Decubitus ulcers • Orthopedic concerns • Urinary tract infections • Poor nutrition The goal of therapy for adults with CP should be to maximize function even if accomplished through the use of assistive technology so that these individuals can achieve their life goals Adult providers should familiarize themselves with the treatments for the neuromuscular complications of CP, be comfortable medically managing dystonia and spasticity with oral medications, and identify referral sources for more invasive treatments if required

Resources for Family with Cerebral Palsy

- United Cerebral Palsy: www.ucp.org.
- Centers for Independent Living: http://www.ilru.org/projects/cil-net/cil-center-and-association-directory.
- The CP Group—A Group for Adults with Cerebral Palsy: http://www.thecpgroup.org/home.

Suggested Reading

- Colver A, Fairhurst C, Pharoah PO. *Cerebral palsy*. Lancet, 2014. 383 (9924): p. 1240–9.
- Glew GM, Bennett FC. *Cerebral palsy grown up*. J Dev Behav Pediatr, 2011. 32 (6): p. 469–5.

References

1. Colver A, Fairhurst C, Pharoah PO. Cerebral palsy. Lancet. 2014;383(9924):1240–9.
2. Palisano R, Rosenbaum P, Walter S, Russell D, Wood E, Galuppi B. Development and reliability of a system to classify gross motor function in children with cerebral palsy. Dev Med Child Neurol. 1997;39(4):214–23.
3. Stevenson CJ, Pharoah PO, Stevenson R. Cerebral palsy—the transition from youth to adulthood. Dev Med Child Neurol. 1997;39(5):336–42.
4. Organization WH. International classification of functioning, disability, and health. Geneva, Switzerland: World Health Organization; 2001.
5. Turk MA. Health, mortality, and wellness issues in adults with cerebral palsy. Dev Med Child Neurol. 2009;51(Suppl 4):24–9.
6. Strauss D, Cable W, Shavelle R. Causes of excess mortality in cerebral palsy. Dev Med Child Neurol. 1999;41(9):580–5.
7. Strauss D, Ojdana K, Shavelle R, Rosenbloom L. Decline in function and life expectancy of older persons with cerebral palsy. NeuroRehabilitation. 2004;19(1):69–78.
8. Blair E, Watson L, Badawi N, Stanley FJ. Life expectancy among people with cerebral palsy in western Australia. Dev Med Child Neurol. 2001;43(8):508–15.
9. Glew GM, Bennett FC. Cerebral palsy grown up. J Dev Behav Pediatr. 2011;32(6):469–75.
10. Haak P, Lenski M, Hidecker MJ, Li M, Paneth N. Cerebral palsy and aging. Dev Med Child Neurol. 2009;51(Suppl 4):16–23.
11. Liptak GS. Health and well being of adults with cerebral palsy. Curr Opin Neurol. 2008;21(2):136–42.
12. Mezaal MA, Nouri KA, Abdool S, Safar KA, Nadeem AS. Cerebral palsy in adults consequences of non progressive pathology. Open Neurol J. 2009;3:24–6.
13. Henderson CM, Rosasco M, Robinson LM, Meccarello J, Janicki MP, Turk MA, et al. Functional impairment severity is associated with health status among older persons with intellectual disability and cerebral palsy. J Intellect Disabil Res. 2009;53(11):887–97.
14. Young NL, Rochon TG, McCormick A, Law M, Wedge JH, Fehlings D. The health and quality of life outcomes among youth and young adults with cerebral palsy. Arch Phys Med Rehabil. 2010;91(1):143–8.
15. Tan SS, van Meeteren J, Ketelaar M, Schuengel C, Reinders-Messelink HA, Raat H, et al. Long-term trajectories of health-related quality of life in individuals with cerebral palsy: a multicenter longitudinal study. Arch Phys Med Rehabil. 2014;95(11):2029–39.
16. Morgan PE, Soh SE, McGinley JL. Health-related quality of life of ambulant adults with cerebral palsy and its association with falls and mobility decline: a preliminary cross sectional study. Health Qual Life Outcomes. 2014;12:132.
17. Jovanovic M, Lakicevic M, Stevanovic D, Milic-Rasic V, Slavnic S. Community-based study of health-related quality of life in spinal cord injury, muscular dystrophy, multiple sclerosis, and cerebral palsy. Disabil Rehabil. 2012;34(15):1284–90.
18. Usuba K, Oddson B, Gauthier A, Young NL. Changes in gross motor function and health-related quality of life in adults with cerebral palsy: an 8-year follow-up study. Arch Phys Med Rehabil. 2014;95(11):2071–2077.e1.
19. Morgan P, McGinley J. Gait function and decline in adults with cerebral palsy: a systematic review. Disabil Rehabil. 2014;36(1):1–9.
20. Tarsuslu T, Livanelioglu A. Relationship between quality of life and functional status of young adults and adults with cerebral palsy. Disabil Rehabil. 2010;32(20):1658–65.
21. Groff DG, Lundberg NR, Zabriskie RB. Influence of adapted sport on quality of life: perceptions of athletes with cerebral palsy. Disabil Rehabil. 2009;31(4):318–26.
22. Roebroeck ME, Jahnsen R, Carona C, Kent RM, Chamberlain MA. Adult outcomes and lifespan issues for people with childhood-onset physical disability. Dev Med Child Neurol. 2009;51(8):670–8.
23. Hergenroder H, Blank R. Subjective well-being and satisfaction with life in adults with spastic cerebral

palsy: a pilot study of a randomized sample. Dev Med Child Neurol. 2009;51(5):389–96.
24. Young NL. The transition to adulthood for children with cerebral palsy: What do we know about their health care needs? J Pediatr Orthop. 2007;27(4):476–9.
25. Cassidy C, Campbell N, Madady M, Payne M. Bridging the gap: the role of physiatrists in caring for adults with cerebral palsy. Disabil Rehabil. 2015;20:1–6.
26. Kibele A. Occupational therapy's role in improving the quality of life for persons with cerebral palsy. Am J Occup Ther. 1989;43(6):371–7.
27. Orlin MN, Cicirello NA, O'Donnell AE, Doty AK. The continuum of care for individuals with lifelong disabilities: role of the physical therapist. Phys Ther. 2014;94(7):1043–53.
28. Schor NF. Life at the interface: adults with "pediatric" disorders of the nervous system. Ann Neurol. 2013;74(2):158–63.
29. Young NL, Barden WS, Mills WA, Burke TA, Law M, Boydell K. Transition to adult-oriented health care: perspectives of youth and adults with complex physical disabilities. Phys Occup Ther Pediatr. 2009;29(4):345–61.
30. Merrick H, McConachie H, Le Couteur A, Mann K, Parr JR, Pearce MS, et al. Characteristics of young people with long term conditions close to transfer to adult health services. BMC Health Serv Res. 2015;15:435.
31. Linroth R. Meeting the needs of young people and adults with childhood-onset conditions: gillette lifetime specialty healthcare. Dev Med Child Neurol. 2009;51(Suppl 4):174–7.
32. Tsybina I, Kingsnorth S, Maxwell J, Bayley M, Lindsay S, McKeever P, et al. Longitudinal evaluation of transition services ("lets study"): protocol for outcome evaluation. BMC Pediatr. 2012;12:51.
33. Watson R, Parr JR, Joyce C, May C, Le Couteur AS. Models of transitional care for young people with complex health needs: a scoping review. Child Care Health Dev. 2011;37(6):780–91.
34. Colver AF, Merrick H, Deverill M, Le Couteur A, Parr J, Pearce MS, et al. Study protocol: longitudinal study of the transition of young people with complex health needs from child to adult health services. BMC Public Health. 2013;13:675.
35. Binks JA, Barden WS, Burke TA, Young NL. What do we really know about the transition to adult-centered health care? A focus on cerebral palsy and spina bifida. Arch Phys Med Rehabil. 2007;88(8):1064–73.
36. Lariviere-Bastien D, Bell E, Majnemer A, Shevell M, Racine E. Perspectives of young adults with cerebral palsy on transitioning from pediatric to adult healthcare systems. Semin Pediatr Neurol. 2013;20(2):154–9.
37. Blackman JA, Conaway MR. Adolescents with cerebral palsy: transitioning to adult health care services. Clin Pediatr (Phila). 2014;53(4):356–63.
38. Moll LR, Cott CA. The paradox of normalization through rehabilitation: growing up and growing older with cerebral palsy. Disabil Rehabil. 2013;35(15):1276–83.
39. Donkervoort M, Wiegerink DJ, van Meeteren J, Stam HJ, Roebroeck ME, Transition Research Group South West N. Transition to adulthood: validation of the rotterdam transition profile for young adults with cerebral palsy and normal intelligence. Dev Med Child Neurol. 2009;51(1):53–62.
40. Bjorquist E, Nordmark E, Hallstrom I. Parents' experiences of health and needs when supporting their adolescents with cerebral palsy during transition to adulthood. Phys Occup Ther Pediatr. 2015;7:1–13.
41. Maggs J, Palisano R, Chiarello L, Orlin M, Chang HJ, Polansky M. Comparing the priorities of parents and young people with cerebral palsy. Disabil Rehabil. 2011;33(17–18):1650–8.
42. Andersson C, Mattsson E. Adults with cerebral palsy: a survey describing problems, needs, and resources, with special emphasis on locomotion. Dev Med Child Neurol. 2001;43(2):76–82.
43. Frisch D, Msall ME. Health, functioning, and participation of adolescents and adults with cerebral palsy: a review of outcomes research. Dev Disabil Res Rev. 2013;18(1):84–94.
44. Bottos M, Feliciangeli A, Sciuto L, Gericke C, Vianello A. Functional status of adults with cerebral palsy and implications for treatment of children. Dev Med Child Neurol. 2001;43(8):516–28.
45. Tosi LL, Maher N, Moore DW, Goldstein M, Aisen ML. Adults with cerebral palsy: a workshop to define the challenges of treating and preventing secondary musculoskeletal and neuromuscular complications in this rapidly growing population. Dev Med Child Neurol. 2009;51(Suppl 4):2–11.
46. Bragg DC, Sharma N. Update on treatments for dystonia. Curr Neurol Neurosci Rep. 2014;14(6):454.
47. Nair KP, Marsden J. The management of spasticity in adults. BMJ. 2014;349:g4737.
48. Charles PD, Gill CE, Taylor HM, Putman MS, Blair CR, Roberts AG, et al. Spasticity treatment facilitates direct care delivery for adults with profound intellectual disability. Mov Disord. 2010;25(4):466–73.
49. Grunt S, Becher JG, Vermeulen RJ. Long-term outcome and adverse effects of selective dorsal rhizotomy in children with cerebral palsy: a systematic review. Dev Med Child Neurol. 2011;53(6):490–8.
50. Hasnat MJ, Rice JE. Intrathecal baclofen for treating spasticity in children with cerebral palsy. Cochrane Database Syst Rev. 2015;11:CD004552.
51. Burns F, Stewart R, Reddihough D, Scheinberg A, Ooi K, Graham HK. The cerebral palsy transition clinic: administrative chore, clinical responsibility, or opportunity for audit and clinical research? J Child Orthop. 2014;8(3):203–13.

52. Moreau M, Drummond DS, Rogala E, Ashworth A, Porter T. Natural history of the dislocated hip in spastic cerebral palsy. Dev Med Child Neurol. 1979;21(6):749–53.
53. Bohtz C, Meyer-Heim A, Min K. Changes in health-related quality of life after spinal fusion and scoliosis correction in patients with cerebral palsy. J Pediatr Orthop. 2011;31(6):668–73.
54. Watanabe K, Lenke LG, Daubs MD, Watanabe K, Bridwell KH, Stobbs G, et al. Is spine deformity surgery in patients with spastic cerebral palsy truly beneficial?: A patient/parent evaluation. Spine (Phila Pa 1976). 2009;34(20):2222–32.
55. Kedem P, Scher DM. Foot deformities in children with cerebral palsy. Curr Opin Pediatr. 2015;27(1):67–74.
56. Davids JR. The foot and ankle in cerebral palsy. Orthop Clin North Am. 2010;41(4):579–93.
57. Karamitopoulos MS, Nirenstein L. Neuromuscular foot: spastic cerebral palsy. Foot Ankle Clin. 2015;20(4):657–68.
58. Horstmann HM, Hosalkar H, Keenan MA. Orthopaedic issues in the musculoskeletal care of adults with cerebral palsy. Dev Med Child Neurol. 2009;51(Suppl 4):99–105.
59. Jaffe JS, Timell AM. Prevalence of low bone density in institutionalized men with developmental disabilities. J Clin Densitom. 2003;6(2):143–7.
60. Smeltzer SC, Zimmerman VL. Usefulness of the score index as a predictor of osteoporosis in women with disabilities. Orthop Nurs. 2005;24(1):33–9.
61. Sheridan KJ. Osteoporosis in adults with cerebral palsy. Dev Med Child Neurol. 2009;51(Suppl 4):38–51.
62. Henderson RC, Lark RK, Kecskemethy HH, Miller F, Harcke HT, Bachrach SJ. Bisphosphonates to treat osteopenia in children with quadriplegic cerebral palsy: a randomized, placebo-controlled clinical trial. J Pediatr. 2002;141(5):644–51.
63. Allington N, Vivegnis D, Gerard P. Cyclic administration of pamidronate to treat osteoporosis in children with cerebral palsy or a neuromuscular disorder: a clinical study. Acta Orthop Belg. 2005;71(1):91–7.
64. Batch JA, Couper JJ, Rodda C, Cowell CT, Zacharin M. Use of bisphosphonate therapy for osteoporosis in childhood and adolescence. J Paediatr Child Health. 2003;39(2):88–92.
65. Grissom LE, Kecskemethy HH, Bachrach SJ, McKay C, Harcke HT. Bone densitometry in pediatric patients treated with pamidronate. Pediatr Radiol. 2005;35(5):511–7.
66. Plotkin H, Coughlin S, Kreikemeier R, Heldt K, Bruzoni M, Lerner G. Low doses of pamidronate to treat osteopenia in children with severe cerebral palsy: a pilot study. Dev Med Child Neurol. 2006;48(9):709–12.
67. Vogtle LK. Pain in adults with cerebral palsy: impact and solutions. Dev Med Child Neurol. 2009;51(Suppl 4):113–21.
68. Schwartz L, Engel JM, Jensen MP. Pain in persons with cerebral palsy. Arch Phys Med Rehabil. 1999;80(10):1243–6.
69. Engel JM, Jensen MP, Hoffman AJ, Kartin D. Pain in persons with cerebral palsy: extension and cross validation. Arch Phys Med Rehabil. 2003;84(8):1125–8.
70. Jensen MP, Engel JM, Schwartz L. Coping with cerebral palsy pain: a preliminary longitudinal study. Pain Med. 2006;7(1):30–7.
71. Vogtle LKMD, Denton B. Outcomes of an aquatic intervention for adults with cerebral palsy. Phys Ther Case Rep. 1998;1:250–9.
72. Vogtle LK ML, editor. Exercise as an antidote for pain in adults with CP. Annual Meeting of the American Academy of Cerebral Palsy and Developmental Medicine. 2008; Atlanta, GA.
73. Pohl JFCA. Gastrointestinal and nutritional issues in cerebral palsy. Pract Gastroenterol. 2006;30(6):14–22.
74. Rogers B. Feeding method and health outcomes of children with cerebral palsy. J Pediatr. 2004;145(2 Suppl):S28–32.
75. Sood MR, Rudolph CD. Gastroesophageal reflux in adolescents. Adolesc Med Clin. 2004;15(1):17–36, vii–viii.
76. Park ES, Park CI, Cho SR, Na SI, Cho YS. Colonic transit time and constipation in children with spastic cerebral palsy. Arch Phys Med Rehabil. 2004;85(3):453–6.
77. Agnarsson U, Warde C, McCarthy G, Clayden GS, Evans N. Anorectal function of children with neurological problems. Ii: Cerebral palsy. Dev Med Child Neurol. 1993;35(10):903–8.
78. Green LGG, Hurwitz E. Primary care of children with cerebral palsy. Clin Fam Pract. 2003;5:467.
79. Murphy KP, Molnar GE, Lankasky K. Medical and functional status of adults with cerebral palsy. Dev Med Child Neurol. 1995;37(12):1075–84.
80. Murphy KP, Boutin SA, Ide KR. Cerebral palsy, neurogenic bladder, and outcomes of lifetime care. Dev Med Child Neurol. 2012;54(10):945–50.
81. Silva JA, Gonsalves Mde C, Saverio AP, Oliveira IC, Carrerette FB, Damiao R. Lower urinary tract dysfunction and ultrasound assessment of bladder wall thickness in children with cerebral palsy. Urology. 2010;76(4):942–5.
82. Marciniak C, O'Shea SA, Lee J, Jesselson M, Dudas-Sheehan D, Beltran E, et al. Urinary incontinence in adults with cerebral palsy: prevalence, type, and effects on participation. PM&R. 2014;6(2):110–20 (quiz 120).
83. Goldfarb RA, Pisansky A, Fleck J, Hoversten P, Cotter KJ, Katorski J, et al. Neurogenic lower urinary tract dysfunction in adults with cerebral palsy: outcomes following a conservative management approach. J Urol. 2015;195(4P1):1009–13.
84. Grigoryan L, Trautner BW, Gupta K. Diagnosis and management of urinary tract infections in the

outpatient setting: a review. JAMA. 2014;312 (16):1677–84.
85. Ailey SH, Johnson TJ, Fogg L, Friese TR. Factors related to complications among adult patients with intellectual disabilities hospitalized at an academic medical center. Intellect Dev disabil. 2015;53 (2):114–9.
86. Chidambaran V, Gentry C, Ajuba-Iwuji C, Sponsellar PD, Ain M, Lin E, et al. A retrospective identification of gastroesophageal reflux disease as a new risk factor for surgical site infection in cerebral palsy patients after spine surgery. Anesth Analg. 2013;117(1):162–8.
87. Giuglea C, Marinescu S, Florescu IP, Jecan C. Pressure sores—a constant problem for plegic patients and a permanent challenge for plastic surgery. J Med Life. 2010;3(2):149–53.
88. Bass MJ, Phillips LG. Pressure sores. Curr Probl Surg. 2007;44(2):101–43.
89. National Pressure Ulcer Advisory Panel EPUA-PaPP, Alliance PI. Prevention and treatment of pressure ulcers: quick reference guide. Perth, Australia: Cambridge Media; 2014.
90. Rimmer JH, Yamaki K, Lowry BM, Wang E, Vogel LC. Obesity and obesity-related secondary conditions in adolescents with intellectual/developmental disabilities. J Intellect Disabil Res. 2010;54(9):787–94.
91. Bhaumik S, Watson JM, Thorp CF, Tyrer F, McGrother CW. Body mass index in adults with intellectual disability: distribution, associations and service implications: a population-based prevalence study. J Intellect Disabil Res. 2008;52(Pt 4):287–98.
92. Ryan JM, Crowley VE, Hensey O, Broderick JM, McGahey A, Gormley J. Habitual physical activity and cardiometabolic risk factors in adults with cerebral palsy. Res Dev Disabil. 2014;35(9):1995–2002.
93. Hurvitz EA, Green LB, Hornyak JE, Khurana SR, Koch LG. Body mass index measures in children with cerebral palsy related to gross motor function classification: a clinic-based study. Am J Phys Med Rehabil. 2008;87(5):395–403.
94. Rogozinski BM, Davids JR, Davis RB, Christopher LM, Anderson JP, Jameson GG, et al. Prevalence of obesity in ambulatory children with cerebral palsy. J Bone Joint Surg Am. 2007;89(11):2421–6.
95. Kwon DG, Kang SC, Chung CY, Lee SH, Lee KM, Choi IH, et al. Prevalence of obesity in ambulatory patients with cerebral palsy in the korean population: a single institution's experience. Clin Orthop Surg. 2011;3(3):211–6.
96. Peterson MD, Gordon PM, Hurvitz EA. Chronic disease risk among adults with cerebral palsy: the role of premature sarcopoenia, obesity and sedentary behaviour. Obes Rev. 2013;14(2):171–82.
97. Wingo BC, Mehta T, Qu P, Vogel LC, Rimmer JH. Exploratory study examining clinical measures of adiposity risk for predicting obesity in adolescents with physical disabilities. Am J Phys Med Rehabil. 2015;94(8):585–94.
98. Ryan JM, Crowley VE, Hensey O, McGahey A, Gormley J. Waist circumference provides an indication of numerous cardiometabolic risk factors in adults with cerebral palsy. Arch Phys Med Rehabil. 2014;95(8):1540–6.
99. Nieuwenhuijsen C, van der Slot WM, Beelen A, Arendzen JH, Roebroeck ME, Stam HJ, et al. Inactive lifestyle in adults with bilateral spastic cerebral palsy. J Rehabil Med. 2009;41(5):375–81.
100. Thorpe D. The role of fitness in health and disease: status of adults with cerebral palsy. Dev Med Child Neurol. 2009;51(Suppl 4):52–8.
101. Flanagan L Jr. Is bariatric surgery effective in the treatment of the neurological motor deficit syndromes? Obes Surg. 1997;7(5):420–3.
102. Livingston MH, Rosenbaum PL, Russell DJ, Palisano RJ. Quality of life among adolescents with cerebral palsy: What does the literature tell us? Dev Med Child Neurol. 2007;49(3):225–31.
103. Donkervoort M, Roebroeck M, Wiegerink D, van der Heijden-Maessen H, Stam H, Transition Research Group South West N. Determinants of functioning of adolescents and young adults with cerebral palsy. Disabil Rehabil. 2007;29(6):453–63.
104. van der Slot WM, Nieuwenhuijsen C, van den Berg-Emons RJ, Wensink-Boonstra AE, Stam HJ, Roebroeck ME, et al. Participation and health-related quality of life in adults with spastic bilateral cerebral palsy and the role of self-efficacy. J Rehabil Med. 2010;42(6):528–35.
105. Balandin S, Berg N, Waller A. Assessing the loneliness of older people with cerebral palsy. Disabil Rehabil. 2006;28(8):469–79.
106. Boucher N, Dumas F, Maltais DB, Richards CL. The influence of selected personal and environmental factors on leisure activities in adults with cerebral palsy. Disabil Rehabil. 2010;32(16):1328–38.
107. Horsman M, Suto M, Dudgeon B, Harris SR. Ageing with cerebral palsy: psychosocial issues. Age Ageing. 2010;39(3):294–9.
108. Verhoef JA, Bramsen I, Miedema HS, Stam HJ, Roebroeck ME, Transition Research Group Southwest N, et al. Development of work participation in young adults with cerebral palsy: a longitudinal study. J Rehabil Med. 2014;46(7):648–55.
109. Wiegerink DJ, Stam HJ, Ketelaar M, Cohen-Kettenis PT, Roebroeck ME. Personal and environmental factors contributing to participation in romantic relationships and sexual activity of young adults with cerebral palsy. Disabil Rehabil. 2012;34(17):1481–7.
110. Wiegerink DJ, Stam HJ, Gorter JW, Cohen-Kettenis PT, Roebroeck ME, Transition Research Group Southwest N. Development of romantic relationships and sexual activity in young adults with

cerebral palsy: a longitudinal study. Arch Phys Med Rehabil. 2010;91(9):1423–8.
111. Wiegerink DJ, Roebroeck ME, van der Slot WM, Stam HJ, Cohen-Kettenis PT, South West Netherlands Transition Research G. Importance of peers and dating in the development of romantic relationships and sexual activity of young adults with cerebral palsy. Dev Med Child Neurol. 2010;52 (6):576–82.
112. Wiegerink D, Roebroeck M, Bender J, Stam H, Cohen-Kettenis P, Transition Research Group South West N. Sexuality of young adults with cerebral palsy: experienced limitations and needs. Sex Disabil. 2011;29(2):119–28.
113. Wiegerink DJ, Roebroeck ME, Donkervoort M, Cohen-Kettenis PT, Stam HJ, Transition Research Group South West N. Social, intimate and sexual relationships of adolescents with cerebral palsy compared with able-bodied age-mates. J Rehabil Med. 2008;40(2):112–8.
114. Iezzoni LI, Wint AJ, Smeltzer SC, Ecker JL. Effects of disability on pregnancy experiences among women with impaired mobility. Acta Obstet Gynecol Scand. 2015;94(2):133–40.
115. Tanqueray TA, Dob DP. Spinal anaesthesia for caesarean section in a patient with cerebral palsy. Int J Obstet Anesth. 2010;19(2):238.

6 Childhood and Adolescent Cancer Survivors

Nirupa Jaya Raghunathan, Larissa Nekhlyudov and Linda S. Overholser

Case Presentation

AD is a 25-year-old female who presents for evaluation in the process of transitioning to an adult primary care provider. She reports that she was previously diagnosed with acute lymphoblastic leukemia (ALL). She is not sure about the details of her history, but she brought with her a copy of her treatment records that her mother previously obtained for her. At 5 years of age she presented with irritability and bruising noted by her parents. She was found to have an elevated white blood cell count (WBC) with blasts on peripheral smear. Bone marrow biopsy was consistent with ALL. A lumbar puncture was negative for leukemia. Records indicate that she was treated on a regimen that included doxorubicin (cumulative dose of 350 mg/m^2), dexamethasone, vincristine, intravenous and intrathecal methotrexate, ara-C, L-asparaginase, and 6-mercaptopurine, all administered over a 2-year time period. Based on a high WBC count, she was considered to be at high risk for recurrence and was treated additionally with cranial radiation at a total dose of 2400 cGy. Complications during therapy included neutropenia, cellulitis, and pancreatitis thought to be secondary to L-asparaginase. She received several blood product transfusions during her treatment. She finished treatment at the age of 7 years.

Her medical concerns since her treatment include cataracts in both eyes for which she follows with ophthalmology, with no surgery planned at this time. She reports irregular menses, currently managed on oral contraceptive pills. She also has intermittent headaches for which she takes an occasional ibuprofen.

During her 2-year treatment, her mother drove her to the Boston area from Maine. She was often away from her friends and school. She has two sisters, who are 4 and 6 years older than her. They lived at home with their father during her treatment. After her treatment was completed, she returned to elementary school but experienced difficulties in school and required additional assistance. During her teenage years, she continued to struggle in school and also in social situations. While her sisters understood her illness, she felt that they were a bit distant. She was aware that as she got older, she did not look like her sisters, who were taller and thinner than she was. She began using alcohol around age 15. At this time, psychological

N.J. Raghunathan (✉)
Department of Medicine, Memorial Sloan Kettering Cancer Center, 485 Lexington Ave, 2nd Floor, New York City, NY 10017, USA
e-mail: raghunan@mskcc.org

L. Nekhlyudov
Harvard Medical School, Brigham and Women's Hospital, 800 Huntington Avenue, 3rd Floor, Boston, MA 02115, USA
e-mail: lnekhlyudov@partners.org

L.S. Overholser
Department of General Internal Medicine, University of Colorado Denver/University of Colorado Health, 12631 E 17th Avenue, Mail Stop B180, 8th Floor, Aurora, CO 80045, USA
e-mail: Linda.Overholser@ucdenver.edu

M. Pilapil et al. (eds.), *Care of Adults with Chronic Childhood Conditions*,
DOI 10.1007/978-3-319-43827-6_6

counseling was suggested and this was thought to have been helpful. She began focusing on artwork, finding this to be a great way for her to express herself and her emotions.

She has not been followed in oncology for about 5 years as she has found it to be quite difficult to travel to Boston to continue to receive her follow-up there. She is working as a receptionist in a gym in Maine. She is single and denies tobacco or alcohol use. She is planning to move to New York City to pursue art studies. She does not currently have a job lined up in New York but plans to search for one when she relocates.

At her mother's request, she presents for this initial evaluation just to "make sure all is okay" before she relocates. She is not sure about insurance as she will be leaving home and may not be able to remain on her parents' health insurance plan. On further questioning, she was not aware that she can remain on her parents' insurance under the Affordable Care Act (ACA).

Review of systems reveals no additional concerns. There is no family history of malignancy, though family history is notable for diabetes mellitus and hypertension on her maternal side.

On physical examination, she is a well-appearing woman in no acute distress. You note microcephaly in relation to her body size, with thinning hair and alopecia. Her height is 4 ft. 10 in., and her body mass index (BMI) is 30 kg/m^2. She has small cataracts bilaterally, her throat is clear, and her ears are normal. Her neck is supple with no palpable thyromegaly, thyroid masses, nor lymphadenopathy. Heart rhythm is regular, with no murmurs, and carotid arteries are without bruits. Her lungs are clear to ascultation. Her abdomen is soft and nondistended with no palpable masses nor hepatosplenomegaly. Extremities are without edema, and she has normal distal pulses. Neurological examination is unremarkable with a normal sensory and motor exam. She completed a screening psychosocial instrument that suggests depression and anxiety. Gynecological examination is unremarkable.

Laboratory evaluation reveals normal blood count, serum creatinine, electrolytes, and thyroid-stimulating hormone, with a borderline elevation of serum glucose and total cholesterol level.

Case Discussion

This patient is a long-term survivor of childhood cancer, treated with multiagent chemotherapy as well as cranial radiation. This evaluation allows for an initial discussion of survivorship care planning and the importance of long-term follow-up and health promotion, setting the stage for risk-based care. Because treatment information is available for review, some recommendations can already be made.

Current issues are as follows.

Risk and Surveillance for Recurrence of Primary Cancer

The patient is close to 20 years postdiagnosis and 18 years out from completion of her therapy. Though she had a high WBC count on initial presentation (which is a risk factor for recurrence), given she is more than 10 years since therapy completion, her risk of recurrence of ALL at this time is low. Though there are no current specific recommendations for surveillance of her original ALL and her current risk for recurrence is low, she is advised to continue to be vigilant and report any new or unusual symptoms to a healthcare provider.

Management and Surveillance for Late Effects of Therapy

The late effects of chemotherapy will first be considered. Her regimen included doxorubicin, which is an anthracycline chemotherapeutic agent and as such is associated with cardiomyopathy. This is an example of a *late effect*, a medical condition that develops some time after the original exposure. Based on current guidelines, given the age of the patient and dose of her exposure, yearly echocardiograms would be recommended. Closer monitoring is also recommended during pregnancy, as will be discussed in greater detail later in this chapter. Her regimen also included vincristine, which may be associated with peripheral neuropathy, though not likely to develop at this time as this is more typically a *long-term effect*, a medical condition that arises at the time of treatment exposure and persists over time. Intrathecal methotrexate may be associated with neurocognitive late effects. Hepatitis is also associated with methotrexate, though typically earlier in the course of treatment. She received steroids, which may be associated with bone loss as well as cataract formation. Her cataracts should be closely monitored by an ophthalmologist. While an assessment of bone density may be considered, unless management may change based on results, it is not routinely recommended. The patient had pancreatitis as a treatment complication of L-asparaginase, but this condition should not be recurrent after completion of treatment. Her other chemotherapeutic agents are not typically associated with late effects.

She also received cranial radiation. Radiation therapy is associated with a number of potential late effects including secondary malignancies in the area of radiation involving the skin, subcutaneous tissue, and organs. As such, she is at risk for skin cancer as well as precancerous skin lesions and should be monitored for this as well as advised to take precautions such as using sunscreen diligently. She is also at risk for soft tissue and other malignancies in the involved field of radiation; benign or malignant meningiomas are examples of this with cranial radiation. Close attention should be paid to her headaches, and if any worsening of headaches or development of associated neurologic symptoms is noted, consideration should be given to imaging with magnetic resonance imaging (MRI) of the brain. Vascular complications, such as strokes arising from damage to the carotid arteries, could occur as well. Oral contraceptives, if considered, should be used with caution. Thyroid dysfunction, thyroid nodules, and thyroid cancer are all associated with cranial radiation that could have included the neck region. Further, central endocrinopathies, including derangements in growth hormone, thyroid function, and the glucocorticoid axis, may occur over time due to radiation effects on the pituitary gland. Individuals with a history of ALL and specifically a history of cranial radiation therapy traditionally used as part of ALL treatment are at a higher risk of metabolic syndrome compared with their peers. A consultation with an endocrinologist could be considered. She can also be referred for hearing evaluation if clinically indicated. Radiation therapy further increases her risk for cataracts.

She received blood products, though in an era after routine testing of blood products for human immunodeficiency virus (HIV), hepatitis C, and hepatitis B was implemented. It might be reasonable to consider screening for hepatitis C as well as an assessment for iron overload with a serum ferritin level.

Psychosocial Concerns

She has had a number of issues related to academic progress in school as well as concerns with family and social functioning since her diagnosis and treatment. She has been to therapy in the past and is currently still having depressive symptoms and anxiety. These are common in young adult survivors of cancer and should be recognized and closely monitored. She may benefit from medication management, referral to a mental health provider, or other strategies for self-management. Since she is moving to a new city, she might be at risk for worsening of her functioning in the absence of a support network. She may benefit from connecting with others who have experienced cancer at an early age, perhaps at a local cancer center or through online resources. She may have already undergone neuropsychological testing and, if so, those records could help shed some light on clarifying diagnoses and planning a strategy for management. If not already done, this could be considered at this point.

Under the ACA, she can remain on her parents insurance until the age of 26 years. She should be sure to get appropriate information from her parents or from another trusted resource in the practice or in the community such as a social worker.

Health Promotion

The patient is at risk for a number of medical conditions including obesity and metabolic syndrome. Healthy lifestyle habits and close monitoring of serum glucose, lipids, blood pressure, and body mass index are recommended. She will need regular follow-up with a primary care provider, routine dermatologic evaluation, and regular dental care.

Overview

Definition and Epidemiology of Childhood Cancers

Childhood and adolescent cancer is defined as any malignancy diagnosed before the age of 20 and treated with cancer therapy [1]. The number of survivors of pediatric cancers in the US and worldwide has grown significantly over the past half century, largely due to the development of increasingly effective treatments. Surveillance, epidemiology, and end results (SEER) data show that patients diagnosed before age 20 years of age now have a 5-year (5-yr) survival of more than 80 % in contrast to only 50 % just 35 years ago [2]. This improved survival has translated into more than 380,000 childhood and adolescent cancer survivors living in the US as of January 1, 2010 [3]. With the improved survival in this population has come a growing recognition of treatment-related late effects. These late effects confer an increased rate of mortality as well as morbidity in the form of chronic health conditions [4].

The Institute of Medicine (IOM) considers childhood cancer according to 12 different categories. They are, briefly, leukemias, central nervous system tumors, lymphomas, carcinomas/malignant epithelial neoplasms, germ cell/gonadal neoplasms, soft tissue sarcomas, malignant bone tumors, sympathetic nervous system tumors, renal tumors, retinoblastoma, hepatic tumors and, last, other unspecified cancers. The characteristics of each of these cancer types are described further in the IOM report "Childhood Cancer Survivorship: Improving Care and Quality of Life" [5]. Cancer therapy may include chemotherapy, radiation therapy, surgery, and bone marrow transplant. There is also growing use of immunotherapies for certain cancer types. The spectrum of cancer therapy also includes blood products, supportive medication for side effects including steroids as well as anti-infective and marrow-stimulating medications. While cancer therapies halt the progression of cancer, among those who survive cancer, chronic medical conditions arise due to late and long-term effects of such therapies. To review, late and long-term effects are medical conditions, including psychosocial comorbidity, that develop acutely during treatment and persist (long-term effects), or that develop many years after treatment exposure (late effects).

Pathophysiology of Chronic Conditions Among Cancer Survivors

In considering the varied therapies that a cancer patient might receive, the conferred late effects are largely related to a "field" effect—the tissues exposed (such as skin, subcutaneous tissue, and underlying organs) to therapy, whether normal or cancerous, are at highest risk for late effects [5]. Host factors such as the age of exposure, gender, pubertal status, family history of illness, or current health behaviors may affect the presentation and/or severity of the late effect. Cytotoxic chemotherapy is intended to kill cancer cells; its systemic administration often leads to effects on normal cells as well. Some classic examples include cardiomyocyte damage due to anthracyclines such as doxorubicin, peripheral neuropathy from platinum-based therapies, and gastroenteritis at the time of chemotherapy administration [6–11]. Radiotherapy is generally administered only to cancer tissue; still, even with advances in radiotherapy modeling, local normal tissue often receives high doses of radiation through scatter, leading to inflammation, fibrosis, and/or tissue destruction [5]. Hormone therapies are used frequently with hormone-sensitive cancers such as breast cancer. This treatment modality is much less commonly used in pediatric cancers, noting that when they are, hormone therapies can lead to disruptions of the endocrine system [1].

Surgical resection of cancer can lead to anatomical disruption of normal structure and scarring. For example, in a patient with resection of brain cancer, there can be significant residual neurological complications. For a patient with significant lymphatic and bone resection for a pelvic sarcoma there can be remnant lymphedema and musculoskeletal abnormalities [1]. Targeted therapies, like immunotherapies, were largely created to minimize systemic effects; still, some of the targeted pathways are nonspecific. For example, therapy targeting vascular endothelial growth factor (VEGF) receptors on cancer cells can have the additional effect of inducing thrombosis in normal vessels [6, 12].

Common Chronic Adult Conditions in this Population

Over the past three decades, several cohort studies, such as the Childhood Cancer Survivor Study (CCSS) [13], the St. Jude's Life cohort study [14], and the British Columbia cohort [15], have provided instrumental information about the effects of cancer treatment on the development of chronic conditions among adult survivors of childhood cancer. This forms the basis for much of what we have learned about long-term survivorship in this population.

Childhood cancer survivors are at risk for premature morbidity [4, 16]. It has been estimated that by 45 years of age, 95 % of childhood cancer survivors have at least one chronic health condition, and 80 % have a condition described as serious or life-threatening [17]. While the risk of primary cancer recurrence decreases as on children and adolescents age, their risk for other medical morbidities outpaces their peers without a history of cancer. Examples of such conditions include important endocrine, cardiac, pulmonary, and neurocognitive conditions discussed in this section [4, 17–22]. In addition to medical morbidity, individuals with a history of childhood cancer are considered to have higher risks of premature death, with the most likely causes being from secondary cancers as well as cardiac and pulmonary conditions [23–26]. Studies in this population indicate that survivors are 3.3 times more likely than their siblings without cancer to have any chronic condition and 8.2 times more likely to have a severe condition, [4] and recent evidence suggests that this disparity in health risks persists as individuals age [27].

In this chapter, a few of the more prevalent conditions that may be identified and are relevant to the presented case are discussed. This chapter is not meant to be inclusive of all potential chronic medical conditions among adult survivors of childhood cancer. Further, the field of cancer survivorship continues to evolve as new data emerges. We provide resources that clinicians will be able to use for future reference as survivorship research advances. A most valuable resource is the Children's Oncology Group *Long-term Follow-up Guidelines for Survivors of Childhood, Adolescent, and Young Adult Cancers* (COG LTFU Guidelines), found online at www.survivorshipguidelines.org [28]. This set of recommendations reviews potential late effects as organized by treatment exposure, such as chemotherapy and radiation. The use of these guidelines is further described in the following sections.

Endocrine Concerns

Endocrinopathies occurring as late and long-term effects of childhood cancer are prevalent and varied. Effects on various hormonally active organs can be related to direct effects, for example direct tumor invasion or surgery, radiation directly to the affected organ systems (i.e., pituitary gland), or chemotherapeutic agents. Thyroid hormone derangements, growth hormone deficiency, and risks for premature menopause are examples. A discussion of the endocrine late effects as it relates to fertility and reproduction follows in the "Special Issues in Adolescent and Young Adult Transition" section appearing later in this chapter. Long-term follow-up studies in this population to date indicate that radiation therapy exposure, including total body irradiation in preparation for bone marrow transplant, and alkylating agents appear to confer the highest risk for various endocrinopathies [29, 30].

In regard to disorders of the hypothalamic-pituitary axis (HPA), growth hormone deficiency, precocious puberty, and central hypothyroidism are the most prevalent. Cranial radiation therapy is considered to be the primary risk factor. Total dose of cranial radiation therapy and increasing time after exposure appeared to be the most important pieces of information to consider when evaluating risk [31, 32]. Growth hormone deficiency is known to be associated with undesirable body fat composition, dyslipidemia, and reduced bone density and is important to recognize as a potential contributing risk factor for morbidity in adults [33]. The benefits of growth hormone replacement in adults with a history of childhood cancer has not yet been proven to reduce long-term morbidity or mortality but may improve both quality of life and risk factors for disease such as osteoporosis or metabolic syndrome [34–36]. Consultation with an endocrinologist would be prudent if such therapy is being considered.

Disorders of the thyroid gland are common in adults with a history of pediatric cancer. Radiation appears to be the major culprit, whether it is cranial irradiation resulting in central hypothyroidism or primary hypothyroidism related to direct effects on the thyroid gland. As a late or long-term effect, primary hypothyroidism occurs more frequently than central hypothyroidism [29]. The risk for hypothyroidism approaches 50 % at 20 years of follow-up in individuals who were treated for Hodgkin's lymphoma, where radiation to the neck and chest area are common modalities for treatment [37]. Risk does not appear to plateau over time. Hyperthyroidism can also occur but is less frequent than hypothyroidism [38]. In addition to functional thyroid disorders, both thyroid nodules and thyroid cancer are seen more commonly in individuals with a history of treatment for childhood cancer. When completing an evaluation for thyroid disease in an adult with a history of radiation exposure to the head/neck area, thyroid function tests—including a free T4 level if central hypothyroidism is being considered—in addition to a careful neck exam yearly is recommended according to the COG LTFU Guidelines [28]. While thyroid ultrasound should be considered in the workup of thyroid nodules, a prospective observational study of survivors of Hodgkin's lymphoma suggested no benefit to routine ultrasound screening for thyroid cancer [39].

The endocrine risks described previously may overlap with other risk factors for the development of cardiovascular disease—a major cause of morbidity and mortality in the general adult population. For reasons that have not yet been fully elucidated, among individuals treated for cancer as on children, the risk of being overweight or obese over time is most strongly correlated with treatment for ALL or brain tumors [29]. Individuals with a history of childhood cancer were about twice as likely as their siblings without cancer to develop diabetes mellitus, even after adjustment for body mass index [40]. Notably, survivors also developed diabetes at significantly younger ages than their sibling counterparts. In multivariate analysis, important risk factors included abdominal radiation therapy, total body radiation, treatment under the age of 5 years, physical inactivity, and BMI above 25 kg/m^2 [41]. A later study indicated that overall childhood cancer survivors were not more likely to be obese, but were more likely over time to be taking medications for hypertension, dyslipidemia, or diabetes [42]. The prevalence of metabolic syndrome in small studies of adult survivors of childhood cancer ranges from 12.6–33 % with 17–25 years of follow-up [43–45].

Cardiovascular Concerns

Many long-term follow-up studies have now described the ongoing risks of cardiovascular disease related to childhood cancer treatment [46]. The risk of cardiovascular morbidity and mortality is significant [26]. A well-recognized late effect includes the development of cardiomyopathy related to anthracyclines. Anthracycline-associated cardiomyopathy as a late effect in childhood cancer survivors appears to be dose-related and knowing the cumulative dose impacts the surveillance strategy [46]. Concomitant therapy with chest irradiation can further increase the risk for cardiomyopathy as well as the risk of myocardial infarction, valvular heart disease, and pericardial disease [47]. A threshold for anthracycline exposure of 250 mg/m^2 increases risk for congestive heart failure, pericardial disease, and valvular heart disease [48]. Radiation exposure above 1500 cGy increases risk for all of the above cardiovascular outcomes in addition to myocardial infarction [48]. Risk factors for toxicity include younger age at exposure, higher cumulative doses of chemotherapy, and increasing time since exposure, which means that symptoms may develop years, sometimes decades, later [49]. Cardiovascular disease is not limited to diseases affecting the heart, and stroke could also be a consequence associated with childhood cancer treatment, with cranial and mantle radiation therapy being significant risk factors [19]. Guidelines describe recommended surveillance for individuals exposed to these risk factors with an algorithm that takes into account the age at exposure and combinations of past treatment [28].

Of note, pregnancy can exacerbate an underlying subclinical heart failure. It is recommended that women exposed to anthracyclines have an echocardiogram during the third trimester and possibly postpartum and should be managed accordingly by a high-risk obstetric or maternal-fetal medicine specialist.

Pulmonary Disease

Though onset of disease and symptoms can be very subtle, late effects related to pulmonary disease are a major source of morbidity, with a prevalence rivaling that of long-term cardiovascular disease after 25 years of follow-up [17]. Pulmonary issues are typically associated with radiation, with select chemotherapeutic agents (bleomycin, carmustine, methotrexate), or as a result of lung or chest surgery. Radiation can lead to interstitial inflammation and progress to fibrosis with development of restrictive lung disease over time. This may not only impact an individual's quality of life and physical functioning, but could also impact the ability to utilize procedures that involve radiation from a diagnostic testing perspective [i.e., use of computed tomography (CT) scanning to follow lung nodules] or from a therapeutic perspective (such as the use of radiation therapy for breast cancer in later years). It is important to have a sense of the cumulative dose of radiation received. Of the chemotherapy agents that lead to pulmonary toxicity, bleomycin has been well described. Bleomycin therapy can lead to pneumonitis and fibrosis. Damage with bleomycin is believed to occur via damage to the pulmonary vasculature and production of free radicals in the lungs. Pulmonary complications may occur in response to the use of high-dose oxygen in lungs that have been exposed to bleomycin, such as that used during prolonged surgical procedures or with activities such as scuba diving. If any surgery is being planned in an adult with a history of bleomycin exposure, the anesthesiologist should be alerted for proper planning. Pulmonary function testing, with evaluation of diffusion capacity [diffusion capacity of the lungs for carbon monoxide (DLCO)], is a useful modality to screen for lung dysfunction in general in pediatric cancer survivors [19, 50]. Such testing is not recommended on a routine basis (in the COG LFTU Guidelines) but rather at baseline, generally upon entry into long-term follow-up, and as needed if symptoms arise [28]. These recommendations have been found to have high yield for surveillance [51]. For the primary care provider, it is especially important to assess individuals at risk for pulmonary complications for smoking and to reinforce the importance of smoking cessation.

Neurocognitive Issues

Neurocognitive deficits related to cancer treatment can have long-lasting consequences; they can affect schooling, employment opportunities, and social interactions. Well-described risk factors that impact neurologic functioning include cranial radiation therapy, intrathecal chemotherapy, and high-dose steroids. The types of childhood cancer most commonly associated with long-term neurologic deficits, other than primary childhood brain tumors, include Hodgkin lymphoma and ALL, most likely due to the use of radiation or intrathecal chemotherapy in treatment. In ALL alone, specific deficits described include impaired attention, decreased executive functioning, visual-spatial deficits, and impaired mathematic abilities, with those treated before the age of 5 years being most sensitive to late and long-term effects [52, 53]. Behavior could be affected as well; self-reported behavior problems increase with each passing year after treatment [53].

Secondary Malignancies

The late effect with the highest rate of mortality in childhood cancer survivors is the finding of second cancers [24, 25]. This is attributed to the effects of treatment but also to possible inherited cancer predispositions syndromes, such as Li–Fraumeni syndrome. With regard to treatment-related cancers, alkylating agents can be associated with secondary blood cancers up to 10–15 years following administration. Radiation-induced cancers tend to have a slower course with the risk increasing many years after therapy and not appearing to plateau [54]. Importantly, secondary malignancies tend to occur in the field of radiation. Classic examples include the development of breast cancer following chest or mantle radiation, increased risk for colon cancer following abdominal/pelvic radiation, meningiomas following cranial radiation, sarcomas following radiation to the extremities or soft tissues, and skin cancer in any involved field. For those cancers that have screening guidelines available (breast and colorectal cancer), a history of radiation exposure can significantly alter both the age at and frequency with which screening and testing should occur; such guidance is again provided in the COG LTFU guidelines. For less common cancers for which no screening recommendations in the general population exist, additional screening may be advised; for example, consider MRI screening for brain meningiomas in patients who received cranial radiation therapy. In individuals for whom radiation has been a significant part of past therapy or past cumulative doses are unknown, consultation with a radiation oncologist can be valuable to help assess potential risks and guide recommended surveillance.

Genetic Considerations

With any of the aforementioned late and long-term effects, obtaining a multigenerational family history is important. Having been diagnosed with and treated for childhood cancer does not in itself appear to confer an increased risk of congenital abnormalities or cancer in offspring outside of a hereditary cancer syndrome, based on early observational studies [55, 56]. Childhood cancer can, however, be an important clue to inherited cancer syndromes, such as the Li–Fraumeni syndrome. Individuals with suggestive family histories for hereditary cancer syndromes should be considered for genetic counseling, and those that are found to carry typical hereditary mutations may require careful and aggressive surveillance for the development of secondary cancers as adults [57]. Family history can also further clarify potential future risks for important health conditions such as cardiovascular disease or predisposition to psychiatric illness.

Special Issues in Adolescent and Young Adult Transition

Access to Care

The adolescent and young adult age is one of transition–transition from childhood to adulthood, from school to work, from dependent to independent. This transition can include changes in financial security, location, and support structure. With the previously described late effects noted, this flux can lead to inconsistent access to health care in a population at high risk of chronic disease.

Many survivors of childhood cancer are not fully aware of their therapies and the risk of sequelae [58, 59]. Also, this is a mobile patient population at risk for inconsistent follow-up. In one study from CCSS data, during at 2-year study period, only 31 % had received any survivor-focused care and 11 % had received no medical care at all [60].

The IOM recommends the use of survivorship care plans (SCP) to facilitate the transfer of information to all providers [61]. The survivorship care plan includes the cancer diagnosis, a summary of the treatment received, any complications related to therapy, and potential long-term and late effects of which to be aware [62]. A survivorship visit allows for review of treatment as well as development of a care plan for follow-up. The education, both in person and on paper through the SCP, may help patients understand their cancer history and treatment and allows for outlining a plan for follow-up. Patients can share these treatment summaries and SCP documents with any provider as they navigate the medical system. A patient may also seek care from a survivorship clinic.

Primary care providers may need guidance on gathering treatment information and formulation of a plan for monitoring long-term survivors of childhood cancer. Such guidance may be derived by a "survivorship care planning visit," which may be offered by oncologists, a local cancer center, or specialized pediatric oncology long-term follow-up program. Novel models of survivorship care planning are emerging and may be available in primary care settings (see Box 6.1).

Box 6.1 Elements of survivorship care planning

- Surveillance for recurrence
- Monitoring for and managing psychosocial and medical late effects
- Providing screening recommendations for second cancers
- Providing health education to survivors regarding their diagnoses, treatment exposures, and potential late and long-term effects
- Providing referrals to specialists and resources as indicated
- Familial genetic risk assessment (as appropriate)
- Guidance about diet, exercise, and health promotion activities
- Providing resources to assist with financial and insurance issues
- Empowering survivors to advocate for their own health care needs

Fertility

Any young adult who was treated for cancer as a child should have a thorough assessment of fertility status, reproductive history and especially future plans for childbearing as young adulthood represents a phase of life that is especially pertinent to these topics and cancer treatment can significantly impact risk. In both women and men, consideration should be given to both reproductive hormone functioning and direct treatment effects to reproductive organs (i.e., ovaries, testes) as well as the stage of pubertal development at the time of exposure. Cranial irradiation can lead to derangements of the reproductive gonadotropins luteinizing hormone (LH) and follicle-stimulating hormone (FSH), but generally this is seen at higher doses [63].

Premature ovarian failure is seen at a significantly increased rate in females with a history of childhood cancer compared with their female siblings and may reduce the span of time that a woman has to consider bearing children. Use of certain chemotherapy agents and radiation exposure to the ovaries appear to be risk factors [64]. Chemotherapeutic agents most commonly described to have an adverse effect on ovarian function includes alkylating agents (cyclophosphamide, ifosfamide, procarbazine, busulfan, melphelan, thiotepa), nitrosureas (BCNU, CCNU), and cisplatin [65, 66]. The cyclophosphamide equivalent dosage (CED) score can assist in quantifying the exposure to alkylating agents and the potential risk for infertility [61, 67, 68]. Ovarian radiation exposure as low as 10 Gy, but especially greater than 20 Gy, has been associated with acute ovarian failure, which may become permanent [69, 70]. For those women who received a combination of pelvic irradiation and alkylating agents, the cumulative incidence of developing premature ovarian failure may approach 30 % [66]. In women, the resumption of menstrual cycles after chemotherapy does not necessarily signify a return to normal fertility.

For both men and women who are sexually active and are uncertain of their fertility status, it is important to reinforce that infertility should not be assumed based on prior cancer treatment and to use recommended methods of contraception if pregnancy is not desired. Evaluation in men includes a semen analysis. In women, testing can include traditional measures of fertility, luteinizing hormone (LH) and follicle-stimulating hormone (FSH) levels, as well as more advanced testing such as anti-Mullerian hormone (AMH) levels and antral follicle counts [28, 71]. Much of this should be done with the assistance of a reproductive medicine specialist. In the absence of a genetic or hereditary basis for the original cancer, it is also important to know that cancer treatment is not associated with an increased risk of birth defects [72, 73]. In women, direct radiation to the pelvic field involving the uterus, cervix, or birth canal could result in scarring, which can pose an increased risk for pregnancy complications.

Psychosocial Considerations

Research suggests that depression, anxiety, and posttraumatic stress disorder (PTSD) are seen in survivors at disproportionately high numbers [74, 75]. Newer studies indicate that this increased risk is in certain subsets of patients. In those with depression, a cluster of poor physical health, cancer-related pain, and emotional concerns can place these patients at higher risk for suicidal ideation [76]. Anxiety is shown to be associated with survivors who are female, unmarried, unemployed, have low household income, lower educational attainment, a chronic health condition, or lack health insurance [77].

The prevalence of anxiety and PTSD appears to be related to family functioning. Literature shows that of a sample of adolescent survivors with PTSD, 75 % came from families with poor family functioning [78, 79].

While there is certainly distress seen in survivorship, there are studies showing positive outcomes of the cancer experience such as resiliency, posttraumatic growth, and benefit finding [80–82]. Optimism, a leukemia diagnosis (compared to central nervous system or solid tumors), and belief that the illness still affected their lives were associated with a tendency toward benefit finding. Many survivors speak toward positive changes in self, relationships, and life goals as a result of the traumatic experience of cancer and cancer therapy [80].

It is also important to remember that significant illness in childhood can affect the achievement of developmental milestones. As such, the childhood cancer survivor can be found to have less satisfaction in social functioning and emotional health [83]. This can play a role in future academic achievement, vocational success, and personal relationships.

Conclusion

There are a host of considerations when taking care of the adult survivor of childhood cancer, particularly during the transitional period of adolescence and young adulthood. With knowledge of the medical, psychological, and social complications of cancer therapy, as well as access to supportive resources, providers can be instrumental in helping childhood cancer survivors navigate the seas of young adulthood and optimize their future health and wellbeing (Appendix).

Appendix

Childhood cancer survivor fact sheet	
Definitions	A childhood cancer survivor is defined as a someone diagnosed and treated for cancer before the age of 20 years with at least 5 years of being cancer-free Survivors are at risk for cancer therapy related chronic medical conditions (long-term and late effects): • Long-term effects are adverse effects as a result of therapy that develop during treatment and persist for several years • Late effects are adverse effects related to cancer therapy that may only develop many years later
Epidemiology	• If diagnosed with cancer before age 20 years, now have a 5-year survival of more than 80 % [2] • Improved survival has translated into more than 380,000 childhood and adolescent cancer survivors living in the US [3] • During a 2-year study period, only 31 % of CCS had received any survivor-focused care and 11 % had received no medical care at all [60]
Common chronic conditions (pathophysiology)	Survivors are at risk for complications related to underlying organ damage from cancer therapy; these therapies include chemotherapy, radiation therapy, surgery, bone marrow transplant, targeted therapies, and transfusions Survivors are particularly at increased risk for the following conditions: • Diabetes/insulin resistance • Radiation-induced endocrinopathies (e.g., growth hormone, thyroid) • Cardiovascular disease including cardiomyopathy and atherosclerotic disease • Restrictive and/or obstructing pulmonary disease • Neurocognitive issues including memory, concentration • Secondary malignancies, particularly in the radiation field • Hypogonadism and reduced fertility
Challenges in transition	• Population is mobile and may have inconsistent follow-up • Changing insurance status can make care for chronic conditions difficult • Psychological needs that may require specialized counseling
Resources	Provider resources • COG Guidelines: http://www.survivorshipguidelines.org/ • ASCO Practice Guidelines: http://www.instituteforquality.org/practice-guidelines • National Cancer Institute: http://www.cancer.gov/cancertopics/aya/survivorship • SurvivorLink CME modules: http://www.cancersurvivorlink.org/CME/Index.aspx?v=HCP Patient resources: • Cancer.Net: http://www.cancer.net/survivorship • Stupid Cancer: http://stupidcancer.org/ • Planet Cancer: http://myplanet.planetcancer.org/ • Cancer and Careers: http://www.cancerandcareers.org/en • Fertility Resources: http://www.myoncofertility.org/ • First Descents: https://firstdescents.org/

References

1. Cleeland CS, Allen JD, Roberts SA, Brell JM, Giralt SA, Khakoo AY, et al. Reducing the toxicity of cancer therapy: recognizing needs, taking action. Nat Rev Clin Oncol. 2012;9(8):471–8.
2. Howlader NNA, Krapcho M, Garshell J, Miller D, Altekruse SF, Kosary CL, et al., editors. SEER cancer statistics review, 1975–2011. Bethesda, MD: National Cancer Institute; 2014.
3. Ward E, DeSantis C, Robbins A, Kohler B, Jemal A. Childhood and adolescent cancer statistics, 2014. CA Cancer J Clin. 2014;64(2):83–103.
4. Oeffinger KC, Mertens AC, Sklar CA, Kawashima T, Hudson MM, Meadows AT, et al. Chronic health conditions in adult survivors of childhood cancer. N Engl J Med. 2006;355(15):1572–82.
5. Hewitt M, Weiner SL, Simone JV, National Cancer Policy Board, Institute of Medicine, National Research Council, editors. Childhood cancer survivorship: improving care and quality of life. Washington, DC: National Academies Press; 2003.
6. Albini A, Pennesi G, Donatelli F, Cammarota R, De Flora S, Noonan DM. Cardiotoxicity of anticancer drugs: the need for cardio-oncology and cardio-oncological prevention. J Natl Cancer Inst. 2010;102(1):14–25.
7. Curigliano G, Mayer EL, Burstein HJ, Winer EP, Goldhirsch A. Cardiac toxicity from systemic cancer therapy: a comprehensive review. Prog Cardiovasc Dis. 2010;53(2):94–104.
8. Sonis ST. Regimen-related gastrointestinal toxicities in cancer patients. Curr Opin Support Palliat Care. 2010;4(1):26–30.
9. Sul JK, Deangelis LM. Neurologic complications of cancer chemotherapy. Semin Oncol. 2006;33(3):324–32.
10. Mohty B, El-Cheikh J, Yakoub-Agha I, Moreau P, Harousseau JL, Mohty M. Peripheral neuropathy and new treatments for multiple myeloma: background and practical recommendations. Haematologica. 2010;95(2):311–9.
11. Hagiwara H, Sunada Y. Mechanism of taxane neurotoxicity. Breast Cancer (Tokyo, Japan). 2004;11(1):82–5.
12. Force T, Kerkela R. Cardiotoxicity of the new cancer therapeutics—mechanisms of, and approaches to, the problem. Drug Discov Today. 2008;13(17–18):778–84.
13. Robison LL, Mertens AC, Boice JD, Breslow NE, Donaldson SS, Green DM, et al. Study design and cohort characteristics of the Childhood Cancer Survivor Study: a multi-institutional collaborative project. Med Pediatr Oncol. 2002;38(4):229–39.
14. Hudson MM, Ness KK, Nolan VG, Armstrong GT, Green DM, Morris EB, et al. Prospective medical assessment of adults surviving childhood cancer: study design, cohort characteristics, and feasibility of the St. Jude Lifetime Cohort study. Pediatr Blood Cancer. 2011;56(5):825–36.
15. McBride ML, Rogers PC, Sheps SB, Glickman V, Broemeling AM, Goddard K, et al. Childhood, adolescent, and young adult cancer survivors research program of British Columbia: objectives, study design, and cohort characteristics. Pediatr Blood Cancer. 2010;55(2):324–30.
16. Hudson MM, Mertens AC, Yasui Y, Hobbie W, Chen H, Gurney JG, et al. Health status of adult long-term survivors of childhood cancer: a report from the Childhood Cancer Survivor Study. JAMA. 2003;290(12):1583–92.
17. Hudson MM, Ness KK, Gurney JG, Mulrooney DA, Chemaitilly W, Krull KR, et al. Clinical ascertainment of health outcomes among adults treated for childhood cancer. JAMA. 2013;309(22):2371–81.
18. Diller L, Chow EJ, Gurney JG, Hudson MM, Kadin-Lottick NS, Kawashima TI, et al. Chronic disease in the Childhood Cancer Survivor Study cohort: a review of published findings. J Clin Oncol. 2009;27(14):2339–55.
19. Hudson MM, Mulrooney DA, Bowers DC, Sklar CA, Green DM, Donaldson SS, et al. High-risk populations identified in Childhood Cancer Survivor Study investigations: implications for risk-based surveillance. J Clin Oncol. 2009;27(14):2405–14.
20. Lipshultz SE, Adams MJ, Colan SD, Constine LS, Herman EH, Hsu DT, et al. Long-term cardiovascular toxicity in children, adolescents, and young adults who receive cancer therapy: pathophysiology, course, monitoring, management, prevention, and research directions: a scientific statement from the American Heart Association. Circulation. 2013;128(17):1927–95.
21. Robison LL, Hudson MM. Survivors of childhood and adolescent cancer: life-long risks and responsibilities. Nat Rev Cancer. 2014;14(1):61–70.
22. Oeffinger KC, Mertens AC, Sklar CA, Yasui Y, Fears T, Stovall M, et al. Obesity in adult survivors of childhood acute lymphoblastic leukemia: a report from the Childhood Cancer Survivor Study. J Clin Oncol. 2003;21(7):1359–65.
23. Yeh JM, Nekhlyudov L, Goldie SJ, Mertens AC, Diller L. A model-based estimate of cumulative excess mortality in survivors of childhood cancer. Ann Intern Med. 2010;152(7):409–17.
24. Armstrong GT, Liu Q, Yasui Y, Neglia JP, Leisenring W, Robison LL, et al. Late mortality among 5-year survivors of childhood cancer: a summary from the Childhood Cancer Survivor Study. J Clin Oncol. 2009;27(14):2328–38.
25. Mertens AC, Liu Q, Neglia JP, Wasilewski K, Leisenring W, Armstrong GT, et al. Cause-specific late mortality among 5-year survivors of childhood cancer: the Childhood Cancer Survivor Study. J Natl Cancer Inst. 2008;100(19):1368–79.
26. Mertens AC, Yasui Y, Neglia JP, Potter JD, Nesbit ME, Ruccione K, et al. Late mortality experience in five-year survivors of childhood and adolescent cancer: the Childhood Cancer Survivor Study. J Clin Oncol. 2001;19(13):3163–72.

27. Armstrong GT, Kawashima T, Leisenring W, Stratton K, Stovall M, Hudson MM, et al. Aging and risk of severe, disabling, life-threatening, and fatal events in the Childhood Cancer Survivor Study. J Clin Oncol. 2014;32(12):1218–27.
28. Children's Oncology Group. Long-term follow-up guidelines for survivors of childhood, adolescent, and young adult cancers, 2016. Available from: http://www.survivorshipguidelines.org/. Accessed 9 Jan 2016.
29. Chemaitilly W, Sklar CA. Endocrine complications in long-term survivors of childhood cancers. Endocr Relat Cancer. 2010;17(3):R141–59.
30. Gurney JG, Kadan-Lottick NS, Packer RJ, Neglia JP, Sklar CA, Punyko JA, et al. Endocrine and cardiovascular late effects among adult survivors of childhood brain tumors. Cancer. 2003;97(3):663–73.
31. Mulder RL, Kremer LCM, Santen HMv, Ket JL, Trotsenburg ASPv, Koning CCE, et al. Prevalence and risk factors of radiation-induced growth hormone deficiency in childhood cancer survivors: a systematic review. Cancer Treat Rev. 2009;35(7):616–32.
32. Tonorezos ES, Hudson MM, Edgar AB, Kremer LC, Sklar CA, Wallace WHB, et al. Screening and management of adverse endocrine outcomes in adult survivors of childhood and adolescent cancer. Lancet Diabetes Endocrinol. 2015;3(7):545–55.
33. Link K, Moëll C, Garwicz S, Cavallin-Ståhl E, Björk J, Thilén U, et al. Growth hormone deficiency predicts cardiovascular risk in young adults treated for acute lymphoblastic leukemia in childhood. J Clin Endocrinol Metab. 2004;89(10):5003–12.
34. Murray RD, Shalet SM. Adult growth hormone replacement: lessons learned and future direction. J Clin Endocrinol Metab. 2002;87(10):4427–8.
35. Mukherjee A, Tolhurst-Cleaver S, Ryder WDJ, Smethurst L, Shalet SM. The characteristics of quality of life impairment in adult growth hormone (GH)-deficient survivors of cancer and their response to GH replacement therapy. J Clin Endocrinol Metab. 2005;90(3):1542–9.
36. Follin C, Thilén U, Ahrén B, Erfurth EM. Improvement in cardiac systolic function and reduced prevalence of metabolic syndrome after two years of growth hormone (GH) treatment in GH-deficient adult survivors of childhood-onset acute lymphoblastic leukemia. J Clin Endocrinol Metab. 2006;91(5):1872–5.
37. Sklar C, Whitton J, Mertens A, Stovall M, Green D, Marina N, et al. Abnormalities of the thyroid in survivors of Hodgkin's Disease: data from the Childhood Cancer Survivor Study. J Clin Endocrinol Metab. 2000;85(9):3227–32.
38. Chow EJ, Friedman DL, Stovall M, Yasui Y, Whitton JA, Robison LL, et al. Risk of thyroid dysfunction and subsequent thyroid cancer among survivors of acute lymphoblastic leukemia: a report from the Childhood Cancer Survivor Study. Pediatr Blood Cancer. 2009;53(3):432–7.
39. Metzger ML, Howard SC, Hudson MM, Gow KW, Li C-S, Krasin MJ, et al. Natural history of thyroid nodules in survivors of pediatric Hodgkin lymphoma. Pediatr Blood Cancer. 2006;46(3):314–9.
40. Meacham LR, Sklar CA, Li S, Liu Q, Gimpel N, Yasui Y, et al. Diabetes mellitus in long-term survivors of childhood cancer. Increased risk associated with radiation therapy: a report for the Childhood Cancer Survivor Study. Arch Intern Med. 2009;169(15):1381–8.
41. Armstrong GT, Oeffinger KC, Chen Y, Kawashima T, Yasui Y, Leisenring W, et al. Modifiable risk factors and major cardiac events among adult survivors of childhood cancer. J Clin Oncol. 2013;31(29):3673–80.
42. Meacham LR, Chow EJ, Ness KK, Kamdar KY, Chen Y, Yasui Y, et al. Cardiovascular risk factors in adult survivors of pediatric cancer–a report from the Childhood Cancer Survivor Study. Cancer Epidemiol Biomarkers Prev. 2010;19(1):170–81.
43. Gurney JG, Ness KK, Sibley SD, O'Leary M, Dengel DR, Lee JM, et al. Metabolic syndrome and growth hormone deficiency in adult survivors of childhood acute lymphoblastic leukemia. Cancer. 2006;107(6):1303–12.
44. Hoffman KE, Derdak J, Bernstein D, Reynolds JC, Avila NA, Gerber L, et al. Metabolic syndrome traits in long-term survivors of pediatric sarcoma. Pediatr Blood Cancer. 2008;50(2):341–6.
45. van Waas M, Neggers SJCMM, Pieters R, van den Heuvel-Eibrink MM. Components of the metabolic syndrome in 500 adult long-term survivors of childhood cancer. Ann Oncol. 2010;21(5):1121–6.
46. de Ville de Goyet M, Moniotte S, Brichard B. Cardiotoxicity of childhood cancer treatment: update and current knowledge on long-term follow-up. Pediatr Hematol Oncol. 2012;29(5):395–414.
47. van der Pal HJH, van Dalen EC, Kremer LCM, Bakker PJM, van Leeuwen FE. Risk of morbidity and mortality from cardiovascular disease following radiotherapy for childhood cancer: a systematic review. Cancer Treat Rev. 2005;31(3):173–85.
48. Mulrooney DA, Yeazel MW, Kawashima T, Mertens AC, Mitby P, Stovall M, et al. Cardiac outcomes in a cohort of adult survivors of childhood and adolescent cancer: retrospective analysis of the Childhood Cancer Survivor Study cohort. BMJ. 2009;339:b4606.
49. Lipshultz SE, Alvarez JA, Scully RE. Anthracycline associated cardiotoxicity in survivors of childhood cancer. Heart. 2008;94(4):525–33.
50. Landier W, Bhatia S, Eshelman DA, Forte KJ, Sweeney T, Hester AL, et al. Development of risk-based guidelines for pediatric cancer survivors: the Children's Oncology Group Long-Term Follow-Up Guidelines From the Children's Oncology Group Late Effects Committee and Nursing Discipline. J Clin Oncol. 2004;22(24):4979–90.
51. Landier W, Armenian SH, Lee J, Thomas O, Wong FL, Francisco L, et al. Yield of screening for long-term complications using the children's oncology group long-term follow-up guidelines. J Clin Oncol. 2012;30(35):4401–8.

52. Edelstein K, D'Agostino N, Bernstein LJ, Nathan PC, Greenberg ML, Hodgson DC, et al. Long-term neurocognitive outcomes in young adult survivors of childhood acute lymphoblastic leukemia. J Pediatr Hematol Oncol. 2011;33(6):450–8.
53. Krull KR, Brinkman TM, Li C, Armstrong GT, Ness KK, Srivastava DK, et al. Neurocognitive outcomes decades after treatment for childhood acute lymphoblastic leukemia: a report from the St Jude lifetime cohort study. J Clin Oncol. 2013;31(35):4407–15.
54. Schaapveld M, Aleman BMP, van Eggermond AM, Janus CPM, Krol ADG, van der Maazen RWM, et al. Second cancer risk up to 40 years after treatment for Hodgkin's Lymphoma. N Engl J Med. 2015;373(26):2499–511.
55. Hawkins MM. Is there evidence of a therapy-related increase in germ cell mutation among childhood cancer survivors? J Natl Cancer Inst. 1991;83(22):1643–50.
56. Madanat-Harjuoja LM, Malila N, Lahteenmaki P, Pukkala E, Mulvihill JJ, Boice JD Jr, et al. Risk of cancer among children of cancer patients—a nationwide study in Finland. Int J Cancer. 2010;126(5):1196–205.
57. McBride KA, Ballinger ML, Killick E, Kirk J, Tattersall MH, Eeles RA, et al. Li–Fraumeni syndrome: cancer risk assessment and clinical management. Nat Rev Clin Oncol. 2014;11(5):260–71.
58. Kadan-Lottick NS, Robison LL, Gurney JG, Neglia JP, Yasui Y, Hayashi R, et al. Childhood cancer survivors' knowledge about their past diagnosis and treatment: Childhood Cancer Survivor Study. JAMA. 2002;287(14):1832–9.
59. Oeffinger KC, Wallace WH. Barriers to follow-up care of survivors in the United States and the United Kingdom. Pediatr Blood Cancer. 2006;46(2):135–42.
60. Nathan PC, Greenberg ML, Ness KK, Hudson MM, Mertens AC, Mahoney MC, et al. Medical care in long-term survivors of childhood cancer: a report from the Childhood Cancer Survivor Study. J Clin Oncol. 2008;26(27):4401–9.
61. Hewitt M, Greenfield S, Stovall E, editors. From cancer patient to cancer survivor: lost in transition. Washington, DC: Institute of Medicine and National Research Council; 2005.
62. ASCO Survivorship Guidelines [cited 9 Jan 2016]. Available from: http://www.instituteforquality.org/practice-guidelines.
63. Green DM, Kawashima T, Stovall M, Leisenring W, Sklar CA, Mertens AC, et al. Fertility of female survivors of childhood cancer: a report from the Childhood Cancer Survivor Study. J Clin Oncol. 2009;27(16):2677–85.
64. Green DM, Sklar CA, Boice JD, Mulvihill JJ, Whitton JA, Stovall M, et al. Ovarian failure and reproductive outcomes after childhood cancer treatment: results from the Childhood Cancer Survivor Study. J Clin Oncol. 2009;27(14):2374–81.
65. Bath LE, Wallace WHB, Critchley HOD. Late effects of the treatment of childhood cancer on the female reproductive system and the potential for fertility preservation. BJOG Int J Obstetr Gynaecol. 2002;109(2):107–14.
66. Sklar C. Maintenance of ovarian function and risk of premature menopause related to cancer treatment. JNCI Monogr. 2005;2005(34):25–7.
67. Green DM, Liu W, Kutteh WH, Ke RW, Shelton KC, Sklar CA, et al. Cumulative alkylating agent exposure and semen parameters in adult survivors of childhood cancer: a report from the St Jude Lifetime Cohort Study. Lancet Oncol. 2014;15(11):1215–23.
68. Green DM, Nolan VG, Goodman PJ, Whitton JA, Srivastava D, Leisenring WM, et al. The cyclophosphamide equivalent dose as an approach for quantifying alkylating agent exposure: a report from the Childhood Cancer Survivor Study. Pediatr Blood Cancer. 2014;61(1):53–67.
69. Thomson AB, Critchley HOD, Kelnar CJH, Wallace WHB. Late reproductive sequelae following treatment of childhood cancer andoptions for fertility preservation. Best Pract Res Clin Endocrinol Metab. 2002;16(2):311–34.
70. Chemaitilly W, Mertens AC, Mitby P, Whitton J, Stovall M, Yasui Y, et al. Acute ovarian failure in the Childhood Cancer Survivor Study. J Clin Endocrinol Metab. 2006;91(5):1723–8.
71. Metzger ML, Meacham LR, Patterson B, Casillas JS, Constine LS, Hijiya N, et al. Female reproductive health after childhood, adolescent, and young adult cancers: guidelines for the assessment and management of female reproductive complications. J Clin Oncol. 2013;31(9):1239–47.
72. Sankila R, Olsen JH, Anderson H, Garwicz S, Glattre E, Hertz H, et al. Risk of cancer among offspring of childhood-cancer survivors. Association of the Nordic Cancer Registries and the Nordic Society of Paediatric Haematology and Oncology. N Engl J Med. 1998;338(19):1339–44.
73. Signorello LB, Mulvihill JJ, Green DM, Munro HM, Stovall M, Weathers RE, et al. Congenital anomalies in the children of cancer survivors: a report from the Childhood Cancer Survivor Study. J Clin Oncol. 2012;30(3):239–45.
74. Zebrack BJ, Zeltzer LK, Whitton J, Mertens AC, Odom L, Berkow R, et al. Psychological outcomes in long-term survivors of childhood leukemia, Hodgkin's disease, and non-Hodgkin's lymphoma: a report from the Childhood Cancer Survivor Study. Pediatrics. 2002;110(1 Pt 1):42–52.
75. Hobbie WL, Stuber M, Meeske K, Wissler K, Rourke MT, Ruccione K, et al. Symptoms of posttraumatic stress in young adult survivors of childhood cancer. J Clin Oncol. 2000;18(24):4060–6.
76. Recklitis CJ, Diller LR, Li X, Najita J, Robison LL, Zeltzer L. Suicide ideation in adult survivors of childhood cancer: a report from the Childhood Cancer Survivor Study. J Clin Oncol. 2010;28(4):655–61.

77. Langeveld NE, Grootenhuis MA, Voûte PA, de Haan RJ. Posttraumatic stress symptoms in adult survivors of childhood cancer. Pediatr Blood Cancer. 2004;42(7):604–10.
78. Ozono S, Saeki T, Mantani T, Ogata A, Okamura H, S-i Nakagawa, et al. Psychological distress related to patterns of family functioning among Japanese childhood cancer survivors and their parents. Psycho-Oncology. 2010;19(5):545–52.
79. Alderfer MA, Navsaria N, Kazak AE. Family functioning and posttraumatic stress disorder in adolescent survivors of childhood cancer. J Fam Psychol. 2009;23(5):717–25.
80. Barakat LP, Alderfer MA, Kazak AE. Posttraumatic growth in adolescent survivors of cancer and their mothers and fathers. J Pediatr Psychol. 2006;31(4):413–9.
81. Zebrack BJ, Stuber ML, Meeske KA, Phipps S, Krull KR, Liu Q, et al. Perceived positive impact of cancer among long-term survivors of childhood cancer: a report from the Childhood Cancer Survivor Study. Psycho-Oncology. 2012;21(6):630–9.
82. Michel G, Taylor N, Absolom K, Eiser C. Benefit finding in survivors of childhood cancer and their parents: further empirical support for the Benefit Finding Scale for Children. Child Care Health Dev. 2010;36(1):123–9.
83. Zeltzer LK, Lu Q, Leisenring W, Tsao JCI, Recklitis C, Armstrong G, et al. Psychosocial outcomes and health-related quality of life in adult childhood cancer survivors: a report from the Childhood Cancer Survivor Study. Cancer Epidemiol Biomark Prev. 2008;17(2):435–46.

Congenital Heart Disease

7

Joseph Truglio and Barry Love

Case Presentations

R.A. is a 20-year-old female with repaired Tetralogy of Fallot (ToF) presenting to an adult medical practice for follow-up. She was diagnosed prenatally with ToF and had a surgical correction at 2 years of age. A workup for syndromes associated with ToF was unrevealing. After her repair she demonstrated age-appropriate growth but mild developmental delay, and was followed regularly by her pediatrician and pediatric cardiologist. She received speech therapy, physical therapy, and occupational therapy in grade school. She started college 2 years ago. She is now sexually active with 1 male partner. She is using condoms for sexually transmitted infection protection and is interested in discussing additional contraception options. She has not seen a doctor since the year before starting college. On review of symptoms she reports intermittent dizziness when exercising. During high school she ran regularly, but she now becomes short of breath and dizzy after around 5 min of jogging. She denies any syncopal episodes. She last saw her pediatric cardiologist 5 years ago.

E.W. is a 52-year-old man with a history of atrioventricular (AV) canal and Down syndrome presenting to an adult medical practice for preoperative assessment for dental rehabilitation under general anesthesia. He had an AV canal repair as an infant and was followed by his pediatric cardiology team well into adulthood. He lived with his mother until his 30s. He has since lived in a group home. Eight years ago he was diagnosed with type 2 diabetes mellitus and hypertension. He takes metformin and glipizide for his diabetes. His most recent hemoglobin A1c was 9, but he has been unable to reliably take insulin. His hypertension is well controlled on lisinopril and chlorthalidone. He has moderate developmental delay and is accompanied by an aid from the group home where he has lived for the past 15 years.

Case Discussions

Over the past 3 decades there has been an epidemiological shift wherein the majority of patients with congenital heart disease (CHD) are now adults. More recently, there has been a significant increase in the number of adults over 40 years of age with CHD. Successes in repairing and managing even highly complex CHD have thus created a large, ever-growing, and

J. Truglio (✉)
Departments of Internal Medicine, Pediatrics and Medical Education, Icahn School of Medicine at Mount Sinai, 1 Gustave Levy Place, New York NY 10129, USA
e-mail: joseph.truglio@mssm.edu

B. Love
Department of Pediatrics, Icahn School of Medicine at Mount Sinai, New York, NY, USA
e-mail: barry.love@mssm.edu

M. Pilapil et al. (eds.), *Care of Adults with Chronic Childhood Conditions*,
DOI 10.1007/978-3-319-43827-6_7

heterogeneous population of adults with congenital heart disease (ACHD).

The above cases illustrate the wide variety of common themes presented to primary care clinicians of ACHD. R.A. is a young woman in college, transitioning from pediatric to adult care. She had a complex heart lesion repaired as a child. Despite a successful surgical repair and a lack of associated syndromes, R.A. experienced developmental delay. A 2014 prospective, longitudinal study found that 75 % of children with congenital heart disease had developmental delay, despite only 19 % of patients in this study having a genetic syndrome [1]. After a period of very close follow-up, R.A. had a significant lapse in care, and she now presents with dizziness, concerning for potential complications of her cardiac repair. A recent study of adults with complex congenital heart disease found that 63 % had a lapse in care while transitioning from pediatric to adult care. The median lapse was 10 years in duration. Unfortunately, those patients with a lapse in care were more than 3 times more likely to require urgent cardiac intervention [2]. R.A. is also in need of sexual and reproductive health counseling as well as guidance regarding appropriate physical activity. Finally, although R.A. underwent genetic testing as a child, it would be reasonable to offer genetic counseling and possible re-testing, as new tests have become available and new syndromes have been recognized in the past 20 years.

E.W. also has a history of CHD requiring repair as a child. Unlike R.A. he has a diagnosed syndrome—Down syndrome—associated with his CHD. E.W.'s Down syndrome has manifested as moderate developmental delay resulting in him living in a group home. It has been estimated that as many as 25 % of patients with congenital heart disease have an associated genetic syndrome with comorbid conditions [3, 4]. For E.W. his care should be provided in the context of his chronological and developmental age. At 52 years of age, E.W. has developed comorbid cardiovascular conditions including diabetes and hypertension. A 2015 American Heart Association (AHA) Scientific Paper is dedicated to the unique needs of the growing population of adults with congenital heart disease over the age of 40 [5]. As seen in E.W., many patients over 40 years of age with ACHD are at increased risk for acquired cardiovascular disease in addition to the late complications of their underlying CHD. The screening and management of acquired cardiovascular disease and cardiovascular risk factors in ADCH should take into account the patient's underlying CHD lesion and should be done in partnership with an ACHD specialist. E.W. has a repaired AV canal. His diabetes and hypertension do not require any special management from a cardiac perspective. E.W. presents in need of perioperative management for non-cardiac surgery. Performing a preoperative assessment for this patient will require consideration of his CHD, his more recent acquired conditions, and his overall developmental status. A thorough history and physical exam should focus on any changes in his cardiac status with special attention paid to his risk for hemodynamic compromise and infective endocarditis risk related to the surgery. A baseline electrocardiogram (EKG) is indicated, given the risk of arrhythmias associated with his underlying lesion. If no murmur is noted on physical exam, an AV canal repaired more than 6 months ago with no evidence of subsequent complication is a low-risk lesion that does not require any particular perioperative management and should not require endocarditis prophylaxis. Additionally, beyond E.W.'s cardiac condition, his underlying genetic syndrome and any associated conditions should be addressed. Common associated conditions related to Down syndrome that may require special attention perioperatively include atlanto-axial instability, potential endocrine disorders such as diabetes and hypothyroidism, and any immune dysfunction.

Definition and pathophysiology

Congenital heart disease refers to a wide range of structural defects of the heart and major blood vessels that are present at birth. The pathophysiology of congenital heart disease is incredibly complex, with numerous genetic mutations, chromosomal abnormalities, epigenetic insults, and environmental exposures implicated in abnormal cardiogenesis [4]. An identifiable genetic or environmental cause is found in approximately 20–30 % of cases of congenital heart disease. As many as 18–25 % of congenital heart defects are associated with a congenital syndrome or chromosomal abnormality, most commonly Down syndrome and 22q11.2 deletion, and less commonly Williams syndrome, Noonan syndrome, and Turner syndrome [3, 4].

Epidemiology

The prevalence of congenital heart disease at birth ranges from 6 to 13 per 1000 live births [6–8]. While there are no national adult congenital heart disease registries, current estimates are that there are ~ 1,250,000 adults in the United States with CHD. More than 50 % of these patients had a moderate-to-severe complexity heart lesion at birth. Survival rates into adulthood for children with CHD vary, from 98 % for mild and 96 % for moderate to 56 % for severe complexity lesions [9]. Due to such high survival rates and improved care for adults with CHD, the ACHD population is currently growing at a rate of approximately 5 % annually [5].

Common Adult Conditions in This Population

Adult conditions associated with congenital heart disease depend upon the presence of an associated congenital syndrome or chromosomal abnormality, the complexity of the underlying CHD lesion, and the age of the patient. Associated syndromes will often require the primary care clinician to coordinate with several subspecialists as well as ancillary services such as physical and occupational therapy. Complications directly related to CHD should be managed in conjunction with an ACHD specialist. These include heart failure, arrhythmia (often atrial tachycardias), vascular complications (pulmonary hypertension, aortic root dilation, aneurysm formation, venous insufficiency), and risk for sudden cardiac death. Such complications can occur at any age. As ACHD patients age they may also develop risk factors for acquired heart disease, most notably hypertension, diabetes, and hyperlipidemia. The diagnosis and management of these risk factors may vary from that in the general population depending on the underlying CHD and any associated syndromes. Primary care clinicians should be comfortable managing such risk factors in most ACHD and should be able to recognize when co-management with an ACHD specialist is indicated. Subsequent acquired heart disease, including coronary artery disease and ischemic heart failure, should be co-managed with a cardiologist experienced in ACHD.

Finally, several themes commonly arise when caring for ACHD regardless of the patient's age or physical condition. These include counseling around physical activity and employment, sexual and reproductive health, genetic counseling, and antibiotic prophylaxis for infective endocarditis.

Screening, Diagnosis, and Management of Cardiovascular Risk Factors

Adults with congenital heart disease may be at higher risk for the development of ventricular dysfunction, arrhythmias, and heart failure. The management of acquired heart disease in ACHD should be managed in conjunction with an ACHD specialist. However, primary care clinicians should be comfortable identifying and managing cardiovascular risk factors in ACHD, including hypertension, diabetes, and hyperlipidemia. National and international guidelines for these risk factors can usually be applied to ACHD, but there are several notable exceptions.

Hypertension

There may be an increased prevalence of hypertension in the ACHD population [10]. The approach to screening, diagnosis, and manage-

Table 7.1 Lesion-specific recommendations for management of cardiovascular risk factors in ACHD

Lesion/condition	CV risk factor	Physiology	Management
Unrepaired cyanotic heart disease or persistent cyanosis	Hypertension	Nephropathy from glomerular sclerosis	Avoid nonsteroidal anti-inflammatory drugs Avoid ACE Inhibitors, ARBs and diuretic use if possible
	Diabetes	Risk for decline in renal function with ACEI and ARBs	Avoid ACE Inhibitors and ARBs for renal protection
Coarctation of the Aorta	Hypertension	Increased incidence of hypertension even with repair	Cardiology evaluation for persistent gradient requiring stenting. Consider ACEI or ARB in setting of aneurysm or Marfan's syndrome, but use caution if renal arteries are involved
	Hyperlipidemia	Increased risk for coronary artery atherosclerosis	Consider earlier initiation of statin therapy and an LDL goal of 70 or less
Eisenmenger physiology	Hypertension	Elevated pulmonary pressures with shunting	Avoid vasodilating agents to limit right-to-left shunting
Bioprosthetic valves in aortic position	Hyperlipidemia	Increased risk for coronary artery atherosclerosis	Consider earlier initiation of statin therapy and an LDL goal of 70 or less
Transposition of the great vessels	Hyperlipidemia	Sympathetic nerve injury during arterial switch operation	Consider earlier initiation of statin therapy and an LDL goal of 70 or less

ACE angiotensin-converting enzyme, *ACEI* angiotensin-converting enzyme inhibitor, *ARB* angiotensin receptor blocker, *LDL* low-density lipoprotein

ment of hypertension in adults with CHD is similar to that within the general population with a few exceptions (see Table 7.1). Coarctation of the aorta (CoA) places patients at higher risk for developing hypertension, even after the lesion is repaired [11]. Close monitoring for hypertension, including ambulatory blood pressure monitoring when available, is reasonable for patients with repaired CoA. For patients who have a persistent gradient across the coarctation site on echocardiogram after repair, an ACHD cardiologist should be consulted to evaluate for possible stenting of this lesion. The choice of antihypertensive agent for patients with CoA depends on the presence of associated syndromes and the presence and location of any aortic aneurysm. For patients with Marfan's syndrome or an aortic aneurysm, an angiotensin-converting enzyme (ACE) inhibitor or angiotensin receptor blocker (ARB) should be considered as a first-line agent. If the aneurysm involves the renal arteries, however, ACE inhibitors and ARBs should be used with caution and renal function closely monitored. Patients with unrepaired cyanotic heart disease or those with persistent cyanosis are at high risk for developing nephropathy from glomerular sclerosis [12, 13]. ACE inhibitors and diuretics should therefore be avoided if possible to prevent further decline in renal function. Finally, Eisenmenger physiology—when pulmonary pressures rise above those of systemic pressures—is typically seen in long-standing, unrepaired complex CHD. Management of systemic hypertension in these patients must be done in conjunction with an ACHD specialist, and the use of vasodilating agents should be avoided to prevent further right-to-left shunting.

Diabetes Mellitus

The incidence of diabetes in the overall ACHD population seems to be similar to that of the general population [14]. However, certain syndromes that are also associated with congenital heart disease, such as Down syndrome and William syndrome, may place patients at increased risk for Type 1 or Type 2 diabetes mellitus. A comprehensive review of such syndromes is beyond the scope of this chapter. Clinicians caring for such patients should familiarize themselves with any syndrome-specific screening guidelines. Regardless of any increased incidence of diabetes, adults with CHD are likely at higher risk for complications from diabetes. The American Heart Association therefore recommends considering screening for diabetes in all adults with congenital heart disease who are over 40 years of age with body mass index ≥ 25 kg/m^2, regardless of additional risk factors, with repeat screening every 3 years [5]. The management of diabetes in ACHD is similar to that in the general population. However, in patients with diabetic nephropathy who also have cyanotic lesions, ACE inhibitors and ARBs should be avoided. As is the case for all patients with diabetes, statin therapy should be initiated in ACHD who have diabetes unless contraindicated.

Hyperlipidemia

With the exception of specific lesions that increase a patient's risk for coronary artery disease, the role of statin therapy is the same in ACHD as in the general population. Patients with surgically repaired d-transposition of the great vessels are at increased coronary artery disease risk, likely due to injury of the sympathetic nerves that supply the coronary arteries during the arterial switch operation [15–17]. Patients with coarctation of the aorta and potentially patients with bioprosthetic valves in the aortic position are also at increased risk [18, 19]. It is reasonable therefore to have a lower threshold to initiate statin therapy in these patients, and to aim for a target LDL of 70 mg/dL or less.

Perioperative Management for Non-cardiac Surgeries in Adults with Congenital Heart Disease

Perioperative management of patients involves providing an assessment of the patient's risk of a perioperative cardiac event, optimizing the patient to reduce this and other risks, and providing recommendations for the management of any chronic illnesses around the time of surgery. The vast majority of ACHD may safely undergo non-cardiac surgeries with appropriate perioperative management. However, traditional cardiac risk calculators [20, 21] may not adequately assess the perioperative risk for ACHD. Further, most current recommendations regarding perioperative care of adults with complex congenital heart disease are based on expert opinion or small case series. An effective approach to ACHD perioperative care includes the traditional Revised Cardiac Risk Index used for adults without CHD plus an assessment of the patients' congenital heart disease and any associated conditions.

In general, cardiac surgeries are not "cures" for congenital heart disease. The hemodynamics and electrophysiology may remain dynamic and change over time. It is reasonable even in the absence of symptoms for some workup to be done for nearly all adults with CHD undergoing non-cardiac surgery. Many experts advise routine complete blood counts, chest X-ray, EKG, and echocardiogram [22]. For adults with simple, uncomplicated, repaired lesions such as ventricular septal defects, atrial septal defects, and patent ductus arteriosis who have a normal physical exam and no new symptoms, it is also reasonable to limit the above testing. Conversely, all patients with moderate to high-risk lesions (see Table 7.2) should undergo a risk assessment by an ACHD expert and have a cardiac anesthesiologist involved in the perioperative management, regardless of the stability of their

Table 7.2 Moderate, high and highest risk lesions for perioperative adverse events for non-cardiac surgery

Highest risk lesions	High-risk lesions	Moderate risk lesions
Fontan procedure	Pulmonary hypertension	Prosthetic valve or conduit
Severe pulmonary arterial hypertension	Severe systemic ventricular dysfunction (LVEF < 35 %)	Intra-cardiac shunt
Cyanotic congenital heart disease	NYHA Class III or IV heart failure	Moderate left-sided heart obstruction
Complex CHD with residual heart failure	Severe left-sided obstructive lesions	Moderate systemic ventricular dysfunction
Valvular heart disease with need for anticoagulation		
CHD complicated by malignant arrhythmia		

LVEF left ventricular ejection fraction, *NYHA* New York Heart Association, *CHD* congenital heart disease

symptoms. Consideration should be given to managing patients with the highest risk lesions at an ACHD center [22, 23].

Physical Activity and Employment

Primary care clinicians play a critical role in empowering ACHD to live full and meaningful lives. This includes encouraging all patients to engage in safe physical activity and developmentally appropriate, meaningful employment. Patients with CHD often have their physical activity limited to decrease the risk of sudden cardiac death. Adults with CHD are also far less likely to be employed as compared with otherwise healthy, age-matched adults [24]. This is at times due to patient, caregiver, and clinician fear of adverse events due to physical exertion. Unfortunately, few data are available for routine physical activity or employment restrictions for ACHD. Guidelines for cardiac evaluation of competitive athletes are found in the 2005 36th Bethesda Conference. Task Force 2 of that conference specifically addressed patients with congenital heart disease [25]. The general high-risk lesions outlined by that task force include hypertrophic cardiomyopathy, Marfan syndrome, aortic valve disease, transposition of the great vessels, single ventricle physiology, and pulmonary vascular disease [26–28].

It must be noted, however, that any individual patient's risk must be assessed with consideration of his or her underlying lesion, surgical repairs, complications, acquired conditions, and associated syndromes. When questions exist regarding a particular activity, the Task Force recommends considering exercise testing including monitoring of symptoms, EKG, and blood pressure under conditions similar to the sport or activity in question. Cardiopulmonary stress testing is a well-established method to assess exercise tolerance [29]. Holter monitoring or long-term event monitoring are also reasonable tests when arrhythmias are suspected.

A more recent 2013 AHA Scientific Statement [30] highlights the difference between the competitive, "systematic (and usually intense) training" referred to in the 36th Bethesda Conference and the various types of less intense static and dynamic physical activities in which patients may wish to participate. This statement outlines an approach to safely promote daily physical activity. A holistic understanding of physical activity is outlined, which includes mobility, object manipulation, cognitive function, behavior and social skills, communication and perception and fitness (emotional and physical). This paradigm is more useful when promoting activity in ACHD of all ages, be it "sports or activities of daily living" or meaningful employment.

Sexual and Reproductive Health

Sexual and reproductive health are arguably the most neglected health domains for adults with CHD. Congenital malformations are the most common causes of maternal cardiac morbidity and mortality in the United States [31]. Despite this risk, women with congenital heart disease are often not counseled on pregnancy-related risk or appropriate contraception. A recent study of more than 500 sexually active women with congenital heart disease revealed 1 in 5 women to be using a contraindicated birth control option, 28 % not using any contraception, and nearly half not having received counseling on pregnancy-related risk [32]. Given the genetic risk for CHD in the offspring of ACHD and the impact of functional limitations on sexual activity, sexual and reproductive health should address in all ACHD, regardless of their sexual orientation or gender identity. The role of the primary care clinician is to advocate for appropriate counseling on sexual and reproductive health and identify when patients need to be referred to subspecialists. The most common issues include contraceptive counseling, pregnancy and delivery, genetic counseling, functional limitations that impact sexual activity, and management of perimenopausal symptoms.

Contraceptive Counseling

The vast majority of women with CHD can have their contraception managed by their primary care clinician. This is especially important as young adults transition from pediatric-oriented to adult-oriented care. The Adult Congenital Heart Association advocates that "no matter how complex a woman's heart there is a safe and effective birth control option for her" [33]. The World Health Organization Medical Eligibility Criteria for Contraceptive Use provides guidance for the safety of contraceptive options for a wide variety of underlying medical conditions [34]. The major concern in adults with CHD is the risk of thromboembolism. Estrogen-containing birth control increases the risk of thromboembolism and is therefore not recommended for adults with cyanotic lesions, pulmonary arterial hypertension, prior Fontan procedure, or atrial fibrillation. The risk of thromboembolism in these conditions must be individualized for each patient in conjunction with an ACHD specialist and gynecologist.

Progesterone-only forms of contraception are often the preferred alternative. However, the risk of fluid overload should be discussed in patients with heart failure, and lifestyle factors must be taken into account given the need for strict adherence. Intrauterine devices (IUDs) are also a popular choice and are widely available in a variety of hormone and non-hormone containing versions. There are concerns regarding infections with IUD use, particularly in ACHD who may be at increased risk of infective endocarditis (IE). However, studies have shown only a modest 1.4 times increase risk of IE in women with ACHD using IUDs [22].

Table 7.3 outlines common high-risk conditions for venous thromboemobolism (VTE) with the use of estrogen, as well as possible alternative contraception options [34, 35].

Management of Perimenopausal Symptoms

The use of hormone replacement therapy (HRT) in the general population for management of perimenopausal symptoms remains controversial but is generally accepted for women ages 50–59 for a period of 5 years [36]. For women with ACHD the risk of venous thromboembolism due to their CHD must be considered prior to any HRT. For women with lesions considered high-risk for VTE (see Table 7.3), estrogen-containing HRT should be avoided. Alternative treatments include vaginal estrogen creams and non-hormonal lubricants for vaginal dryness and

Table 7.3 High-risk lesions for thrombosis with the use estrogen-containing birth control or estrogen hormone replacement

High-risk lesions	Alternative contraceptive options
Atrial fibrillation/flutter not on anticoagulation	Non-estrogen intrauterine devices
Bjork–Shiley or Starr–Edwards Valve	Progesterone-only pill ("mini pill")
Dilated left atrium >4 cm	Depot medroxyprogesterone acetate
Cyanotic heart disease	Etonogestrel implant
Pulmonary arteriovenious malformation	Barrier methods
Prior thrombotic event	
Left ventricular dysfunction with ejection fraction <30 %	
Kawasaki disease with coronary involvement	
Complicated valvular heart disease (pulmonary hypertension, risk of a trial fibrillation, history of infective endocarditis)	

selective serotonin reuptake inhibitors for mood disorders and vasomotor symptoms. For women with lower risk lesions in whom HRT is an option, the lowest dose of estrogen for the shortest period of time is recommended [37]. In general transdermal estrogen preparations deliver lower, more consistent doses of estrogen than oral preparations.

Sexual Dysfunction

Sexual dysfunction and anxiety around sexual activity may impact adults of all ages with congenital heart disease, regardless of the severity of the underlying lesion. In a study of ACHD patients ranging in age from 18 to 57 years, 20 % of individuals surveyed responded "yes" when asked the following: "being insecure about having sex," "being afraid of having sex," or "worrying about your sex life" [38]. Ninety-four percent of these patients had mild cardiovascular disease and were New York Heart Association (NYHA) functional class I or II. The American Heart Association recommends that "sexual activity is reasonable for most CHD patients who do not have decompensated or advanced heart failure, severe and/or significantly symptomatic valvular disease, or uncontrolled arrhythmias" [39]. Unfortunately, these guidelines are based predominantly on expert opinion and little data exist to help guide clinicians on counseling ACHD around sexual activity and sexual dysfunction. A reasonable approach takes into account the patient's chronologic age and developmental stage, the severity of his or her underlying CHD lesion, and any subsequent physical and mental conditions (please refer to Chap. 23 on "Sexual and Reproductive Health" of this textbook for a more detailed discussion of sexual and reproductive health considerations for adults with intellectual and developmental disabilities).

Types of sexual dysfunction may vary based on patient age, the severity of the underlying cardiac lesion and any medical and surgical treatments. A study of women aged 18–75 found cardiac symptoms with sexual activity occurred in 6–26 % of women, with presence and severity of symptoms related to the severity of the underlying lesion [40]. Similar studies in men reveal erectile dysfunction (ED) in 10–42 % of patients [41, 42]. However, the likelihood of ED is unrelated to the severity of the underlying condition and similar to rates in the general population. Primary care clinicians for ACHD cannot assume the presence or absence of sexual activity or sexual dysfunction, regardless of age of severity of the underlying cardiac lesion. Rather, assessment of sexual and reproductive health must be included as part of the routine care of any adult patient, regardless of underlying health status.

Genetic Screening

An identifiable genetic or environmental cause is found in approximately 20–30 % of cases of CHD [3, 4]. For patients with CHD, defining a genetic cause may help identify other organ systems at risk for complications [43], may provide prognostic information, and may help clarify the risk of CHD in their offspring and other family members [44]. Guidelines suggest genetic evaluation of patients with CHD, especially complex CHD, and genetic risk factors [45, 46]. Recent guidelines for older ACHD reinforce the importance of such screening and highlight the need to consider re-evaluating patients periodically as new genetic tests become available and new syndromes are recognized [5]. In general, guidelines call for a thorough history and physical exam to identify any non-cardiac manifestations of possible syndromes and a detailed, 3-generation family history with attention to CHD and other birth defects, consanguinity, and spontaneous abortions. Primary care clinicians should work closely with ACHD cardiologists and, when available, cardiovascular geneticists to ensure that ACHD with genetic risks are offered genetic counseling and genetic testing, and that the results of such testing are integrated into their overall care.

Infective Endocarditis Prophylaxis

The use of antibiotics for the prevention of infective endocarditis (IE) balances the risk reduction of IE from antibiotics against the risk of adverse reactions to antibiotics and the development of antibiotic resistant organisms. Adults with CHD may be at higher risk for developing IE and at higher risk for adverse outcomes from IE. In the general population the incidence of infective endocarditis after dental procedures is less than 1 per 100,000. For patients with predisposing conditions, the incidence is 9 per 100,000. In this population, pre-procedural antibiotics reduce this risk to ~2/100,000 [47]. CHD is present in 11–13 % of cases of infective endocarditis [48]. However, studies of adults with certain congenital heart lesions have found the incidence of IE to be 35 times higher than that of the general population [49]. It is therefore critical to recognize the conditions and lesions that place a patient at increased risk for IE. Table 7.4 presents the cardiac conditions that are associated with the highest risk of IE or adverse events from IE [22, 50]. Prior infective endocarditis and a history of heart transplant can be obtained by history. Residual defects near patches or prosthetic devices tend to have high velocity jets, resulting in easily audible murmurs. Prosthetic valves and prosthetic materials used in valve repairs also produce characteristic murmurs. Therefore, a patient's likelihood of having a high-risk condition for IE and need for additional workup can easily be assessed by the primary care clinician through a careful history and physical exam.

An appreciation of high-risk conditions and lesions will help guide the primary care clinician in prescribing appropriate prophylactic antibiotics, expediting treatment of possible sources of IE and raising the index of suspicion for patients presenting with clinical features of IE.

The appropriate prophylactic antibiotics for infective endocarditis are based primarily on the patient's allergies. Table 7.4 also shows the recommended regimens for antibiotic prophylaxis for dental procedures in adults. The 2007

Table 7.4 Recommendations for primary and secondary prevention of infective endocarditis

High-risk lesions for which IE prophylaxis with dental procedures is reasonable	Regiments for antibiotic prophylaxis for dental procedures in adults[a]	Procedures where antibiotic prophylaxis is indicated
Prosthetic cardiac valve or prosthetic material used for cardiac valve repair, including trans-catheter valve replacements	(1) Amoxicillin 2 g orally (2) Amplicillin 2 g IM/IV, cefazolin 1 g IM/IV or ceftriaxone 1 g IM/IV if unable to take PO (3) Cephalexin 2G or clindamycin 600 mg or azithromycin/clarithromycin 500 mg if allergic to PCN or ampicillin (4) Cefazolin, ceftriaxone or clindamycin if allergic to PCN or ampicillin AND unable to take PO	Dental procedures (all high-risk lesions) [22, 50] Consider during complicated vaginal deliveries for patient with unrepaired cyanotic lesions or prosthetic valves [22]
Previous infective endocarditis		
Congenital Heart Disease: • Unrepaired cyanotic CHD, including palliative shunts and conduits • Completely repaired congenital heart defect with prosthetic material or device, whether placed by surgery or by catheter intervention, during the first 6 months after the procedure • Repaired CHD with residual defects at the site or adjacent to the site of a prosthetic device (which inhibit endothelialization)		
Cardiac transplant recipients who develop cardiac valvulopathy		

[a]All antibiotics to be given as a single dose 30–60 min prior to procedure
IE infective endocarditis, *CHD* congenital heart disease, *PCN* penicillin

American Heart Association guidelines advise the use of these antibiotics in patients at high risk for IE prior to dental procedures [50]. Their use prior to genitourinary procedures is no longer recommended. However, the 2008 American College of Cardiology/American Heart Association Guidelines for the Management of Adults with Congenital Heart Disease recommend considering IE prophylaxis with antibiotics in patients with prosthetic valves or unrepaired cyanotic CHD undergoing complex vaginal deliveries, despite lack of evidence of efficacy [22].

Conclusion

The primary care of adults with congenital heart disease requires a patient-centered approach that takes into account the presence of any associated syndrome or chromosomal abnormality, the complexity of the underlying CHD lesion and the chronologic and developmental age of the patient (Appendix). The role of the primary care clinician in caring for ACHD is to partner with and advocate for the patient in understanding his or her heart and the individualized care required.

Appendix

Adult Congenital Heart Disease (ACHD) fact sheet

Definition	Congenital heart disease (CHD) refers to a wide range of structural defects of the heart and major blood vessels that are present at birth
Epidemiology	• The prevalence of congenital heart disease at birth ranges from 6 to 13 per 1000 live births • There are more than 1.2 million adults with congenital heart disease (ACHD) in the United States – 50 % of ACHD had a moderate-to-severe complexity heart lesion at birth. – The total ACHD population is growing at a rate of approximately 5 % per year
Special considerations	ACHD are at risk for complications from their underlying CHD and often require special management for acquired CV risks Common complications of CHD: • Heart failure • Arrhythmia • Vascular complications • Sudden death Cardiovascular risk factors requiring special management: • Diabetes • Hyperlipidemia • Hypertension Perioperative management of ACHD should include traditional Revised Cardiac Risk Index (RCRI) assessments and considering of the patient's CHD and any associated syndromes • Consideration should be given to managing patients with high-risk lesions in a center specialized in perioperative care for patients with ACHD Sexual and reproductive health: • Thrombotic risk should be assessed when considering estrogen-containing medications for contraception or for management of perimenopausal symptoms • ACHD should be assessed for sexual dysfunction in the context of their overall development, the severity of their underlying cardiac lesion and any ongoing cardiovascular therapies Genetic screening: • An identifiable genetic or environmental cause is found in approximately 20–30 % of cases of congenital heart disease • All ACHD with genetic risks should be offered genetic counseling and genetic testing Prevention of infective endocarditis (IE): • High-Risk lesions for IE particular to ACHD include unrepaired cyanotic CHD, repaired lesions within the first 6 months post-procedure, and repaired lesions with residual defects at or adjacent to the site of a prosthetic device

General Resources

- Congenital Heart Disease Clinic Directory—Includes a listing of centers designated as an Adult Congenital Heart Disease clinic: https://www.cardiosmart.org/Heart-Conditions/Congenital-Heart-Defects/CHD
- The International Society for Adults with Congenital Heart Disease http://isachd.org

Clinical Guidelines and Scientific Statements

General Guidelines

- ACC/AHA 2008 Guidelines for the Management of Adults with Congenital Heart Disease. http://circ.ahajournals.org/content/118/23/e714.full.pdf
- AHA Scientific Statement - Congenital Heart Disease in the Older Adult. http://circ.ahajournals.org/content/early/2015/04/20/CIR.0000000000000204.full.pdf
- Report of the National Heart, Lung, and Blood Institute Working Group on Research in Adult Congenital Heart Disease. http://content.onlinejacc.org/article.aspx?articleid=1137284&issueno=4

Prevention of Infectious Endocarditis Guidelines

- American Heart Association Guidelines for the Prevention of Infective Endocarditis. http://circ.ahajournals.org/content/116/15/1736.full.pdf
- AHA/ACC Guideline for the Management of Patients with Valvular Heart Disease. http://content.onlinejacc.org/article.aspx?articleid=1838843
- British Society for Antimicrobial Chemotherapy Guidelines for the Prevention of Infective Endocarditis. http://jac.oxfordjournals.org/content/57/6/1035.full.pdf

Physical Activity

- AHA Scientific Statement - Promotion of Physical Activity for Children and Young Adults with Congenital Heart Disease. http://circ.ahajournals.org/content/127/21/2147.full

Reproductive Health

- AHA Scientific Statement - Sexual Activity and Cardiac Health. http://circ.ahajournals.org/content/125/8/1058.full
- World Health Organization Medical Eligibility Criteria for Contraceptive Use. http://www.who.int/reproductivehealth/publications/family_planning/9789241563888/en/

Genetic Resources

- National Institutes of Health Genetics Home Reference, Congenital Heart Disease: http://ghr.nlm.nih.gov/condition/critical-congenital-heart-disease
- Information on labs for gene testing: www.genetest.org
- Online Mendelian Inheritance in Man. http://www.omim.org

Patient Resources

- Adult Congenital Heart Association. "For the Patient" http://www.achaheart.org/resources/for-patients.aspx
- Adult Congenital Heart Association Free Printable Handouts of Specific Conditions: http://www.achaheart.org/library-education-materials/free-downloads.aspx
- Adult Congenital Heart Association. "Q and A - Birth Control for Women with Congenital Heart Disease." https://www.achaheart.org/Portals/0/pdf/Library%20Education/ACHA-Q-and-A-Birth-Control-for-Women-with-CHD.pdf
- Insurance and the Affordable Care Act. http://www.achaheart.org/resources/for-patients/insurance-and-affordable-care-act.aspx
- American Heart Association. Conditions: Congenital Defects, Adults and Children. http://www.heart.org/HEARTORG/Conditions/CongenitalHeartDefects/Congenital-Heart-Defects_UCM_001090_SubHomePage.jsp

References

1. Mussatto KA, Hoffmann RG, Hoffman GM, Tweddell JS, Bear L, Cao Y, Brosig C. Risk and prevalence of developmental delay in young children with congenital heart disease. Pediatrics. 2014;133(3): e570–7.
2. Yeung E, Kay J, Roosevelt GE, Brandon M, Yetman AT. Lapse of care as a predictor for morbidity in adults with congenital heart disease. Int J Cardiol. 2008;125(1):62–5.
3. Beauchesne LM, Warnes CA, Connolly HM, Ammash NM, Grogan M, Jalal SM, Michels VV. Prevalence and clinical manifestations of 22q11.2 microdeletion in adults with selected conotruncal anomalies. J Am Coll Cardiol. 2005;45:595–8.
4. Cowan JR, Stephanie MW. Genetics and genetic testing in congenital heart disease. Clin Perinatol. 2015;42:373–99.
5. Bhatt AB, Foster E, Kuehl K, Alpert J, Brabeck S, Crumb S, et al. on behalf of the American Heart Association Council on Clinical Cardiology. Congenital heart disease in the older adult: a scientific statement from the American Heart Association. Circulation. 2015;131.
6. Tanner K, Sabrine N, Wren C. Cardiovascular malformations among preterm infants. Pediatrics. 2005;116(6):e833–8.
7. Wren C, Irving CA, Griffiths JA, O'Sullivan JJ, Chaudhari MP, Haynes SR, et al. Mortality in infants with cardiovascular malformations Eur J Pediatr. 2012;17(2):281.
8. Khoshnood B, Lelong N, Houyel, Thieulin AC, Jouannic JM, Magnier S, et al. on behalf of the EPICARD Study Group. Prevalence, timing of diagnosis and mortality of newborns with congenital heart defects: a population-based study. Heart. 2012;98 (22):1667–73.
9. Warnes CA, Liberthson R, Danielson GK, Dore A, Harris L, Hoffman JI, et al. Task force 1: the changing profile of congenital heart disease in adult life. J Am Coll Cardiol. 2001;37:1170–5.
10. Billett J, Cowie MR, Gatzoulis MA, Vonder Muhll IF, Majeed A. Comorbidity, healthcare utilisation and process of care measures in patients with congenital heart disease in the UK: cross-sectional, population-based study with case–control analysis. Heart. 2008;94:1194–9.
11. Kenny D, Hijazi ZM. Coarctation of the aorta: from fetal life to adulthood. Cardiol J. 2011;18:487–95.
12. Flanagan MF, Hourihan M, Keane JF. Incidence of renal dysfunction in adults with cyanotic congenital heart disease. Am J Cardiol. 1991;68:403–6.
13. Perloff JK, Latta H, Barsotti P. Pathogenesis of the glomerular abnormality in cyanotic congenital heart disease. Am J Cardiol. 2000;86:1198–204.
14. Moons P, Van Deyk K, Dedroog D, Troost E, Budts W. Prevalence of cardiovascular risk factors in adults with congenital heart disease. Eur J Cardiovasc Prev Rehabil. 2006;13:612–6.
15. Gagliardi MG, Adorisio R, Crea F, Versacci P, Di Donato R, Sanders SP. Abnormal vasomotor function of the epicardial coronary arteries in children five to eight years after arterial switch operation: an angiographic and intracoronary Doppler flow wire study. J Am Coll Cardiol. 2005;46:1565–72.
16. Kondo C, Nakazawa M, Momma K, Kusakabe K. Sympathetic denervation and reinnervation after arterial switch operation for complete transposition. Circulation. 1998;97:2414–9.
17. Pasquali SK, Marino BS, Powell DJ, McBride MG, Paridon SM, Meyers KE, et al. Following the arterial switch operation, obese children have risk factors for early cardiovascular disease. Congenit Heart Dis. 2010;5:16–24.
18. Gilmanov D, Bevilacqua S, Mazzone A, Glauber M. Do statins slow the process of calcification of aortic tissue valves? Interact Cardiovasc Thorac Surg. 2010;11:297–301.
19. Paraskevas KI, Mikhailidis DP. Statins may not prevent structural valve degeneration of aortic bioprosthetic valves, but should probably be prescribed to patients undergoing heart valve surgery nonetheless. Interact Cardiovasc Thorac Surg. 2010;11:302.
20. Goldman L, Caldera DL, Nussbaum SR, Southwick FS, Krogstad D, Murray B, et al. Multifactorial index of cardiac risk in noncardiac surgical procedures. N Engl J Med. 1977;297(16):845–50.
21. Lee TH, Marcantonio ER, Mangione CM, Thomas EJ, Polanczyk CA, Cook EF, et al. Derivation and prospective validation of a simple index for prediction of cardiac risk of major noncardiac surgery. Circulation. 1999;100(10):1043–9.
22. Warnes CA, Williams RG, Bashore TM, Child JS, Connolly HM, Dearani JA, et al. ACC/AHA 2008 guidelines for the management of adults with congenital heart disease: a report of the American College of Cardiology/American Heart Association Task Force on Practice Guidelines (Writing Committee to Develop Guidelines for the Management of Adults With Congenital Heart Disease). Circulation. 2008;118:e714–833.
23. Ammash NM, Connolly HM, Abel MD, Warnes CA. Noncardiac surgery in Eisenmenger syndrome. J Am Coll Cardiol. 1999;33:222–7.
24. Simko LC, McGinnis KA, Schembri J. Educational needs of adults with congenital heart disease. J Cardiovasc Nurs. 2006;21:85–94.
25. Graham TP Jr, Driscoll DJ, Gersony WM, Newburger JW, Rocchini A, Towbin JA. Task Force 2: congenital heart disease. J Am Coll Cardiol. 2005;45:1326–33.
26. Driscoll DJ, Edwards WD. Sudden unexpected death in children and adolescents. J Am Coll Cardiol. 1985;5:118B–21B.
27. Garson AJ, McNamara DG. Sudden death in a pediatric cardiology population, 1958 to 1983:

relation to prior arrhythmias. J Am Coll Cardiol. 1985;5:134B–7B.
28. Maron BJ. Sudden death in young athletes. N Engl J Med. 2003;349:1064–75.
29. Inuzuka R, Diller GP, Borgia F, Benson L, Tay EL, Alonso-Gonzalez R, et al. Comprehensive use of cardiopulmonary exercise testing identifies adults with congenital heart disease at increased mortality risk in the medium term. Circulation. 2012;125:250–9.
30. Longmuir PE, Brothers JA, de Ferranti SD, Hayman LL, Van Hare GF, Matherne GP, et al. on behalf of the American Heart Association Atherosclerosis, Hypertension and Obesity in Youth Committee of the Council on Cardiovascular Disease in the Young. Promotion of physical activity for children and adults with congenital heart disease: a scientific statement from the American Heart Association. Circulation. 2013;127:2147–59.
31. Siu SC, Sermer M, Colman JM, Alvarez AN, Mercier LA, Morton BC, et al. Prospective multicenter study of pregnancy outcomes in women with heart disease. Circulation. 2001;104:515–21.
32. Vigl M, Kaemmerer M, Seifert-Klauss V, Niggemeyer E, Nagdyman N, Trigas V, et al. Contraception in women with congenital heart disease. Am J Cardiol. 2010;106(9):1317–21.
33. The Adult Congenital Heart Association. ACHA Q and A: birth control for women with congenital heart disease. 2008. https://www.achaheart.org/Portals/0/pdf/Library%20Education/ACHA-Q-and-A-Birth-Control-for-Women-with-CHD.pdf.
34. Berry-Bibee E, Curtis K, Dragoman M, Gaffield ML, Jatlaoui T, Kim C, et al. Medical eligibility criteria for contraceptive use. 5th ed. Geneva: The World Health Organization; 2015.
35. Silversides CK, Sermer M, Siu S. Choosing the best contraceptive method for the adult with congenital heart disease. Curr Cardiol Rep. 2009;11:298–305.
36. Santen RJ, Allred DC, Ardoin SP, Archer DF, Boyd N, Braunstein GD, et al. Endocrine Society. Postmenopausal hormone therapy: an Endocrine Society scientific statement. J Clin Endocrinol Metab. 2010;95(suppl 1):s1–66.
37. Canobbio MM, Perloff JK, Rapkin AJ. Gynecological health of females with congenital heart disease. Int J Cardiol. 2005;98:379–87.
38. Moons P, Van Deyk K, Marquet K, De Bleser L, Budts W, De Geest S. Sexual functioning and congenital heart disease: something to worry about? Int J Cardiol. 2007;121:30–5.
39. Levine GN, Steinke EE, Bakaeen FG, Bozkurt B, Cheitlin MD, Conti JB, et al; on behalf of the American Heart Association Council on Clinical Cardiology, Council on Cardiovascular Nursing, Council on Cardiovascular Surgery and Anesthesia, and Council on Quality of Care and Outcomes Research. Sexual activity and cardiovascular disease: a scientific statement from the American Heart Association. Circulation. 2012;125:1058–72.
40. Vigl M, Kaemmerer M, Niggemeyer E, Nagdyman N, Seifert-Klauss V, Trigas V, et al. Sexuality and reproductive health in women with congenital heart disease. Am J Cardiol. 2010;105:538–41. doi:10.1016/j.amjcard.2009.10.025.
41. Cook SC, Arnott LM, Nicholson LM, Cook LR, Sparks EA, Daniels CJ. Erectile dysfunction in men with congenital heart disease. Am J Cardiol. 2008;102:1728–30.
42. Vigl M, Hager A, Bauer U, Niggemeyer E, Wittstock B, Köhn FM, et al. Sexuality and subjective wellbeing in male patients with congenital heart disease. Heart. 2009;95:1179–83.
43. Burchill L, Greenway S, Silversides CK, Mital S. Genetic counseling in the adult with congenital heart disease: what is the role? Curr Cardiol Rep. 2011;13:347–55.
44. Cowan J, Morales A, Dagua J, Hershberger RE. Genetic testing and genetic counseling in cardiovascular genetic medicine: overview and preliminary recommendations. Congest Heart Fail. 2008;14:97–105.
45. Pierpont ME, Basson CT, Benson DW Jr, Gelb BD, Giglia TM, Goldmuntz E, et al. Genetic basis for congenital heart defects: current knowledge: a scientific statement from the American Heart Association Congenital Cardiac Defects Committee, Council on Cardiovascular Disease in the Young. Circulation. 2007;115:3015–38.
46. Silversides CK, Marelli A, Beauchesne L, Dore A, Kiess M, Salehian O, et al. Canadian Cardiovascular Society 2009 Consensus Conference on the management of adults with congenital heart disease: executive summary. Can J Cardiol. 2010;26:143–50.
47. Duval X, Alla F, Hoen B, Danielou F, Larrieu S, Delahave F, et al. Estimated risk of endocarditis in adults with predisposing cardiac conditions undergoing dental procedures with or without antibiotic prophylaxis. Clin Infect Dis. 2006;42:e102.
48. van der Meer JT, Thompson J, Valkenburg HA, Michel MF. Epidemiology of bacterial endocarditis in The Netherlands, I. Patient characteristics. Arch Intern Med. 1992;152:1863–8.
49. Hayes CJ, Gersony WM, Driscoll DJ, Keane JF, Kidd L, O'Fallon WM, et al. Second natural history study of congenital heart defects. Results of treatment of patients with pulmonary valvar stenosis. Circulation. 1993;87(suppl 2):I28–37.
50. Wilson W, Taubert KA, Gewitz M, Lockhart PB, Baddour LM, Levison M, et al. Prevention of infective endocarditis: guidelines from the American Heart Association: a guideline from the American Heart Association Rheumatic Fever, Endocarditis, and Kawasaki Disease Committee, Council on Cardiovascular Disease in the Young, and the Council on Clinical Cardiology, Council on Cardiovascular Surgery and Anesthesia, and the Quality of Care and Outcomes Research Interdisciplinary W orking Group. Circulation. 2007;116:1736–54.

Cystic Fibrosis

8

Ross C. Klingsberg and Michael Landry

Case Presentation

Dillon T., a 19-year-old young man, presents for his initial visit to establish care with an adult primary care physician. Although he plans to attend a Cystic Fibrosis Foundation-accredited care center, he recognizes that he needs a physician closer to home as he lives 3 h away from the nearest cystic fibrosis (CF) center. Dillon was diagnosed with CF shortly after birth secondary to meconium ileus. His sweat chloride test result was 105 mmol/L, and his genotype is homozygous Phe508del. Up until this visit, Dillon was treated by a pediatric pulmonologist for his healthcare. His parents are divorced, and Dillon is cared for by his mother. He has completed high school and will be starting college in the fall close to home but will be living on campus. He is 1 year delayed in his education secondary to multiple hospitalizations that necessitated his starting kindergarten a year late. At that time, he required a percutaneous endoscopic gastrostomy (PEG) tube for supplemental feeding as he was severely underweight. The PEG tube has since been removed, and his weight is improved on oral pancreatic enzyme supplementation.

His past medical history is also significant for a pneumothorax at age 17 years. This required chest tube placement but resolved without further intervention. When he goes to the beach with family and friends, he is self-conscious about the surgical scars on his chest and abdomen.

Dillon is prescribed daily airway clearance therapy consisting of the following inhaled medications via a nebulizer: a short-acting bronchodilator, hypertonic saline (7 %), dornase alpha, and an antipseudomonal antibiotic. He also has a pneumatic oscillating vest (a.k.a. "The Vest"), which he uses for chest physiotherapy. He has a daily cough, worse in the morning upon awakening, which produces yellow/green sputum. He admits to intermittent noncompliance with doing his airway clearance therapy twice daily as prescribed. He says that he is better on school days. He frequently oversleeps and skips treatments when his routine is unstructured on holidays, during the summer, and on the weekends. He is admitted for intravenous (IV) antibiotics once or twice per year for exacerbations of his CF-related bronchiectasis. Sputum cultures have shown methicillin-resistant *Staphylococcus aureus* (MRSA) and *Pseudomonas aeruginosa*,

R.C. Klingsberg (✉)
Department of Medicine, Tulane/Southeast Louisiana Veteran's Healthcare System, 1430 Tulane Avenue, Box 8509, New Orleans, LA 70112, USA
e-mail: Ross.klingsberg@tulane.edu; rklingsb@tulane.edu

M. Landry
Department of Internal Medicine, Southeast Louisiana Veterans Healthcare System and Tulane University School of Medicine, 1430 Tulane Avenue, SL 16, New Orleans, LA 70112, USA
e-mail: mlandry@tulane.edu

M. Pilapil et al. (eds.), *Care of Adults with Chronic Childhood Conditions*,
DOI 10.1007/978-3-319-43827-6_8

and screening for non-tuberculous mycobacterial respiratory infections has been negative. He takes azithromycin, 500 mg, 3 times per week year round.

He takes pancreatic enzyme replacement therapy with meals to treat exocrine pancreatic insufficiency. Dillon almost never forgets this medication because without pancreatic enzymes, he suffers severe gastrointestinal discomfort and produces oily foul-smelling stools. He has occasionally required osmotic laxatives for constipation. Dillon was also found to have glucose intolerance on an oral glucose tolerance test (OGTT) performed last year. He does not take insulin. He has congenital bilateral absence of the vas deferens (CBAVD). He has had unprotected sex on multiple occasions because he has been told that male CF patients are infertile. He has tried smoking tobacco on a few occasions with his friends but noticed that he suffered dyspneic episodes afterward. He reports occasional alcohol intake but denies binge drinking.

He emphasizes his hope that he will be able to establish with an adult-oriented practice, as his pediatric provider has told him he now needs to start seeing an adult provider. He admits that he was quite apprehensive in making this appointment and has canceled several prior appointments due to anxiety over this transition, as he has been through so much with his pediatrician.

Case Discussion

Dillon has a classic presentation of cystic fibrosis ("Appendix") [1]. He also has the most common genetic cause of CF, two copies of F508del, a deletion of the amino acid phenylalanine at position 508 of the cystic fibrosis transmembrane conductance regulator (CFTR) protein. More than 2000 variations in the CFTR gene have been discovered. Of those, 23 were previously identified by the American College of Medical Genetics as clearly CF-causing (if an individual has one of these mutations on each chromosome inherited from his or her parents, he or she will have CF disease and symptoms).

The remaining 1700 plus mutations vary across a spectrum of CF presentations and symptom manifestations. They may cause CF with a full spectrum of symptoms, CF with variable symptoms, milder forms of CF, or have no effect or association with CF [2]. The clinical spectrum for symptom manifestation in CF ranges from asymptomatic individuals to chronic rhinosinusitis to male infertility to the symptoms classically associated with CF.

The diagnosis of CF is often made soon after birth when there is no meconium passed. As Dillon's case illustrates, abdominal distention, feeding intolerance, and vomiting appear, suggesting a meconium ileus. This is a common initial presentation for patients with CF and occurs in approximately 20 % of newborns that are eventually diagnosed with CF by the sweat chloride test, which is considered the gold standard for diagnosis [3].

Pancreatic dysfunction causes both endocrine and exocrine symptom manifestations in CF patients. Dillon has been diagnosed with CF-related diabetes (CFRD). It is important for primary care physicians to recognize CFRD as the most common comorbidity in people with CF, occurring in $\sim$20 % of adolescents and 40–50 % of adults. Appropriate screening and workup for symptoms related to diabetes presentation should be considered in CF patients [4].

While CFRD shares features of type 1 and type 2 diabetes mellitus, CFRD is a distinct clinical entity. It is primarily caused by insulin insufficiency, although fluctuating levels of insulin resistance related to acute and chronic illness also play a role. Interestingly, there are no documented cases of death from atherosclerotic vascular disease in patients with CFRD, despite the fact that some patients with CFRD now live into their sixth and seventh decades [5].

The diagnosis of CFRD is made by performing an oral glucose tolerance test (OGTT): measurement of fasting glucose followed by a 75 g glucose challenge and a 2-h post-challenge plasma glucose measurement. A plasma glucose $\geq$200 mg/dL is diagnostic of CF-related diabetes. Dillon's glucose tolerance test result was a glucose level of 285 mg/dL. The hemoglobin A1c (HgA1c) test is not sufficiently sensitive for diagnosis of CFRD and thus should not be used as a screening test. A HgA1C level <6.5 % does not rule out CFRD because this value is often spuriously low in CF patients. However, an HgA1C $\geq$6.5 % does confirm the diagnosis of CFRD. Furthermore, a fasting plasma glucose $\geq$126 mg/dL will also confirm the diagnosis [5].

Dillon's history is also notable for the presence of a pneumothorax. This complication, along with hemoptysis, is more common among individuals with CF as compared to the general population, and specific guidelines exist for management. It is critical to note that pleurodesis, a therapy used to treat recurrent pneumothorax, may be deferred after a single pneumothorax in CF. Pleurodesis may have a negative effect on future candidacy for lung transplantation, which may be critical for extending Dillon's life expectancy [6].

Dillon is infertile, as are the majority of men with CF. Naturally, men with CF are subject to the same sexually transmitted infections as men without CF and safe sex practices are to be encouraged. If parenthood is desired, genetic counseling is advised and spermatozoa can be surgically harvested by a urologist. Many men with CF elect to have sperm donated instead. Finally, it must be remembered that women with CF remain fertile and may become pregnant without fertility treatment.

Definition, Epidemiology, and Natural History of Cystic Fibrosis

The association between abnormal sweat chloride, salt loss, and illness in children was made in the nineteenth century as shown by the adage, "Woe to the child who tastes salty from a kiss on the brow, for he is cursed and soon must die." In 1938, Dorothy Anderson made the first association between pancreatic disease, lung disease, and intestinal disease. Dr. Anderson called the disease, "cystic fibrosis of the pancreas." She was the first to utilize pancreatic enzyme replacement therapy (PERT) to treat affected children [7].

In 1952, Paul di Sant'Agnese discovered abnormalities in sweat electrolytes that are associated with CF. A sweat test was subsequently developed and improved over the next decade. This test remains in widespread use for establishing the diagnosis of cystic fibrosis. In 1989, Francis Collins, Lap-Chee Tsui, and John R. Riordan discovered the first gene mutation for CF, F508del (see case discussion). The nomenclature for this mutation has evolved from "delta F508" to "F508del" to "Phe508del" with the latter being the most current and accurate terminology.

For a child to be born with CF, one gene with CFTR abnormalities must be inherited from each parent (CF gene homozygous). People carrying one gene for CF are clinically unaffected but carry the risk of passing on this gene to subsequent offspring (CF gene heterozygous). One out of 25 persons of European descent is a carrier for a CF-causing gene mutation. However, abnormalities in the CFTR gene can be found in all races. CF is the most common lethal genetic mutation in persons of European descent [8].

The cystic fibrosis transmembrane conductance regulator (CFTR) is in an epithelial cell surface chloride channel. Changes in CFTR function have the greatest deleterious effects on the respiratory tract and the pancreas in most patients. Cystic fibrosis causes bronchiectasis and CF has become a paradigm for this condition. Bronchiectasis causes airflow obstruction and a chronic productive cough. Most patients who die from complications of CF do so because of respiratory failure.

The life expectancy for patients living with CF has increased dramatically secondary to therapeutic advances in nutrition, pancreatic enzyme replacement therapy, inhaled airway clearance therapy (mucolytics), anti-inflammatory medications, and aggressive use of antibiotic therapy. In 1970, the median predicted survival was 16 years. Today, the median predicted survival is close to 40 years of age. An increase in survival has led to many patients needing to transition their care from pediatric providers to adult physicians including primary care and specialists [9].

Currently, there are approximately 30,000 patients within the United States and 70,000 worldwide living with CF. Most of the patients in the US participate in the CF Foundation's Data Registry. Patient information is collected by CF care centers that are accredited by the CF Foundation (CFF). There are more than 120 CF care centers that form a nationwide network. These centers are held accountable for informing best practices and infection-control guidelines [1].

Medical and Mental Health Assessment

Living with CF creates tremendous psychological, financial, and physical burdens for patients and their families. Patients with CF are aware of their limited life expectancy. The treatments are expensive and time-consuming. Patients are afflicted with chronic cough that may be disruptive to close personal contacts and in group settings such as classrooms. Exacerbations of bronchiectasis are unpredictable and may disrupt planned activities and employment. Extended hospital stays and frequent clinic visits can become part of a hopeless cycle for some. Disease progression often leads to decreased exercise tolerance and inability to complete activities of daily living.

Given the tremendous psycho-social burden this creates, patients with CF are prone to anxiety, depression, and other psychological disorders such as sleep disturbance, substance abuse, and suicide. These issues fluctuate as patients transit from childhood into adolescence and adulthood. Dramatic differences exist between pediatric and adult healthcare systems including physical location, structure, patient responsibilities, and caregiver's mindsets. Physicians should be sure to screen for mental health issues in addition to treating the acute and chronic conditions associated with CF [10].

Care of Cystic Fibrosis and Associated Medical Conditions

Overview

The routine care of cystic fibrosis is best provided by one of the nationwide CF Foundation (CFF) Accredited Care Centers. Many of the medications require experience with prescribing, prior authorization from third-party payers, and specialty pharmacy dispensing. The time and costs involved in the provision of these services would be prohibitive to a clinic that sees an occasional CF patient. The current guidelines for CF-specific care include quarterly clinic visits with submission of sputum samples for analysis via specialized CF culture. Pulmonary function testing is recommended twice yearly. All accredited CF care centers have multidisciplinary care teams that include social workers, dietitians, respiratory therapists, and clinical coordinators. Another key service delivered by accredited CF centers includes the collection of data, which is submitted to the CF Foundation Registry. This is a valuable resource for tracking the CF population as a whole, leading to improved clinical care delivery and population health management.

The development of the care center network by the CFF occurred in the early 1960s. These centers were established to ensure the rapid adoption of new CF therapies and developments by providers to maximize care for CF patients. In addition to providing care, these centers serve as a focus for CF clinical trials, where new CF therapeutics are first introduced. It is in the best interest of patients with CF to be seen regularly at CFF-accredited care centers [11].

Primary care physicians (PCPs) play an important role in the lives of patients with CF. Even medium to large CF care centers do not have daily clinics. As mentioned, some patients live far from CF care centers. Since many of the CF care needs are chronic and recurring, a simple

Table 8.1 Fundamentals of chronic cystic fibrosis therapy

Airway clearance	Antimicrobials	Nutrition	CFTR modulation
Physical vibration • Manual percussion • Oscillating vest • Flutter valve • Vigorous exercise	• Nebulized tobramycin (alternate months) • Aztreonam lysine • Colistimethate (less common)	• High-caloric/high-salt diet • Fat-soluble vitamin supplementation (A, D, E, and K)	Genotype-specific oral medications • Ivacaftor • Lumacaftor/ivacaftor
Surface hydration • Inhaled hypertonic saline	• Oral azithromycin (anti-inflammatory)		
Mucolysis • Dornase alfa	• Aggressive antibiotic therapy for exacerbations		

Modified with permission from Boyle [12]
Not all patients will perform all therapies listed. Treatments are individualized

clinic visit may be able to address problems early and prevent hospitalization (Table 8.1) [12]. Some examples would be helping with adherence issues, treating minor gastrointestinal disturbances such as constipation, and initiating oral antibiotics for mild exacerbations.

Respiratory System

In CF, the respiratory tract secretions lining the airways are thicker than normal. Thus, the name "mucoviscidosis" is more descriptive of the underlying pathophysiology of CF. Most current therapies are aimed at mobilizing the thick airway secretions and decreasing the overgrowth of characteristic bacteria. A typical CF airway clearance regimen starts with a bronchodilator. All patients with bronchiectasis have airflow obstruction and the current thinking is that subsequent therapies are most effective if they are preceded by a bronchodilator such as albuterol.

Following administration of a bronchodilator, 4 mL of 7 % hypertonic saline is inhaled by nebulization. This agent is inexpensive and is an effective way of drawing water from the lung interstitium into the surface layer of the airway. This will decrease the viscosity and allow easier expectoration of secretions by the patient. Current guidelines recommend hypertonic saline twice daily. Some patients find this therapy highly effective and utilize it more frequently. Nebulized hypertonic saline twice daily has been shown to decrease the frequency of exacerbations and improve pulmonary function in terms of forced vital capacity (FVC) and forced expiratory volume in 1 s (FEV_1) [13]. Unfortunately, a small number of patients do not tolerate 7 % hypertonic saline because of bronchospasm or cough.

Most patients with CF take a mucolytic agent: dornase alfa. This nebulized enzymatic solution cleaves the long nucleic acid chains that accumulate in the mucosal layer from lysed neutrophils found in purulent sputum. It is taken once or twice daily. Combining medications is not advisable because it dilutes the concentration of the solutions and decreases effectiveness. Unlike hypertonic saline, dornase alpha is not associated with bronchospasm.

All patients with CF should participate in some form of vigorous exercise. This not only helps mobilize respiratory secretions, but also helps to strengthen the overall musculature leading to increased efficiency of the cough. Patients with CF experience all of the benefits of exercise that non-CF patients experience and this should be encouraged at all clinical encounters.

Many patients with CF, however, do not exercise regularly. Alternative airway clearance therapies are frequently used. These include high-frequency pneumatic chest wall oscillation devices (such as "The Vest"); Acapella (flutter) valves, which create a vibrating column of air upon forceful exhalation; and manual chest physical therapy. All of these modalities seek to apply vibrating energy to the airways to help mobilize secretions for expectoration.

Following the aforementioned airway clearance techniques, patients with pseudomonas colonization often take a nebulized antipseudomonal antibiotic. Currently, there are commercially available nebulized forms of tobramycin and aztreonam in widespread use among CF patients. Specialized pharmacies may create nebulized forms of colistin and amikacin, although these are less commonly used. Nebulized antibiotics are taken after hypertonic saline and dornase alfa.

Since bronchiectasis is an obstructive disease, many patients with CF also take asthma medications such as long-acting beta-agonists and inhaled corticosteroids. Making a distinction between the obstruction of asthma and the obstruction of bronchiectasis may be difficult and may only be a matter of semantics, as the treatments for airflow obstruction are the same in both conditions [14]. Patients are encouraged to take their inhaled medications in the following order: bronchodilator, hypertonic saline/dornase alfa, inhaled antibiotics, and long-acting beta-agonists/inhaled corticosteroids (if being prescribed).

Gastrointestinal System

The gastrointestinal system can be severely affected despite the use of pancreatic enzyme replacement therapy. Patients may suffer from mild to severe functional bowel disorders and from mild to severe liver cirrhosis.

Adult patients with CF have frequent episodes of diarrhea alternating with constipation and/or the distal intestinal obstruction syndrome (DIOS). Constipation refers to the inability to evacuate the colon, whereas DIOS refers to the inability to evacuate the distal small intestine. Both constipation and DIOS may require hospitalization for IV fluids, nasogastric suctioning, anti-emetics, pain control, and aggressive use of osmotic cathartic agents such as polyethylene glycol to help relieve bowel obstruction.

When CF patients present with acute abdominal pain, physicians must consider a broad differential diagnosis, which includes complications such as intussusception. As with the general population, gallbladder disease and acute appendicitis are common causes of acute abdominal symptoms that should be considered.

The complications from cirrhosis are similar to the complications from other causes of chronic liver disease and include the complications of portal hypertension: esophageal varices, splenomegaly, thrombocytopenia, and gastrointestinal bleeding.

As patients with cystic fibrosis live into their fourth and fifth decade, there is a significantly increased incidence of gastrointestinal malignancies. Although there are no established guidelines, screening for gastrointestinal cancer starts at an earlier age in patients with CF. Many CF centers are now affiliated with gastroenterologists with specialized training and experience with CF to assist in managing CF-related gastrointestinal symptoms.

Endocrine System

The incidence of CF-related diabetes increases with age, as was previously reviewed in the case discussion. CF-related diabetes occurs when patients can no longer produce enough insulin to meet the metabolic demands of a large meal. CFRD should not be confused with type 1 diabetes mellitus. Unlike type 1 diabetics, most CF patients with diabetes can still produce insulin at a basal rate. Consequently, CF patients rarely experience diabetic ketoacidosis (DKA). If a CF patient presents with DKA, one should suspect coexisting type 1 diabetes mellitus.

CF-related diabetes is also different from type 2 diabetes mellitus. Patients with CF often suffer with protein–calorie malnutrition, so there is no insulin resistance as is seen in type 2 diabetes mellitus. Therefore, patients with CF-related diabetes should not be restricted calorically as one would in the treatment of type 2 diabetes mellitus. In fact, a cornerstone of CF care is encouraging and promoting a high calorie/high protein diet. Most CF patients benefit from some form of caloric and nutritional medical food supplementation. Additionally, their diets should be supplemented with the fat-soluble vitamins (A, D, E, and K) due to malabsorption of these vitamins secondary to pancreatic insufficiency.

The treatment of CF-related diabetes starts with moderate aerobic exercise. Pharmacologic treatment consists of insulin therapy. Oral hypoglycemic agents should not be used in CF-related diabetes, as they are not as effective as insulin in improving nutritional and metabolic outcomes [15].

Patients with CF are also at increased risk for reduced bone mineral density, with some studies suggesting 50–75 % of adults with CF have low bone density and increased rates of fractures [16]. Several factors likely contribute to this risk including glucocorticoid therapy, malabsorption of vitamin D, physical inactivity, and poor nutritional status [16]. PCPs can play a vital role in disease prevention by assisting patients in the prevention and treatment of these risk factors.

Acute Care

Unfortunately, since CF is a relatively rare disease, CF care centers often have ambulatory sessions only a few days per week and do not always have availability on the days when patients need to seek acute care. Patients with CF are subject to many of the same acute medical issues as people without CF. They need many of the same medical services that do not require specialized CF knowledge or treatment including preventive healthcare. Some examples include routine immunizations, testing for influenza, routine gynecologic care, and symptomatic treatment for acute medical issues. Ideally, a primary care physician would have an open communication access to a CF care center. It is also optimal for patients to be established with providers in the local healthcare system before needing acute interventions, as CF patients often have complicated medical histories and physical exam findings.

Transplant Evaluation

When patients with CF no longer experience clinical improvement with IV antibiotics, become oxygen-dependent, and have FEV_1 measurements less than 30–35 % of predicted, lung transplantation has become an option for those who meet transplant criteria. These criteria include an adequate social support system to ensure follow-up after hospital discharge. Certain infections, notably *Mycobacterium abscessus* and *Burkholderia cenocepacia,* are contraindications to lung transplantation, as patients tend to have much worse outcomes if these infections are present before transplantation. When patients undergo lung transplantation, they typically transfer care from CF specialists at CF centers to specialists at the lung transplant centers. These patients will still benefit from local established primary, preventive, and acute care management, as the distance from their transplant center may be similar to that from the CF center of care.

Primary and Preventive Care

Persons living with CF are subject to the same non-CF issues as the general population. Having a non-CF specialist general physician can be a valuable asset to the patient and a rewarding collaboration for the physician. Patients who are located greater distances from CF centers often have the greatest need to find local primary care providers and non-CF specialists.

Substance Abuse

The psychological burden of the disease is great, and persons with CF are susceptible to forming destructive dependencies on alcohol, sedatives, and analgesic drugs.[1] The same defense and denial mechanisms may occur as in the non-CF population. Thus, detecting illicit substance abuse and dependency requires a high level of suspicion. Irregular behaviors, difficulty answering and returning phone calls, noncompliance with medication regimens, complaints of sleep disturbances, or missed appointments may provide early clues to substance abuse issues. Avoidance of tobacco use is critical to CF patients given the impact of tobacco smoke on the pulmonary system in these patients.

Medication Management

CF centers are best suited to help patients manage the specialty medications and interventions used for cystic fibrosis. These include dornase alfa, nebulized antibiotics, pneumatic compression devices, and new classes of medication that actually modify and improve the function of CFTR at the cellular level (e.g., ivacaftor and lumacaftor). These new medications may only be prescribed by CF specialists and require prior authorization from third-party payers. However, the regimen does not change frequently and primary physicians are well-suited to reinforce adherence to high calorie/high protein diet exercise, and airway clearance therapy. Primary care providers can play a critical role in reinforcing the need for medication compliance.

Reproductive Health

In general, men with cystic fibrosis are infertile, with rates estimated at 95 % [17]. The abnormal CFTR gene causes absence of the vas deferens during development. Women, on the other hand, remain fertile and must be counseled on appropriate prophylaxis if pregnancy is not desired. Men who desire children may have sperm harvested by a specialty urologist. Many patients seek assisted reproduction and utilize sperm donation. Adolescents and young adults need counseling on safe sex practices even though the chance of pregnancy is low for male CF patients. Female CF patients are considered high-risk pregnancies and often require care by a high-risk obstetrician [18].

Palliative Care

End-of-life care is individualized. Some patients are not eligible or choose not to undergo lung transplant evaluation. This process is best managed by the physician with the best rapport with the patient and family. This may be the CF multidisciplinary team, though the primary care provider may also be suited for engaging in this discussion. When cystic fibrosis progresses to respiratory failure and mechanical ventilation, the prognosis is uniformly poor. Patients with cystic fibrosis rarely recover from respiratory failure requiring mechanical ventilation. Thus, advance planning may prevent days on mechanical ventilation that create anxiety and discomfort for the patient and the family.

Coordinated Care with Cystic Fibrosis Specialists

Although a majority of the routine care can be handled by local physicians, there will be times when clinical conditions arise that necessitate specialty care by physicians trained in CF. Pulmonary complications of CF including bronchiectasis, hemoptysis, and pneumothoraces are life-threatening emergencies that require prompt attention by specialists. Hemoptysis and pneumothorax occur with greater frequency in the patients with CF as compared to the general population.

Bronchiectasis

Patients with CF are prone to frequent exacerbations of bronchiectasis, and these episodes are best treated in care centers with experience

[1]Ross Klingsberg's personal observation.

treating CF. Exacerbations may occur several times per year in the most severely affected patients. Conversely, some patients with CF rarely experience exacerbations. The frequency of exacerbations increases as the disease progresses. Based upon clinical trials and collective experience of experienced CF care physicians, exacerbations are best treated as aggressively as possible as soon as they are recognized. This usually includes either oral antibiotics for mild exacerbations or IV antibiotics for moderate to severe exacerbations. The choice of antibiotic should be based upon the CF respiratory cultures and on the previous antibiotic history of the patient.

When a person with CF presents with acute symptoms of increased productive cough, fatigue, lassitude, and weight loss, physicians not familiar with CF may erroneously attribute symptoms to "bronchitis." Indeed, the chest radiograph may be unchanged, but the loss of lung function that occurs during CF exacerbations may not be recovered unless aggressive treatment regimens are initiated early in the exacerbation.

The determination of when to treat for an exacerbation of cystic fibrosis is a clinical judgment. When symptoms are mild, oral antibiotics may be used at the highest dose tolerable by the patient. A typical regimen for a mild exacerbation in a patient with pseudomonas and MRSA includes ciprofloxacin 750 mg 2 or 3 times daily and trimethoprim/sulfamethoxazole (double strength) 2 or 3 times daily.

Many patients experience exacerbations and more rapid declines in lung function because of lapses in their CF airway clearance regimen. Consequently, reinstitution of airway clearance is a priority during exacerbations, as this is a "teachable moment." Experienced CF providers will observe this phenomenon frequently. Patients drift away from their daily routine of airway clearance and their lung function declines precipitously. Unfortunately, not all decreases in lung function are reversible and so a lifelong program of adherence to airway clearance therapy must be continually, but tactfully, reinforced.

Hemoptysis

For some patients, hemoptysis may occur daily and thus not require acute evaluation. However, when hemoptysis is noted for the first time or increases in severity, it may be associated with an exacerbation of bronchiectasis. Hemoptysis is characterized as either mild/moderate or severe/massive. This distinction is based upon the volume of blood expectorated. As a general rule, any hemoptysis greater than a cup (approximately 8 oz or 240 mL) constitutes "massive" hemoptysis. Massive hemoptysis should be managed in an acute hospital setting with access to interventional radiology.

There are no clear guidelines for the management of hemoptysis. However, expert opinion is that hypertonic saline and dornase alfa should be discontinued in the setting of massive hemoptysis. Bronchoscopy adds little to the acute evaluation and should not be performed routinely. Bronchial arterial imaging in the form of bronchial arterial computed tomography (CT) angiogram is often requested, as it may help the radiologist locate the bleeding vessel. This test requires special coordination with the radiologist, as the timing of contrast administration is different from the timing of contrast administration for a pulmonary artery imaging study.

When hemoptysis continues or escalates despite antibiotic treatment and cessation of hypertonic saline and dornase alfa, bronchial artery embolization should be considered. The most serious complication of this procedure is inadvertent embolization of an anatomical variant spinal-penetrating arterial branch of the bronchial artery. When this variant is present, embolization can lead to irreversible lower extremity paralysis. The bronchial arterial imaging study can aid in identifying this variant.

Pneumothorax

Pneumothorax is encountered less frequently than hemoptysis. Small pneumothoraces in clinically stable patients may be observed for resolution but large pneumothoraces require tube thoracostomy for evacuation. Positive pressure ventilation should be avoided during episodes of pneumothorax. Recurrent pneumothoraces are sometimes referred for pleurodesis. However, in patients with advanced lung disease (FEV1 <40 % of predicted) and large pneumothorax, pleurodesis should be deferred until an evaluation for lung transplantation has been performed. Pleurodesis can make removal of the diseased lung prohibitive during the lung transplant procedure.

Transition Care Management of Cystic Fibrosis Patients

The transition from pediatric to adult medicine can be a stressful time for people with CF and their families. Adult healthcare systems have significant differences in patient care delivery compared with pediatric systems of care, with one of the most significant differences being in care management responsibility. Pediatric systems of care often focus on the parents as the primary focus for healthcare education and care management. Adult healthcare system providers often assume, sometimes incorrectly, that the adult patient is capable of managing their own healthcare independently. The transition process will vary from person to person. Some patients are ready to assume personal responsibility for their care and well-being when they reach age 18 or 19 years, while others are not. Caregivers should keep in mind that maintaining and refilling a long list of medications, keeping follow-up appointments every 3 months, and addressing payment are extremely time-consuming tasks for parents and patients. Some individuals rise to the challenge of independence earlier while others need more help. Many adolescents and young adults have adapted to the "sick role," as their care may have led to extended hospital stays where extra attention and special gifts/care are bestowed upon them. It can be extremely challenging at times for adolescents to transit from this system where they may be coddled, to their own detriment, to a system that they may perceive as uncaring and indifferent.

Pediatricians often arbitrarily develop their own criteria for transitioning their patients to adult care. Some use a specific age cutoff, some wait for the first year of college to conclude, some wait for an acute illness and transition when the patient presents to an emergency room, and some transition after the patient becomes sexually active. Once a pediatrician transitions a patient, they often will never see them again. The transition can be emotionally traumatic for some patients as they may have come to trust and rely on a specific physician for nearly 20 years and often through very serious illnesses. This transition can also be difficult for pediatric care providers as they may have developed special bonds with patients and their families over many years. They may have seen these patients through life-challenging events and share concerns that adult healthcare providers may not exhibit the same depth of understanding regarding their patient's issues as they do. Optimal transitions should be planned and occur during times of well-being in the chronic disease process if at all possible and should be viewed as a well-coordinated process rather than as an event. The stress of transition during a sudden acute medical issue can lead to unnecessary stress for the patient and their family [19].

A particular time of concern is the first year of college for those patients who attend. During the first year of immersion in campus life, CF patients often decrease their adherence to therapy. A therapeutic alliance with providers and patience on the part of providers and caregivers are critical in helping the young adult navigate this difficult life change. Treatment adherence usually improves after the first year of college, once daily routines are established.

To better plan for transition, the pediatric team and parents may begin teaching the responsibility for obtaining medications, adherence, and follow-up to the patient as the patient approaches their teenage years. As a patient approaches the transition to adult medicine, the adult and pediatric teams should meet and discuss the particular needs of each patient. There should be a clear plan prior to the last pediatric visit that delineates the adult physician who will assume care for the person with CF. When the transition occurs smoothly, some of the lapses in treatment can be averted.

Many physicians involved in the care of patients diagnosed with a chronic disease of childhood advocate that transition should begin at diagnosis. Understandably, physical transition will be deferred until the clinically appropriate time. However, early discussions about the process of transitioning to an adult healthcare system help to assure successful experiences and outcomes. In some centers, adult health care providers will meet with parents and pediatric patients during their initial pediatric visits to initiate the concept that a transition plan will need to be enacted at the appropriate time. Care of adolescents and adult CF patients requires a CF-trained specialist. However, the best patient-centered outcomes include the care and input from a multidisciplinary team that will include non-CF-trained physicians in addition to CF care centers.

Conclusion

The progress made to prolong and improve the lives of patients with CF is one of the great success stories of modern medicine. However, with a current life expectancy of around 40 years and with time-consuming and costly therapies that fall far short of a cure, there is much work to be done for this vulnerable and dependent population. Thus, there is an important role for primary care physicians who are part of a care team and can recognize acute situations that require more urgent specialist involvement. What is more, PCPs play vital roles in the lives of people with CF and support both patient and family while increasing patient independence both medically and socially. Caring for patients with CF can be among the most rewarding of doctor–patient relationships.

Appendix

Cystic fibrosis (CF) fact sheet	
Definition and symptoms	**Cystic fibrosis (CF) is an inherited lifelong condition characterized by** • Inherited abnormalities in the cystic fibrosis transmembrane conductance regulator (CFTR), an epithelial cell membrane protein and chloride channel • Abnormal CFTR protein disrupts chloride transport and water movement across secretory epithelial membranes • Thick (viscous) mucus buildup in the lungs, pancreas, and other organs • Bronchiectasis (persistent lung infections and progressive obstructive airway disease) • Persistent coughing, at times with phlegm • Hemoptysis and pneumothorax • Exocrine pancreatic enzyme insufficiency with poor growth or weight gain in spite of good appetite • Frequent greasy, bulky stools or difficulty with bowel movements • Male (not female) infertility • Very salty-tasting skin
Prevalence	In the United States • About 30,000 people are living with cystic fibrosis (70,000 worldwide) • Approximately 1000 new cases of CF are diagnosed each year • More than 75 % of people with CF are diagnosed by age 2 years • Nearly half of the CF population is age 18 or older • Predicted median survival: 39.3 years
Genetics and epidemiology	Epidemiology • CF is the most common disorder of autosomal recessive inheritance in Caucasians

(continued)

	• In general, it occurs in 1/3000 Caucasian, 1/6000 Hispanic, 1/10,000 African-American, and 1/90,000 Asian-American births Genetics: • More than 2000 mutations in the CFTR gene have been identified • The most common CF-causing mutation is Phe508del • The most common CF-causing genes are screened for at birth • People with only one copy of the defective CF gene are called carriers, but they do not have the disease. Each time two CF carriers have a child, the chances are – 25 % (1 in 4) the offspring will have CF – 50 % (1 in 2) the offspring will be a carrier but will not have CF – 25 % (1 in 4) the offspring will not be a carrier and will not have CF
Characteristics of adults with CF 18 years and older	• 7 % Masters/Doctoral Level Degree • 28.8 % College Graduate • 33 % Some College • 24.2 % High School Diploma • 41.2 % Married/Co-habitating • 35.3 % Full-time employment • 99.2 % have Medical Insurance • Phe508del homozygotes—46.4 % of CF population • Phe508del heterozygotes—40.1 % of CF population
Associated conditions	Individuals with cystic fibrosis have high rates of comorbid physical and mental health conditions, including • Bronchiectasis • Airway colonization and chronic infections with *Pseudomonas aeruginosa*, *Staphylococcus aureus*, and *Burkholderia* spp. • Allergic bronchopulmonary aspergillosis • Non-tuberculous mycobacterial infection • Exocrine pancreatic insufficiency • CF-related diabetes • Fat-soluble vitamin (A, D, E, and K) deficiency • Osteopenia/Osteoporosis • Male infertility • Hepatobiliary disease (cirrhosis, gallstones, biliary disease) • Pancreatitis • Intestinal obstruction, intussusception • Chronic pain • Depression, anxiety, substance abuse, and suicide
Challenges in transition	• Learning to manage time, finances, housing, employment, education, medication, and frequent physician visits • Challenges impacting the transition to adulthood include – Parental educational and financial status – Proximity to specialized CF care centers – Financial burden of medications and inability to work due to illness – Unpredictable nature of exacerbations requiring intensification of care and usually IV antibiotics and disruption of usual activities – Reluctance on part of patient and parents/caregivers as well as pediatric providers to initiate transition – Difficulty identifying adult generalist willing to accept patient into practice

Adapted from Cystic Fibrosis Patient Registry Annual Data Report 2014 [1]

References

1. Cystic Fibrosis Foundation. Cystic Fibrosis Patient Registry Annual Data Report 2014. https://www.cff.org/2014_CFF_Annual_Data_Report_to_the_Center_Directors.pdf.
2. United States Cystic Fibrosis Foundation, Johns Hopkins University, The Hospital for Sick Children. Clinical and functional translation of CFTR. 2011. www.cftr2.org.
3. Farrell PM, Rosenstein BJ, White TB, Accurso FJ, Castellani C, Cutting GR, et al. Guidelines for diagnosis of cystic fibrosis in newborns through older adults: cystic fibrosis' foundation consensus report. J Pediatr. 2008;153(2):S4–14.
4. Moran A, Dunitz J, Nathan B, Saeed A, Lolme B, Thomas W. Cystic fibrosis-related diabetes: current trends in prevalence, incidence, and mortality. Diabetes Care. 2009;32(9):1626–31.
5. Moran A, Brunzell C, Cohen RC, Katz M, Marshall BC, Onady G, et al. Clinical care guidelines for cystic fibrosis-related diabetes. Diabetes Care. 2010;33(12):2697–708.
6. Flume PA, Mogayzel PJ, Robinson KA, Rosenblatt RL, Quittell L, Marshall BC. Cystic fibrosis pulmonary guidelines. Pulmonary complications: hemoptysis and pneumothorax. Am J Respir Crit Care Med. 2010;182(3):298–306.
7. Anderson DH. Cystic fibrosis of the pancreas and its relation to celiac disease: a clinical and pathologic study. Am J Dis Child. 1938;56(2):344–99.
8. Tobias E, Connor M, Ferguson-Smith M. Ch 15. Strong family history—typical Mendelian disease. In: Tobias ES, editor. Essential medical genetics, 6E. New Jersey. USA: Wiley; 2011. p. 312.
9. MacKenzie T, Gifford AH, Sabadosa KA, Quinton HB, Knapp EA, Goss CH, Marshall BC. Longevity of patients with cystic fibrosis in 2000 to 2010 and beyond: survival analysis of the cystic fibrosis foundation patient registry. Ann Intern Med. 2014;161(4):233–41.
10. Quittner AL, Abbott J, Georgiopoulos AM, Goldbeck I, Smith B, Hempstead SE, et al. International Committee on Mental Health in Cystic Fibrosis: Cystic Fibrosis Foundation and European Cystic Fibrosis Society consensus statements for screening and treating depression and anxiety. Thorax. 2016;71(1):26–34.
11. Beall RJ. The cystic fibrosis foundation. In: Yankaskas JR, Knowles MR, editors. Cystic fibrosis in adults. Riverwoods. IL. USA: Walters Kluwer Publishers; 1999. p. 477–84.
12. Boyle MP. Adult cystic fibrosis. JAMA. 2007;298(15):1787–93.
13. Donaldson SH, Bennett WD, Zeman KL, Knowles MR, Tarran R, Boucher RC. Mucus clearance and lung function in cystic fibrosis with hypertonic saline. N Engl J Med. 2006;354(3):241–50.
14. Flume PA, Robinson KA, O'Sullivan BP, Finder JD, Vender RL, Willey-Courand DB, et al. Cystic fibrosis pulmonary guidelines: airway clearance therapies. Respir Care. 2009;54(4):522–37.
15. Moran A, Dunitz J, Nathan B, Saeed A, Lolme B, Thomas W. Cystic fibrosis-related diabetes: current trends in prevalence, incidence, and mortality. Diabetes Care. 2009;32(9):1626–31.
16. Aris RM, Merkel PA, Bachrach LK, Borowitz DS, Boyle MP, Elkin SL, et al. Guide to bone health and disease in cystic fibrosis. J Clin Endocrinol Metab. 2005;90(3):1888–96.
17. Popli K, Stewart J. Infertility and its management in men with cystic fibrosis: review of literature and clinical practices in the UK. Hum Fertil (Camb). 2007;10(4):217–21.
18. Yankaskas JR, Marshall BC, Sufian B, Simon RH, Rodman D. Cystic fibrosis adult care. Chest. 2004;125(1 Suppl):1S–39S.
19. Okumur MJ, Kleinhenz ME. Cystic fibrosis transitions of care: lessons learned and future directions for cystic fibrosis. Clin Chest Med. 2016;37(1):119–26.

9 Diabetes Mellitus (Type 1)

Elizabeth O. Buschur and Stephanie Lawrence

Case Presentation

Mark is a 22-year-old young man with type 1 diabetes mellitus diagnosed at age 15. He is being seen at the Diabetes Transition Clinic for the first time after last being seen about 5 months earlier in the pediatric endocrinology clinic. He presents with his mother. Mark admits that he has not been checking blood sugars for several months. He takes basal insulin (glargine) every day and denies missing any doses. He is also prescribed short-acting insulin for meals and correction, but has also not taken this in several months. When asked why, he says he does not care. He denies difficulty affording insulin or supplies. On review of prior records, his hemoglobin A1c has been between 11 % to greater than 14 % since 1–2 years after diagnosis. He complains of blurry vision, polyuria, polydipsia, fatigue, and depression. He has had some skin problems for which he has been seeing a dermatologist. He is embarrassed by his skin and reports feeling depressed and unconfident about his appearance. He is not dating. He is not interested in seeing a counselor regarding his depression. He works the night shift at a warehouse. His mother, with whom he lives, works during the day while Mark sleeps during the day. His eating schedule is somewhat erratic—usually 2 meals per day with the largest before going to work in the evening. He denies smoking and illicit drug use. He occasionally drinks beer, but denies any binge drinking behavior. His mother's main concern that she asks about is how long do complications of diabetes take to occur. She would like her son to change his behavior, but is not sure how to help him, and admits that she does not see him awake much due to their differing work schedules. On exam, Mark appears to be a thin young man, well-groomed, and quiet. He wears a hat covering his eyes. His exam is unremarkable, including his thyroid and foot exam. Skin exam shows no obvious blemishes. Hemoglobin A1c is >14 %.

Case Discussion

The case of Mark illustrates the importance of necessary adherence to glucose checks, insulin injection administration, and careful dietary assessment, which people with diabetes live with on a daily basis. During the pediatric time period,

E.O. Buschur (✉)
Department of Internal Medicine, Division of Endocrinology, Diabetes, and Metabolism, The Ohio State University Wexner Medical Center, 564 McCampbell Hall, 1581 Dodd Drive, Columbus, OH 43210, USA
e-mail: elizabeth.buschur@osumc.edu

S. Lawrence
Department of Internal Medicine, The Ohio State University Wexner Medical Center, 895 Yard Street, Grandview Heights, OH 43212, USA
e-mail: Stephanie.Lawrence@osumc.edu

M. Pilapil et al. (eds.), *Care of Adults with Chronic Childhood Conditions*,
DOI 10.1007/978-3-319-43827-6_9

glucose checks, insulin dosing, and meal planning are often team-based with the individual child, his family, and his teacher and/or school nurse playing helpful roles. During adolescence, teens with diabetes often seek independence and at times will rebel against self-care behaviors. Furthermore, many adolescents and young adults with diabetes have coexisting depression, anxiety, and other mental health disorders that need treatment. During the teenage years, diabetes self-care behaviors should become incorporated into the young adult's normal life.

In the well-known Diabetes Control and Complications Trial (DCCT) of youth and adults with type 1 diabetes, children and adolescents had hemoglobin A1c (HbA1c) values above recommended targets [1–3]. Adolescents in the intensive insulin regimen had better HbA1c values than those in the conventional arm, but these values were still at least 1 percentage point higher than the adults in the trial [4]. Increases in HbA1c are clearly associated with risk of complications of diabetes [4]. For example, a 1 percentage point increase in HbA1c (for instance 9 vs. 8 %) is associated with a 40 % higher risk of developing retinopathy [5, 6].

Adhering to the complex, daily management required to achieve glycemic control is difficult for any person with diabetes, especially for adolescents and young adults with diabetes. Young adults with type 1 diabetes are recommended frequent self-monitoring of blood glucose (4–6 times per day), following a balanced diet and counting carbohydrates, balancing activity levels, and administering insulin by injection or infusion pump. A large meta-analysis of more than 2000 youth with type 1 diabetes showed that increases in adherence parallel increases in glycemic control [7]. Multiple factors have been associated with adherence to diabetes care and glycemic control among children, adolescents, and adults with type 1 diabetes including access to diabetes care professionals and devices (self-monitored blood glucose monitors, insulin pens, insulin infusion pumps, etc.) [8, 9], social support from family and friends [10], peer pressure [11], economic status [12], interactions with diabetes care providers [8], presence of mental health problems such as depression [10], and transition to adolescence [10, 11, 13, 14]. Illness identity has also been identified as a key factor in diabetes care adherence among emerging adults with type 1 diabetes. In a study of more than 575 adolescents and emerging adults (14–25 years of age), illness identity categorized as rejection, engulfment, acceptance, and enrichment was associated with variations in glycemic control (rejection associated with higher HbA1c values), more diabetes-related problems, and better adherence [15].

The case of Mark illustrates that young adults with type 1 diabetes present a challenging patient population for adult health care providers. As discussed earlier, multiple factors influence diabetes care adherence, glycemic control, and ultimately overall health among emerging adults with type 1 diabetes. This chapter discusses the coexisting conditions that may affect adults with type 1 diabetes as well as the factors that influence care adherence and glycemic control.

Definition and Pathophysiology

Type 1 diabetes is one of the most common chronic conditions affecting children. Type 1 diabetes results from autoimmune destruction of the pancreatic beta cells resulting in complete insulin deficiency. It most commonly presents in childhood, although some people are diagnosed as adults. Type 1 diabetes occurs in genetically susceptible individuals and is thought to be triggered by environmental agents. The autoimmune process is thought to occur over months to years before clinical symptoms (polyuria, polydipsia, polyphagia, weight loss) occur and hyperglycemia is diagnosed. The American Diabetes Association/Worldwide Health Organization (ADA/WHO) criteria for the diagnosis of diabetes include fasting blood glucose ≥ 126 mg/dL at least twice, 2-h post 75-g glucose challenge value ≥ 200 mg/dL, any random glucose ≥ 200 mg/dL with symptoms of diabetes, or hemoglobin A1c ≥ 6.5 % [16, 17].

Epidemiology

The incidence of type 1 diabetes is increasing worldwide [18]. In a Swedish registry of 1666 adults, blood samples were obtained from 1630 (97.8 %) patients. The ADA/WHO criteria for diagnosis of diabetes were used. Those subjects with positive autoantibodies—glutamic decarboxylase (GAD) antibody and/or islet cell antibody (ICA)—and/or c-peptide levels less than 0.25 nmol/L (0.7 %) were classified as having type 1 diabetes [19]. In this large Swedish population, the incidence of type 1 diabetes in 0- to 19-year olds was 37.8 per 100,000 per year (36.1–39.6, 95 % confidence interval [CI]) and in 20- to 100-year olds was 27.1 (25.6–27.4) per 100,000 per year [19]. There was a bimodal distribution with equal peaks in 0- to 9-year olds and 50- to 80-year olds. In contrast, the incidence of type 2 diabetes among adults in this population was higher at 378 (375–380, 95 % CI) per 100,000 per year. There were 101 adults that had one or more autoantibodies positive; GAD antibody was the most common in 90 %, ICA in 71 %, and both GAD and ICA in 61 % [19]. There were no significant gender differences in type 1 diabetes in any age group, except for some trends in pediatric subgroups.

A second study examined the time trends and gender differences in incidence and prevalence of type 1 diabetes in Sweden [20]. The Nordic countries have the highest reported incidence rates of type 1 diabetes in the world. The incidence of type 1 diabetes in Sweden is most recently reported to be 43.9 per 100,000 among children less than 15 years of age [21]. The incidence of type 1 diabetes has been increasing over time in Sweden with a mean annual relative increase of 1.7 % between 1978 and 1997 with the most prominent rise among 0–4 years of age (6.3 %) [20].

Several studies have examined the prevalence and trends of diabetes in the United States [22]. Data from the National Survey of Children's Health found an estimated prevalence of diabetes (both types 1 and 2 diabetes) among children in the United States to be 3.2 per 1000 (95 % CI 2.6–3.7) or an estimated 229,240 children [23]. There were differences among race and obesity status: non-Hispanic white children had higher prevalence of diabetes (3.8 per 1000 children) compared with other racial and ethnic categories (2.2 per 1000 children) [23]. In the SEARCH for Diabetes in Youth Study, the prevalence of diabetes (both types 1 and 2) among youth (less than 18 years of age) was 1.82 cases per 1000 youth. There were significant differences in age and gender with lower prevalence among youth 0–9 years of age (0.79 cases per 1000 youth) compared to those 10–19 years of age (2.8 cases per 1000 youth). Non-Hispanic white youth had the highest prevalence in the younger group (1.06 cases per 1000 youth). Among younger children, type 1 diabetes accounted for the majority of cases (more than 80 %), and among the older group, there were higher estimates of type 2 diabetes ranging from 6 to 76 % [24].

Common Adult Conditions in Patients with Type 1 Diabetes

Mood Disorders

Psychosocial challenges commonly occur during periods of transition for young adults. However, they are more pronounced for patients with diabetes due to their associated disease-related emotional distress. At baseline, patients with diabetes report feeling scared, angry, alone, and depressed when thinking about having diabetes. Most patients worry about the future and the possibility of developing serious complications related to their diabetes. Many feel discouraged and overwhelmed by their diabetes regimen. There is often "burnout" from the constant effort to manage diabetes, and guilt and anxiety regarding poor adherence. Patients with diabetes also report concern about reactions and uncomfortable interactions around family, friends, or coworkers who do not have diabetes [25]. This diabetes-related emotional distress can lead to conflict within families, strained relationships with providers, increased risk for depression and anxiety, and ultimately diminished motivation for self-care and poorer glycemic control [26–29].

As a result, the American Diabetes Association's "Standards of Medical Care in Diabetes—2016" position statement recommends routine screening for psychosocial problems including diabetes-related distress, depression, anxiety, and eating disorders so that they can be addressed [17]. Several screening tools have been used to evaluate psychosocial functioning among patients with diabetes, including the Patient Health Questionnaire-2 (PHQ-2), the Diabetes Distress Scale (DDS), and the Problem Areas in Diabetes (PAID)-1 scale [30–32].

Depression has been clearly identified as a common comorbid condition in patients with diabetes. In fact, patients with diabetes are almost twice as likely as those without diabetes to be diagnosed with depression [33]. Recent studies demonstrate that about 10 % of adult patients with type 1 diabetes have comorbid depression [34], while over 20 % of older adolescent females with type 2 diabetes exhibit significant depressive symptoms [35]. Depression has not only been identified as a risk factor for decreased adherence [36] and poor glycemic control [37] but also for increased morbidity and mortality in patients with diabetes [34, 38]. Given the high prevalence of depression in the diabetic population and the serious implications it has for morbidity and mortality, it is very important for the provider to identify and treat this mood disorder. Not only has depression treatment been shown to improve symptoms, but it also has a significant economic benefit by reducing health care costs [39].

Anxiety is the most frequently diagnosed psychiatric disorder in the general adolescent population [40] and poses unique challenges to patients with diabetes. Studies demonstrate that between 13 and 17 % of adolescents with type 1 diabetes have symptoms of anxiety [41]. Similar to depression, symptoms of anxiety have been associated with decreased blood glucose monitoring and poorer glycemic control among adolescents with type 1 diabetes [41]. However, somatic symptoms of anxiety such as increased heart rate and perspiration, dizziness, lightheadedness, and abdominal discomfort [42] are very similar to those associated with hypoglycemia and may make it difficult for patients with diabetes to appropriately understand their glycemic levels [41].

Overweight and Obesity

Typically, young adults with type 1 diabetes are lean in contrast to those with type 2 diabetes who are often obese. However, with the global increases in overweight and obesity, more than 25 % of children under 18 years of age with type 1 diabetes are overweight (body mass index [BMI] $\geq$ 85th to 95th percentile) [43]. In the United States, the SEARCH for Diabetes in Youth Study found 34 % of youth with type 1 diabetes were overweight or obese, similar to the background rate of 33 % of youth without diabetes [43]. Minority youth with type 1 diabetes (African American, Asian or Pacific Islander, American Indian, Hispanic) are at increased risk of obesity [43]. The risk for overweight and obesity also seems to be increased among girls with type 1 diabetes [44], although not all studies have shown this gender difference [45]. Apart from female gender, other risk factors for higher BMI changes during childhood that may lead to overweight and obesity include intensification of insulin regimen (a greater number of injections per day or insulin pump therapy) and higher total daily insulin dose, lower BMI at diabetes onset, pubertal diabetes onset, and long diabetes duration [44]. Children and adolescents with type 1 diabetes should be counseled on the independent risks of overweight and obesity on cardiometabolic complications. Minorities and young girls with type 1 diabetes, especially those diagnosed between ages 10–15 years of age, have been shown to be at highest risk of overweight and obesity and may benefit from targeted counseling and risk factor modification (dietary changes and exercise) for reducing weight gain during the course of diabetes treatment.

Thyroid Disease

Autoimmune thyroid disease is a common coexisting condition among men and women with type 1 diabetes [46, 47]. Autoimmune thyroiditis manifesting as hypothyroidism (Hashimoto's thyroiditis) is more common than autoimmune hyperthyroidism (Graves' disease). An estimated 20 % of patients with type 1 diabetes have positive thyroid antibodies (anti-thyroid peroxidase and anti-thyroglobulin antibodies), while an estimated 2–5 % of patients with type 1 diabetes develop autoimmune primary hypothyroidism [48, 49]. Some estimates report even higher rates of autoimmune thyroiditis among subjects with type 1 diabetes [50, 51]. Autoimmune thyroid disease is more common among women than men with type 1 diabetes [46] as well as more common with increasing age. Coexisting thyroid disease can complicate the management of diabetes, and emerging adults with both type 1 diabetes and an underlying thyroid disease may potentially have more difficulty with transition to adult medical care. Uncontrolled or suboptimally treated thyroid disease can worsen hypoglycemia (for hyperthyroidism), weight changes, depression, anxiety, insomnia, fatigue, and other problems that may be common among adolescents and young adults with diabetes. A study of children aged 8–18 years showed reduced health-related quality of life among those with type 1 diabetes and levothyroxine-treated thyroid disease compared to those patients with diabetes but without thyroid disease [52]. The American Diabetes Association recommends regular screening of children, adolescents, and young adults with type 1 diabetes for development of thyroid disease at diagnosis of diabetes and every 1–2 years or sooner if symptoms of hypothyroidism are seen [17]. In addition to thyroid disease, other autoimmune diseases may also accompany type 1 diabetes including celiac disease, and much less commonly adrenal insufficiency (Addison's disease), pernicious anemia, among others.

Celiac Disease

Along with autoimmune thyroid disease, celiac disease is an additional autoimmune disease that is common among people with type 1 diabetes. Celiac disease is more common among subjects with type 1 diabetes (estimates between 2.3 and 5 % of patients with type 1 diabetes) than those without type 1 diabetes [53, 54]. An estimated 7–10 % of patients with type 1 diabetes have positive anti-endomysial antibodies or tissue transglutaminase antibodies [49]. Risk factors for development of celiac disease include female gender, longer duration of diabetes, and presence of autoimmune thyroid disease [49, 55]. Most patients with type 1 diabetes and celiac disease will not present with classic gastrointestinal symptoms (diarrhea, food intolerance, food avoidance, abdominal cramping, and gastrointestinal discomfort). Most patients with type 1 diabetes and celiac disease will present without symptoms or with vague symptoms including recurrent hypoglycemia, unpredictable glycemic patterns, growth failure, and low bone density or fractures [56]. The American Diabetes Association recommends regular screening of children and adolescents with type 1 diabetes (through age 19 years of age) for celiac disease at diagnosis and every 2–3 years thereafter or if clinically suspected [57]. However, there are fewer guidelines in terms of recommendations for adult screening. Often children and adults with type 1 diabetes have less frequent abdominal symptoms of celiac disease [58]. Adults with type 1 diabetes should be screened if any classic signs or symptoms of celiac disease are present, or if an individual has unexplained hypoglycemia or unusual glycemic patterns, iron deficiency anemia, or low bone density. The American College of Gastroenterology recommends screening of adults with type 1 diabetes if there are any suggestive symptoms [58, 59].

Complications of Diabetes

Multiple longitudinal randomized trials have shown that poor glycemic control is associated with long-term vascular complications of diabetes, including nephropathy, retinopathy, neuropathy, and cardiovascular disease [60, 61]. Typically, vascular complications of diabetes do not clinically manifest until adulthood, but their pathogenesis begins much earlier at disease onset. Furthermore, microvascular complications of diabetes have been diagnosed at times in emerging adulthood. There has been no significant difference in screening for complications of diabetes between pediatric and adult medical care, but one study of 108 subjects with type 1 diabetes showed that background retinopathy increased from 5 to 29 % from age 18 to 24 years [62].

Diabetic nephropathy rates have decreased over the past several decades with improvements in hemoglobin A1c [63]. Subjects with longer duration of diabetes and suboptimal glycemic control are at increased risk of developing albuminuria. Glycemic control is a strong predictor of development of nephropathy, although albuminuria risk by age 20 was approximately 15 % in one large population-based study, even among those with mean hemoglobin A1c $\leq$ 8.5 % [64]. Cumulative prevalence of increased albuminuria was 26 % after a 10-year duration of type 1 diabetes and as high as 51 % after 19 years of diabetes [64]. Tobacco use significantly increases the risk of progression of microalbuminuria to nephropathy, and adult providers should therefore screen and counsel patients with type 1 diabetes regarding tobacco use.

Hypertension is also an independent risk factor for nephropathy [64–66] and is an important risk factor for development of albuminuria [67]. Hypertension is more common among adolescents with type 1 diabetes than teens without diabetes [68]. Therefore, blood pressure measurement and screening for hypertension should be done at each visit for diabetes care. In children and adolescents with diabetes, prehypertension is defined as systolic or diastolic blood pressure between the 90th and 95th percentiles for age, gender, and height or blood pressure $\geq$ 120/80, whichever is higher, at three different time points. Hypertension is defined as systolic or diastolic blood pressure $\geq$ 95th percentile (or $\geq$ 130/80, whichever is higher) at three different time points. Those teens with blood pressure readings in the prehypertension range should be recommended lifestyle changes (diet and exercise). Medical treatment is indicated for adolescents and young adults with blood pressure in the hypertensive range or for those with blood pressures in the prehypertensive range despite lifestyle changes for 3–6 months. An angiotensin-converting enzyme (ACE) inhibitor is the recommended pharmacologic treatment if needed, as this class of drugs has been shown to protect against development of progressive nephropathy in patients with diabetes [17, 69]. If an ACE inhibitor is prescribed to female patients of childbearing age, it is recommended to counsel on the teratogenic potential of this class of medications [17]. The goal blood pressure for patients with diabetes is systolic blood pressure <130 mmHg and diastolic blood pressure <80 mmHg [70] with definition of hypertension as systolic blood pressure above 140 mmHg and diastolic blood pressure above 90 mmHg [17].

Symptomatic neuropathy is uncommon in teens with type 1 diabetes; however, subclinical neurologic impairment has been identified in many youths with type 1 diabetes and in adolescents with type 2 diabetes more often than those with type 1 diabetes [71, 72]. Both peripheral and autonomic nervous systems may be affected with the classic symmetric distal sensory loss in peripheral neuropathy as well as abnormal heart rate variability, postural blood pressure abnormalities, and impairment of pupillary dilation in autonomic dysfunction. Cardiac autonomic dysfunction may be associated with pubertal development and more often occurs in those patients with poor glycemic control [73, 74]. Screening for peripheral neuropathy should be done annually with monofilament and vibratory sensation testing. As in older adults with diabetes, better glycemic control can lead to improvements in nerve function in teens and young adults with diabetes.

Cardiovascular disease and dyslipidemia are common in adults with type 1 diabetes. Cardiovascular disease is much more common among adults with diabetes (both types 1 and 2) compared to matched controls without diabetes. For example, adult men with diabetes have a four times elevated risk of major cardiovascular events (myocardial infarction, stroke, acute coronary heart disease death, and need for coronary revascularization) compared to healthy controls, while adult women with diabetes have an eightfold elevated risk compared with healthy controls [75]. Although very few teens have had cardiovascular disease events, changes in lipids and cardiac function begin to occur in childhood, including reductions in left ventricular size and stroke volume [76], atherosclerotic changes [77], and increases in vascular stiffness [78, 79]. The American Diabetes Association recommends screening children and adolescents with type 1 diabetes with a lipid panel (ideally fasting) at age 10 or older or at puberty. If low-density lipoprotein (LDL) is <100 mg/dL, a lipid screen should be repeated every 5 years. If lipids are abnormal, annual lipid assessments are recommended. If LDL is <100 and hemoglobin A1c is elevated greater than 9 %, screening should occur more often than every 5 years (i.e., every 2 years) [17]. Exercise has been shown to reduce cardiometabolic risk, and should be advised to all children and young adults with diabetes. Diet, exercise, and better glycemic control are recommended if hyperlipidemia is diagnosed. HMG-CoA reductase inhibitors (statins) are recommended if lifestyle changes and improvements in hemoglobin A1c do not achieve target lipid goals: LDL <100 mg/dL, high-density lipoprotein (HDL) >35 mg/dL, and triglycerides <150 mg/dL. If a statin is prescribed to a female of reproductive age, it is recommended to counsel her on discontinuation prior to conception as there have been poor fetal outcomes thought to be related to statins [80].

Disordered Eating

Eating disorders are a well-known problem for patients with diabetes. According to the Diagnostic and Statistical Manual of Mental Disorders, Fifth Edition (DSM-V), an eating disorder is characterized by a persistent disturbance of eating that impairs health or psychosocial functioning. Disturbed eating behavior is common in late adolescent and young adult women in the general population [81]. Adolescent girls with type 1 diabetes are 2.4 times more likely to develop an eating disorder and 1.9 times more likely to develop a subclinical eating disorder than female adolescents without diabetes [82]. In a meta-analysis of adolescents with type 1 diabetes, 7 % had an eating disorder [82]. Subclinical eating disorder symptoms have been noted in more than 30 % of women with type 1 diabetes [83].

Patients with diabetes and eating disorders are less likely to use weight control behaviors such as vomiting, laxatives, or diuretics as their peers without diabetes [84]. The most common weight control method for patients with diabetes is the purposeful insulin omission for the intention of preventing weight gain [82]. This causes catabolism of lipids and induced glycosuria, leading to excretion of calories with urine. This is a behavior unique to patients with diabetes given the role insulin plays in disease management. It has been recognized by the DSM-V as either an inappropriate compensatory feature of bulimia nervosa or as a purging disorder [85]. The prevalence of insulin omission for weight loss increases with age, affecting up to 40 % of young adult females with type 1 diabetes [85].

Many factors specific to diabetes have been shown to predispose patients to developing eating disorders. The age of onset of diabetes in adolescence [86] as well as the cycle of weight loss at disease onset and subsequent weight gain with the initiation of insulin therapy [82] correlate with later development of an eating disorder. It has been proposed that intensive insulin therapy also puts patients at risk for eating disorders because it can cause weight gain, negative feelings around body image, and fear of further gain [87]. The dietary restraint demanded by diabetes management is thought to contribute by leading to craving and then binging "forbidden foods" without appropriate insulin coverage [88]. Similarly, episodes of hypoglycemia may trigger disordered eating because the associated intense hunger can lead to binging on "forbidden foods" and subsequent guilt about over-eating [89].

Eating disorders are especially serious for patients with diabetes because they are associated with increased morbidity and mortality. Multiple studies have shown worse metabolic control with higher hemoglobin A1c in patients with diabetes who have an eating disorder compared to those who do not [82, 85]. Consequently, research has also demonstrated an accelerated rate of long-term microvascular complications including retinopathy [90] and nephropathy [91] as well as hypertension and dyslipidemia [92] in patients with diabetes and disordered eating compared to diabetic patients without eating disorders. Due to insulin omission and disturbed eating, patients with diabetes and an eating disorder have significantly higher rates of severe hypoglycemia, hypoglycemia with coma, and diabetic ketoacidosis (DKA) with hospitalization than those without an eating disorder [92]. Multiple studies have shown an increased risk of death among this group of patients, with one study citing a 3.2-fold increase in the risk of death in women with diabetes and an eating disorder compared to those without an eating disorder [91].

To avoid the severe consequences of an eating disorder, it is important for healthcare providers to prevent and identify eating disorders. They should be sensitive to a preoccupation with body weight and to minimize risk factors that have been shown to lead to an eating disorder by promoting flexibility with treatment and a non-depriving diet [93]. A high index of suspicion is required to identify an eating disorder in patients with diabetes, as they frequently conceal and deny that they have a problem and do not often use the unhealthy weight control behaviors such as vomiting, laxatives, skipping meals as their peers without diabetes do, but rather often omit insulin. The following clinical signs should alert physicians of a possible eating disorder: poor glycemic control, recurrent episodes of DKA, recurrent hypoglycemic episodes, frequently missed medical appointments, refusal to be weighed, and preoccupation with appearance [85].

Special Issues that Arise with Transition to Adulthood

Alcohol, Tobacco, and Illicit Drug Use

The prevalence of tobacco, alcohol, and illicit drug use in young adults with diabetes approximates that of the general population [94]. In general, substance abuse has negative effects on adolescent health, but it can affect patients with type 1 diabetes to a more significant degree by increasing their risk for acute and chronic complications of diabetes [95].

Cigarette smoking is associated with increased development and progression of neuropathy, microalbuminuria, and impairment of renal function [96]. It is also a well-known risk factor for cardiovascular disease. Because diabetes itself is a cardiovascular risk factor, cigarette smoking significantly heightens the risk of premature death due to stroke and coronary artery disease [96]. Prevention and cessation of cigarette smoking is an important goal for providers caring for patients with diabetes.

It is well known that alcohol is a risk factor for hypoglycemia in patients with type 1 diabetes, likely due to inhibition of gluconeogenesis in the liver [97]. This can be especially dangerous as moderate alcohol intake has been shown to cause decreased awareness of hypoglycemia in patients with type 1 diabetes despite exaggerated physiological changes [98]. Physicians should routinely educate these patients about the risk of nocturnal hypoglycemia with alcohol.

Substance abuse has been shown to be a significant contributing factor for noncompliance in patients with diabetes [99]. Cocaine has been found to be a risk factor for diabetic ketoacidosis, either due to its association with insulin therapy omission or its effects on counter-regulatory hormones [100].

Sexual Health, Contraception, and Preconception Planning

The number of women with pre-existing diabetes (both types 1 and 2) who become pregnant and deliver babies is increasing [101]. Unfortunately, unplanned pregnancy is a major concern. More than one-half of women with diabetes have experienced unplanned pregnancies [102]. Contraceptive use is lower in women with diabetes than in women without diabetes [102]. Only half of young adults with diabetes who reported being sexually active had ever used birth control to prevent pregnancy [103].

It is critical to include reproductive and sexual health in the care of the young adult with type 1 diabetes to prevent unplanned pregnancy and to optimize the health outcomes of diabetic women and their infants. Multiple studies have demonstrated high rates of spontaneous abortions and major congenital malformations in infants of mothers with type 1 diabetes who have poor glycemic control during pregnancy [104].

To minimize the risk of devastating malformations, the American Diabetes Association recommends that all women of childbearing potential receive preconception counseling [105]. Despite this recommendation, most women do not. Less than half of teenagers with diabetes had discussed birth control with a health care professional and 31 % reported that they would not feel comfortable bringing up the subject [103]. Sixty-five percent of young adults (age 16–20) reported knowing nothing about preconception counseling and more than 75 % were not aware of the maternal and fetal risks in women with diabetes and the need for good glycemic control [106].

In a survey of primary care physicians who care for adolescents with chronic health conditions, all agreed that reproductive and sexual health is one of the most important issues, but many did not feel prepared to discuss it with their patients [107]. To help clarify goals of preconception care, the American Diabetes Association has outlined two key objectives:

1. Educate patients on the risk of malformations associated with unplanned pregnancies and poor glycemic control.
2. Provide effective contraception to all women with diabetes who are at childbearing age (unless the patient has good metabolic control and is trying to conceive).

Contraceptive choice should focus on which is the most effective method for the patient as there are no specific contraindications to particular contraceptive methods in patients with diabetes. The Centers for Disease Control has also developed recommendations for preconception care that can help in the development of a reproductive health plan [10].

Americans with Disabilities Act and School/Work Accommodations

The Americans with Disabilities Act [108] protects teens and young adults with diabetes against workplace discrimination. An employer cannot fail to hire or fail to promote a young adult due to diabetes, nor can they terminate an individual because of diabetes and must not discriminate with regard to employer-paid health insurance. An employer should provide reasonable accommodations if requested by the employee. Similarly, in educational settings, teens and young adults with diabetes may request reasonable accommodations for learning, if needed. Directing undergraduate students to register with their Disabilities Services Office is the first step in requesting accommodations. At many universities, the Disabilities Services Office will provide an accommodation letter that the student can provide to each of his/her instructors at the beginning of the semester. Both the American Diabetes Association's Going Away to College [109] and the College Diabetes Network website [13] have resources about standardized testing and asking for possible testing accommodations.

Financial Issues

Financial concerns may pose a significant barrier to successful transition from pediatric to adult medical care for patients with diabetes. Patients with diabetes may have difficulty affording supplies, including glucometer test strips, insulin syringes or insulin pen needles, insulin itself, and possibly insulin pump or continuous glucose monitoring supplies. Government programs and medication assistance programs may be able to help. Patients should be encouraged to check if they are eligible for the hospital's financial assistance program, the Bureau for Children with Medical Handicaps for their state, and also prescription assistance programs. The College Diabetes Network website has several resources on obtaining and affording diabetes supplies and health insurance [13].

Changing Living Situations

As patients with diabetes move away from home, it is very important that they inform the people with whom they will be living about their diabetes. If they are going to college, this would include their roommate and residence hall advisor. It is helpful to provide some basic information to these people on what diabetes entails in order to clear up any possible misconceptions. It may be useful to demonstrate how supplies, including glucagon, work. Most importantly, the roommate should be made aware of the dangers of hypoglycemia, how to recognize it, and what to do if the patient becomes confused or unarousable. This would entail calling 911 and administering glucose gel or glucagon [110]. Because patients may find starting a conversation about their diabetes challenging, the College Diabetes Network has developed tools and tips on how to talk with friends and roommates about diabetes [13]. The Juvenile Diabetes Research Foundation (JDRF) has also developed a letter that can be used to facilitate this discussion [15]. Similarly, the College Diabetes Network has resources for preparing to talk to one's roommate about having diabetes [13].

Family-Oriented Care to Self-Care Behaviors and Adherence

Fundamental differences between pediatric "family-oriented" care and adult care are well recognized. In the pediatric setting, care is provided in a family-focused model that tries to accommodate the child and family's needs with significant support. Parents are highly involved because children do not have the cognitive skills to independently manage their diabetes. In the adult model, patients are treated as autonomous individuals, provided with information and recommendations, and expected to independently make decisions about their disease management. Visits tend to be shorter, less holistic, and more focused on medical problems. The contrast between these two models can be upsetting for young adults with diabetes as they transition to adult models of care [95]. Furthermore, patients struggle with self-care and adherence as they attempt to manage their diabetes in a model that demands independence during transition. Over the 2-year period following transition to adult care, research demonstrates a significant deterioration in treatment adherence as well as glycemic control in young adults with type 1 diabetes [13].

Conclusion

Adolescents and young adults with type 1 diabetes present a challenging patient population for primary care providers. In addition to focusing on glycemic control and screening for long-term microvascular and macrovascular complications of diabetes, young adults with type 1 diabetes need screening for associated mental health conditions, including depression, anxiety, disordered eating, and diabetes distress (see Table 9.1) [17]. Furthermore, all women of reproductive age with type 1 diabetes need

Table 9.1 Screening for complications and coexisting conditions of diabetes [17]

Condition	Test	Frequency
Blood glucose control	Hemoglobin A1c	At least 2 times a year in patients who meet treatment goals (and have stable glycemic control) Quarterly in patients whose therapy has changed or who are not meeting glycemic goals
Retinopathy	Dilated eye exam by a trained eye services professional	Patients *with* evidence of retinopathy should be screened annually Patients *without* evidence of retinopathy should be screened every 2 years
Nephropathy	Urine spot microalbumin/creatinine ratio	Annually
Autonomic Neuropathy	Ask about symptoms of sexual dysfunction and gastroparesis	Annually
Peripheral Neuropathy	Physical exam focused on ankle reflexes, dorsalis pedis pulses, vibratory sensation, and 5.07 monofilament touch sensation	Patients at *very high risk* should be seen every 3 months by a wound care nurse Patients at *increased risk* and *average risk* should be screened annually
Hypertension	Blood pressure measurement by a trained professional	Every visit
Hyperlipidemia	Lipids	At the time of diabetes diagnosis or at initial medical evaluation. If LDL is <100 mg/dL, recheck lipids every 5 years. If lipids are abnormal, check annually. If HbA1c is >9 %, check more often (i.e., every 2 years)
Electrolyte and chemistry abnormalities	Serum creatinine and potassium	At least annually
Depression and diabetes-related distress	Patient Health Questionnaire (PHQ-2) and either the Diabetes Distress Scale (DDS) or Problem Areas in Diabetes (PAID)-1 scale	Screen at each visit (quarterly)
Celiac disease	Anti-tissue transglutaminase antibody	Regular screening of children at diagnosis and also every 2–3 years or if clinically suspected. Screening in adults with signs or symptoms of celiac disease, unexplained hypoglycemia, glycemic patterns, or low bone density
Thyroid disease	TSH	Every 1–2 years or sooner if symptoms of hypothyroidism
Obesity	BMI	Quarterly
Periodontal disease	Routine dental exam	Every 6 months
Unplanned pregnancy	Counsel on reproductive and sexual health	Every visit (quarterly)
Immunizations	Hepatitis B vaccine	3-dose series ages 19–59. Age 60 and older depending on risk
	Pneumococcal polysaccharide (PPSV23) vaccine	Once between age 19 and 64 years Booster after age 65 (at least 5 years after previous dose)
	Influenza vaccine	Annually

LDL low-density lipoproteins, *TSH* thyroid-stimulating hormone, *BMI* body mass index preconception planning and education. Transitioning to adulthood is a challenging time period for emerging adults with type 1 diabetes, and longitudinal support from a team of health care providers is needed ("Appendix").

Appendix

Type 1 diabetes condition fact sheet

Definition	Type 1 diabetes is an autoimmune condition that affects the pancreas' ability to make insulin needed to break down food (sugar) into energy needed for survival. It is defined by any of the following criteria: • Fasting plasma glucose $\geq$ 126 mg/dL (7.0 mmol/L). Fasting is defined as no caloric intake for at least 8 h • 2-hour plasma glucose $\geq$ 200 mg/dL (11.1 mmol/L) during an oral glucose tolerance test • A1C $\geq$ 6.5 % (48 mmol/mol) • In a patient with classic symptoms of hyperglycemia or hyperglycemic crisis, a random plasma glucose $\geq$ 200 mg/dL (11.1 mmol/L)
Epidemiology	• Prevalence of diabetes (both types 1 and 2 diabetes) among children in the United States is 3.2 per 1000 • Non-Hispanic white children have higher prevalence of diabetes (3.8 per 1000 children) compared with other racial and ethnic categories (2.2 per 1000 children)
Special considerations	• *Depression and anxiety* are more common and more pronounced in patients with diabetes due to the associated disease-related emotional distress • *Disordered eating* is 2.4 times more common in adolescent women with diabetes than those without, and the prevalence of insulin omission for weight loss affects up to 40 % of young adult females with type 1 diabetes • *Reproductive health* is critical to discuss to prevent unplanned pregnancy and to optimize the health outcomes of diabetic women and their infants. More than one-half of women with diabetes have experienced unplanned pregnancies and more than 75 % were not aware of the maternal and fetal risks and the need for good glycemic control • *Long-term vascular complications* are associated with poor glycemic control and should be routinely screened for to identify any nephropathy, retinopathy, neuropathy, and cardiovascular disease • *Obesity* in patients with diabetes disproportionally affects minorities and young girls, especially those diagnosed between ages 10–15 years of age • *Associated autoimmune diseases* that should be routinely screened for include thyroid disease and celiac disease • *Alcohol, tobacco, and illicit drug use* can increase the risk for complications in patients with type 1 diabetes; Physicians should routinely educate patients about the risk of cigarettes and nocturnal hypoglycemia with alcohol
Recommended screening	See Table 9.1

Suggested Reading List

- American Diabetes Association Standards of Medical Care in Diabetes—2015 and Diabetes Care for Emerging Adults: Recommendations for Transition from Pediatric to Adult Diabetes Care Systems
- Endocrine Society Managing the Transition of Care for Patients with Type 1 Diabetes (including A Recommended Approach to

Planning for Pediatric Practices and A Recommended Approach to the Adolescent Transitioning to Adult Practice) https://www.endocrine.org/education-and-practice-management/quality-improvement-resources/clinical-practice-resources/transition-of-care
- Juvenile Diabetes Research Foundation
- National Diabetes Education Program—Transition Resources Pediatric to Adult Health Care
- American Association of Clinical Endocrinologists: Find an endocrinologist
- Hormone Health Network: Find an Endocrinologist.

Patient/Caregiver Resources

- American Diabetes Association's Going to College with Diabetes: A Self Advocacy Guide for Students
- Juvenile Diabetes Research Foundation "Letter to My Roommate" (https://hscweb3.hsc.usf.edu/wp-content/uploads/2012/02/Dear_Roommate.pdf) and Type 1 Diabetes Teen Toolkit (http://typeonenation.org/resources/type-1-toolkits/)
- American Association of Clinical Endocrinologists
- Endocrine Society Transitions of Care for Diabetes Resources https://www.endocrine.org/education-and-practice-management/quality-improvement-resources/clinical-practice-resources/transition-of-care
- College Diabetes Network—Preparing for College, Life on Campus, Between Visits and other resources (http://www.collegediabetesnetwork.org)
- National Diabetes Education Program http://ndep.nih.gov/transitions/resourceslist.aspx
- Americans with Disabilities Act http://www.dol.gov/dol/topic/disability/ada.htm
- Hormone Health Network—Find an Endocrinologist.

References

1. Mortensen HB, Hougaard P. Comparison of metabolic control in a cross-sectional study of 2,873 children and adolescents with IDDM from 18 countries. The Hvidore Study Group on childhood diabetes. Diabetes Care. 1997;20(5):714–20.
2. Springer D, Dziura J, Tamborlane WV, Steffen AT, Ahern JH, Vincent M, et al. Optimal control of type 1 diabetes mellitus in youth receiving intensive treatment. J Pediatr. 2006;149(2):227–32.
3. Danne T, Mortensen HB, Hougaard P, Lynggaard H, Aanstoot HJ, Chiarelli F, et al. Persistent differences among centers over 3 years in glycemic control and hypoglycemia in a study of 3,805 children and adolescents with type 1 diabetes from the Hvidore Study Group. Diabetes Care. 2001;24(8):1342–7.
4. Anonymous. Effect of intensive diabetes treatment on the development and progression of long-term complications in adolescents with insulin-dependent diabetes mellitus: DIABETES control and complications trial. Diabetes control and complications trial research group. J Pediatr. 1994;125(2):177–188.
5. Anonymous. The relationship of glycemic exposure (HbA1c) to the risk of development and progression of retinopathy in the diabetes control and complications trial. Diabetes. 1995;44(8):968–983.
6. Lachin JM, Genuth S, Nathan DM, Zinman B, Rutledge BN, Group DER. Effect of glycemic exposure on the risk of microvascular complications in the diabetes control and complications trial–revisited. Diabetes. 2008;57(4):995–1001.
7. Hood KK, Peterson CM, Rohan JM, Drotar D. Association between adherence and glycemic control in pediatric type 1 diabetes: a meta-analysis. Pediatrics. 2009;124(6):e1171–9.
8. Schwartz DD, Cline VD, Hansen JA, Axelrad ME, Anderson BJ. Early risk factors for nonadherence in pediatric type 1 diabetes: a review of the recent literature. Curr Diabetes Rev. 2010;6(3):167–83.
9. Nyomba BL, Berard L, Murphy LJ. Facilitating access to glucometer reagents increases blood glucose self-monitoring frequency and improves glycaemic control: a prospective study in insulin-treated diabetic patients. Diabet Med. 2004;21(2):129–35.
10. Malerbi FE, Negrato CA, Gomes MB, Brazilian Type 1 Diabetes Study G. Assessment of psychosocial variables by parents of youth with type 1 diabetes mellitus. Diabetol Metab Syndr. 2012;4(1):48.
11. Borus JS, Laffel L. Adherence challenges in the management of type 1 diabetes in adolescents: prevention and intervention. Curr Opin Pediatr. 2010;22(4):405–11.

12. Gomes MB, de Mattos Matheus AS, Calliari LE, Luescher JL, Manna TD, Savoldelli RD, et al. Economic status and clinical care in young type 1 diabetes patients: a nationwide multicenter study in Brazil. Acta Diabetol. 2013;50(5):743–52.
13. Rausch JR, Hood KK, Delamater A, Shroff Pendley J, Rohan JM, Reeves G, et al. Changes in treatment adherence and glycemic control during the transition to adolescence in type 1 diabetes. Diabetes Care. 2012;35(6):1219–24.
14. Viana LV, Gomes MB, Zajdenverg L, Pavin EJ, Azevedo MJ, Brazilian Type 1 Diabetes Study G. Interventions to improve patients' compliance with therapies aimed at lowering glycated hemoglobin (HbA1c) in type 1 diabetes: systematic review and meta-analyses of randomized controlled clinical trials of psychological, telecare, and educational interventions. Trials. 2016;17(1):94.
15. Oris L, Rassart J, Prikken S, Verschueren M, Goubert L, Moons P, et al. Illness identity in adolescents and emerging adults with type 1 diabetes: Introducing the illness identity questionnaire. Diabetes Care. 2016 May;39(5):757–63.
16. Anonymous. Available from: http://www.who.int/diabetes/publications/Definition%20and%20diagnosis%20of%20diabetes_new.pdf.
17. Anonymous. Standards of medical care in diabetes-2016: summary of revisions. Diabetes Care. 2016;39(Suppl 1):S4–5.
18. Group DP. Incidence and trends of childhood type 1 diabetes worldwide 1990–1999. Diabetic Med. 2006;23(8):857–66.
19. Thunander M, Petersson C, Jonzon K, Fornander J, Ossiansson B, Torn C, et al. Incidence of type 1 and type 2 diabetes in adults and children in Kronoberg, Sweden. Diabetes Res Clin Pract. 2008;82(2):247–55.
20. Wandell PE, Carlsson AC. Time trends and gender differences in incidence and prevalence of type 1 diabetes in Sweden. Curr Diabetes Rev. 2013;9(4):342–9.
21. Berhan Y, Waernbaum I, Lind T, Mollsten A, Dahlquist G, Swedish Childhood Diabetes Study G. Thirty years of prospective nationwide incidence of childhood type 1 diabetes: the accelerating increase by time tends to level off in Sweden. Diabetes. 2011;60(2):577–81.
22. Menke A, Casagrande S, Geiss L, Cowie CC. Prevalence of and trends in diabetes among adults in the United States, 1988–2012. JAMA. 2015;314(10):1021–9.
23. Lee JM, Herman WH, McPheeters ML, Gurney JG. An epidemiologic profile of children with diabetes in the U.S. Diabetes Care. 2006;29(2):420–1.
24. Group SfDiYS, Liese AD, D'Agostino RB Jr, Hamman RF, Kilgo PD, Lawrence JM, et al. The burden of diabetes mellitus among us youth: prevalence estimates from the search for diabetes in youth study. Pediatrics. 2006;118(4):1510–8.
25. Polonsky WH, Anderson BJ, Lohrer PA, Welch G, Jacobson AM, Aponte JE, et al. Assessment of diabetes-related distress. Diabetes Care. 1995;18(6):754–60.
26. Jacobson AM, Adler AG, Wolfsdorf JI, Anderson B, Derby L. Psychological characteristics of adults with IDDM. Comparison of patients in poor and good glycemic control. Diabetes Care. 1990;13(4):375–81.
27. Konen JC, Summerson JH, Dignan MB. Family function, stress, and locus of control. Relationships to glycemia in adults with diabetes mellitus. Arch Fam Med. 1993;2(4):393–402.
28. Delamater AM, Kurtz SM, Bubb J, White NH, Santiago JV. Stress and coping in relation to metabolic control of adolescents with type 1 diabetes. J Dev Behav Pediatr. 1987;8(3):136–40.
29. Lustman PJ, Griffith LS, Clouse RE, Cryer PE. Psychiatric illness in diabetes mellitus. Relationship to symptoms and glucose control. J Nerv Ment Dis. 1986;174(12):736–42.
30. Peyrot M, Rubin RR. Behavioral and psychosocial interventions in diabetes: a conceptual review. Diabetes Care. 2007;30(10):2433–40.
31. Fisher L, Glasgow RE, Mullan JT, Skaff MM, Polonsky WH. Development of a brief diabetes distress screening instrument. Ann Fam Med. 2008;6(3):246–52.
32. McGuire BE, Morrison TG, Hermanns N, Skovlund S, Eldrup E, Gagliardino J, et al. Short-form measures of diabetes-related emotional distress: the problem areas in diabetes scale (paid)-5 and paid-1. Diabetologia. 2010;53(1):66–9.
33. Anderson RJ, Freedland KE, Clouse RE, Lustman PJ. The prevalence of comorbid depression in adults with diabetes: a meta-analysis. Diabetes Care. 2001;24(6):1069–78.
34. Trief PM, Xing D, Foster NC, Maahs DM, Kittelsrud JM, Olson BA, et al. Depression in adults in the T1D exchange clinic registry. Diabetes Care. 2014;37(6):1563–72.
35. Anderson BJ, Edelstein S, Abramson NW, Katz LE, Yasuda PM, Lavietes SJ, et al. Depressive symptoms and quality of life in adolescents with type 2 diabetes: baseline data from the today study. Diabetes Care. 2011;34(10):2205–7.
36. Gonzalez JS, Safren SA, Cagliero E, Wexler DJ, Delahanty L, Wittenberg E, et al. Depression, self-care, and medication adherence in type 2 diabetes: relationships across the full range of symptom severity. Diabetes Care. 2007;30(9):2222–7.
37. Lustman PJ, Anderson RJ, Freedland KE, de Groot M, Carney RM, Clouse RE. Depression and poor glycemic control: a meta-analytic review of the literature. Diabetes Care. 2000;23(7):934–42.
38. Sullivan MD, O'Connor P, Feeney P, Hire D, Simmons DL, Raisch DW, et al. Depression predicts all-cause mortality: epidemiological evaluation from

the accord HRQL substudy. Diabetes Care. 2012;35 (8):1708–15.
39. Simon GE, Katon WJ, Lin EHB, Rutter C, Manning WG, Von Korff M, et al. Cost-effectiveness of systematic depression treatment among people with diabetes mellitus. Arch Gen Psychiatry. 2007;64 (1):65–72.
40. Dierker LC, Albano AM, Clarke GN, Heimberg RG, Kendall PC, Merikangas KR, et al. Screening for anxiety and depression in early adolescence. J Am Acad Child Psychiatry. 2001;40(8):929–36.
41. Herzer M, Hood KK. Anxiety symptoms in adolescents with type 1 diabetes: association with blood glucose monitoring and glycemic control. J Pediatr Psychol. 2010;35(4):415–25.
42. Ginsburg GS, Riddle MA, Davies M. Somatic symptoms in children and adolescents with anxiety disorders. J Am Acad Child Psychiatry. 2006;45 (10):1179–87.
43. Liu LL, Lawrence JM, Davis C, Liese AD, Pettitt DJ, Pihoker C, et al. Prevalence of overweight and obesity in youth with diabetes in USA: the search for diabetes in youth study. Pediatr Diabetes. 2010;11 (1):4–11.
44. Frohlich-Reiterer EE, Rosenbauer J, Bechtold-Dalla Pozza S, Hofer SE, Schober E, Holl RW, et al. Predictors of increasing BMI during the course of diabetes in children and adolescents with type 1 diabetes: data from the German/Austrian DPV Multicentre Survey. Arch Dis Child. 2014;99 (8):738–43.
45. Conway B, Miller RG, Costacou T, Fried L, Kelsey S, Evans RW, et al. Temporal patterns in overweight and obesity in type 1 diabetes. Diabet Med. 2010;27(4):398–404.
46. Wagner AM, Santana A, Hernndez M, Wiebe JC, Novoa J, Mauricio D, et al. Predictors of associated autoimmune diseases in families with type 1 diabetes: results from the type 1 diabetes genetics consortium. Diabetes Metab Res Rev. 2011;27 (5):493–8.
47. Hanukoglu A, Mizrachi A, Dalal I, Admoni O, Rakover Y, Bistritzer Z, et al. Extrapancreatic autoimmune manifestations in type 1 diabetes patients and their first-degree relatives: a multicenter study. Diabetes Care. 2003;26(4):1235–40.
48. Kordonouri O, Klinghammer A, Lang EB, Gruters-Kieslich A, Grabert M, Holl RW. Thyroid autoimmunity in children and adolescents with type 1 diabetes: a multicenter survey. Diabetes Care. 2002;25(8):1346–50.
49. Warncke K, Frohlich-Reiterer EE, Thon A, Hofer SE, Wiemann D, Holl RW, et al. Polyendocrinopathy in children, adolescents, and young adults with type 1 diabetes: a multicenter analysis of 28,671 patients from the German/Austrian DPV-WISS database. Diabetes Care. 2010;33 (9):2010–2.
50. Buschur E, Sarma AV, Pietropaolo M, Dunn RL, Braffett BH, Cleary PA, et al. Self-reported autoimmune disease by sex in the diabetes control and complications trial/epidemiology of diabetes interventions and complications (DCCT/EDIC) study. Diabetes Care. 2014;37(2):e28–9.
51. Kordonouri O, Hartmann R, Deiss D, Wilms M, Gruters-Kieslich A. Natural course of autoimmune thyroiditis in type 1 diabetes: association with gender, age, diabetes duration, and puberty. Arch Dis Child. 2005;90(4):411–4.
52. Spirkova A, Dusatkova P, Peckova M, Kolouskova S, Snajderova M, Obermannova B, et al. Treated autoimmune thyroid disease is associated with a decreased quality of life among young persons with type 1 diabetes. Int J Endocrinol. 2015;2015:185859.
53. Dogan B, Oner C, Bayramicli OU, Yorulmaz E, Feyizoglu G, Oguz A. Prevalence of celiac disease in adult type 1 patients with diabetes. Pak J Med Sci. 2015;31(4):865–8.
54. Aktay AN, Lee PC, Kumar V, Parton E, Wyatt DT, Werlin SL. The prevalence and clinical characteristics of celiac disease in juvenile diabetes in Wisconsin. J Pediatr Gastroenterol Nutr. 2001;33 (4):462–5.
55. Cerutti F, Bruno G, Chiarelli F, Lorini R, Meschi F, Sacchetti C, et al. Younger age at onset and sex predict celiac disease in children and adolescents with type 1 diabetes: an italian multicenter study. Diabetes Care. 2004;27(6):1294–8.
56. Verkasalo M, Kuitunen P, Leisti S, Perheentupa J. Growth failure from symptomless celiac disease. A study of 14 patients. Helvetica Paediatrica Acta. 1978;33(6):489–95.
57. Silverstein J, Klingensmith G, Copeland K, Plotnick L, Kaufman F, Laffel L, et al. Care of children and adolescents with type 1 diabetes: a statement of the American Diabetes Association. Diabetes Care. 2005;28(1):186–212.
58. DeMelo EN, McDonald C, Saibil F, Marcon MA, Mahmud FH. Celiac disease and type 1 diabetes in adults: Is this a high-risk group for screening? Can J Diabetes. 2015;39(6):513–9.
59. Rubio-Tapia A, Hill ID, Kelly CP, Calderwood AH, Murray JA, American College of G. ACG clinical guidelines: diagnosis and management of celiac disease. Am J Gastroenterol. 2013;108(5):656–76 quiz 677.
60. Anonymous. The effect of intensive treatment of diabetes on the development and progression of long-term complications in insulin-dependent diabetes mellitus. The diabetes control and complications trial research group. The New Engl J Med. 1993;329(14):977–86.
61. Pambianco G, Costacou T, Ellis D, Becker DJ, Klein R, Orchard TJ. The 30-year natural history of type 1 diabetes complications: The Pittsburgh epidemiology of diabetes complications study experience. Diabetes. 2006;55(5):1463–9.
62. Sparud-Lundin C, Ohrn I, Danielson E, Forsander G. Glycaemic control and diabetes care utilization in

young adults with type 1 diabetes. Diabet Med J Br Diabet Assoc. 2008;25(8):968–73.
63. Nordwall M, Bojestig M, Arnqvist HJ, Ludvigsson J, Linkoping Diabetes Complications S. Declining incidence of severe retinopathy and persisting decrease of nephropathy in an unselected population of type 1 diabetes-the Linkoping diabetes complications study. Diabetologia. 2004;47(7):1266–72.
64. Amin R, Widmer B, Prevost AT, Schwarze P, Cooper J, Edge J, et al. Risk of microalbuminuria and progression to macroalbuminuria in a cohort with childhood onset type 1 diabetes: prospective observational study. BMJ. 2008;336(7646):697–701.
65. Scott LJ, Warram JH, Hanna LS, Laffel LM, Ryan L, Krolewski AS. A nonlinear effect of hyperglycemia and current cigarette smoking are major determinants of the onset of microalbuminuria in type 1 diabetes. Diabetes. 2001;50(12):2842–9.
66. Svensson M, Nystrom L, Schon S, Dahlquist G. Age at onset of childhood-onset type 1 diabetes and the development of end-stage renal disease: a nationwide population-based study. Diabetes Care. 2006;29(3):538–42.
67. Guntsche Z, Saravi FD, Reynals EA, Rauek B, Rauek M, Guntsche EM. Parental hypertension and 24 h-blood pressure in children prior to diabetic nephropathy. Pediatr Nephrol. 2002;17(3):157–64.
68. Theochari MA, Vyssoulis GP, Toutouzas PK, Bartsocas CS. Arterial blood pressure changes in children and adolescents with insulin-dependent diabetes mellitus. J Pediatr. 1996;129(5):667–70.
69. Hilgers KF, Dotsch J, Rascher W, Mann JF. Treatment strategies in patients with chronic renal disease: ace inhibitors, angiotensin receptor antagonists, or both? Pediatr Nephrol. 2004;19(9):956–61.
70. Handelsman Y, Bloomgarden ZT, Grunberger G, Umpierrez G, Zimmerman RS, Bailey TS, et al. American association of clinical endocrinologists and american college of endocrinology—clinical practice guidelines for developing a diabetes mellitus comprehensive care plan—2015. Endocr Pract. 2015;21(Suppl 1):1–87.
71. Solders G, Thalme B, Aguirre-Aquino M, Brandt L, Berg U, Persson A. Nerve conduction and autonomic nerve function in diabetic children. A 10-year follow-up study. Acta Paediatr. 1997;86(4):361–6.
72. Jaiswal M, Lauer A, Martin CL, Bell RA, Divers J, Dabelea D, et al. Peripheral neuropathy in adolescents and young adults with type 1 and type 2 diabetes from the search for diabetes in youth follow-up cohort: a pilot study. Diabetes Care. 2013;36(12):3903–8.
73. Barkai L, Kempler P, Vamosi I, Lukacs K, Marton A, Keresztes K. Peripheral sensory nerve dysfunction in children and adolescents with type 1 diabetes mellitus. Diabet Med J Br Diabet Assoc. 1998;15(3):228–33.
74. Karavanaki K, Baum JD. Prevalence of microvascular and neurologic abnormalities in a population of diabetic children. J Pediatr Endocrinol Metab. 1999;12(3):411–22.
75. Soedamah-Muthu SS, Fuller JH, Mulnier HE, Raleigh VS, Lawrenson RA, Colhoun HM. High risk of cardiovascular disease in patients with type 1 diabetes in the U.K.: a cohort study using the general practice research database. Diabetes Care. 2006;29(4):798–804.
76. Gotzsche O, Darwish A, Gotzsche L, Hansen LP, Sorensen KE. Incipient cardiomyopathy in young insulin-dependent diabetic patients: a seven-year prospective doppler echocardiographic study. Diabet Med. 1996;13(9):834–40.
77. Jarvisalo MJ, Putto-Laurila A, Jartti L, Lehtimaki T, Solakivi T, Ronnemaa T, et al. Carotid artery intima-media thickness in children with type 1 diabetes. Diabetes. 2002;51(2):493–8.
78. Maahs DM, Maniatis AK, Nadeau K, Wadwa RP, McFann K, Klingensmith GJ. Total cholesterol and high-density lipoprotein levels in pediatric subjects with type 1 diabetes mellitus. J Pediatr. 2005;147(4):544–6.
79. Maahs DM, Dabelea D, D'Agostino RB Jr, Andrews JS, Shah AS, Crimmins N, et al. Glucose control predicts 2-year change in lipid profile in youth with type 1 diabetes. J Pediatr. 2013;162(1):101–107e101.
80. Petersen EE, Mitchell AA, Carey JC, Werler MM, Louik C, Rasmussen SA, et al. Maternal exposure to statins and risk for birth defects: a case-series approach. Am J Med Genetics Part A. 2008;146A(20):2701–5.
81. Fairburn CG, Beglin SJ. Studies of the epidemiology of bulimia nervosa. Am J Psychiatry. 1990;147(4):401–8.
82. Jones JM, Lawson ML, Daneman D, Olmsted MP, Rodin G. Eating disorders in adolescent females with and without type 1 diabetes: cross sectional study. BMJ. 2000;320(7249):1563–6.
83. Polonsky WH, Anderson BJ, Lohrer PA, Aponte JE, Jacobson AM, Cole CF. Insulin omission in women with IDDM. Diabetes Care. 1994;17(10):1178–85.
84. Ackard DM, Vik N, Neumark-Sztainer D, Schmitz KH, Hannan P, Jacobs DR Jr. Disordered eating and body dissatisfaction in adolescents with type 1 diabetes and a population-based comparison sample: comparative prevalence and clinical implications. Pediatric Diabetes. 2008;9(4 Pt 1):312–9.
85. Pinhas-Hamiel O, Hamiel U, Levy-Shraga Y. Eating disorders in adolescents with type 1 diabetes: challenges in diagnosis and treatment. World J Diabetes. 2015;6(3):517–26.
86. Takii M, Uchigata Y, Kishimoto J, Morita C, Hata T, Nozaki T, et al. The relationship between the age of onset of type 1 diabetes and the subsequent development of a severe eating disorder by female patients. Pediatr Diabetes. 2011;12(4 Pt 2):396–401.
87. Goebel-Fabbri AE. Disturbed eating behaviors and eating disorders in type 1 diabetes: clinical

significance and treatment recommendations. Curr DiabRep. 2009;9(2):133–9.
88. Rodin GM, Daneman D. Eating disorders and IDDM. A problematic association. Diabetes Care. 1992;15(10):1402–12.
89. Verrotti A, Catino M, De Luca FA, Morgese G, Chiarelli F. Eating disorders in adolescents with type 1 diabetes mellitus. Acta Diabetol. 1999;36(1–2):21–5.
90. Rydall AC, Rodin GM, Olmsted MP, Devenyi RG, Daneman D. Disordered eating behavior and microvascular complications in young women with insulin-dependent diabetes mellitus. New Engl J Med. 1997;336(26):1849–54.
91. Goebel-Fabbri AE, Fikkan J, Franko DL, Pearson K, Anderson BJ, Weinger K. Insulin restriction and associated morbidity and mortality in women with type 1 diabetes. Diabetes Care. 2008;31(3):415–9.
92. Scheuing N, Bartus B, Berger G, Haberland H, Icks A, Knauth B, et al. Clinical characteristics and outcome of 467 patients with a clinically recognized eating disorder identified among 52,215 patients with type 1 diabetes: a multicenter German/Austrian study. Diabetes Care. 2014;37(6):1581–9.
93. Rodin G, Olmsted MP, Rydall AC, Maharaj SI, Colton PA, Jones JM, et al. Eating disorders in young women with type 1 diabetes mellitus. J Psychosom Res. 2002;53(4):943–9.
94. Martinez-Aguayo A, Araneda JC, Fernandez D, Gleisner A, Perez V, Codner E. Tobacco, alcohol, and illicit drug use in adolescents with diabetes mellitus. Pediatr Diabetes. 2007;8(5):265–71.
95. Peters A, Laffel L, American Diabetes Association Transitions Working G. Diabetes care for emerging adults: recommendations for transition from pediatric to adult diabetes care systems: a position statement of the American Diabetes Association, with representation by the American College of Osteopathic Family Physicians, the American Academy of Pediatrics, the American Association of Clinical Endocrinologists, the American Osteopathic Association, the Centers for Disease Control and Prevention, Children with Diabetes, the Endocrine Society, the International Society for Pediatric and Adolescent Diabetes, Juvenile Diabetes Research Foundation International, the National Diabetes Education Program, and the Pediatric Endocrine Society (formerly Lawson Wilkins Pediatric Endocrine Society). Diabetes Care. 2011;34(11):2477–85.
96. Haire-Joshu D, Glasgow RE, Tibbs TL. Smoking and diabetes. Diabetes Care. 1999;22(11):1887–98.
97. Lange J, Arends J, Willms B. Alcohol-induced hypoglycemia in type i diabetic patients. Med Klin. 1991;86(11):551–4.
98. Kerr D, Macdonald IA, Heller SR, Tattersall RB. Alcohol causes hypoglycaemic unawareness in healthy volunteers and patients with type 1 (insulin-dependent) diabetes. Diabetologia. 1990;33(4):216–21.
99. Umpierrez GE, Kelly JP, Navarrete JE, Casals MM, Kitabchi AE. Hyperglycemic crises in urban blacks. Arch Intern Med. 1997;157(6):669–75.
100. Warner EA, Greene GS, Buchsbaum MS, Cooper DS, Robinson BE. Diabetic ketoacidosis associated with cocaine use. Arch Intern Med. 1998;158(16):1799–802.
101. Lawrence JM, Contreras R, Chen W, Sacks DA. Trends in the prevalence of preexisting diabetes and gestational diabetes mellitus among a racially/ethnically diverse population of pregnant women, 1999–2005. Diabetes Care. 2008;31(5):899–904.
102. Vahratian A, Barber JS, Lawrence JM, Kim C. Family-planning practices among women with diabetes and overweight and obese women in the 2002 national survey for family growth. Diabetes Care. 2009;32(6):1026–31.
103. Schwarz EB, Sobota M, Charron-Prochownik D. Perceived access to contraception among adolescents with diabetes: barriers to preventing pregnancy complications. Diabetes Educ. 2010;36(3):489–94.
104. Kitzmiller JL, Buchanan TA, Kjos S, Combs CA, Ratner RE. Pre-conception care of diabetes, congenital malformations, and spontaneous abortions. Diabetes Care. 1996;19(5):514–41.
105. American Diabetes A. Preconception care of women with diabetes. Diabetes Care. 2004;27(Suppl 1):S76–8.
106. Charron-Prochownik D, Sereika SM, Wang SL, Hannan MF, Fischl AR, Stewart SH, et al. Reproductive health and preconception counseling awareness in adolescents with diabetes: what they don't know can hurt them. Diabetes Educ. 2006;32(2):235–42.
107. Scal P. Transition for youth with chronic conditions: primary care physicians' approaches. Pediatrics. 2002;110(6 Pt 2):1315–21.
108. Peyrot MF. Theory in behavioral diabetes research. Diabetes Care. 2001;24(10):1703–5.
109. Gary TL, Genkinger JM, Guallar E, Peyrot M, Brancati FL. Meta-analysis of randomized educational and behavioral interventions in type 2 diabetes. Diabetes Educ. 2003;29(3):488–501.
110. Mellinger DC. Preparing students with diabetes for life at college. Diabetes Care. 2003;26(9):2675–8.

Down Syndrome 10

Kristin M. Jensen and Peter D. Bulova

Case Presentations

Susan and Jonathan were each referred to the adult Down syndrome center for evaluation of a decline in skills and possible Alzheimer's type dementia.

Susan is a 33-year-old female with Down syndrome with a history of hypothyroidism and a ventricular septal defect repaired during early childhood. She completed high school and her post-high school transition program. Since then she has been employed by a clothing shop several days per week. She recently moved from her family home to a group home, as the health of her parents was failing. Since moving to the group home, Susan has shown little interest in leaving the house and has had a decline in productivity in her work at the clothing shop. Concurrently, she has had an increase in self-talking and compulsive behaviors, making piles of her belongings and refusing to throw out old magazines or papers. She is less social and spends more time in her room. Susan's parents remain involved in her life and visit her at the group home regularly.

Upon review of systems, Susan has had no changes in her medications, and her weight has been stable despite a slight decrease in her appetite. She has been sleeping more than normal without any complaints of snoring. Susan has no known conflicts with any of the staff or other residents in her group home or place of employment. During examination, her vital signs are within normal limits, body mass index (BMI) is 27. She is awake and alert, but rather withdrawn, frequently engaging in self-talk throughout the encounter from which she can be redirected. Neurologic examination is significant for 2+/4 deep tendon reflexes with mild hypotonia. There were no significant findings on the remainder of her examination.

Jonathan is a 52-year-old male with Down syndrome with a history of congenital heart disease, difficulty swallowing, and several previous bouts of aspiration pneumonia. He has been living in the same group home for the past 5 years. Over the past 6 months, Jonathan has shown a gradual decline in skills, with new issues of balance disturbance and recent urinary incontinence. He demonstrates persistent forgetfulness, often having trouble remembering previous skills such as how to set the table or brush his teeth. He was found to have a new tonic-clonic seizure

K.M. Jensen (✉)
Departments of Pediatrics and Internal Medicine, Adult and Child Consortium for Outcomes Research and Delivery Science, University of Colorado School of Medicine, 13199 E Montview Blvd, Suite 300, Mailstop F-443, Aurora, CO 80045, USA
e-mail: kristin.jensen@ucdenver.edu

P.D. Bulova
Department of Internal Medicine, General Internal Medicine, Montefiore Hospital, University of Pittsburgh Medical Center, 200 Lothrop Street, Pittsburgh, PA 15213, USA
e-mail: bulovapd@upmc.edu

M. Pilapil et al. (eds.), *Care of Adults with Chronic Childhood Conditions*,
DOI 10.1007/978-3-319-43827-6_10

5 months ago and is now on levetiracetam. He has had no further seizure episodes.

Upon examination, Jonathan is a frail, 52-year-old male with a 10-lb weight loss over the past year. He has difficulty ambulating without assistance. Jonathan cannot participate in answering questions from his provider as well as he did previously, and often responds with blank stares or non-specific phrases, such as "you know." Urinalysis and thyroid studies were normal. His neurologic examination was significant for slowed gait, prolonged time to rise from seated to standing position, and difficulty standing without holding onto his caregiver for support.

Case Discussion

Decline in Skills in Down Syndrome

While the case of Jonathan describes a common presentation of Alzheimer's dementia in an adult with Down syndrome, Susan's case is a "masquerader" of dementia—in this case, depression.

A great deal of attention is paid to the development of dementia in adults with Down syndrome. This is due to the fact that the pathogenesis of Alzheimer's dementia is linked to excess amyloid protein, the gene for which is found on chromosome 21 [1]. Despite the fact that autopsy specimens of adults with Down syndrome over age 35 years show neurofibrillary plaques and tangles [2], Alzheimer's dementia is a clinical diagnosis and does not develop universally in this population. Current estimates of the prevalence of Alzheimer's dementia among individuals with Down syndrome are 10 % in those ages 40–49 years, 20 % in those ages 50–60 years, and 40 % in those over 60 years of age. There are very few cases of true Alzheimer's dementia before age 40 years [3].

Because Alzheimer's dementia is a clinical diagnosis, most of the data used rely on the first-hand descriptions provided by caregivers, who tend to focus on patient behaviors that impact the caregivers. This can lead to an overestimation of the diagnosis when compared to results from direct assessment. Additionally, clinicians are predisposed to over-diagnose dementia, as the clinical diagnosis of dementia is difficult to make and the inevitability of dementia is presumed in adults with Down syndrome [4]. Traditional tools such as the mini-mental status exam are unreliable and unusable in nearly half of adults with Down syndrome [4]. There is a recent study using the Rapid Assessment for Developmental Disabilities (RADD)-2 questionnaire that has shown good sensitivity and specificity in identifying dementia and takes approximately 15 min to perform [5]. A dementia assessment must include a medical and psychiatric evaluation, as multiple conditions can mimic the decline in skills of Alzheimer's. One must assess emotional and motivational change in addition to memory changes.

There are distinguishing differences between the presentations of Alzheimer's dementia in those with Down syndrome compared to those without Down syndrome. The incidence of adult-onset seizure development is much higher in those with dementia and Down syndrome [6]. They often develop incontinence, sleep disturbance, apathy, gait changes, and personality changes [4]. At this time, the treatments available for adults with Down syndrome and dementia are mainly supportive. There are several Cochrane database reviews of medications for the treatment of dementia in adults with Down syndrome, none of which support their use [7–11]. The largest trial of pharmaceutical intervention used memantine, which showed no benefit and actually showed a trend toward worse behaviors in the treatment group [12]. Current recommendations focus on interventions to minimize caregiver burden, including respite care and creating an environment for the patient to maintain function.

The differential diagnosis of a decline in skills is complex and requires a comprehensive approach to care, as there are several masqueraders of dementia. The most common are psychiatric issues, including depression, anxiety, obsessive–compulsive disorder, adjustment disorder, attention deficit disorder, and psychosis [13]. There have been many patients referred for an evaluation of dementia who were later diagnosed with depression [14]. The differentiation between true Alzheimer's dementia and other causes is difficult as there are several overlapping causes of behavioral changes, such as urinary changes, mood changes, irritability, and decline in skills [15]. There is a description in the literature of "pseudo-dementia" in persons with Down syndrome, which resolves after starting an antidepressant [16]. The most common endocrine cause for a decline in skills is hypothyroidism [13], which is described later in this chapter. Therefore, the traditional workup of reversible causes of dementia in those without Down syndrome includes a thyroid-stimulating hormone (TSH). Additionally, a vitamin B12 level is also recommended. The other issues particular to Down syndrome and decline in skills include sensory impairment, urinary infections, menopause, seizure disorder, and obstructive sleep apnea [13].

In summary, the differential diagnosis for a decline in skills in an adult with Down syndrome is broad and includes dementia, depression, hypothyroidism, sleep apnea, hearing loss, vision loss, seizure disorder, infection, menopause, and developmental regression [17].

Background: Definition and Epidemiology

Occurring in 1 in 700 to 1 in 1000 live births, Down syndrome is the most common identifiable genetic cause of intellectual disability [18–20]. Due to dramatic improvements in clinical care during early childhood, nearly 90 % of persons with Down syndrome now survive to 20 years old with a median life expectancy in their mid-50s [21–29]. This is a dramatic improvement compared to their life expectancy of less than 10 years of age in the 1970s [21–29]. The World Health Organization (WHO) currently estimates 250,000 persons with Down syndrome in the United States [19]. Down syndrome is caused by extra material on chromosome 21, with 93–95 % of karyotypes displaying trisomy 21, 3–4 % having a translocation involving chromosome 21, and 1–3 % displaying mosaic trisomy 21 [30–32]. In addition to the risk of comorbidities discussed in this chapter, persons with Down syndrome are universally affected by moderate to severe intellectual disability, which may be less severe in persons with mosaic trisomy 21 [32]. With appropriate medical, social, and educational support, persons with Down syndrome can live long, fulfilling lives.

Special Issues in the Care of the Adult with Down Syndrome

Additional Neurologic and Behavioral Issues

While dementia is the most common neurologic condition in adults with Down syndrome (as discussed in the case), there are several other issues that adult providers should consider. Seizures are much more common than in the general population, with a bimodal distribution—usually occurring in childhood or after the third decade of life. Up to 84 % of adults with dementia develop seizures [33]. This is particularly important, as untreated seizures in the setting of dementia have been shown to hasten decline [34]. While there is an association between Down syndrome and Moyamoya disease as a cause of cerebrovascular events, this is still a rare finding [35]. Adults are at higher risk for strokes than the general population, and these can be ischemic, hemorrhagic, or cardio-embolic in etiology [36]. Adults are also found to have micro- and macro-hemorrhages in association with amyloid deposition [37].

Concurrent mental health conditions are common in persons with Down syndrome, particularly depression, anxiety, obsessive–compulsive tendencies, and behavioral issues [38, 39]. Mental illness can present with a decline in skills or urinary incontinence, which can be mislabeled as Alzheimer's dementia [39]. Depression can be triggered by a stressful life event, such as separation from a parent or a death in the family. As depression is often responsive to medical therapy in those with Down syndrome [40], differentiating it from dementia is vital. Recent epidemiologic data indicate that adolescents and young adults with Down syndrome have similar rates of anxiety (18 %) and depression (15 %) with lower rates of bipolar (4 %) and impulse control (20 %) disorders when compared to persons with other forms of intellectual disability in this age group [41]. Hyperactivity and impulsive behaviors have been observed in children with Down syndrome as young as 3 years of age [42]. These can be treated with both behavioral modifications and traditional attention deficit/hyperactivity disorder medications. In particular, persons with Down syndrome tend to thrive in systems incorporating routine and a stable environment, which is theorized to increase feelings of competence, reduce anxiety, and free up cognitive capacity [43]. There is evidence to suggest an increased prevalence of psychosis (35 %) in adolescents and young adults with Down syndrome compared to peers with other etiologies of intellectual disability [41]. This finding needs to be interpreted with caution, however, as it is quite common for persons with Down syndrome to engage in self-talk as a mechanism to guide problem solving or revisit previous conversations and activities, which can be unrelated to behavioral problems [41].

Individuals with Down syndrome have increased risk of concurrent autistic spectrum disorder compared to the general population, with estimated prevalence rates of 5–39 % [38, 44, 45]. However, many individuals with Down syndrome display symptoms of autism spectrum disorder without a true diagnosis, especially in those with more severe expressive language difficulties. Concurrent Down syndrome and autism spectrum disorder can be extremely difficult to treat, often requiring a specialist who works with adolescents and adults with special needs [38]. Medical therapies, behavioral management, maintenance of a stable environment, communication supports, and reduction of stressors are all accepted forms of therapy [38, 45].

Persons with Down syndrome are also at risk for a rare developmental regression during young adulthood involving rapid, atypical loss of previously acquired skills in activities of daily living, cognition, and socialization with an increase in maladaptive behaviors [46–48]. Clinical experience suggests this regression may develop in response to transitions, hormonal/menstrual changes, or significant life events [46], with early data suggesting a link between this condition and the pathogenesis of dementia later in life [48]. Given the rarity of this phenomenon, little evidence exists to recommend standard treatment modalities [46]. Evaluation of developmental regression in persons with Down syndrome should include all causes of loss of skills as discussed previously.

Cardiology

Congenital heart disease is present in 40–60 % of persons with Down syndrome [49–53]. The most common forms of congenital heart disease within Down syndrome are atrioventricular septal defects, atrial septal defects, and ventricular septal defects, followed by patent ductus arteriosus, coarctation of the aorta, tetralogy of Fallot, and other forms of congenital heart disease [53–55]. Previously, congenital heart disease was responsible for high mortality rates during early childhood in Down syndrome. Now, these lesions are routinely surgically corrected with similar 5-year survival rates to non-Down syndrome children with congenital heart disease [55, 56]. Older adult patients with Down syndrome and congenital heart disease were born in an era during which surgical repair for congenital heart disease was not universal [57]. Consequently, primary care providers may encounter patients with Eisenmenger syndrome due to their now-unrepairable defects [58]. Recently published data analyzing 10 years of a nationally representative sample of U.S. hospital admissions indicates increased inpatient mortality for adults with Down syndrome and congenital heart disease compared to adults with congenital heart disease without Down syndrome [59]. It is unclear whether this mortality difference results from differing approaches to the care of adults with Down syndrome currently versus long-term sequelae of differences in the care of their congenital heart disease during early childhood versus other causes. All persons with congenital heart disease should be followed by a cardiologist trained in the care of adults with congenital heart disease. Subsequent follow-up will be dictated by the nature of their lesion, repair status, and associated complications [50].

Outside of their congenital heart disease status, adults with Down syndrome are at risk for developing *acquired valve disease*, most commonly mitral valve prolapse followed by aortic regurgitation and tricuspid valve prolapse [53, 60, 61, 62]. In many cases, murmurs may not be detectable. Current evidence supports obtaining an echocardiogram for those who did not have one in childhood and for patients presenting with a new murmur or any clinical signs of heart failure [53]. Likewise, electrocardiograms should be obtained for any concerns of arrhythmia [63].

Down syndrome was previously believed to be protective against the development of *atherosclerosis* and subsequently ischemic heart disease or cerebrovascular accidents [64]. However, autopsy studies from the 1980s demonstrate similar levels of atherosclerosis in persons with Down syndrome compared to non-Down syndrome institutionalized peers [65]. More recent studies confirm increased adverse lipid profiles among individuals with Down syndrome as compared to their siblings [66]. Although the incidence of ischemic heart disease is lower in adults with Down syndrome compared to the general population, longitudinal population studies in Denmark, Sweden, and Australia report a higher prevalence than previously documented [36, 25, 67] at 6.9 % of the overall Down syndrome population [25] and 13.2 % of those >50 years of age [25]. Despite the aforementioned discussion on cardiac risk factors in Down syndrome, adults with Down syndrome tend to have decreased risks for hypertension, with blood pressure measurements averaging approximately 10 points lower than their age-matched peers [68].

Pulmonology

Due to both congenital malformations (e.g., pulmonary hypoplasia, laryngomalacia, hypotonia, pulmonary hypertension) and deficiencies in their innate and adaptive immunity, *respiratory illnesses* such as influenza, pneumonia, and aspiration pneumonia are common in persons with Down syndrome [69–72]. Many individuals with Down syndrome also experience recurrent wheeze that is thought to be related to airway malacia, generalized hypotonia, or recurrent gastroesophageal reflux disease (GERD), given often suboptimal responsiveness to traditional asthma medications [71, 73]. Pneumonia is the leading cause of hospital admission and the second leading cause of death in adults with Down syndrome, after congenital heart disease [25, 74, 75]. As the rate of death from congenital heart disease decreases in adults with Down syndrome, the proportion of deaths attributable to pneumonia increases with age [25]. Therefore, primary care providers should be vigilant in identifying and treating respiratory illnesses in persons with Down syndrome. Primary care providers should immunize adults with Down syndrome against influenza, pneumonia, and pertussis according to the current vaccine schedule published by Centers for Disease Control and Prevention [76].

Obstructive sleep apnea (OSA) is among the more common comorbidities in persons with Down syndrome, with estimated prevalence rates at 30–50 % during childhood and >90 % in adults [73, 77, 78, 79, 80, 81, 82, 83]. This increased risk of OSA in Down syndrome is multifactorial. Persons with Down syndrome have many physical attributes that predispose them to OSA including midface and maxillary hypoplasia, relative macroglossia, hypertrophy of the tonsils and adenoids, laryngomalacia, and generalized hypotonia [69, 73, 77, 78, 82]. Persons with Down syndrome also have increased risks for developing hypothyroidism and obesity, both of which are associated with OSA [73, 78]. Obstructive sleep apnea can present at any age in persons with Down syndrome, with symptoms such as snoring, fatigue, restless sleep, hyperactivity, behavioral or mood changes, decline in skills, daytime sleepiness, nocturnal gasping or choking episodes, or unusual sleep postures [73, 77, 84, 85]. The consequences of untreated OSA range from behavioral disturbances, decreased executive function, and learning difficulties

[73, 86] to neuronal changes in the brain, pulmonary hypertension, and right-sided heart failure [80, 87]. Overnight pulse oximetry has poor sensitivity to diagnose obstructive sleep apnea in Down syndrome, so providers should strongly consider formal polysomnography for diagnosis [73]. Treatment options range from traditional positive airway pressure modalities (CPAP or BiPAP), weight loss, or dental appliances to surgical interventions, such as tonsillectomy and adenoidectomy [73].

Gastroenterology

The primary issues of the gastrointestinal (GI) tract pertinent to adults with Down syndrome are celiac disease, dysphagia, and gastroesophageal reflux.

While routine screening for *celiac disease* in asymptomatic individuals is not recommended [49], one should be vigilant for signs and symptoms of the condition, as individuals with Down syndrome are greater than 6 times more likely than the general population to develop celiac disease [88]. In most cases, the presentation of celiac disease among those with Down syndrome is no different from that of the general population, with abdominal pain, diarrhea, and weight loss as the more common symptoms. In addition, celiac disease can present as new or challenging behavioral problems [49]. The only effective treatment is a gluten-free diet [89]. While the establishment of a restrictive diet can be difficult, it is generally well tolerated in most adults with Down syndrome.

Dysphagia is one of the most common conditions in adults with Down syndrome, especially in older adults. One study found the condition in more than 50 % of those over 50 years old, with increasing prevalence associated with advancing age [90]. This is of particular importance due to a high risk of aspiration. Dysphagia can also lead to malnutrition and dehydration [91]. This condition needs to be managed symptomatically with interventions ranging from dietary restrictions on easily aspirated foods, thickening liquids, strengthening exercises, and mealtime supervision to normalize eating rate. Many patients eat very quickly, which will increase the risk for aspiration [92].

Gastroesophageal reflux is also common, occurring in 20 % of patients over 50 years old [90]. The true prevalence of gastroesophageal reflux is likely underestimated, however, as it is often treated empirically. It can present as chest pain, involuntary weight loss, or a variety of behavioral changes.

Endocrinology

Hypothyroidism is among the more common comorbidities in persons with Down syndrome, presenting with fatigue, weight gain, decreased interest in activities, a decline in skills, cold intolerance, constipation, dry skin, and growth impairment [17, 51, 93, 94, 95]. Prevalence estimates for hypothyroidism range from 9 to 45 % of persons with Down syndrome of all ages [17, 51, 94, 95, 96, 97]. Moreover, 1–6 % of children with Down syndrome are born with congenital hypothyroidism [49, 98]. An additional 25–60 % of persons with Down syndrome demonstrate subclinical hypothyroidism [95], which can be transitory and does not definitively predict progression to clinical hypothyroidism [95, 98]. The risks for acquired hypothyroidism correlate with age in persons with Down syndrome, with onset of autoimmune thyroid disease starting in puberty and increasing with age [98, 99]. Thyroid antibodies (thyroid peroxidase [TPO] antibody, thyroglobulin antibody) are found in approximately one-third of persons with Down syndrome [98, 99]. Prior to age 12 years, hypothyroidism in persons with Down syndrome is thought to be due to poor development or hypoplasia of the thyroid gland [93, 99]. Untreated hypothyroidism can contribute to decreased cognitive function and is thus important to identify and treat. Current consensus guidelines recommend testing thyroid function at birth, 6 months, 12 months, and then annually throughout the lifespan for persons with Down syndrome [17, 49, 94, 100].

Hyperthyroidism is slightly more common in the Down syndrome population (0.65–3 %) than the general population but is still relatively uncommon [98, 101, 102]. This typically presents with heat intolerance, irritability, weight loss, tachycardia, and palpitations and appears to be the result of autoimmune thyroiditis [93, 98]. Autoimmune thyroiditis can have a fluctuating course in persons with Down syndrome between hypo- and hyperthyroidism [93]. Definitive therapy for hyperthyroidism is iodine-131 with surgical treatment reserved for patients requiring rapid resolution of thyrotoxicosis or for those with serious side effects from the anti-thyroid medications [98].

There is also an increased prevalence of *diabetes mellitus* (DM) among children and adults with Down syndrome compared to the general population [94, 100, 103, 104, 105, 106], with a higher predominance of type 1 diabetes than type 2 diabetes [107]. More typically, type 1 diabetes presents in a bimodal distribution during childhood, with peaks at less than 2 years old and again in early adolescence [108]. Reports from Denmark demonstrate a fourfold increase in the presence of Down syndrome in persons <20 years old with type 1 diabetes (0.38 %) compared to the prevalence of Down syndrome in the background Danish population [106]. Similarly, a Scottish study demonstrated a prevalence of type 1 DM in adults with Down syndrome ranging from 1.4 to 10.6 % [104]. Within a population-based study of persons with intellectual disability of all ages in Ireland, 23 % of those with type 1 diabetes and intellectual disabilities had Down syndrome, compared to 8 % of those with type 2 diabetes and intellectual disabilities [107]. There is additional evidence to suggest co-existing autoimmune disease with type 1 diabetes in persons with Down syndrome, with one study reporting 74 % with co-existing thyroid autoimmunity, 14 % with celiac disease, and 8 % with combined diabetes, thyroid autoimmunity, and celiac disease [108]. Overall, the literature suggests a slightly higher prevalence of diabetes mellitus in persons with Down syndrome (Type 1 > Type 2), with a younger age of onset than the general population [104–109]. Primary care providers should have a low threshold to screen for diabetes based on symptoms and risk factors.

Obesity is widespread among persons with intellectual disabilities but disproportionately affects more persons with Down syndrome compared to other causes of intellectual disability [94, 110, 111, 112, 113]. It has been reported that 25–55 % of persons with Down syndrome are overweight with roughly another one-third meeting criteria for obesity [110, 112, 113, 114]. Women with Down syndrome tend to have slightly higher rates of overweight and obesity than men [110, 115]. Additionally, overweight and obesity tend to be associated with milder forms of intellectual disability [110, 115]. Likely reasons for the high prevalence of obesity within Down syndrome include lower levels of physical activity [116], lower resting metabolic rate [115, 117], and poor nutritional choices [114], especially among the more independent and ambulatory populations [114]. Compared to non-Down syndrome peers, persons with Down syndrome tend to have higher fat and lower lean mass in their body composition, making traditional measurements of adiposity (e.g., BMI) less helpful [113, 118, 119]. Due to differences such as limb length, those with Down syndrome have a different distribution of body mass. One can use the 2015 growth charts, recently published in *Pediatrics,* that continue to age 20 as a good approximation for adults [120]. As with the non-Down syndrome population, overweight and obesity increase the risk of musculoskeletal complications, insulin resistance, and overall mortality in persons with Down syndrome [113, 121, 122, 123]. However, overweight and obesity in persons with Down syndrome do not seem to translate into metabolic syndrome [122]. To combat overweight and obesity in Down syndrome, experts have found the greatest success using a multidisciplinary approach involving physical exercise, nutrition counseling, caloric restriction, and a comprehensive behavioral management program involving the patient's family [114, 124, 125]. While regular exercise in moderate intervals does improve muscle strength and core balance in the Down syndrome population, persons with Down syndrome appear to need longer training durations (45–60 min) to improve their overall aerobic fitness [124].

Musculoskeletal

The issues of primary concern in adults with Down syndrome are osteoporosis, osteoarthritis, and rarely atlantoaxial instability. The classic skeletal association with Down syndrome is atlantoaxial instability; however, this is typically more of a concern with children than adults. The more common condition in the spine of adults with Down syndrome is osteoarthritis. One study showed a prevalence of osteoarthritis of the cervical spine to be 64 % in people with Down syndrome between the ages of 21 and 60 years. In comparison, atlantoaxial instability was found in only 8 % of this population [126]. In addition, while atlantoaxial instability may be present on a radiologic study, it does not mean that subluxation and clinical symptoms will follow. It is estimated that 2 % of people with Down syndrome are at risk for spinal cord compression from atlantoaxial instability [127]. Although rare, it is still prudent to evaluate for atlantoaxial instability in adults with new neurologic symptoms, as prompt intervention is necessary. Symptoms can vary, with presentations ranging from cervical pain, torticollis, hyperreflexia, ataxia, quadriparesis, syncope, vertigo, and change in handedness to ear pain [94, 100, 128, 129, 130, 131, 132, 133, 134, 135, 136, 137]. One recent review estimated symptom prevalence for atlantoaxial dislocation as follows: 50 % presented with neck pain or restriction of neck movement, 70 % with numbness and/or weakness, and 90 % presented with pyramidal signs [138]. Neurosurgical evaluation would be recommended prior to any athletic participation with the aforementioned symptoms of atlantoaxial dislocation. Providers should confirm the cervical spine is in neutral position prior to any anesthesia, surgical, or radiographic procedures. Otherwise, screening for atlantoaxial instability is recommended during childhood, with neurologic changes, and for participation in the Special Olympics [131].

Osteoporosis is common in Down syndrome. In one study, 43 % of adults over 50 were found to have this condition [90]. Down syndrome is an independent risk factor for low bone mineral density [139–141], with the incidence of reported fracture as high as 55 % (long bones) or 30 % (vertebral bodies) in adults with Down syndrome over 50 years old [17, 142, 143]. Persons with Down syndrome have multiple risk factors for lower bone integrity due to decreased muscle tone/hypermobility leading to decreased physical activity and increased risk of joint dislocation, delayed puberty, hormonal factors, thyroid abnormalities, epilepsy, high risk medication use, low intake of calcium, vitamin D insufficiency, and autoimmune diseases [139, 144, 145]. In addition, bone formation and resorption were suppressed in a study of a cohort of adults with Down syndrome compared to controls, which suggests a Down syndrome-specific mechanism responsible for decreased bone mineral density [143]. Persons with Down syndrome should be regularly screened for risk factors of low bone mineral density, including annual thyroid function tests and intermittent screening for celiac disease, while addressing high risk medication use, ensuring adequate levels of calcium and vitamin D, along with increased physical activity [139, 144]. Data is not yet available to guide evidence-based preventive therapeutic interventions among young adults with Down syndrome [139]. Given the increased risk of osteoporotic fractures in adults with Down syndrome, general consensus recommends screening adults for osteoporosis starting in their 40s or with their first fracture if earlier than 40 years old [17]. A study in children with Down syndrome ages 7–12 years demonstrated that weight-bearing exercise and calcium intake have a synergistic effect on femoral neck bone mineral density [146]. This suggests that prevention plays an important role.

Reproductive Health

Reproductive health for persons with Down syndrome is an area that is often poorly addressed by healthcare providers [147]. Both men and women with Down syndrome can experience delays in puberty and have decreased fertility compared to the general population [148–151].

Women with Down syndrome can have regular ovulatory menstrual cycles, although there is evidence to suggest ovarian hypoplasia and gonadal dysfunction with decreased follicular growth, decreased number of oocytes, and decreased ovarian sensitivity to follicle-stimulating hormone (FSH) [151, 152]. Women with Down syndrome typically go through menopause at younger ages than women with other forms of intellectual disability (median reported age of menopause in Down syndrome: 47.1 years) [147, 153]. However, many women with Down syndrome are able to conceive and bear children [148, 149, 154]. Approximately, 50 % of their children will have Down syndrome, and these children are at increased risk for other congenital malformations [155].

Men with Down syndrome are typically considered sterile, with evidence for germ cell hypoplasia demonstrated by elevated luteinizing hormone (LH) and FSH hormone levels, lower testosterone levels, and smaller testicular volume [152, 156]. However, there have been case reports of children being fathered by men with complete trisomy 21 [157]. Additionally, persons with intellectual disability, such as Down syndrome, are at increased risk for sexual exploitation and abuse [158]. Consequently, it is important to educate persons with Down syndrome about their reproductive capacity, to assess their sexual practices and/or desires, to screen for abuse, and to address these concerns clinically [158]. Primary care providers should consider contraceptive methods to prevent undesired pregnancy and should routinely offer age-, gender-, and risk factor appropriate reproductive health screenings in a disability-friendly manner [17, 158].

Visual and Hearing Issues

The disability caused by people with Down syndrome with ophthalmologic pathology cannot be underestimated. Especially in adults who often have compromised hearing and balance issues, poor vision can manifest with an Alzheimer's-like picture of withdrawal from social situations and a decline in skills. Many patients will not complain of visual loss, and will instead only exhibit behavioral changes. This issue and the high prevalence of visual change makes routine screening a necessity. While there is not unanimous consensus of the frequency of screening, our review of the literature suggests a routine ophthalmologic exam every 2 years in adults [17].

All structures of the eye are at increased risk of abnormalities: the cornea, retina, iris, and lens as well as the eyelid. The prevalence is much higher in those with more severe cognitive limitations. The overall incidence of some vision compromise is as high as 75 % in people 30 years and older [159]. Of note, those with mosaic Down syndrome are also at significantly increased risk for structural abnormalities [160]. The most common abnormalities in adults are cataracts, strabismus, refractive errors, and presbyopia, all of which are more common compared to the general population. In one large study, 42 % of 455 adults with Down syndrome were found to have cataracts, with incidences of 37.8 % in the 40–49 year age range and 100 % in the 70–79 year age range [159]. This is of particular significance, as many physicians are wary of recommending cataract surgery for this population. In actuality, the benefits of surgery are mixed. The surgical outcomes are generally good, but the patients' visual abilities often remained compromised, due to other ocular comorbidities [161].

Caring for the ophthalmologic issues in adults with Down syndrome is often challenging. Visual impairments in those with intellectual disabilities can lead to behavioral changes such as self-injurious behavior. This may manifest as self-stimulatory behaviors such as eye poking/pressing or staring into bright lights. Finding an ophthalmic specialist experienced with intellectual disabilities can be invaluable as problems with cooperation with the exam is common and creative solutions with more engaging visual tests may be necessary. There are several forms of testing that have been successful in these settings [162].

According to one source, approximately 40–77 % of adults with Down syndrome have disabling hearing loss [163]. The incidence of hearing loss increases sharply after age 40. It is at this point when the incidence differs dramatically from the general population [29]. The importance of recognizing and treating sensory impairments is critical, as they can present as a decline in skills, thereby being misdiagnosed as dementia, as well as diminished quality of life.

Hematology–Oncology

Persons with Down syndrome have increased risks for hematologic conditions, ranging from idiopathic macrocytosis and mild polycythemia [164] to myelodysplastic syndrome [165] to actual leukemias [67, 166, 167]. Studies show a high frequency of leukopenia, idiopathic macrocytosis, and mild polycythemia in the Down syndrome population, often without underlying disease [164]. Elevations in mean corpuscular volume (MCV) are frequently found in infants with Down syndrome and can persist throughout their lives [168]. In one observational study, approximately two-thirds of persons with Down syndrome had an elevated mean corpuscular volume and one-third had mild leukopenia [168]. Although myelodysplastic syndrome is often transient in individuals with Down syndrome, this can progress to leukemia and/or marrow failure in both children and adults [168, 169].

Leukemia in Down syndrome is predominantly found in the pediatric population, with >90 % of cases occurring before age 20 years [123, 165]. Acute myeloid leukemia and acute lymphoblastic leukemia seem to occur with equal frequencies within the Down syndrome population [167]. Although leukemia in Down syndrome is generally associated with a poor prognosis [170], childhood acute megakaryoblastic leukemia is unusually sensitive to chemotherapy with excellent outcomes [165, 171].

Persons with Down syndrome have a decreased—but not zero—risk of developing most solid tumors compared to the general population [67, 167]. However, combined analyses of nearly 30 years of cancer registry data from Denmark and Sweden observed a modest increased risk of liver, testicular, and male penile cancers among adults with Down syndrome compared to non-Down syndrome rates in these countries [67]. These same registries documented the presence of solid tumor neoplasms in persons with Down syndrome in numerous organ systems, including cancers of the colon, testes, breast, liver, penis, stomach, brain, endometrium, parathyroid, kidney, and small intestine [67]. There have been additional case reports of male breast cancer in adults with Down syndrome [172, 173].

Primary care providers of adults with Down syndrome should retain a high index of suspicion for underlying hematologic or solid tumor neoplasms. Solid tumor screening should be dictated by clinical symptoms, family history, and risk factors. Providers should follow complete blood counts in situations that would raise one's suspicions for hematologic processes, such as easy bruising, petechiae, fatigue, or change in feeding patterns, and refer to specialty providers as appropriate [49, 166].

Conclusion

While every person with Down syndrome is unique, there are several issues that are common throughout the population ("Appendix"). It is important to have a systematic approach to both health maintenance and active medical issues, as multiple organ systems can be involved. One must take a comprehensive approach to the diagnosis of decline in skills, paying particular attention to mental health issues. While all people with Down syndrome may develop amyloid deposition in the brain, not all will develop clinical dementia. In addition, a medical workup is warranted for unexplained behavioral changes, as common conditions such as hypothyroidism, sleep apnea, and sensory changes may present this way.

Appendix

Suggested Reading List

- Bull MJ. Health supervision for children with Down syndrome. Pediatrics. 2011;128 (2):393–406.
- Jensen KM, Bulova PD. Managing the care of adults with Down syndrome. BMJ. 2014;349: g5596.
- Smith DS. Health care management of adults with Down syndrome. Am Fam Physician. 2001;64(6):1031–8.

Down syndrome (DS) condition fact sheet

Definition	Down syndrome is a genetic condition resulting from triplication of all or a portion of chromosome 21 (Trisomy 21). Down syndrome is characterized by • Intellectual disability, ranging from mild to profound • Common physical findings include hypotonia, epicanthal folds, flat nasal bridge, upward-slanting palpebral fissures, high arched palate, narrow ear canals, short stature, single transverse palmar crease, and wide-spacing between the first and second toes Persons with Down syndrome have increased risks for congenital and acquired conditions involving most organ systems as described below
Epidemiology	In the United States, Down syndrome occurs in 1/700–1/1000 live births, affecting approximately 250,000 persons Karyotypes for persons with Down syndrome are as follows: • 93–95 % of persons with Down syndrome have complete trisomy 21 •3–4 % have a chromosomal translocation involving chromosome 21 •1–3 % have mosaic trisomy 21
Special considerations	In addition to intellectual and developmental disabilities, adults with Down syndrome have high rates of comorbid physical and mental health conditions, including • Congenital heart disease • Obesity • Hypothyroidism • Obstructive sleep apnea • Hearing abnormalities • Behavioral/mental health disorders • Vision abnormalities • Acquired cardiac valve disease • Gastroesophageal reflux • Cervical spinal instability • Celiac disease Adults with Down syndrome also experience accelerated aging, which can involve • Early Dementia • Osteoarthritis • Osteoporosis • Dysphagia
Recommended Screening	In addition to appropriate age and gender primary health screenings, we recommend the following screenings for adults with Down syndrome: Yearly: • Hypothyroidism • Obesity Every 1–2 years: • Hearing • Vision As directed by comorbidities, risk factors, and clinical presentation: • Echocardiogram • Cervical spine imaging • Sleep study • Celiac disease screening labs • Bone densitometry

- Steingass KJ, Chicoine B, McGuire D, Roizen NJ. Developmental disabilities grown up: Down syndrome. J Dev Behav Pediatr. 2011;32(7):548–58.

Patient/Caregiver Resources

- The ARC: http://www.thearc.org/
- Canadian Down Syndrome Society: http://www.cdss.ca/
- National Down Syndrome Congress: https://www.ndsccenter.org/
- National Down Syndrome Society: http://www.ndss.org/
- DS-Connect: https://dsconnect.nih.gov/
- University of Pittsburgh, Down Syndrome Center: http://www.chp.edu/our-services/down-syndrome/online-resources
- Down Syndrome Education International: https://www.dseinternational.org/en-us/
- Alzheimer's and Down Syndrome: http://alzheimers.gov/down_syndrome.html

Medical Providers

- American Academy of Developmental Medicine and Dentistry: http://aadmd.org/
- Down Syndrome Australia: http://www.downsyndrome.org.au/
- Down Syndrome Medical Interest Group of the United Kingdom & Ireland: http://www.dsmig.org.uk/
- Down Syndrome Medical Interest Group—USA: http://dsmig-usa.wildapricot.org/
- Vanderbilt University: Health Watch Table—Down syndrome: http://vkc.mc.vanderbilt.edu/etoolkit/physical-health/health-watch-tables-2/down-syndrome/

References

1. Zigman WB, Devenny DA, Krinsky-McHale SJ, Jenkins EC, Urv TK, Wegiel J, et al. Alzheimer's disease in adults with Down syndrome. Int Rev Res Ment Retard. 2008;36:103–45.
2. Lott IT, Head E. Alzheimer disease and Down syndrome: factors in pathogenesis. Neurobiol Aging. 2005;26(3):383–9.
3. Livingston G, Strydom A. Improving Alzheimer's disease outcomes in Down's syndrome. Lancet. 2012;379(9815):498–500.
4. Nieuwenhuis-Mark RE. Diagnosing Alzheimer's dementia in Down syndrome: problems and possible solutions. Res Dev Disabil. 2009;30(5):827–38.
5. Walsh DM, Doran E, Silverman W, Tournay A, Movsesyan N, Lott IT. Rapid assessment of cognitive function in down syndrome across intellectual level and dementia status. J Intellect Disabil Res. 2015;59(11):1071–9.
6. Menendez M. Down syndrome, Alzheimer's disease and seizures. Brain Dev. 2005;27(4):246–52.
7. Mohan M, Bennett C, Carpenter PK. Memantine for dementia in people with Down syndrome. Cochrane Database Syst Rev. 2009;1:CD007657.
8. Mohan M, Bennett C, Carpenter PK. Galantamine for dementia in people with Down syndrome. Cochrane Database Syst Rev. 2009;1:CD007656.
9. Mohan M, Bennett C, Carpenter PK. Rivastigmine for dementia in people with Down syndrome. Cochrane Database Syst Rev. 2009;1:CD007658.
10. Mohan M, Carpenter PK, Bennett C. Donepezil for dementia in people with Down syndrome. Cochrane Database Syst Rev. 2009;1:CD007178.
11. Livingstone N, Hanratty J, McShane R, Macdonald G. Pharmacological interventions for cognitive decline in people with Down syndrome. Cochrane Database Syst Rev. 2015;10:CD011546.
12. Hanney M, Prasher V, Williams N, Jones EL, Aarsland D, Corbett A, et al. Memantine for dementia in adults older than 40 years with Down's syndrome (MEADOWS): a randomised, double-blind, placebo-controlled trial. Lancet. 2012;379(9815):528–36.
13. Chicoine B, McGuire D, Rubin SS. Specialty clinic perspectives. In: Janicki MP, Dalton AJ, editors. Dementia, aging, and intellectual disabilities: a handbook. London: Routledge; 1999.
14. Warren AC, Holroyd S, Folstein MF. Major depression in Down's syndrome. Br J Psychiatry. 1989;155:202–5.
15. Burt DB. Dementia and depression. In: Janicki MP, Dalton AJ, editors. Dementia, aging, and intellectual disabilities: a handbook. London: Routledge; 1999.
16. Tsiouris JA, Patti PJ. Drug treatment of depression associated with dementia or presented as 'pseudodementia' in older adults with Down syndrome. J Appl Res Intellect. 1997;10(4):312–22.
17. Jensen KM, Bulova PD. Managing the care of adults with Down's syndrome. BMJ. 2014;349:g5596.
18. Centers for Disease Control and Prevention. Data and statistics: occurence of down syndrome [updated October 21, 2014; October 12, 2015]. http://www.cdc.gov/ncbddd/birthdefects/downsyndrome/data.html.

19. World Health Organization. Genes and human disease 2012 [April 9, 2012]. http://www.who.int/genomics/public/geneticdiseases/en/print.html.
20. Parker SE, Mai CT, Canfield MA, Rickard R, Wang Y, Meyer RE, et al. Updated national birth prevalence estimates for selected birth defects in the United States, 2004–2006. Birth Defects Res A. 2010;88(12):1008–16.
21. Lose EJ, Robin NH. Caring for adults with pediatric genetic diseases: a growing need. Curr Opin Pediatr. 2007;19(6):611–2.
22. Centers for Disease Control and Prevention. Racial disparities in median age at death of persons with Down syndrome—United States, 1968–1997. MMWR Morb Mortal Wkly Rep. 2001;50(22):463–5.
23. Glasson EJ, Sullivan SG, Hussain R, Petterson BA, Montgomery PD, Bittles AH. The changing survival profile of people with Down's syndrome: implications for genetic counselling. Clin Genet. 2002;62(5):390–3.
24. Presson AP, Partyka G, Jensen KM, Devine OJ, Rasmussen SA, McCabe LL, et al. Current estimate of down syndrome population prevalence in the United States. J Pediatr. 2013 Oct;163(4):1163–8. doi: 10.1016/j.jpeds.2013.06.013. Accessed 23 Jul 2013.
25. Englund A, Jonsson B, Zander CS, Gustafsson J, Anneren G. Changes in mortality and causes of death in the Swedish Down syndrome population. Am J Med Genet A. 2013;161A(4):642–9.
26. Zhu JL, Hasle H, Correa A, Schendel D, Friedman JM, Olsen J, et al. Survival among people with Down syndrome: a nationwide population-based study in Denmark. Genet Med. 2013;15(1):64–9.
27. Wu J, Morris JK. The population prevalence of Down's syndrome in England and Wales in 2011. Eur J Hum Genet. 2013;21(9):1016–9.
28. Kucik JE, Shin M, Siffel C, Marengo L, Correa A, Congenital Anomaly Multistate P, et al. Trends in survival among children with Down syndrome in 10 regions of the United States. Pediatrics. 2013;131(1):e27–36.
29. Glasson EJ, Dye DE, Bittles AH. The triple challenges associated with age-related comorbidities in Down syndrome. J Intellect Disabil Res. 2014;58(4):393–8.
30. Mutton D, Alberman E, Hook EB. Cytogenetic and epidemiological findings in Down syndrome, England and Wales 1989 to 1993. National Down Syndrome Cytogenetic Register and the Association of Clinical Cytogeneticists. J Med Genet. 1996;33(5):387–94.
31. Mulcahy MT. Down's syndrome in Western Australia: cytogenetics and incidence. Hum Genet. 1979;48(1):67–72.
32. Bittles AH, Glasson EJ. Clinical, social, and ethical implications of changing life expectancy in Down syndrome. Dev Med Child Neurol. 2004;46(4):282–6.
33. Lott IT. Neurological phenotypes for Down syndrome across the life span. Prog Brain Res. 2012;197:101–21.
34. Lott IT, Doran E, Nguyen VQ, Tournay A, Movsesyan N, Gillen DL. Down syndrome and dementia: seizures and cognitive decline. J Alzheimer's Dis. 2012;29(1):177–85.
35. Hwang SW, Jea A. A review of the neurological and neurosurgical implications of Down syndrome in children. Clin Pediatr (Phila). 2013;52(9):845–56.
36. Sobey CG, Judkins CP, Sundararajan V, Phan TG, Drummond GR, Srikanth VK. Risk of major cardiovascular events in people with Down syndrome. PLoS ONE. 2015;10(9):e0137093.
37. Wilcock DM, Schmitt FA, Head E. Cerebrovascular contributions to aging and Alzheimer's disease in Down syndrome. Biochim Biophys Acta. 2016 May;1862(5):909–14. doi: 10.1016/j.bbadis.2015.11.007. Accessed 26 Nov 2015.
38. Capone G, Goyal P, Ares W, Lannigan E. Neurobehavioral disorders in children, adolescents, and young adults with Down syndrome. Am J Med Genet C Semin Med Genet. 2006;142C(3):158–72.
39. Mantry D, Cooper SA, Smiley E, Morrison J, Allan L, Williamson A, et al. The prevalence and incidence of mental ill-health in adults with Down syndrome. J Intellect Disabil Res. 2008;52(Pt 2):141–55.
40. Walker JC, Dosen A, Buitelaar JK, Janzing JG. Depression in Down syndrome: a review of the literature. Res Dev Disabil. 2011;32(5):1432–40.
41. Dykens EM, Shah B, Davis B, Baker C, Fife T, Fitzpatrick J. Psychiatric disorders in adolescents and young adults with Down syndrome and other intellectual disabilities. J Neurodev Disord. 2015;7(1):9.
42. Capone GT, Brecher L, Bay M. Guanfacine Use in Children With Down Syndrome and Comorbid Attention-Deficit Hyperactivity Disorder (ADHD) With Disruptive Behaviors. J Child Neurol. 2016 Jul; 31(8):957–64. doi: 10.1177/0883073816634854. Accessed 2 Mar 2016.
43. Glenn S, Cunningham C, Nananidou A, Prasher V, Glenholmes P. Routinised and compulsive-like behaviours in individuals with Down syndrome. J Intellect Disabil Res. 2015;59(11):1061–70.
44. Lott IT, Dierssen M. Cognitive deficits and associated neurological complications in individuals with Down's syndrome. Lancet Neurol. 2010;9(6):623–33.
45. Channell MM, Phillips BA, Loveall SJ, Conners FA, Bussanich PM, Klinger LG. Patterns of autism spectrum symptomatology in individuals with Down syndrome without comorbid autism spectrum disorder. J Neurodev Disord. 2015;7(1):5.

46. Devenny D, Matthews A. Regression: atypical loss of attained functioning in children and adolescents with down syndrome. In: Hodapp RM, editor. International review of research in developmental disabilities. Oxford: Academic Press; 2011. p. 233–64.
47. Prasher VP. Disintegrative syndrome in young adults. Ir J Psychol Med. 2002;19(3):101.
48. Tamasaki A, Saito Y, Ueda R, Ohno K, Yokoyama K, Satake T, et al. Effects of donepezil and serotonin reuptake inhibitor on acute regression during adolescence in Down syndrome. Brain Dev. 2016;38(1):113–7.
49. Bull MJ. Health supervision for children with down syndrome. Pediatrics. 2011;128(2):393–406.
50. Warnes CA, Liberthson R, Danielson GK, Dore A, Harris L, Hoffman JI, et al. Task force 1: the changing profile of congenital heart disease in adult life. J Am Coll Cardiol. 2001;37(5):1170–5.
51. Maatta T, Maatta J, Tervo-Maatta T, Taanila A, Kaski M, Iivanainen M. Healthcare and guidelines: a population-based survey of recorded medical problems and health surveillance for people with Down syndrome. J Intellect Dev Disabil. 2011;36(2):118–26.
52. Tan M, Xu C, Sim SK, Seow AL, Tan TH, Quek SC. Types and distribution of congenital heart defects associated with trisomy 21 in Singapore. J Paediatr Child Health. 2013;49(3):223–7.
53. Lin AE, Basson CT, Goldmuntz E, Magoulas PL, McDermott DA, McDonald-McGinn DM, et al. Adults with genetic syndromes and cardiovascular abnormalities: clinical history and management. Genet Med. 2008;10(7):469–94.
54. Stoll C, Dott B, Alembik Y, Roth MP. Associated congenital anomalies among cases with Down syndrome. Eur J Med Genet. 2015 Dec;58(12):674–80. doi: 10.1016/j.ejmg.2015.11.003. Accessed 11 Nov 2015.
55. Ko JM. Genetic Syndromes associated with congenital heart disease. Korean Circ J. 2015;45(5):357–61.
56. Pierpont ME, Basson CT, Benson DW Jr, Gelb BD, Giglia TM, Goldmuntz E, et al. Genetic basis for congenital heart defects: current knowledge: a scientific statement from the American Heart Association Congenital Cardiac Defects Committee, Council on Cardiovascular Disease in the Young: endorsed by the American Academy of Pediatrics. Circulation. 2007;115(23):3015–38.
57. Champagne CR, Lewis M, Gilchrist DM. Should we mend their broken hearts? The history of cardiac repairs in children with Down syndrome. Pediatrics. 2014;134(6):1048–50.
58. Diller GP, Alonso-Gonzalez R, Kempny A, Dimopoulos K, Inuzuka R, Giannakoulas G, et al. B-type natriuretic peptide concentrations in contemporary Eisenmenger syndrome patients: predictive value and response to disease targeting therapy. Heart. 2012;98(9):736–42.
59. Baraona F, Gurvitz M, Landzberg MJ, Opotowsky AR. Hospitalizations and mortality in the United States for adults with Down syndrome and congenital heart disease. Am J Cardiol. 2013;111(7):1046–51.
60. Geggel RL, O'Brien JE, Feingold M. Development of valve dysfunction in adolescents and young adults with Down syndrome and no known congenital heart disease. J Pediatr. 1993;122(5 Pt 1):821–3.
61. Goldhaber SZ, Brown WD, Sutton MG. High frequency of mitral valve prolapse and aortic regurgitation among asymptomatic adults with Down's syndrome. JAMA. 1987;258(13):1793–5.
62. Goldhaber SZ, Rubin IL, Brown W, Robertson N, Stubblefield F, Sloss LJ. Valvular heart disease (aortic regurgitation and mitral valve prolapse) among institutionalized adults with Down's syndrome. Am J Cardiol. 1986;57(4):278–81.
63. Majdalany DS, Burkhart HM, Connolly HM, Abel MD, Dearani JA, Warnes CA, et al. Adults with Down syndrome: safety and long-term outcome of cardiac operation. Congenit Heart Dis. 2010;5(1):38–43.
64. Murdoch JC, Rodger JC, Rao SS, Fletcher CD, Dunnigan MG. Down's syndrome: an atheroma-free model? Br Med J. 1977;2(6081):226–8.
65. Chaney RH. Neurogenic atherosclerosis in mentally retarded persons. J Ment Defic Res. 1987;31(Pt 3):235–40.
66. Adelekan T, Magge S, Shults J, Stallings V, Stettler N. Lipid profiles of children with Down syndrome compared with their siblings. Pediatrics. 2012;129(6):e1382–7.
67. Hill DA, Gridley G, Cnattingius S, Mellemkjaer L, Linet M, Adami HO, et al. Mortality and cancer incidence among individuals with Down syndrome. Arch Intern Med. 2003;163(6):705–11.
68. Rodrigues AN, Coelho LC, Goncalves WL, Gouvea SA, Vasconcellos MJ, Cunha RS, et al. Stiffness of the large arteries in individuals with and without Down syndrome. Vasc Health Risk Manag. 2011;7:375–81.
69. McDowell KM, Craven DI. Pulmonary complications of Down syndrome during childhood. J Pediatr. 2011;158(2):319–25.
70. Ram G, Chinen J. Infections and immunodeficiency in Down syndrome. Clin Exp Immunol. 2011;164(1):9–16.
71. Weijerman ME, Brand PL, van Furth MA, Broers CJ, Gemke RJ. Recurrent wheeze in children with Down syndrome: is it asthma? Acta Paediatr. 2011;100(11):e194–7.
72. Broers CJ, Gemke RJ, Weijerman ME, Kuik DJ, van Hoogstraten IM, van Furth AM. Frequency of lower respiratory tract infections in relation to adaptive immunity in children with Down syndrome compared to their healthy siblings. Acta Paediatr. 2012;101(8):862–7.
73. Lal C, White DR, Joseph JE, van Bakergem K, LaRosa A. Sleep-disordered breathing in Down syndrome. Chest. 2015;147(2):570–9.

74. Tenenbaum A, Chavkin M, Wexler ID, Korem M, Merrick J. Morbidity and hospitalizations of adults with Down syndrome. Res Dev Disabil. 2012;33 (2):435–41.
75. Bittles AH, Bower C, Hussain R, Glasson EJ. The four ages of Down syndrome. Eur J Public Health. 2007;17(2):221–5.
76. Centers for Disease Control and Prevention. Recommended adult immunization schedule—United States, 2014 [February 27, 2014]. http://www.cdc.gov/vaccines/schedules/hcp/imz/adult.html.
77. Ono J, Chishaki A, Ohkusa T, Sawatari H, Nishizaka M, Ando S. Obstructive sleep apnea-related symptoms in Japanese people with Down syndrome. Nurs Health Sci. 2015;17(4):420–5.
78. Trois MS, Capone GT, Lutz JA, Melendres MC, Schwartz AR, Collop NA, et al. Obstructive sleep apnea in adults with Down syndrome. J Clin Sleep Med. 2009;5(4):317–23.
79. Shott SR. Down syndrome: common otolaryngologic manifestations. Am J Med Genet C Semin Med Genet. 2006;142C(3):131–40.
80. Marcus CL, Keens TG, Bautista DB, von Pechmann WS, Ward SL. Obstructive sleep apnea in children with Down syndrome. Pediatrics. 1991;88 (1):132–9.
81. de Miguel-Diez J, Villa-Asensi JR, Alvarez-Sala JL. Prevalence of sleep-disordered breathing in children with Down syndrome: polygraphic findings in 108 children. Sleep. 2003;26(8):1006–9.
82. Pandit C, Fitzgerald DA. Respiratory problems in children with Down syndrome. J Paediatr Child Health. 2012;48(3):E147–52.
83. Rosen D. Management of obstructive sleep apnea associated with Down syndrome and other craniofacial dysmorphologies. Curr Opin Pulm Med. 2011;17(6):431–6.
84. Capone GT, Aidikoff JM, Taylor K, Rykiel N. Adolescents and young adults with Down syndrome presenting to a medical clinic with depression: co-morbid obstructive sleep apnea. Am J Med Genet Part A. 2013;161(9):2188–96.
85. Myers KA, Mrkobrada M, Simel DL. Does this patient have obstructive sleep apnea? The rational clinical examination systematic review. JAMA. 2013;310(7):731–41.
86. Breslin J, Spano G, Bootzin R, Anand P, Nadel L, Edgin J. Obstructive sleep apnea syndrome and cognition in Down syndrome. Dev Med Child Neurol. 2014;56(7):657–64.
87. Halbower AC, Degaonkar M, Barker PB, Earley CJ, Marcus CL, Smith PL, et al. Childhood obstructive sleep apnea associates with neuropsychological deficits and neuronal brain injury. PLoS Med. 2006;3(8):e301.
88. Marild K, Stephansson O, Grahnquist L, Cnattingius S, Soderman G, Ludvigsson JF. Down syndrome is associated with elevated risk of celiac disease: A nationwide case–control study. J Pediatr. 2013;163(1):237–42.
89. Mooney PD, Hadjivassiliou M, Sanders DS. Coeliac disease. BMJ. 2014;348:g1561.
90. Hermans H, Evenhuis HM. Multimorbidity in older adults with intellectual disabilities. Res Dev Disabil. 2014;35(4):776–83.
91. Lazenby T. The impact of aging on eating, drinking, and swallowing function in people with Down's syndrome. Dysphagia. 2008;23(1):88–97.
92. Smith CH, Teo Y, Simpson S. An observational study of adults with down syndrome eating independently. Dysphagia. 2014;29(1):52–60.
93. Popova G, Paterson WF, Brown A, Donaldson MD. Hashimoto's thyroiditis in Down's syndrome: clinical presentation and evolution. Horm Res. 2008;70 (5):278–84.
94. Steingass KJ, Chicoine B, McGuire D, Roizen NJ. Developmental disabilities grown up: down syndrome. J Dev Behav Pediatr. 2011;32 (7):548–58.
95. Prasher V, Gomez G. Natural history of thyroid function in adults with Down syndrome—10-year follow-up study. J Intellect Disabil Res. 2007;51(Pt 4):312–7.
96. Jensen KM, Taylor LC, Davis MM. Primary care for adults with Down syndrome: adherence to preventive healthcare recommendations. J Intellect Disabil Res. 2013;57(5):409–21.
97. Brodtmann A. Hashimoto encephalopathy and Down syndrome. Arch Neurol. 2009;66(5):663–6.
98. King K, O'Gorman C, Gallagher S. Thyroid dysfunction in children with Down syndrome: a literature review. Ir J Med Sci. 2014;183(1):1–6.
99. Ivarsson SA, Ericsson UB, Gustafsson J, Forslund M, Vegfors P, Anneren G. The impact of thyroid autoimmunity in children and adolescents with Down syndrome. Acta Paediatr. 1997;86 (10):1065–7.
100. Smith DS. Health care management of adults with Down syndrome. Am Fam Physician. 2001;64 (6):1031–8.
101. Goday-Arno A, Cerda-Esteva M, Flores-Le-Roux JA, Chillaron-Jordan JJ, Corretger JM, Cano-Perez JF. Hyperthyroidism in a population with Down syndrome (DS). Clin Endocrinol (Oxf). 2009;71 (1):110–4.
102. Londhey VA, Rajadhyaksh GC, Barhate KS, More AV, Dedhia CR. Hyperthyroidism in a case of Down syndrome. J Assoc Physicians India. 2010;58:568–9.
103. Roizen NJ, Patterson D. Down's syndrome. Lancet. 2003;361(9365):1281–9.
104. Anwar AJ, Walker JD, Frier BM. Type 1 diabetes mellitus and Down's syndrome: prevalence, management and diabetic complications. Diabet Med. 1998;15(2):160–3.

105. Schmidt F, Kapellen TM, Wiegand S, Herbst A, Wolf J, Frohlich-Reiterer EE, et al. Diabetes mellitus in children and adolescents with genetic syndromes. Exp Clin Endocrinol Diabetes. 2012;120(10):579–85.
106. Bergholdt R, Eising S, Nerup J, Pociot F. Increased prevalence of Down's syndrome in individuals with type 1 diabetes in Denmark: a nationwide population-based study. Diabetologia. 2006;49(6):1179–82.
107. Taggart L, Coates V, Truesdale-Kennedy M. Management and quality indicators of diabetes mellitus in people with intellectual disabilities. J Intellect Disabil Res. 2013;57(12):1152–63.
108. Aitken RJ, Mehers KL, Williams AJ, Brown J, Bingley PJ, Holl RW, et al. Early-onset, coexisting autoimmunity and decreased HLA-mediated susceptibility are the characteristics of diabetes in Down syndrome. Diabetes Care. 2013;36(5):1181–5.
109. Hoorn EJ, de Vogel S, Zietse R. Insulin resistance in an 18-year-old patient with Down syndrome presenting with hyperglycaemic coma, hypernatraemia and rhabdomyolysis. J Intern Med. 2005;258(3):285–8.
110. Stancliffe RJ, Lakin KC, Larson S, Engler J, Bershadsky J, Taub S, et al. Overweight and obesity among adults with intellectual disabilities who use intellectual disability/developmental disability services in 20 U.S. States. Am J Intellect Dev Disabil. 2011;116(6):401–18.
111. Rimmer JH, Yamaki K, Davis BM, Wang E, Vogel LC. Obesity and overweight prevalence among adolescents with disabilities. Prev Chronic Dis. 2011;8(2):A41.
112. Rimmer JH, Yamaki K, Lowry BM, Wang E, Vogel LC. Obesity and obesity-related secondary conditions in adolescents with intellectual/developmental disabilities. J Intellect Disabil Res. 2010;54(9):787–94.
113. Real de Asua D, Parra P, Costa R, Moldenhauer F, Suarez C. Evaluation of the impact of abdominal obesity on glucose and lipid metabolism disorders in adults with Down syndrome. Res Dev Disabil. 2014;35(11):2942–9.
114. Wong C, Dwyer J, Holland M. Overcoming weight problems in adults with down syndrome. Nutr Today. 2014;49(3):109–19.
115. de Winter CF, Bastiaanse LP, Hilgenkamp TI, Evenhuis HM, Echteld MA. Overweight and obesity in older people with intellectual disability. Res Dev Disabil. 2012;33(2):398–405.
116. Hsieh K, Rimmer JH, Heller T. Obesity and associated factors in adults with intellectual disability. J Intellect Disabil Res. 2014 Sep;58(9):851–63. doi: 10.1111/jir.12100. Accessed 20 Nov 2013.
117. Allison DB, Gomez JE, Heshka S, Babbitt RL, Geliebter A, Kreibich K, et al. Decreased resting metabolic rate among persons with Down syndrome. Int J Obes Relat Metab Disord. 1995;19(12):858–61.
118. Gonzalez-Aguero A, Ara I, Moreno LA, Vicente-Rodriguez G, Casajus JA. Fat and lean masses in youths with Down syndrome: gender differences. Res Dev Disabil. 2011;32(5):1685–93.
119. Gonzalez-Aguero A, Vicente-Rodriguez G, Ara I, Moreno LA, Casajus JA. Accuracy of prediction equations to assess percentage of body fat in children and adolescents with Down syndrome compared to air displacement plethysmography. Res Dev Disabil. 2011;32(5):1764–9.
120. Zemel BS, Pipan M, Stallings VA, Hall W, Schadt K, Freedman DS, et al. Growth charts for children with Down syndrome in the United States. Pediatrics. 2015;136(5):e1204–11.
121. Pau M, Galli M, Crivellini M, Albertini G. Relationship between obesity and plantar pressure distribution in youths with Down syndrome. Am J Phys Med Rehabil. 2013;92(10):889–97.
122. Real de Asua D, Parra P, Costa R, Moldenhauer F, Suarez C. A cross-sectional study of the phenotypes of obesity and insulin resistance in adults with down syndrome. Diabetes Metab J. 2014;38(6):464–71.
123. Yang Q, Rasmussen SA, Friedman JM. Mortality associated with Down's syndrome in the USA from 1983 to 1997: a population-based study. Lancet. 2002;359(9311):1019–25.
124. Li C, Chen S, Meng How Y, Zhang AL. Benefits of physical exercise intervention on fitness of individuals with Down syndrome: a systematic review of randomized-controlled trials. Int J Rehabil Res. 2013;36(3):187–95.
125. Curtin C, Bandini LG, Must A, Gleason J, Lividini K, Phillips S, et al. Parent support improves weight loss in adolescents and young adults with Down syndrome. J Pediatr. 2013;163(5):1402–8.
126. Maclachlan RA, Fidler KE, Yeh H, Hodgetts PG, Pharand G, Chau M. Cervical-spine abnormalities in institutionalized adults with Down's syndrome. J Intellect Disabil Res. 1993;37:277–85.
127. Cohen WI. Current dilemmas in Down syndrome clinical care: celiac disease, thyroid disorders, and atlanto-axial instability. Am J Med Genet C Semin Med Genet. 2006;142C(3):141–8.
128. Lott IT, editor. Dementia in Down syndrome. In: Down Syndrome Medical Interest Group National Symposium; June 2015; Phoenix, AZ.
129. Pueschel SM, Scola FH. Atlantoaxial instability in individuals with Down syndrome: epidemiologic, radiographic, and clinical studies. Pediatrics. 1987;80(4):555–60.
130. Cohen WI. Down syndrome preventive medical check list. Down Syndr Q. 1999;4(3):1–16.
131. Vanderbilt Kennedy Center for Research on Human Development. Health care for adults with intellectual and developmental disabilities—toolkit for primary care providers: checklist—Down syndrome 2014

[cited 2014 February 14, 2014]. http://vkc.mc.vanderbilt.edu/etoolkit/physical-health/health-watch-tables-2/down-syndrome/.
132. Van Riper M, Cohen WI. Caring for children with Down syndrome and their families. J Pediatr Health Care. 2001;15(3):123–31.
133. Roizen NJ. Medical care and monitoring for the adolescent with Down syndrome. Adolesc Med. 2002;13(2):345–58, vii.
134. Pueschel SM, Anneren G, Durlach R, Flores J, Sustrova M, Verma IC. Guidelines for optimal medical care of persons with Down syndrome. International League of Societies for Persons with Mental Handicap (ILSMH). Acta Paediatr. 1995;84(7):823–7.
135. Davidson MA. Primary care for children and adolescents with Down syndrome. Pediatr Clin North Am. 2008;55(5):1099–111, xi.
136. Taggard DA, Menezes AH, Ryken TC. Treatment of Down syndrome-associated craniovertebral junction abnormalities. J Neurosurg. 2000;93(2 Suppl):205–13.
137. Radcliff K, Kepler C, Reitman C, Harrop J, Vaccaro A. CT and MRI-based diagnosis of craniocervical dislocations: the role of the occipitoatlantal ligament. Clin Orthop Relat Res. 2012;470(6):1602–13.
138. Sun YY, Boniello AJ, Poorman CE, Chang AL, Wang S, Passias PG. A review of the diagnosis and treatment of atlantoaxial dislocations. Global Spine J. 2014;4:197–210.
139. Hawli Y, Nasrallah M, El-Hajj Fuleihan G. Endocrine and musculoskeletal abnormalities in patients with Down syndrome. Nat Rev Endocrinol. 2009;5(6):327–34.
140. Dreyfus D, Lauer E, Wilkinson J. Characteristics associated with bone mineral density screening in adults with intellectual disabilities. J Am Board Fam Med. 2014;27(1):104–14.
141. Geijer JR, Stanish HI, Draheim CC, Dengel DR. Bone mineral density in adults with Down syndrome, intellectual disability, and nondisabled adults. Am J Intellect Dev Disabil. 2014;119(2):107–14.
142. Van Allen MI, Fung J, Jurenka SB. Health care concerns and guidelines for adults with Down syndrome. Am J Med Genet. 1999;89(2):100–10.
143. McKelvey KD, Fowler TW, Akel NS, Kelsay JA, Gaddy D, Wenger GR, et al. Low bone turnover and low bone density in a cohort of adults with Down syndrome. Osteoporos Int. 2013;24(4):1333–8.
144. Srikanth R, Cassidy G, Joiner C, Teeluckdharry S. Osteoporosis in people with intellectual disabilities: a review and a brief study of risk factors for osteoporosis in a community sample of people with intellectual disabilities. J Intellect Disabil Res. 2011;55(1):53–62.
145. Stagi S, Iurato C, Lapi E, Cavalli L, Brandi ML, de Martino M. Bone status in genetic syndromes: a review. Hormones (Athens). 2015;14(1):19–31.
146. Reza SM, Rasool H, Mansour S, Abdollah H. Effects of calcium and training on the development of bone density in children with Down syndrome. Res Dev Disabil. 2013;34(12):4304–9.
147. Toler F. Females with Down syndrome: lost opportunities in primary care. J Am Assoc Nurse Pract. 2015;27(7):356–62.
148. McGuire DE, Chicoine BA. Life issues of adolescents and adults with down syndrome. In: Cohen WI, Nadel L, Madnick ME, editors. Down syndrome: visions for the 21st century. New York, NY: Wiley-Liss, Inc; 2002. p. 221–45.
149. Edwards J. Sexuality, marriage, and parenting for persons wtih down syndrome. In: Pueschel SM, editor. The young person with down syndrome: transition from adolescence to adulthood. Baltimore, MD: Paul H. Brookes Publishing Company; 1988. p. 187–204.
150. Pueschel SM, Orson JM, Boylan JM, Pezzullo JC. Adolescent development in males with Down syndrome. Am J Dis Child. 1985;139(3):236–8.
151. Cento RM, Proto C, Guido M, Lanzone A. Post-menarchal Down's syndrome: a theoretical model of growth hormone action on ovarian function. Gynecol Endocrinol. 2001;15(1):81–8.
152. Hsiang YH, Berkovitz GD, Bland GL, Migeon CJ, Warren AC. Gonadal function in patients with Down syndrome. Am J Med Genet. 1987;27(2):449–58.
153. Schupf N, Zigman W, Kapell D, Lee JH, Kline J, Levin B. Early menopause in women with Down's syndrome. J Intellect Disabil Res. 1997;41(Pt 3):264–7.
154. Angelopoulou N, Souftas V, Sakadamis A, Matziari C, Papameletiou V, Mandroukas K. Gonadal function in young women with Down syndrome. Int J Gynaecol Obstet. 1999;67(1):15–21.
155. Bovicelli L, Orsini LF, Rizzo N, Montacuti V, Bacchetta M. Reproduction in Down syndrome. Obstet Gynecol. 1982;59(6 Suppl):13S–7S.
156. Suzuki K, Nakajima K, Kamimura S, Takasugi K, Suzuki Y, Sekine H, et al. Eight case reports on sex-hormone profiles in sexually mature male Down syndrome. Int J Urol. 2010;17(12):1008–10.
157. Pradhan M, Dalal A, Khan F, Agrawal S. Fertility in men with Down syndrome: a case report. Fertil Steril. 2006;86(6):1765 e1–3.
158. Scheepers M, Kerr M, O'Hara D, Cooper S-A, Davis R, Fujiura G, et al. Reducing health disparity in people with intellectual disabilities: A report from Health Issues Special Interest Research Group of the International Association for the Scientific Study of Intellectual Disabilities. J Policy Pract Intellect Disabil. 2005;2(3/4):249–55.
159. Krinsky-McHale SJ, Jenkins EC, Zigman WB, Silverman W. Ophthalmic disorders in adults with down syndrome. Curr Gerontol Geriatr Res. 2012;2012:974253.
160. Motley WW 3rd, Saltarelli DP. Ophthalmic manifestations of mosaic Down syndrome. J AAPOS. 2011;15(4):362–6.

161. Li EY, Chan TC, Lam NM, Jhanji V. Cataract surgery outcomes in adult patients with Down's syndrome. Br J Ophthalmol. 2014;98(9):1273–6.
162. Li J, Wong K, Park AS, Fricke TR, Jackson AJ. The challenges of providing eye care for adults with intellectual disabilities. Clin Exp Optom. 2015;98 (5):420–9.
163. Keiser H, Montague J, Wold D, Maune S, Pattison D. Hearing loss of Down syndrome adults. Am J Ment Defic. 1981;85(5):467–72.
164. Akin K. Macrocytosis and leukopenia in Down's syndrome. JAMA. 1988;259(6):842.
165. Seewald L, Taub JW, Maloney KW, McCabe ER. Acute leukemias in children with Down syndrome. Mol Genet Metab. 2012;107(1–2):25–30.
166. McLean S, McHale C, Enright H. Hematological abnormalities in adult patients with Down's syndrome. Ir J Med Sci. 2009;178(1):35–8.
167. Hasle H, Clemmensen IH, Mikkelsen M. Risks of leukaemia and solid tumours in individuals with Down's syndrome. Lancet. 2000;355(9199):165–9.
168. Dixon N, Kishnani PS, Zimmerman S. Clinical manifestations of hematologic and oncologic disorders in patients with Down syndrome. Am J Med Genet C Semin Med Genet. 2006;142C (3):149–57.
169. Roizen NJ, Amarose AP. Hematologic abnormalities in children with Down syndrome. Am J Med Genet. 1993;46(5):510–2.
170. Cheng YZ, Wang HF, Wang HP, Chen ZM, Jin J. Trisomy 21 in patients with acute leukemia. Am J Hematol. 2009;84(3):193–5.
171. Malinge S, Izraeli S, Crispino JD. Insights into the manifestations, outcomes, and mechanisms of leukemogenesis in Down syndrome. Blood. 2009;113 (12):2619–28.
172. Devata S, Pfiefer K. Doubly unexpected: down syndrome and male breast cancer. Society of General Internal Medicine Annual Meeting; June 2010; Minneapolis, MN: Journal of General Internal Medicine; 2010. p. S508.
173. Bratman SV, Horst KC, Carlson RW, Kapp DS. Solid malignancies in individuals with Down syndrome: a case presentation and literature review. J Natl Compr Canc Netw. 2014;12(11):1537–45.

Human Immunodeficiency Virus (HIV) 11

Kimberly Carter Bates

Case Presentation

Jane is a 23-year-old-female with perinatal human immunodeficiency virus (HIV) infection who presents to her primary care physician (PCP) to discuss preconception care. She has been relatively healthy since her diagnosis of HIV at age 2, when she was found to be HIV-positive after a hospitalization for *Pneumocystis* pneumonia. She was placed on trimethoprim-sulfamethoxazole prophylaxis at age 2 after her hospitalization and followed with a pediatric HIV specialist until recently. She reports taking various medications as a child and teenager for her HIV disease and noted variable adherence to therapy during her childhood years. She knows that she had problems with drug resistance that required changes in medications during her childhood but is not sure to which agents her virus has developed resistance. Jane reports that her mother managed her medications until about age 16, when she began taking them on her own. She became aware of her diagnosis at age 12, when her family disclosed her HIV status to her, and she admits to refusing medications around that time due to difficulty adjusting to the diagnosis. She attended counseling from age 14–16 to help her cope with the stigma associated with her disease and the challenges she felt as she became interested in dating and sexual activity. She became active in a youth-with-HIV support group and learned to become more responsible for her own health care. Jane has managed her own medications since age 16, and has been on her current antiretroviral (ARV) regimen since age 19. She has maintained viral suppression (viral load <200 on HIV RNA testing) for the past 4 years with her current regimen of tenofovir, emtricitabine, darunavir, and ritonavir.

Her current medical problems include obesity with a body mass index (BMI) of 32, history of major depression in remission on fluoxetine, and asthma, which is currently well controlled on a moderate-dose inhaled corticosteroid and as-needed inhaled short-acting bronchodilator. She has a history of sexually transmitted infection (STI) with *Chlamydia trachomatis* at age 18, but has had no further STI since that time and her most recent testing 6 months ago was negative. She has kept up to date with all health screenings that she has been informed she needed, including cervical cancer screening, which she started at age 19 and has annually. Jane reports that her routine vaccinations are "up to date" and mentioned that she completed the entire human papillomavirus (HPV) vaccination series "several years ago." She is a lifelong nonsmoker, but was exposed to passive smoke as a child due to her

K.C. Bates (✉)
Internal Medicine Residency, Department of Graduate Medical Education, Gwinnett Medical Center, 1000 Medical Center Blvd, Lawrenceville, GA 30046, USA
e-mail: kibates@gwinnettmedicalcenter.org

M. Pilapil et al. (eds.), *Care of Adults with Chronic Childhood Conditions*,
DOI 10.1007/978-3-319-43827-6_11

mother's cigarette usage. Jane drinks about 2–4 alcoholic beverages per month and denies all illicit drug use, including marijuana.

Jane has had four lifetime sexual partners and had her first sexual activity at age 17, with an older male she met through friends. She admits to intermittent condom usage as a teenager, but has used condoms with every sexual encounter with her current partner. She has never been pregnant, and is not currently on birth control. One year ago, she began dating her current sexual partner, whom she met while in college. They became sexually active 10 months ago, after she disclosed her HIV status to him, and they have used barrier contraceptives (male condom) faithfully without evidence of malfunction. The couple were recently married and have started to discuss having children. Her husband has been tested serially during their relationship and has remained HIV-negative. Jane is here to establish primary care with an adult care provider, as she has only followed up with her pediatric HIV team until now. She wants to discuss strategies to prevent HIV transmission during sexual activity and possible pregnancy, as well as chronic disease management and health maintenance now that she has made it to adulthood with her perinatal HIV infection. She is very concerned about life expectancy, as her mother died at age 40 from HIV-related end-stage renal disease (ESRD), despite being on combination antiretroviral therapy (cART). She wants to discuss how to remain healthy in adulthood with HIV.

Case Discussion

Preconception Counseling in HIV-Infected Women

Although it would have been unthinkable only a few decades ago, children born with HIV are living well into adulthood—life expectancy improving every year [1, 2]. With the advances in prevention of maternal-to-child transmission decreasing the risk of HIV transmission to less than 2 %, primary care providers should expect to offer counseling in patients with HIV infection interested in conception.

Consideration for preconception counseling to couples where at least one partner has HIV include:

1. Prevention of maternal-to-child transmission (MTCT) of HIV by HIV-infected women
2. Prevention of HIV transmission in serodiscordant couples
3. Medical concerns in HIV-infected pregnant women, including perinatally infected women.

Prevention of Maternal-to-Child Transmission of HIV

Women who are well controlled on combination antiretroviral therapy (cART) and continue to be adherent to care during conception and pregnancy are unlikely to vertically transmit HIV to their offspring. Untreated women with HIV have approximately a 12–40 % chance of transmission, but this risk can be decreased to 2 % or less with antepartum treatment with ARVs, postexposure prophylaxis of the infant, and avoidance of breastfeeding [3]. These three strategies are responsible for the dramatic decrease in MTCT in developed countries such as the United States. Nevertheless, annually, between 150 and 200 infants born to HIV-infected women in the United States are perinatally infected with HIV. Most are born to women who are either unaware of their HIV status or not engaged in HIV care [4]. For Jane, the major predictor of the ability to prevent transmission of HIV to her offspring is her adherence to cART during her pregnancy and maintenance of an undetectable viral load. Preconception counseling should include discussion of continued adherence to her current therapy. Her current regimen is one of several preferred regimens for prevention of MTCT (PMTCT), and, per current guidelines for PMTCT she should remain on her current regimen as her HIV disease is stable and she has maintained viral suppression for the preceding 12 months [5].

Prevention of Horizontal Transmission of HIV in Serodiscordant Couples

When counseling serodiscordant couples on conception, providers should stress the low (but not zero) risk of HIV transmission when the HIV-infected partner maintains an undetectable viral load. In this case, Jane's viral load is below the level of detection on the HIV RNA assay used, and has been that way for several years. An additional strategy to minimize risk to her new husband would be to engage in unprotected sexual intercourse only during ovulation, to maximize her chances of conception during the unprotected encounter [5]. Using methods such as home ovulation prediction kits can help the couple decide on an optimal time for unprotected intercourse. Artificial insemination (either in a medical setting or at home using a syringe method) is the safest option for Jane and other HIV-positive women in serodiscordant couples to ensure zero risk of HIV transmission to sexual partners during fertility attempts. Studies are currently underway to look at the use of pre-exposure prophylaxis (PrEP) in HIV-positive females in heterosexual, serodiscordant couples who are actively trying to conceive. Currently, the only U.S. Food and Drug Administration (FDA)-approved medication for use in PrEP is tenofovir-emtricitabine single-dose combination pill.

PrEP is taken 1 tablet daily by the HIV-negative partner to decrease risk of HIV transmission. PrEP has been shown in numerous studies to be safe and effective in decreasing HIV transmission. The PartnersPrEP study enrolled HIV-negative women in heterosexual, serodiscordant couples to use PrEP daily compared to placebo and showed significant reduction in HIV transmission risk to HIV-negative women with persistently detectable levels of PrEP drug in the bloodstream during the study period [6]. Incidence of pregnancies in the PartnersPrEP study was 10 %. Women who became pregnant had high medication adherence (97 % of prescribed doses overall), had similar adherence in the periconception period, and did not vary from total adherence overall, suggesting PrEP use was sustainable in women wishing to conceive [7]. Mothers who had received PrEP in the study were no more likely to experience preterm birth, congenital anomalies, or growth suppression in their infants than those who received placebo [8]. In addition, the Antiretroviral (use in) Pregnancy Registry has not shown any evidence of increases in birth defects in infants exposed to tenofovir-emtricitabine during gestation [9].

There are no studies looking at the efficacy of PrEP in HIV-infected patients on cART with viral suppression, but PrEP appears to be a useful tool to decrease HIV transmission among serodiscordant couples attempting to conceive. A recent study looking at intermittent use of PrEP immediately before and after sexual activity to prevent HIV transmission also adds to the body of evidence of PrEP efficacy, with an 82 % relative risk reduction in HIV acquisition [10]. In this study of PrEP in men who have sex with men (MSM) without HIV infection, detection of serum blood levels of tenofovir and emtricitabine were over 80 %, and the median use of medication was 15 pills per month [10]. It is unclear if the same level of protection would be possible with less frequent dosing.

Chronic Medical Conditions in Women with HIV Infection

Both prolonged HIV infection and medications used to treat the disease can lead to medical issues. This will need to be discussed with Jane and her husband prior to conception. Primary care physicians are well equipped to assist Jane's HIV care team in screening and management of comorbidities. With her current cART regimen, there are several medical risks to be considered. Protease inhibitors, while among the preferred agents for use during pregnancy, increase the risk of metabolic disorders, such as hyperlipidemia and hyperglycemia. Pregnant women on protease inhibitor therapy should be considered for early screening with oral glucose tolerance testing and should receive dietary counseling to prevent gestational diabetes [5]. Tenofovir has been associated with decreased bone density in women and men on therapy [11]. Instructions on strategies to improve bone health during pregnancy and beyond should be included in her preconception counseling.

In addition, Jane has a higher risk of HIV-related chronic disease due to prolonged HIV infection. Adults with perinatal infection of HIV are at risk for end-organ damage related to prolonged periods of HIV viremia throughout their lifetimes. Presumably, in Jane's case, she has been in care for at least the previous 7 years, and she should have received screening for chronic medical conditions related to HIV such as renal insufficiency, diabetes, hyperlipidemia, and mental health disorders. If such screening has not been done, it may be helpful to screen prior to conception. With the consideration of pregnancy, it will also be important for her to establish an adult care team, including an adult HIV provider (infectious disease trained subspecialist or generalist with HIV expertise) and obstetrical provider with experience in the care of HIV-infected women. Given her perinatal HIV infection and young age, her care may still be under her pediatric HIV care team, and she should ideally transition to an adult care team prior to her pregnancy.

Pathophysiology of HIV and Its Effects on Immunity

HIV is a non-oncogenic virus of the Retroviridae family, and belongs to the *Lentivirus* genus. There are two types of HIV (HIV-1 and HIV-2), with the vast majority of disease caused by HIV-1. HIV-2 exists primarily in West Africa, and HIV-1 is the predominant virus type in the Western world. HIV invades helper T (CD4) lymphocytes, integrates its viral DNA into the host DNA as part of the replication process, and destroys the host cell. CD4 cells help CD8 cells activate into cytotoxic T cells and help B cells produce antibodies (humoral immunity). Specialized CD4 cells, called Th17 cells, assist in the recruitment of neutrophils to the site of bacterial infections and are a key component of mucosal immunity as well. The loss of CD4 T cells (through both direct HIV infection and cytotoxic T cell-mediated destruction), monocytes and macrophages, as well as suppressed mucosal immunity predispose HIV-infected patients to opportunistic infections, fungal infections, severe infections with enteric organisms, and malignancies.

HIV is transmitted through transmission of infected blood and/or bodily fluids. Infection with HIV may predate clinical symptoms by 5–10 years, and progression from infection to disease tends to be slow, with the exception of children who are infected with HIV, who tend to progress more rapidly. In the first few weeks of early infection, HIV viremia is high and CD4 cells dramatically decline as infected cells are cleared by cytotoxic T cells. Over the following months to years, CD4 cells rebound and HIV viremia stabilizes until immunodeficiency is present, and viremia is able to proceed unchecked. During the period of clinical latency after acute HIV infection, reservoirs of HIV-infected cells develop, and these reservoirs are resistant to treatment with antiviral agents. Latent HIV infection in resting T cells and other reservoirs is responsible for the chronic nature of the disease and the requirement for lifelong antiretroviral therapy for control of the HIV disease.

Epidemiology of HIV Infection in U.S. Young Adults

HIV surveillance data from the Centers for Disease Control (CDC) show youth ages 13–24 living with HIV infection in the U.S. totaled over 64,000 by the end of 2012. In 2010, youth accounted for 26 % of new HIV infections (estimated at 12,200), despite constituting only 17 % of the U.S. population. Underrepresented minority groups are overrepresented in the HIV epidemic among youth. African-American youth made up 57 % of newly infected youth, and young men who have sex with men (YMSM) constituted 72 % of new HIV infections among adolescents and young adults. Eighty percent (80 %) of these new diagnoses are in the 20- to 24-year-old age group [12].

Year-end 2013 estimates of HIV prevalence in the 20- to 24-year-old age group report 33,000 young adults with HIV living in the U.S., with only 50 % being aware of their diagnosis. The highest rates of HIV prevalence are in the southern United States, District of Columbia, and urban areas in the northeastern U.S., with rates higher than the U.S. average (0.8 % prevalence among 20- to 24-year-olds in D.C. vs 0.3 % U.S average) [12]. Expanded HIV testing among high-risk groups such as youth ages 20–24 and African-American YMSM have helped to increase the number of young people who are newly aware of their HIV status. As these persons become linked to care and begin to access the healthcare system, primary care physicians will likely participate in their care as they transfer into the adult healthcare system.

Nearly 11,000 youth and young adults in the U.S. and U.S. territories as of 2010 were living with perinatal HIV infection, constituting approximately 18 % of the HIV-infected population. More than 40 % of perinatally infected youth have been diagnosed with acquired immunodeficiency syndrome (AIDS) at some point during their lifetimes, representing a population with high potential for early comorbidity [13]. As these patients continue to age and transition to adult care, adult providers will need to be attentive to the medical challenges of this group, particularly as data on long-term prognosis and long-term health concerns are just becoming available.

Characteristics of Perinatally Versus Behaviorally Infected Youth and Young Adults

Most youth and young adults living with HIV were infected through horizontal/behavioral transmission [12]. Sexually active youth are at risk of HIV infection due to behaviors such as decreased condom usage compared to older adults, substance abuse, and multiple sexual partners—particularly older partners [14, 15]. Centers for Disease Control and Prevention data from 2014 report that youth and young adults aged 13–24 had the second highest incidence of new HIV infection in the U.S., and youths representing ethnic and sexual minorities are overrepresented. As young adults with horizontally transmitted HIV transition to adult health care, it is important to recognize that they may still engage in high-risk behaviors and may be unaware of their risks, therein increasing their exposure to other sexually transmitted infections (STIs). Data from a sample of 143 sexually active HIV-positive youth showed that there was no difference in sexual risk behaviors between perinatally infected and heterosexually infected youth, suggesting that secondary STI prevention is an essential component of primary care for all HIV-infected youth, not just those with horizontal transmission [16].

Some notable differences have been observed in young adults vertically (vHIV+) and horizontally (hHIV+) infected with HIV. When compared to uninfected and hHIV+ cohorts, young adult vHIV+ have a higher incidence of mental health conditions as well as lower academic achievement and are less likely to have sustained viral suppression [14]. The reasons for these differences are not completely clear but are likely in part due to the stress and challenges of chronic disease management in vHIV+ youth. In those vHIV+ youth who were on cART therapy early (by age 5), prevention of HIV encephalopathy appears to provide protection against cognitive delays. However, for those perinatally infected who were not on early therapy or for those with a history of HIV encephalopathy, neurological comorbidities are not uncommon [17]. These young adults may present with cognitive delays, history of stroke with resultant disability, learning disabilities, and other neurological disorders [18]. Such neurocognitive effects present additional challenges for disease self-management and engagement in care and may require a different approach from the adult provider, including inclusion of immediate family, extended family, and friends to help with medical decision-making and medication adherence.

Although data on young adults with perinatal HIV infection is minimal, existing data point to other potential concerns due to long-term HIV infection and prolonged exposure to antiretroviral medications. Issues such as hyperlipidemia and insulin resistance that develop during early childhood may predispose vHIV+ young adults to early cardiac disease [19]. Typically vHIV+ youth have higher drug resistance than behaviorally infected counterparts due to lapses in treatment during adolescence and varied ART options in early childhood, including single ART therapy. Thus, they may have more complicated medical regimens and experience higher side effects. This may also negatively affect adherence to therapy [20]. Finally, for many young adults with perinatal HIV infection, issues such as sexual and reproductive health may not have been adequately addressed during adolescence due to caregiver fear of HIV transmission. Timing of disclosure of their disease by providers or family varies but often occurs during early adolescence for most with perinatal HIV infection [21, 22]. For many HIV-positive youth, abstinence-based counseling may have been their only reproductive health education, and awareness of contraceptive options may be minimal. Primary care providers should not assume that even by early adulthood, vHIV+ patients are aware of and practicing "safe" sexual practices and have discussed contraceptive options that are available for prevention of pregnancy. Similar to age-matched cohorts, pregnancies in perinatally infected women are most commonly unplanned [23].

Special Populations

Young MSM of Color

Minority populations in the U.S. are overrepresented in the HIV epidemic and none more so than young men who have sex with men (YMSM). African-American YMSM account for more than 50 % of YMSM infected with HIV, and YMSM account for more than 80 % of HIV infections in males between 13 and 24 years of age [24]. Young males tend to have older sexual partners, putting themselves at increased risk for coercive sexual practices [24]. In addition, studies have shown MSM of color tend to have relatively small, homogenous sexual networks and that HIV and other STIs can rapidly spread throughout these networks [25, 26]. Providers should frequently screen HIV-positive YMSM for intimate partner violence and coercive sexual activity, since YMSM of color tend to engage older partners and may be at a power disadvantage in the relationship. Discussion of current sexual practices as well as risk assessment and screening for STIs should be a part of primary care for YMSM with HIV. PrEP for HIV-negative partners of HIV-infected YMSM may also be a powerful tool to prevent continued spread of HIV in the sexual networks of YMSM of color. Generalists caring for HIV-positive YMSM (as well as at risk HIV-negative men) should be aware of PrEP and consider prescribing PrEP to decrease transmission among this group of patients.

African-American Women

Young African-American women have high rates of HIV infection in the U.S., primarily through heterosexual activity with older men [27]. A small case-control study conducted in 2003–2004 of HIV-infected black women and matched controls (black women at risk for HIV infection) in North Carolina showed HIV-infected women were more likely to exchange basic needs or drugs for sex (p value = 0.01) and were more likely to have sexual partners with a prior history of incarceration (p value = 0.04) [28]. This suggests that economic disadvantage and reliance on a partner for substantive needs increase the risk for HIV infection among African-American women. A component of patient-centered care for young African-American women with HIV should include evaluation of their current living situation to screen for transactional sex that may increase the risk for other STIs as well as intimate partner violence and loss of power arising from such relationships.

Socioeconomically Disadvantaged Youth

Despite improved access to health care through both the Ryan White Care Act, which provides HIV primary care services for HIV-infected men, women, and children, as well as the Affordable Care Act (ACA), young adults with HIV continue to face difficulty engaging in HIV care and being retained in treatment. Poverty remains an independent risk factor for HIV infection and failure to be retained in HIV care [29]. Socioeconomically disadvantaged youth and young adults have unique challenges remaining in HIV care, including lack of transportation, unemployment, and lack of health insurance. As a result, they may require additional strategies to maintain viral suppression. In order to better engage young adults with HIV, it is vital for providers to address social issues such as high unemployment rates, HIV stigma and disclosure, and lack of social supports. Young adults living in poverty also have less opportunity to learn key self-management skills that may help them cope with chronic disease. Special attention should be placed on educating young adults about their disease and the importance of self-care in preventing additional HIV-related comorbidities.

Common Comorbidities in HIV-Infected Adolescents

Sexually Transmitted Infections

Youth with HIV infection (through either horizontal or vertical transmission) commonly acquire other STIs, noted either at the time of initial diagnosis or during routine follow-up visits. Analyses of perinatally infected patients in the Pediatric HIV/AIDS Cohort Study (PHACS) registry showed that 62 % of sexually active HIV-positive youth reported unprotected sexual activity [30]. A single-center, retrospective analysis of urban HIV-infected youth (primarily via horizontal transmission) also documented evidence of unprotected sexual activity as measured by STI acquisition. In this cohort, 76 % of youth reported using barrier contraceptive methods "intermittently," yet during the 3-year period studied, 67 % contracted an STI. Risk factors for STI acquisition in this cohort included lack of HIV virological control and number of sexual partners. Notably, sexual preference was not seen to be an indicator of risk for STI in this cohort [31]. Some studies have shown that HIV-positive youth use barrier contraception less often than HIV-negative youth, particularly those with higher numbers of sexual partners [32]. Further review of longitudinal data from the most recent National Youth Risk Behavioral Survey in 2013 shows that the percentage of youth who used a condom during their last sexual intercourse has not topped 65 % since 1991 and has actually declined over the last decade (2003–2013) [33]. For the adult provider, it is important to recognize that STI risk reduction has not been as effective as it should be for the current generation of adolescents. HIV-infected young adults are no more likely to utilize STI risk reduction strategies, such as condom usage, and should therefore be counseled on secondary risk reduction for HIV transmission and STIs at every visit. Providers should screen for *Neisseria gonorrhoeae* (rectal, pharyngeal, and urethral), *C. trachomatis* (urethral) and syphilis in young men and women with risk factors, and Hepatitis C in young MSM and people who inject drugs (PWID). All those not immunized against Hepatitis B should be vaccinated. Risk factors for new STI acquisition include high-risk sexual behaviors, such as lack of condom usage, sexual intercourse while intoxicated, anal intercourse, MSM, and multiple or new sexual partners.

Mental Illness and Substance Abuse

Mental health disorders are not uncommon for healthy adolescents and young adults, and those with HIV are at even higher risk for development of mental health conditions and substance abuse. The Substance Abuse and Mental Health Services Administration (SAMHSA) National Survey on Drug Use and Health report from 2014 recorded that one in five young adults aged 18–25 reported a mental illness in the previous year and that 4 % were diagnosed with a serious illness [34]. More than 40 % of youth have experienced a behavioral health problem by the time they reach seventh grade. Despite the fact that an estimated 2.8 million adolescents had at least one major depressive episode in the year prior to being surveyed, only 41 % actually received treatment for their condition [34]. Disparities exist in the general population of youth and young adults with mental health disorders, and these disparities are even more profound for those with HIV infection.

A study of predominantly African-American youth living with HIV in New York City showed that 24 % reported clinically significant levels of depressive symptoms using a validated tool for screening for depression [35]. A meta-analysis of youth with perinatal HIV infection noted parental or caregiver health was associated with depression and anxiety in the youth, with those patients in homes with caregivers with functional limitations due to mental health conditions having higher risks of developing mental health disorders themselves. This same study also noted various other issues that impacted mental health of youth living with perinatal HIV infection, including death of parents and peers, stigma, concerns over disclosure, and development of healthy identity [36]. Perinatally infected youth are, by definition, the offspring of an HIV-infected parent (or 2) and represent failure of preventive strategies for maternal-to-child transmission of HIV. Risks for lack of adherence to MTCT prevention, such as substance abuse, lack of HIV care, psychiatric conditions in the mother, poverty, and insecurity of food and housing, represent the conditions in which many of these youth lived. These young adults have often experienced significant trauma related to chronic illness, disability, and potential loss of a parent, and they may have been subject to instability in their home environment from these or other issues such as parental substance abuse, involvement in the foster care system, and lack of social supports. HIV-infected youth also have a higher incidence of experiencing or witnessing violence. A cohort study of inner city HIV-positive youth from 2009 described high percentages of youth with a history of sexual or physical abuse as well as intimate partner violence. These experiences were also associated with psychological disorders such as major depression, posttraumatic stress disorder, and generalized anxiety [37].

When compared to other adults, transitional age persons (ages 21–25) have some of the highest rates of high-risk drinking behavior, with 43 % of young adults in this age range reporting binge drinking [34]. Youth living with HIV are similarly likely to report high-risk substance abuse behaviors, such as binge drinking, use of marijuana and other drugs, as well as use of drugs during sexual activity. In addition, among youth living with HIV, substance abuse is associated with decreased adherence to cART and risky sexual behaviors. Screening for substance abuse in persons living with HIV is recommended at least yearly and more often if issues of adherence to therapy arise.

HIV-Associated Neurocognitive Conditions

Perinatally infected young adults with increased HIV severity (at any point during their childhood) are at risk for neurocognitive effects of HIV infection. Risk factors for neurocognitive disease include history of HIV encephalopathy, higher peak viral load, and earlier nadir CD4 count [17]. Behaviorally infected youth have also been found to exhibit impairments in neurocognitive function, although it is unclear if these are premorbid impairments or are due directly to HIV infection. Abnormalities include psychomotor and cognitive slowing, deficits in learning and memory and executive function, as well as fine motor impairments [17]. A meta-analysis of studies looking at cognitive deficits in children with HIV (most via perinatal transmission) have shown lower performance on standardized tests of cognition and IQ when compared to healthy controls, as well as poorer academic performance of varying types (learning disabilities, failing, or repeating grade levels) among HIV-infected youth [18]. There is little data on prevention of neurocognitive impairment in this patient population, and risk factors for development are not consistent among studies. However, most studies of pediatric HIV patients suggest that although disease severity is associated with worse performance on measures of cognition, cART alone does not slow or prevent cognitive impairment and psychosocial wellbeing of the youth, and caregivers may be vitally important to diminishing any negative impact of HIV infection and treatment on cognitive development in youth and adolescents [18]. Some adult providers may not consider issues such as home environment and prior parental or caregiver mental health as predictors of neurocognitive development in their patient population, but they should address these issues with their young adult patients who are living with HIV. In addition, providers should have a strong index of suspicion regarding potential neurocognitive deficits in these patients and how these deficits may affect the ability of patients to engage in adult activities such as employment and post-secondary education as well as their engagement with the health care system.

Metabolic Disease in HIV Infection

Several metabolic complications associated with cART have been documented in youth and young adults living with HIV, including lipodystrophy, hyperlipidemia, poor bone health, micronutrient deficiencies, and insulin resistance [19]. Protease inhibitors increase the risk of metabolic disorders, such as hyperlipidemia and hyperglycemia. Patients on protease inhibitor therapy should be screened early and often for the development of diabetes, particularly in those who are also obese. However, there are no long-term studies of outcomes of metabolic complications of therapy in this age group, and no recommendations on screening for metabolic disease exist for adolescents and young adults. Care for these patients are extrapolated from care of adults with HIV infection [38]. As a result of cART-associated lipodystrophy and HIV effects on pancreatic function, some youth and young adults with HIV develop elevated serum triglyceride and low-density lipoprotein (LDL) cholesterol levels as well as insulin resistance. Because these conditions have been associated with an increased risk of cardiovascular disease among adults with HIV, concern for similar outcomes among youth and young adults with HIV is raised. The effects of ART on bone development and bone mineral density in HIV-infected youth are unknown, but among HIV-infected adults, decreases in bone mineral density are associated with increased risk of fractures in Caucasian and African-American patients [39]. However, decreases in bone density with specific ARVs, such as tenofovir, appear to be reversible and bone density has been shown to return to normal after cessation. More importantly, uncontrolled HIV viremia has also been shown to adversely affect bone health in adults with HIV. HIV has been associated with increased fracture risk in men. There are no evidence-based recommendations on use of dual-energy X-ray absorptiometry (DEXA) scanning for osteopenia and osteoporosis screening in young adults with HIV.

Special Topics in Youth and Young Adults Living with HIV Infections

Reproductive Health in Young Women Living with HIV

HIV does not appear to affect fertility for young women with HIV, and pregnancies are common in this group. As in all women of reproductive age, the primary care physician should counsel young women with HIV on their options for pregnancy prevention. Because ARVs have multiple drug–drug interactions, previously there were concerns regarding both the effectiveness of hormonal contraception as well as a possible association with injectable hormonal contraception and HIV transmission among women receiving ARVs. However, the U.S. Guidelines for the Medical Eligibility for Contraception reaffirmed that women with HIV can use any form of hormonal contraception (both progesterone only and combination estrogen-progesterone regimens) without restriction [40]. Women who are interested in pregnancy prevention should be started on hormonal contraception (oral, injectable, or preferably long-acting reversible contraception [LARC]) immediately to prevent unwanted pregnancy. Additionally, they do not require dosing adjustment of ARV medication or drug-level monitoring after the initiation of hormonal contraception.

Retention in Care for Youth with HIV

The National HIV/AIDS Strategy has listed five major components of the HIV Care Continuum: (1) diagnosis, (2) linkage to care, (3) retention and engagement in care, (4) prescription of antiretroviral therapy, and (5) viral suppression. In every aspect of the care continuum, youth and young adults lag behind the general population of those with HIV. Approximately 50 % of youth with HIV are undiagnosed [24]. Of those ages 13–24 living with HIV in 2011, only 73 % were linked to care, compared to 80 % overall [41]. Of the approximately 13,000 youth linked to HIV care, only 56 % of them have achieved viral suppression [42]. Primary care providers caring for this group of patients should expect that retention in care and viral suppression will continue to be challenging and should screen for barriers to adherence to therapy at each visit, even if they are not providing HIV care themselves. Identifying and addressing potential threats to adherence may decrease likelihood of development of drug-resistant virus and HIV-related comorbidities.

Immunization Needs of Young Adults with HIV

All patients with HIV should receive vaccination against influenza yearly as well as one-time vaccination with 13-valent conjugate pneumococcal vaccine and 23-valent polysaccharide pneumococcal vaccine. In addition, patients with HIV infection are at high risk of human papillomavirus (HPV)-related cancers, and so both men and women under the age of 26 should receive vaccination against HPV (2-valent HPV for women or 4-valent or 9-valent for either women or men). HIV is also an indication for vaccination against Hepatitis B virus for all individuals and for Hepatitis A virus for men who have sex with men. HIV is not an independent risk factor for meningococcal disease but young adults should receive age-appropriate vaccination against meningococcal A, C, W, and Y disease during late adolescence if not addressed previously [42].

HPV-Related Cancer Screening

HPV-related cancers include cervical, many anogenital cancers, and some oropharyngeal cancers. Patients with HIV are at higher risk of HPV-related cancers, and this risk is present for both men and women, regardless of type of sexual activity. HIV-infected individuals have a higher prevalence of cancer risk factors, including smoking and oncogenic HPV infection of the oral and genital track, compared to the general U.S. population, which may have an additive effect when combined with immunosuppression from HIV [43–45]. Due to the elevated risk of HPV-related cancers, there are specific recommendations regarding screening for HPV-related disease in women (see Table 11.1) [46, 47].

People with HIV infection have a 30-fold increase in lifetime risk for anal cancer and a fourfold increase in 5-year mortality from invasive anal cancer compared to HIV-unaffected individuals. This disparity continues to exist even when controlling for history of receptive anal intercourse [48]. Although there are no current guidelines for HPV-related anal cancer screening, several studies reviewed the use of anal cytology and high-resolution anoscopy (HRA) as a tool for screening for anal dysplasia and invasive anal cancer in HIV-infected persons. A retrospective cohort analysis of the development of incident invasive anal cancer in HIV-positive

Table 11.1 Recommendations for cervical cancer screening in HIV-infected women compared to general population

	Age < 30		Age 30 or greater	
	HIV (+)	HIV (−)	HIV (+)	HIV (−)
Initiation of Screening	Within 1 year of first sexual activity but no later than age 21[a,b]	Age 21	At time of HIV diagnosis	At initial evaluation if not previously screened
Type of Screening	Pap Test (Cytology) Only	Pap Test (Cytology) Only	Pap (Cytology) + HPV co-testing	Pap (Cytology) + HPV co-testing (age 35 and older)
Screening Interval	Initial: Every 12 months[c]	Initial: Every 3 years	Negative cytology with negative HPV: 3 years Negative cytology with positive HPV (non-16/18): Pap and HPV co-testing in 12 months Negative cytology with positive HPV (16/18): referral for colposcopy	Negative cytology with negative HPV: 5 years Negative cytology with positive HPV (non-16/18): pap and HPV co-testing in 12 months Negative cytology with positive HPV (16/18): referral for colposcopy
	Every 3 years after 3 consecutive negative tests[d,e]	Every 3 years[d,e]	Every 3 years[e,f]	Every 5 years[e,f] until age 65

Adapted from [46, 47]
[a]Women 21–29 years newly infected with HIV should be tested at time of initial HIV diagnosis
[b]Regardless of mechanism of HIV transmission (perinatal or acquired)
[c]Some centers recommend repeat Pap in 6 months after initial Pap in HIV-positive women
[d]Until age 30. After age 30, women should receive co-testing if available
[e]Assuming previous testing negative for abnormal cytology and/or high-risk HPV
[f]Acceptable to have Pap test alone every 3 years after 3 annual consecutive negative tests if co-testing not available

persons after baseline anal cytology demonstrated an association between initial high-grade squamous epithelial lesion (HSIL) and the development of invasive anal cancer (IAC). After a median of 4 years of follow-up, 1.65 % of persons with initial HSIL on baseline cytology developed IAC, with a hazard ratio of 2.92 for development of IAC compared to those without HSIL on baseline cytology [49]. A 2013 study of HIV-positive men with and without a history of receptive anal intercourse (RAI) demonstrated a link between HPV infection and abnormal anal cytology and histology irrespective of RAI history, suggesting that sexual behaviors are not predictive of risk for anal cancer [50]. Reviews of current practices worldwide for anal cancer screening show a mixture of the use of anal cytology and/or high-resolution anoscopy for screening in HIV-positive men and women, and HIV-positive MSM are more likely to be screened than other populations [51]. In the same review, more than 50 % of respondents recommended screening every 2 years with HRA in immunosuppressed patients. While waiting for full recommendations to be developed, the primary care physician should at a minimum discuss anal cancer screening with HIV-infected patients and identify a high-quality referral center performing high volumes of HRA screening to refer to should the patient be interested in screening.

Non-HPV-Related Cancer Screening

Kaposi sarcoma and non-Hodgkin's Lymphoma, the two AIDS-defining malignancies, have decreased in the cART era, due to improvements in immunodeficiency status in patients on cART. However, adults who were diagnosed with AIDS during childhood continue to be at risk for development of AIDS-defining malignancies, although at a much lower incidence than prior to

Table 11.2 Health maintenance screening guidelines for primary care of patients with HIV. Adapted from [38]

Screening	Interval	Reason for recommendation
Digital rectal exam	Consider annually	Examination for anal lesions, anal warts and other HPV-related changes
Depression screening	Annually	Depression is the most common mental health co-morbidity in PLWH
Fasting glucose or HgA1c	Annually	Screening for diabetes due to metabolic dysfunction in HIV infection
Fasting lipid profile	Annually	Screening for hyperlipidemia due to metabolic dysfunction in HIV infection
Trichomoniasis	Annually in women	Increased risk of STI acquisition in women with untreated trichomoniasis
Tobacco use screening and cessation counseling	Annually, and at each visit for active tobacco users	Association with smoking and disease progression in HIV and HIV-associated co-morbidities
STI testing-syphilis, gonorrhea and chlamydia	Annually for those at risk for STIs	Increased incidence of non-HIV STI infection in youth and young adults with HIV due to continued high-risk sexual practices
Alcohol and drug screening	Annually, and at each visit for active users	Increased incidence of alcohol and drug use as part of high-risk sexual behaviors in young adults with HIV
Secondary HIV prevention	At each visit if possible	Prevention of HIV transmission
Medication adherence	At each visit if possible	Maintenance of viral suppression
Intimate Partner Violence screening	At least annually and more often if needed	Patients with HIV are at higher risk of intimate partner violence than general population

HPV human papilloma virus, *PLWH* people living with HIV, *STI* sexually transmitted infection

the cART era [52]. A systematic review also showed an increase in non-AIDS-defining cancers after the introduction of cART, particularly HPV-related anal cancer [53]. A review of cancer registries shows a lower than average risk for prostate and breast cancers but a statistically significant increase in HPV-related cancers as well as Hodgkin's lymphoma, lung, liver, leukemia, and poorly specified cancers [54].

HIV Primary Care Screening

Health maintenance screening is also necessary in young adults transitioning to adult medical care. Young adults with HIV should have yearly preventative medicine visits to address chronic disease management and screening for common comorbidities. The Infectious Diseases Society of America (IDSA) and HIV Medicine Association (HIVMA) released updated guidelines in 2013 for primary care for adults with HIV. Health maintenance activities that are specific to young adults with HIV infection which could be delivered in a primary care practice have been summarized below (see Table 11.2) [38].

Conclusion

Youth and young adults are living with HIV, and life expectancy continues to approach that of non-HIV infected individuals. The majority of HIV-infected adults, regardless of route of transmission, will live with HIV as a chronic medical condition and will need providers skilled in chronic disease management to help them lead healthy lives. Primary care physicians are essential in the care of all patients with chronic disease, but perhaps more so in a population for which their survival is so dependent on strict medication adherence and chronic disease self-management. As more data on the natural history of adolescents and young adults with HIV develop, physicians will need to remain up to date on recommendations for disease screening and chronic disease management for those living with HIV (Appendix). As these patients transition to adult services, special attention should be given to the challenges unique to HIV-infected patients, including mental health concerns, secondary HIV prevention, increased risk for secondary cancers, and lifelong medication adherence.

Appendix

Human immunodeficiency virus (HIV) condition fact sheet

Definition	Human immunodeficiency virus (HIV) is a retrovirus that infects helper T lymphocytes and causes CD4 cell depletion resulting in a chronic immunodeficiency • HIV causes AIDS (acquired immunodeficiency syndrome) • Due to advances in treatment, HIV infection is now a chronic disease which is manageable with combination antiretroviral therapy (cART)
Epidemiology	• Advances in cART have resulted in extended life expectancy for those living with HIV disease • Youth and young adults with perinatal HIV infection make up 18 % of cases of persons with HIV • More than 40 % of perinatally infected persons have been diagnosed with AIDS during their lifetime • Approximately 1 in 4 new HIV infections are in persons age 13–24, and sexual and ethnic minorities are significantly over-represented
Special considerations	Adolescents and young adults with HIV are at risk for the following conditions related to HIV disease and treatment • Neurocognitive effects of prolonged HIV disease in perinatally infected persons • Metabolic disease, such as diabetes and hyperlipidemia • HPV-related malignancies • Stigma and concerns with HIV disclosure • Disease progression related to non-adherence to therapy • Body image concerns from lipodystrophy • Secondary HIV prevention • Higher incidence of STI infection and substance abuse in certain populations, such as young men who have sex with men Individuals are at heightened risk for chronic conditions, including • Non-AIDS-defining malignancies such as HPV-related cancers (particularly anal cancers), lung cancers, and Hodgkin's lymphoma • Diabetes and hyperlipidemia • Depression and anxiety
Recommended screening	Annual screening for • Diabetes • Sexually transmitted infections (STI) • Mental health disorders and substance abuse • Hyperlipidemia • Cervical cancer in women (every 3 years after three consecutive normal screenings)

References

1. Samji H, Cescon A, Hogg RS, Modur SP, Athoff KN, Buchacz K, for the North American AIDS Cohort Collaboration on Research and Design, et al. Closing the gap: increases in life expectancy among treated HIV-positive individuals in the United States and Canada. PLoS ONE. 2013;8(12):e81355.
2. Brady MT, Oleske JM, Williams PL, Elgie C, Mofenson LM, Dankner WM, et al. Declines in mortality rates and changes in causes of death in HIV-1-infected children during the HAART era. J Acquir Immune Defic Syndr. 2010;53(1):86–94.
3. Mofenson L, Taylor AW, Rogers M, Campsmith M, Ruffo NM, Clark J, Centers for Disease Control, et al. Achievements in public health: reduction in perinatal transmission of HIV infection—United States, 1985–2005. MMWR. 2006;55(21):592–7.
4. Branson BM, Handsfield HH, Lampe MA, Janssen RS, Taylor AW, Lyss SB, Centers for Disease Control and Prevention, et al. Revised recommendations for HIV testing of adults, adolescents, and pregnant women in health-care settings. MMWR. 2006;55(RR14):1–17.
5. Panel on Treatment of HIV-Infected Pregnant Women and Prevention of Perinatal Transmission. Recommendations for Use of Antiretroviral Drugs in Pregnant HIV-1-Infected Women for Maternal Health and Interventions to Reduce Perinatal HIV Transmission in the United States. http://aidsinfo.nih.gov/contentfiles/lvguidelines/PerinatalGL.pdf. Accessed 29 Feb 2016.
6. Baeten JM, Celum C. Antiretroviral prophylaxis for HIV prevention in heterosexual men and women. N Engl J Med. 2013;368(1):399–410.
7. Matthews LT, Heffron R, Mugo NR, Cohen CR, Hendrix CW, Celum C. High medication adherence during periconception periods among HIV-1 Uninfected women participating in a clinical trial of antiretroviral pre-exposure prophylaxis. J Acquir Immune Defic Syndr. 2014;67(1):91–7.
8. Mugo NR, Hong T, Celum C, Donnell D, Bukusi EA, John-Stewart G, et al. Pregnancy incidence and outcomes among women receiving preexposure prophylaxis for HIV prevention: a randomized clinical trial. JAMA. 2014;312(4):362–71.
9. Lampe MA, Smith DK, Anderson GJ, Edwards AE, Nesheim SR. Achieving safe conception in HIV-discordant couples: the potential role of oral preexposure prophylaxis (PrEP) in the United States. Am J Obstet Gynocol. 2011;204(6):488.e1–8.
10. Molina JM, Capitant C, Spire B, Pialoux G, Cotte L, Charreau I, et al. On demand preexposure prophylaxis in men at high risk for HIV-1 infection. N Engl J Med. 2015;373:2237–46.
11. Walker Harris V, Brown TT. Bone loss in the HIV-infected patient: evidence, clinical implications, and treatment strategies. J Infect Dis. 2012;205(S3):S391–8.
12. Division of HIV/AIDS Prevention, National Center for HIV/AIDS, Viral Hepatitis, Sexual Transmitted Diseases and Tuberculosis Prevention, Centers for Disease Control and Prevention. HIV Surveillance in Adolescents and Young Adults (through 2014) [Online]. http://www.cdc.gov/hiv/pdf/statistics_surveillance_adolescents.pdf. Accessed 29 Feb 2016.
13. Division of HIV/AIDS Prevention, National Center for HIV/AIDS, Viral Hepatitis, Sexual Transmitted Diseases and Tuberculosis Prevention, Centers for Disease Control and Prevention. Pediatric HIV Surveillance [Online] http://www.cdc.gov/hiv/pdf/statistics_surveillance_Pediatric.pdf. Accessed 29 Feb 2016.
14. Spiegel H, Futterman DC. Adolescents and HIV: prevention and clinical care. Curr HIV/AIDS Rep. 2009;6:100–7.
15. Centers for Disease Control and Prevention. Vital signs: HIV infection, testing, and risk behaviors among youths—United States. MMWR. 2012;27(61):1–6.
16. Renaud TC, Bocour A, Tsega A, Sepkowitz KA, Udeagu CC, Shepard CW. Do sexual risk behaviors differ between heterosexual youth infected with HIV perinatally vs sexually? J Adolesc Health. 2013;53(2):222–7.
17. Nichols SL, Brummel SS, Smith RA, Garvie PA, Hunter SJ, Malee KL, et al. Executive functioning in children and adolescents with perinatal HIV infection. Pediatr Infect Dis J. 2015;334:969–75.
18. Laughton B, Cornell M, Boivin M, Van Rie A. Neurodevelopment in perinatally HIV-infected children: a concern for adolescence. J Int AIDS Soc. 2013;16:18603.
19. Barlow-Mosha L, Eckard AR, McComsey GA, Musoke PM. Metabolic complications and treatment of perinatally HIV infected children and adolescents. J Int AIDS Soc. 2013;16:1–11.
20. Chandwani S, Koenig L, Sill AM, Abramowitz S, Conner LC, D'Angelo L. Predictors of antiretroviral medication adherence among a diverse cohort of adolescents with HIV. J Adolesc Health. 2012;51:242–51.
21. Lee S, Yamazaki M, Harris DR, Harper GW, Ellen J. Social Support and Human Immunodeficiency Virus-Status Disclosure to friends and family: implications for human immunodeficiency virus-positive youth. J Adolesc Health. 2015;57:73–80.
22. Santamaria EK, Dolezal C, Marhefka SL, Hoffman S, Ahmed Y, Elkington K, Mellins CA. Psychosocial implications of HIV serostatus disclosure to youth with perinatally acquired HIV. AIDS Patient Care STDS. 2011;25(4):257–64.
23. Agwu AL, Jang SS, Korthuis PT, Araneta MR, Gebo K. Pregnancy incidence and outcomes in vertically and behaviorally HIV infected youth. JAMA. 2011;305(5):468–70.
24. Division of HIV/AIDS Prevention, National Center for HIV/AIDS, Viral Hepatitis, Sexual Transmitted

Diseases and Tuberculosis Prevention, Centers for Disease Control and Prevention. HIV in Youth. 2015 June 30. [Online] Accessed 29 Feb 2016.
25. Hernandex-Romieu AC, Sullivan PS, Rothenberg R, Grey J, Luisi N, Kelley CF, Rosenberg ES. Heterogeneity of HIV prevalence among the sexual networks of black and white men who have sex with men in Atlanta: illuminating a mechanism for increased HIV risk for young black men who have sex with men. Sex Transm Dis. 2015;42(9):505–12.
26. Tieu HV, Liu TY, Hussen S, Connor M, Wang L, Buchbinder S, et al. Sexual networks and HIV risk among black men who have sex with men in 6 U.S. cities. PLoS ONE. 2015;10(8):e0134085.
27. Division of HIV/AIDS Prevention, National Center for HIV/AIDS, Viral Hepatitis, Sexual Transmitted Diseases and Tuberculosis Prevention, Centers for Disease Control and Prevention. HIV Among African Americans. 2013 February; 1–2.
28. Centers for Disease Control and Prevention. HIV transmission among black women-North Carolina, 2004. MMWR. 2005;54(4):89–94.
29. Centers for Disease Control and Prevention. Social determinants of health among adults with diagnosed HIV in 11 states, the District of Columbia and Puerto Rico, 2013. HIV Surveil Suppl Rep. 2015;20(5):1–38.
30. Tassiopoulos K, Moscicki AB, Mellins C, Kacanek D, Malee K, Allison S, Hazra R, et al. Sexual risk behavior among youth with perinatal HIV infection in the United States: predictors and implications for intervention development. Clin Infect Dis. 2013;56(2):283–90.
31. Brownstein PS, Gillespie SE, Leong T, Chahroudi A, Chakraborty R, Camacho-Gonzalez AF. The association of uncontrolled HIV infection and other sexually transmitted infections in metropolitan Atlanta youth. Pediatr Infect Dis J. 2015;34(5):e119–24.
32. Hein K, Dell R, Futterman D, Rotheram-Borus MJ, Shaffer N. Comparison of HIV+ and HIV− adolescents: risk factors and social determinants. Pediatrics. 1995;95(1):96–104.
33. Centers for Disease Control and Prevention. Youth risk behavior surveillance-United States, 2013. MMWR. 2014;63(4):1–168.
34. Center for Behavioral Health Statistics and Quality. Behavioral health trends in the United Stats: results from the 2014 National survey on drug use and health. HHS Publication No. SMA15-4927, NSDUH Series H-50. 2015. Retrieved from http://www.samhsa.gov/data/.
35. Salama C, Morris M, Armistead L, Koenig LJ, Demas P, Ferdon C, Bachanas P. Depressive and conduct disorder symptoms in youth living with HIV: the independent and interactive roles of coping and neuropsychological functioning. AIDS Care. 2013;25(2):160–8.
36. Mellins CA, Malee KM. Understanding the mental health of youth living with perinatal HIV infection: lessons learned and current challenges. J Int AIDS Soc. 2013;18(16):18593.
37. Martinez J, Hosek SG, Carleton RA. Screening and assessing violence and mental health disorders in a cohort of inner city HIV-positive youth between 1998–2006. AIDS Patient Care STDs. 2009;23(6):469–75.
38. Aberg JA, Gallant JE, Ghanem KG, Emmanuel P, Zingman BS, Horberg MA. Primary care guidelines for the management of persons infected with HIV: 2013 update by the HIV Medicine Association of the Infectious Diseases Society of America. Clin Inf Dis. 2014;58(1):e1–34.
39. Triant VA, Brown TT, Lee H, Grinspoon SK. Fracture prevalence among human immunodeficiency virus (HIV)-infected versus non-HIV-infected patients in a large US healthcare system. J Clin Endocrinol Medab. 2008;93(9):3499–504.
40. Centers for Disease Control and Prevention. Update to CDC's U.S. Medical eligibility criteria for contraceptive use, 2010: revised recommendations for the use of hormonal contraception among women at high risk for HIV infection or infected with HIV. MMWR 2012;61(24):449–452.
41. Centers for Disease Control and Prevention. Vital signs: HIV diagnosis, care, and treatment among persons living with HIV—United States, 2011. MMWR. 2014;63(47):1113–7.
42. Centers for Disease Control and Prevention. Advisory committee on immunization practices recommended immunization schedule for adults aged 19 years or older—United States, 2016. National Center for Immunization and Respiratory Diseases, 2016.
43. Park LS, Hernandez-Ramirez RU, Silverberg MJ, Crothers K, Dubrow K. Prevalence of non-HIV cancer risk factors in persons living with HIV/AIDS: a meta-analysis. AIDS. 2016;30(2):273–91.
44. Shiels MS, Cole SR, Kirk GD, Poole C. A meta-analysis of the incidence of non-AIDS cancers in HIV-infected individuals. J Acquir Immune Defic Syndr. 2009;52(5):611–22.
45. Leeds IL, Fang SH. Anal cancer and intraepithelial neoplasia screening: a review. World J Gastrointest Surg. 2016;8(1):41–51.
46. Panel on Opportunistic Infections in HIV-Infected Adults and Adolescents. Guidelines for the prevention and treatment of opportunistic infections in HIV-infected adults and adolescents: recommendations from the Centers for Disease Control and Prevention, the National Institutes of Health, and the HIV Medicine Association of the Infectious Diseases Society of America. http://aidsinfo.nih.gov/contentfiles/lvguidelines/adult_oi.pdf. Accessed 5 Mar 2016.
47. Saslow D, Solomon D, Lawson HW, Killackey M, Kulasingam S, Cain J, et al. American Cancer Society, American Society for Colposcopy and Cervical Pathology, and American Society for Clinical Pathology Screening Guidelines for the Prevention

and Early Detection of Cervical Cancer. CA Cancer J Clin. 2012;62(3):147–72.
48. Cachay E, Agmas W, Matthews C. Five-year cumulative incidence of invasive anal cancer among HIV-infected patients according to baseline anal cytology results: an inception cohort analysis. HIV Med. 2015;16(3):191–5.
49. Darwich L, Videla S, Canadas MP, Pinol M, Garcia-Cuyas F, Vela S, et al. Distribution of human papillomavirus genotypes in anal cytological and histological specimens from HIV-infected men who have sex with men and men who have sex with women. Dis Colon Rectum. 2013;56(9):1043–52.
50. Patel J, Salit IE, Berry MJ, de Pokomandy A, Nathan M, Fishman F, et al. Environmental scan of anal cancer screening practices: worldwide survey results. Cancer Med. 2014;3(4):1052–61.
51. Centers for Disease Control and Prevention. Monitoring selected national HIV prevention and care objectives by using HIV surveillance data—United States and 6 dependent areas—2012 HIV Surveillance Supplemental Report. 2014 November;19(3).
52. Simard ED, Shiels MS, Bhatia K, Engels EA. Long-term cancer risk among people diagnoses with AIDS during childhood. Cancer Epidemiol Biomarkers Prev. 2012;21(1):148–54.
53. Cobucci RN, Lima PH, de Souza PC, Costa VV, da Cornetta MC, Fernandes JV, Goncalves AK. Assessing the impact of HAART on the incidence of defining and non-defining AIDS cancers among patients with HIV/AIDS: a systematic review. J Infect Public Health. 2015;8(1):1–10.
54. Simard EP, Pfeiffer RM, Engels EA. Spectrum of cancer risk late after AIDS onset in the United States. Arch Intern Med. 2010;170(15):1337–45.

12 Inflammatory Bowel Disease

Elana Maser and Anish Patel

Case Presentation

Michelle is an 18-year-old woman with Crohn's disease who presents for initial evaluation to an adult internal medicine office accompanied by her parents. She was diagnosed at age 12 years. She had severe disease, requiring two small bowel resections by ages 14 and 15 years due to recurrent Crohn's strictures. She has been maintained on biologic therapy since her last surgery and is planning on leaving for college out of state in 6 months. Her parents wanted her to establish care prior to her departure as was recommended by their pediatrician.

Michelle is a well-groomed, well-mannered patient. She is slightly timid and quiet. Her parents speak the majority of the time. She only speaks when spoken to directly, with frequent interjections by her parents. She reports good compliance with her medication, but her mother notes "missed timing" of doses on frequent occasions. She appears healthy, is an appropriate weight, and has almost reached the height of her parents. There are no abnormalities on physical exam other than well-healed abdominal surgical scars.

Michelle's parents have voiced three concerns: They are uneasy about leaving their lifelong and beloved pediatrician, they have concerns about their daughter's compliance with medications, and they are worried about their daughter having reduced access to the appropriate care while in college.

Case Discussion

Transition is a very difficult and often fearful time for families, especially for patients with severe Crohn's disease [1]. Pediatric gastroenterologists often develop strong bonds with their patients and families. However, limited time is spent on the preparation for transition to adult providers [2, 3]. Difficulties arise in the transition to adult care as adult providers are often faced with patients who have limited knowledge of their complicated medical, surgical, and drug history.

This case is a common scenario in the adult medicine realm. Michelle has severe Crohn's disease requiring multiple surgeries at an early age and requires biologic drugs to maintain remission. Her parents are apprehensive about letting her go alone to an out-of-state college where access to specialists or generalists who

E. Maser
Division of Gastroenterology, Mt. Sinai Hospital, 17 East 102nd Street, 5th Floor, New York, NY 10029, USA
e-mail: elana.maser@mountsinai.org

A. Patel (✉)
Department of Gastroenterology/Hepatology, Carl R. Darnall Army Medical Center, 36000 Darnall Loop, Ft. Hood, TX 76544, USA
e-mail: anishpa81@gmail.com

M. Pilapil et al. (eds.), *Care of Adults with Chronic Childhood Conditions*,
DOI 10.1007/978-3-319-43827-6_12

understand Crohn's disease may be scarce and access to biologic drugs may be difficult as well.

For Michelle, developing a good rapport with and trust in her adult doctor is critical to a successful transition and ongoing care. Discussions need to focus on adherence to medication and risks to her health and quality of life if regimens are not maintained. As new generations of adolescents are more involved with technology, discussions about maintaining communication, whether via email and/or patient portals, could help reduce the stress experienced by patients and their parents. To alleviate fears about Michelle's relocation out of state, identifying a local physician for emergency purposes would be helpful. She should contact her insurance provider to find a local infusion center that is able to administer biologics unless she is able to make arrangements to come home for infusions. Switching biologics (often from infusion to self injection) should be avoided if Michelle is in remission. Switching biologics puts patients at risk of a flare, which would be undesirable during this stressful period [4].

Overview

Epidemiology

Crohn's disease (CD) and ulcerative colitis (UC) affect more than 5 million people worldwide, with more than 1.7 million in the United States and about 3 million in Europe [5]. Higher rates occur in industrialized countries [6, 7]. The lifetime risk of developing inflammatory bowel disease (IBD), including both CD and UC, is approximately 1 %.

Over one-quarter of all patients will first be diagnosed in childhood or adolescence. While the incidence in adults seems to be stabilizing, the incidence rates in pediatrics are currently rising [8]. The annual incidence has doubled over an 11-year span from 1.1/100,000 to 2.4/100,000 in the pediatric population [9]. Following childhood, the diagnosis of IBD can occur at any age but there are two peaks of higher incidence around ages 20 and 50 years [7, 10].

There are no significant gender differences found in the prevalence of UC, but there is a slightly higher incidence of CD among women as compared to men [11, 12].

IBD is thought to be a disease that affects mostly Ashkenazi Jews, however, Sephardic Jews are affected as well, albeit with a lower incidence [13]. IBD is not a disease reserved only for those of Jewish descent though. While these populations have the highest incidence, IBD can occur in any race [13].

Pathophysiology

The term IBD includes Crohn's disease (CD) and ulcerative colitis (UC). IBD is characterized by chronic, relapsing inflammation within the gastrointestinal tract. One has to have a genetic predisposition and be exposed to an environmental trigger in order to develop the disease. There have been more than 100 genes identified in the pathogenesis of IBD, and numerous environmental factors including smoking, the use of oral contraceptives, and exposure to antibiotics have been suggested, though none have been clearly implicated [14, 15].

Current literature suggests that the inflammation is a result of inappropriate and ongoing activation of the innate immune system of the gut mucosa, driven by the commensal luminal flora in a genetically susceptible host [16, 17]. Once the inflammation has been initiated, it has difficulty resolving without the help of medication. It is not yet clear which commensal flora are responsible; however, a more limited variation in gut bacteria is typically seen in an IBD host [18]. Current understanding is that both CD and UC have a similar pathogenesis, but clinically they have varying characteristics. The characteristic features are summarized in Table 12.1.

Table 12.1 Comparison of Crohn's disease and ulcerative colitis

Feature	Crohn's disease	Ulcerative colitis
Site of origin	Terminal ileum (can occur anywhere in gastrointestinal tract)	Colon
Pattern of progression	"Skip" lesions/irregular	Contiguous
Histopathology	Transmural disease Deep ulcers, granulomas, "cobblestoning"	Submucosa/mucosa
Complications	Fistulas/abscesses/obstruction	Bleeding/toxic megacolon
Radiographic findings	String sign	Lead pipe colon
Clinical features	Crampy abdominal pain	Bloody diarrhea

Clinical Definition, Presentation, and Natural History of IBD

Ulcerative Colitis

UC is a chronic inflammatory disease affecting the mucosal layer of the colon and rectum. The disease is relapsing and remitting. When the disease is active, also called "flaring," patients typically suffer from urgent and frequent bouts of bloody diarrhea. Flares are intermittent, unpredictable, and vary in severity. Most commonly, UC is painless unless the disease is severe. Endoscopically, inflammation is continuous from the anal verge extending proximally. One-third of patients have mild disease requiring minimal medication, one-third of patients require chronic maintenance medication, and 20–30 % will need colectomy [19]. Patients with UC develop colorectal cancer at twice the population risk. Therefore, guidelines suggest screening patients with annual colonoscopies, as is further discussed later in this chapter [20]. Patients with proctitis do not have an increased risk of colon cancer and therefore should not be screened more frequently than the general population. This disease can affect quality of life but not duration of life. A normal life span should be expected [5].

Crohn's Disease

CD is also a chronic inflammatory condition with periods of wellness interspersed with flares. In contrast to UC, CD affects all layers of the bowel and can occur in any part of the gastrointestinal tract from mouth to anus. The most common presentation is terminal ileitis. A child may present with weight loss or poor growth and have no other symptoms. Pain is more commonly seen in patients with CD as compared to those with UC. Symptoms can range from mild abdominal cramping to severe diarrhea or symptoms of intestinal obstruction. Perianal disease is common and can manifest as abnormal anal skin tags, deep anal fissures, and fistulae. Endoscopically, inflammation can occur in patches with normal mucosa interspersed with inflamed mucosa. There is no single test to diagnose CD, however, rarely granulomas are seen on histopathology. When these are seen, CD can be differentiated from UC.

The disease course can range from mild intermittent flares to the more severe cases that are difficult to control. Up to 70 % of patients with CD will require at least 1 surgery [21]. Risk of colon cancer is also increased in patients with CD, and like patients with UC, patients with colonic Crohn's should have annual colonoscopies, again as will be further discussed later in this chapter [22]. Patients with CD are also at higher risk for nutritional deficiencies and should be monitored for deficiencies in folate and vitamins B12 and D. In severe cases, total parenteral nutrition (TPN) may be required. Like UC, quality of life may be affected, however, the vast majority of patients with CD have a normal life span.

Risk Factors

The etiology for the development of mucosal inflammation is multifactorial. Current theories focus on genetic factors, immunoregulatory defects, microbial exposure, and environmental triggers [23].

Microbial Exposure

The epithelial layer of intestinal mucosa plays an essential role in maintaining functional equilibrium within the lumen from the spectrum of microbial species and their byproducts. Barrier defects within the mucosa increase microbial and antigen presentation, leading to perturbations in the immune response causing IBD. Growing evidence suggests a significant dysbiosis or imbalance among protective and harmful species of microbiota within the intestinal lumen [24]. IBD patients have demonstrated a lack of diversity among species, but no specific species has been implicated as a causative agent in IBD [25]. Identifying the key factors and/or species that shape microbiota-host interactions in the structure and function of the immune response will be a key to the further understanding of the pathogenesis of IBD.

Immunoregulatory Defects

The loss of barrier function can lead to microbial and antigen penetration into the intestinal mucosa, causing immune activation. Both the innate and acquired immune systems are activated with antigen presentation, but differences have been demonstrated within the IBD subtypes. CD results in Th1 and/or Th17 responses with subsequent production of proinflammatory cytokines (i.e., IL-12, IL-18, IFN-γ[gamma]) [26]. The cascade of proinflammatory mediators with CD leads to activation of proteases and metalloproteinases causing tissue destruction and sustained chronic inflammation. The mediator response with UC was previously theorized as a Th2 response, but this is still under investigation [26].

Genetics

Epidemiological and clinical data from Europe and North America have provided strong evidence that CD and UC are related polygenic disorders, and genetic factors play a role in susceptibility to IBD [27, 28]. Up to 14 % of patients with IBD will report a family history of either CD or UC [29]. The relative risk of developing IBD for a first-degree relative is up to 8 % for CD and 5 % for UC, but the risk is increased to 30 % for offspring of parents both affected with IBD [30, 31]. Familial studies have demonstrated a significant genetic link with IBD; however, it appears that IBD is not inherited in simple Mendelian fashion. Rather, it has a complex genetic basis with multiple contributing genes [32].

Genetic linkage studies have demonstrated numerous IBD loci overlapping between UC and CD, with one of the earliest and clearest linkages on chromosome 16 for nucleotide-binding oligomerization domain 2 (NOD2), also known as caspase activation and recruitment domain 15 (CARD15) [33, 34]. NOD2/CARD15 defects have been associated with up to 25 % of CD cases [35]. Homozygosity is associated with a >20-fold increased risk of the development of CD, with heterozygosity conferring a two- to fourfold increased risk [35, 36]. Despite having significant advances in identifying genetic risk factors, genetics may account for <25 % of the pathogenesis of IBD, further suggesting the strong role played by environmental factors [29].

Environmental

Hygiene Similar to other autoimmune diseases such as rheumatoid arthritis, IBD confers an inverse-relationship with sanitation. In other words, poor sanitation appears to protect against

IBD [23]. A 1989 study citing the rising incidence of autoimmune diseases, such as IBD, in developing countries was the first to propose the "hygiene hypothesis." [37] Factors including number of siblings, larger family size, living on a farm, and pet exposures in childhood have been implicated with a reported decreased risk of developing IBD, but such studies were limited in size and subject to significant bias [38, 39]. Less robust associations have been made on the mode of childbirth (potential increased risk with cesarean delivery) and role of breastfeeding (decreased risk) in the development of IBD [40, 41].

Smoking One of the strongest environmental risk factors is smoking tobacco. Patients with CD who smoke have a more aggressive disease course. They typically require more immunosuppression, earlier surgery, and have a higher risk of disease recurrence after ileocecal resection [42]. A 2006 meta-analysis demonstrated an almost twofold increased risk of developing CD associated with smoking; conversely, a strong inverse association with active smoking and UC was seen [43]. Current smoking appears to reduce the risk of developing UC. In a cohort of female nurses, there was an increased risk of developing UC within 5 years of smoking cessation. This risk remained elevated for up to 20 years [44]. Passive smoking had similar effects [45]. While it appears that smoking can reduce inflammation in patients with UC, it is not a recommended habit due to the other well-described health concerns.

Medications Antibiotics have been implicated as a potential risk factor for IBD due to the alteration of the gut flora. A 2014 study reported an almost twofold increased risk for developing CD from prior antibiotic exposure, though the same risk did not apply to UC [46]. The association of IBD with antibiotics has also been shown to be stronger with exposure in the first year of life compared with later use [47]. However, conflicting evidence from Asia has demonstrated a protective association of antibiotic exposure with the development of IBD [48]. Nonsteroidal anti-inflammatory drugs (NSAIDs) can increase the risk of IBD, but the absolute risk is small [49, 50]. The association was strongest with higher doses and longer duration of therapy. The conferred risk was similar for both CD and UC [51, 52]. Avoidance of NSAIDs is recommended; however, occasional use likely presents an acceptable risk.

Prior case reports have suggested an association between IBD and isotretinoin, used in the treatment of acne vulgaris [53, 54]. However, in a meta-analysis, pooled results from the United States claims database did not support this association [55]. Therefore, clinicians should not avoid prescribing retinoic acid when other drugs fail. Acne carries a high psychosocial burden and the association between retinoic acid and IBD has not been confirmed.

Current oral contraceptive use poses a very minor increased risk for developing CD, and the risk is even lower for past users [56, 57]. The same risk was not seen with UC. Lower-estrogen formulations of contraception may be safer. Because the overall risk is so low, avoidance of oral contraceptive use cannot be recommended.

Stress Most patients with IBD note that their disease often flares during stressful events. Large observational studies support an association between major life stressors, anxiety, depression, and the risk of IBD development [58–61]. Due to the unpredictable nature of IBD, anxiety is a major concern, especially for adolescents. Working with a psychologist is often helpful. Newer cognitive behavioral techniques and mindfulness training are currently being investigated in patients with IBD.

Obesity An association between IBD and obesity still remains unclear [62, 63]. In CD patients, the accumulation of intra-abdominal fat may play a role in mucosal inflammation and progression of disease [64]. Obese patients have been shown to have higher rates of hospitalizations and are more likely to require IBD-related surgery [65, 66]. A 2013 prospective study demonstrated that intense physical activity had a >40 % risk reduction in the development of CD, but there was no significant association with UC [67].

Sleep Sleep quality and duration can have an impact on IBD. Sleep deprivation has been associated with an increased risk of UC, and poor sleep quality was implicated with higher risk of relapse [68, 69].

Clinical Considerations in Individuals with IBD

The role of the primary care provider (PCP) in the co-management of IBD with the subspecialist is essential in optimizing the clinical care of the IBD patient.

Sexual and Reproductive Health

Ideally, dialogue about the impact that IBD has on intimacy, reproduction, and pregnancy should have already been initiated by the patient's pediatric or adolescent provider. However, this is not always the case. Conversations with an adult provider about intimacy and sexuality may therefore be welcome [70]. In fact, this may be a useful way for the young adult to separate from his or her parents and develop an independent relationship with the adult provider.

One-third of CD patients say IBD has a major impact on their sexual life. Impaired body image has been reported in 35 % of women and 13 % of men [71]. There may be disfiguration of the rectovaginal area, abdominal scars, or the presence of an ostomy. About 58 % of patients report decreased libido caused by diarrhea, fever, and/or abdominal pain [72]. Patients need a safe place to discuss these issues. They may want to know how and when to disclose their chronic condition to their partners. Unfortunately, 1 study reported that 40 % of IBD patients feel that the disease prevents an intimate relationship altogether [73]. While it may not be practical for the adult physician to provide extensive counseling, the acknowledgement that these are important quality-of-life issues can help patients feel comfortable with their new adult doctor.

Fecundity, the probability of becoming pregnant per month by unprotected intercourse, is normal in female IBD patients. The exceptions are active disease and pelvic surgery—most commonly the creation of an ileal pouch after total colectomy [74]. There is, however, a decrease in fertility by as much as 14–36 % due to voluntary childlessness among both male and female patients with IBD. They may be afraid of passing on the disease to their offspring, be concerned about medication teratogenicity, or be worried about the difficulty of raising a child when they themselves have active and unpredictable disease [75, 76]. By establishing a positive relationship with young adult patients, adult physicians can educate patients and help them overcome these barriers.

Pregnancy outcomes have been well studied in IBD patients. A majority of the literature demonstrates a slightly higher risk of IBD-related pregnancy complications that include preterm birth and low birth weight, but there is not a significant increased risk of congenital abnormalities [77–79]. Patients should understand that these risks are caused by active inflammation and not by their medications. The majority of medications, including the thiopurines and biologics, are safe for use during pregnancy with the exception of methotrexate, which is a category X agent. Patients should be encouraged to continue to take their medications throughout their pregnancy in order to allow for the best outcome. Pregnancy has not shown a higher likelihood to induce flares, but active disease at conception has been associated with higher rates of disease worsening throughout pregnancy [80, 81].

The role of the PCP is to acknowledge the need to discuss the impact of IBD on intimacy, sexuality, and fertility with both male and female patients. It is important to maintain good communication with the patient's gastroenterologist so that the same messages are conveyed and reinforced. Conflicting messages can be harmful to patients and may cause unnecessary anxiety.

The strong bond between the PCP and patient allows for open discussion of these delicate yet important topics.

Preventive Care

Preventive care has traditionally been in the domain of the PCP. With the increased use of immunomodulators and biologics, the task of providing proper preventive measures can be daunting. Important preventive health considerations for individuals with IBD include cancer screening and prevention, osteoporosis screening and prevention, and immunizations.

Cancer Screening and Prevention

In patients with IBD, the risk of colon cancer is much higher than in the general population. General population screening without risk factors begins at age 50 years. For patients with IBD, it is recommended that patients with 8–10 years of Crohn's colitis (Crohn's that involves the large bowel) or UC have an annual or biannual surveillance colonoscopy with multiple biopsies [20]. For patients with concomitant primary sclerosing cholangitis, colonoscopic surveillance should begin immediately. Patients with isolated ulcerative proctitis (colitis involving the rectum only) do not have an increased risk of colon cancer beyond that of the general population. Therefore, increased screening is not required.

Women with IBD, especially those requiring use of immunomodulators and biologics, have a higher prevalence of abnormal Pap smears [82, 83]. The American College of Obstetrics and Gynecology (ACOG) recommends screening of women starting at 21 years of age with Pap smears and then every 3 years thereafter [84]. However, due to the increased risk among women on immunosuppressive therapy, expert recommendations are for yearly screening with Pap smears in patients on immunomodulator and/or biologic therapy once sexual activity has begun [85].

IBD patients, especially those on immunomodulators and/or biologics, have an increased risk of skin cancers compared to the general population. Thiopurine use is associated with an increased risk of nonmelanoma skin cancers, particularly basal cell carcinoma and squamous cell carcinoma, with an incidence rate of 1.1 cases per 1000 person-years [86]. With respect to melanoma, patients exposed to tumor necrosis factor-alpha (TNF-α[alpha]) antagonists have a twofold higher risk than in unexposed patients, with an incidence rate of about 0.5 cases per 1000 person-years [87]. Experts recommend yearly visual skin exam by a dermatologist for patients on immunomodulators and/or TNF-α(alpha) antagonists in combination with appropriate sun exposure precautions.

Osteoporosis Screening and Prevention

IBD itself, along with an increased use of corticosteroids, puts this population at risk for osteoporosis. Nutritional assessments, such as vitamin D testing, are recommended to be performed at least annually, with appropriate repletion for those individuals with a deficiency. Bone density assessment is in line with the U.S. Preventative Services Task Force recommendations, but with additional considerations:

1. Steroid use >3 months
2. Inactive disease but past chronic steroid use of at least 1 year within the past 2 years
3. Inactive disease but maternal history of osteoporosis
4. Inactive disease but malnourished or very thin
5. Inactive disease but amenorrhiec.

Consideration should be made to screen patients earlier than normal if such risk factors exist [85, 88].

Immunizations

As the rates of use for immunosuppressive drugs in IBD increases, optimal preventable measures, such as vaccinations, can help limit the risk of infectious complications. Patients often turn to their PCP who had been responsible for administering vaccines throughout their life. Therefore, the role of the PCP in managing vaccine administration is pivotal.

Adult patients are often unaware of the recommended adult immunization schedule, and this may be especially concerning for those who

Table 12.2 Live and inactivated adult vaccines in the United States

Live	Inactivated
Live attenuated influenza vaccine (LAIV)	Inactivated Influenza Vaccine (IIV)
Varicella (chicken pox)	Tetanus/diphtheria/pertussis (Tdap)
Zoster (shingles)	Pneumococcal 13 valent (PCV-13)
Measles, mumps, and rubella (MMR)	Pneumococcal polysaccharide (PPSV23)
Yellow fever	Meningococcal
	Hepatitis A and B
	Human papilloma virus

are immunosuppressed and may require additional vaccinations. Patients with IBD have a higher risk of pneumonia [89]. Therefore, if the pneumococcal 13-valent and 23-valent vaccines were not administered during childhood, they should be offered to adult patients. Unfortunately, current vaccination rates in IBD populations are suboptimal with <90 % of patients receiving yearly influenza vaccinations and <50 % receiving pneumococcal vaccinations [90, 91]. To help improve these rates, patients should be advised to bring updated vaccination records to their adult provider.

There are special considerations for vaccinating patients who are on immunosuppressive therapy. Administering a live vaccine to an immunosuppressed patient can be life threatening [92]. All live vaccines that are available in the United States are listed in Table 12.2. Ideally, live vaccines should be administered more than 4 weeks before immunosuppression is initiated. However, there are some exceptions. For IBD patients on low levels of immunosuppression—defined as methotrexate <0.4 mg/kg per week, azathioprine <3 mg/kg per day, and 6-mercaptopurine <1.5 mg/kg per day—live vaccines, such as the varicella vaccination, can be considered. For highly immunosuppressed patients—defined as individuals with primary immunodeficiency disorder, cancer chemotherapy, within 2 months of solid organ transplant, human immunodeficiency virus (HIV) infection with a CD4 T-cell count <200/mm^3, systemic corticosteroid >20 mg/day for more than 14 days, anti-TNF agent use or rituximab use—live vaccines should be avoided altogether [93]. Unlike live vaccines, inactivated vaccines can be administered at any point while on immunosuppression. To allow adequate time for development of protective antibodies, inactivated vaccines should be administered at least 2 weeks prior to initiation of immunosuppression. Therefore, it is good practice to vaccinate patients with IBD when they are well, even if they are not on immunosuppressive therapy. This will allow for the immediate initiation of treatment should a flare occur. A complete vaccine dosing schedule can be found through the Centers for Disease Control and Prevention [94].

There have been many newly licensed vaccines, and the recommendations for vaccine administration for immunosuppressed patients are rapidly evolving. Having both the PCP and the gastroenterologist offer these important vaccines in comanagement of patients could increase the vaccination rates.

Diet

It would be clearly beneficial if following a specific diet could cure or improve symptoms in patients with IBD. However, because strictly controlling diet is difficult, prospective studies are limited. It is known, though, that food plays an important role. Strict enteral nutrition has shown benefits in the induction and maintenance of remission in IBD, particularly in children [95].

Patients frequently scour the Internet for special diets, hoping to manage their disease without the use of medication. Popular diets include the specific carbohydrate diet; the low fermentable oligosaccharides, disaccharides, and monosaccharides (FODMAP) diet; a paleolithic (paleo) diet; or a vegan diet [96]. For some, these diets work tremendously well. For the majority, they do not. Currently there is no diet that can be prescribed for everyone. The most important point to emphasize is that a balanced healthy diet be followed. Many of these well-meaning diets cause weight loss, which can be dangerous. Some are so difficult to follow that it leads to unnecessary stress.

Avoiding dairy is also a popular fad diet, but this puts patients at an even higher risk for osteoporosis and there is no current evidence to support this practice. A vegan diet increases the risk for vitamin D and vitamin B12 deficiency.

There is scientific evidence that particular dietary factors may influence the risk of developing IBD. Dietary fiber intake has been associated with a lower risk of developing CD, but not UC [97]. The consumption of greater amounts of red meat and fats, particularly polyunsaturated fatty acids (PUFAs) and omega-6 (n-6) fatty acids, increases the risk of developing IBD as opposed to a diet high in fiber, fruits, and vegetables [98]. Ingested iron, particularly iron sulfate, has been directly linked with intestinal inflammation; however, the effects of iron from red meat is unknown [99]. Dietary calcium and vitamin D are important for IBD patients, not only for bone health but also because vitamin D is involved in anti-inflammatory pathways [100].

Some specific dietary recommendations can include reducing red meat and saturated fats, and increasing dietary fiber, such as oatmeal. For patients with known stenosis or those in the first 6 weeks after a partial bowel resection, a low residue diet is recommended to avoid the risk of possible obstruction. Following a low residue diet means avoiding peanuts, popcorn, raw vegetables, skins of vegetables, and high fiber foods.

At this time, there is no diet that can cure or reduce existing inflammation. The role of the PCP is to recommend eating a healthy balanced diet, replenish possible nutrient deficiencies, and encourage avoidance of extreme, possibly stressful diets. If the patient is at risk of poor nutrient intake, a multivitamin can be supplemented.

Drug Monitoring/Side Effect Management

Over the last decade, a large number of therapeutic options has become available for the treatment of IBD. These drugs include mesalamines, thiopurines, and, more recently, biological agents with multiple different mechanisms of action. The majority of such medications will be under the management of a gastroenterologist, but the PCP can still play a key role when drug side effects arise or in routine lab monitoring.

One of the first-line class choices for treatment of IBD is the mesalamine-based (5-ASA) drugs. Mesalamine has an advantage in UC, but there is limited data to support its use in CD [101, 102]. There are minimal side effects associated with the newer generation 5-ASA drugs. However, headaches, hair loss, and, rarely, pancreatitis have been reported. Because there is a small but real risk of developing interstitial nephritis, routine assessment of renal function every 6–12 months and a yearly urinalysis are recommended [103].

Corticosteroids are often needed to provide immediate relief for patients with UC. They are used in UC when mesalamines do not control the inflammation and in CD when the symptoms are severe or a biologic is not available. Steroid use is typically recommended for shorter durations due to the significant side effect profile. Along with the known side effects of corticosteroids, patients with CD can develop fistulae or opportunistic infections. Because patients with IBD are often on steroids along with other immunosuppressive agents, prophylaxis against *Pneumocystis* pneumonia, which can be initiated by the PCP, is important. Management of side effects requires the use of steroid-sparing drugs.

Immunomodulators are steroid-sparing drugs that work by inhibiting the proliferation and activation of lymphocytes. Common drugs in this class include azathioprine (AZA), 6-mercaptopurine

(6-MP), and methotrexate (MTX). AZA and 6MP are also called thiopurines and follow weight-based dosing. Gastroenterologists can optimize the dose by using biomarkers such as thiopurine methyltransferase (TPMT) activity and drug metabolites such as 6-thioguanine (6-TG) and 6-methylmercaptopurine (6-MMP). Side effects include agranulocytosis and hepatotoxicity [104]. Other complications include autoimmune hepatitis, fatigue, and pancreatitis. Severe effects such as myelosuppression and pancreatitis can be managed with discontinuation of therapy and supportive care. To minimize complications, routine lab monitoring with complete blood count (CBC) with differential and hepatic function should be performed every 3 months. A reduction in the white blood cell (WBC) count is desired, but if it falls to $<4.0 \times 10^3$ cells/μ(mu)L, the drug should be held and restarted at a lower dose once the WBC count returns to normal. Methotrexate is an alternative to the thiopurines and is used more commonly in CD. Major complications include hepatotoxicity, myelosuppression, and pneumonitis, which occur in <10 % of patients [105]. This agent should always be taken in conjunction with folic acid to avoid anemia. Chest X-ray and baseline liver function tests, followed by an assessment of CBC with differential and hepatic function every 3 months, are recommended. Consideration for liver biopsy is suggested for patients with liver enzymes that remain persistently elevated for more than 12 months [106].

The use of biologic drugs, such as anti-TNFα (alpha), has had a significant impact on the treatment of IBD. The medications included in this class are infliximab, adalimumab, and certolizumab. Numerous clinical trials have demonstrated efficacy for use in moderate to severe CD and UC [107–109]. These drugs are very well tolerated and have minimal side effects. Side effects include infusion or injection site reactions, opportunistic infections, autoimmune hepatitis, and psoriasis. Rarely, there are neurological side effects including unmasking of underlying multiple sclerosis. The most feared side effect is hepatosplenic T-cell lymphoma. This occurs rarely, seen in approximately 4–5/10,000 patients. The demographic most often affected are men under the age of 35 years [110]. A thorough exam for lymphadenopathy and splenomegaly is required at every visit. Prior to drug initiation, latent tuberculosis infection and hepatitis B virus infection should be ruled out to prevent dissemination. The PCP can assist with routine lab testing, which should be drawn every 3–6 months.

Extraintestinal Manifestations

An extraintestinal manifestation (EIM) is a disease that occurs outside of the bowel and is associated with IBD. At least 25 % of patients with IBD are affected [111]. While there are numerous EIMs, the most common include arthropathy, cutaneous lesions, and ocular inflammation (see Table 12.3). Unfortunately, the underlying pathogenesis of EIM development

Table 12.3 Common extraintestinal manifestations (EIM) and relationship to IBD activity

EIM	Paralleling disease activity	Independent of disease activity	Either parallel or independent of activity
Axial arthropathy		X	
Peripheral arthropathy	X (Type I)	X (Type II)	
Erythema nodosum	X		
Pyoderma gangrenosum			X
Oral apthous ulcers	X		
Episcleritis	X		
Uveitis			X
Primary sclerosing cholangitis			X

in IBD is not well understood. EIMs can either parallel or be independent of disease activity. They can be the first presenting feature of IBD, and the finding of 1 of these conditions should trigger a referral to a gastroenterologist. Pediatric patients have been shown to have a higher prevalence of EIMs in comparison to adult patients [112]. Furthermore, because patients with IBD are often unaware of EIM, they may first seek care for them from their PCP. It is critical that the PCP coordinate appropriate evaluation with the gastroenterologist when this occurs.

Arthropathy

Joint pain or inflammation is the most common EIM in IBD, occurring in up to 40 % of IBD patients [113]. Peripheral arthralgia can occur in up to 10 % of UC patients and 20 % of CD patients. It is characterized as seronegative, and classified into 2 distinct categories. Type I (pauciarticular) involves <5 large joints and is dependent on disease activity. Type II (polyarticular) involves >5 large joints, and its severity is independent of disease activity. Knees tend to be the most commonly affected joints, but differentiation of Type I versus Type II is seldom clinically relevant. Treating the underlying bowel inflammation can help in the control of joint symptoms, but further evaluation by rheumatology is recommended in refractory cases. The use of NSAIDs is discouraged due to the potential for worsening of underlying IBD [114].

Skin/Mucosal Lesions

Cutaneous disorders associated with IBD can occur in up to 15 % of patients [115]. Erythema nodosum (EN) is characterized as raised, tender, red/violet subcutaneous nodules measuring up to 5 cm in diameter. They are typically located on the anterior surface of the lower extremities (Fig. 12.1) [116]. EN usually resolves when the bowel inflammation is treated. Pyoderma gangrenosum (PG), on the other hand, has an unpredictable course and does not parallel disease activity. It is characterized initially with an erythematous pustule/nodule, followed by rapid local spread and development into a burrowing ulcer with irregular violaceous edges (Fig. 12.2) [117]. The same drugs used to treat IBD are used to treat PG. However, refractory cases have shown benefit with intralesional steroids and/or cyclosporine [118]. PG typically involves expert consultation with a dermatologist.

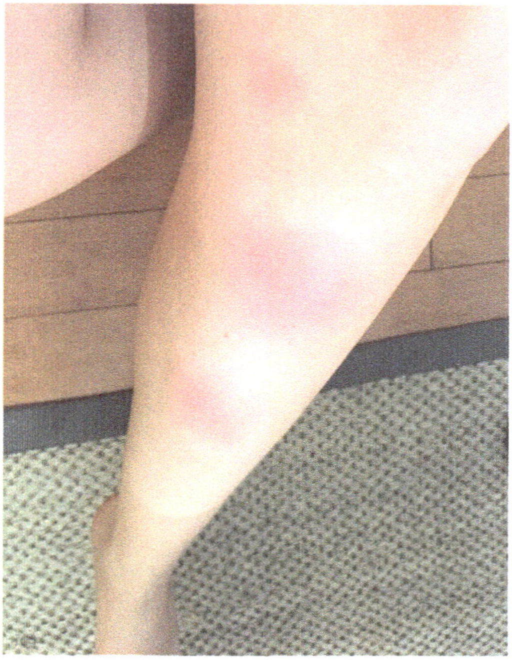

Fig. 12.1 Erythema nodosum of the anterior left leg in a patient with ulcerative colitis. (Courtesy of Dr. Elana Maser)

Apthous ulcers in the oral cavity typically occur in conjunction with IBD activity and are localized to the buccal mucosa, with occasional appearances on the tongue. Treatment typically involves therapy of underlying IBD in combination with antiseptic mouthwashes and topical steroid dental paste.

Ophthalmologic Manifestations

Up to 5 % of IBD patients will present with ocular manifestations [119]. Episcleritis is characterized as a painless hyperemia of the conjunctiva and often parallels IBD activity. Treatment of the underlying bowel inflammation, along with topical steroids, is used to relieve symptoms. Alternatively, the temporal correlation of uveitis with IBD is unpredictable. Uveitis

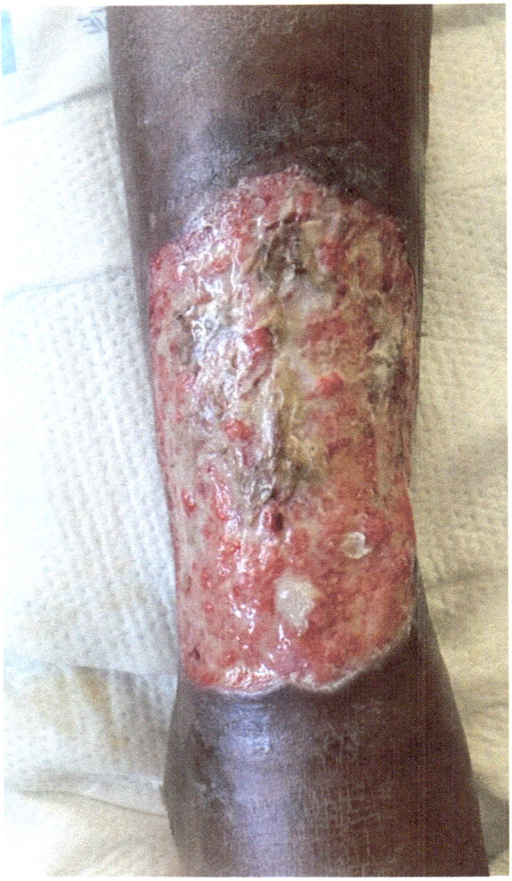

Fig. 12.2 Pyoderma gangrenosum of the anterior left leg in a patient with ulcerative colitis. Note the "violaceous" hue along the borders. (Courtesy of Dr. David Faleck and Dr. Serre-yu Wong)

may present as ocular pain, blurred vision, or photophobia. Uveitis can progress to blindness, thus all patients with IBD who present with any ocular symptoms should be immediately referred to an ophthalmologist in addition to annual ophthalmological evaluation.

Special Issues in the Transition to Adult Care

With the rising incidence of pediatric IBD, a larger number of young patients are transitioning to adult care. Adult providers need to be ready to manage young adults who may lack the readiness to cope with their illness independently. With evidence from chronic disease models, poorer outcomes have been demonstrated in young adults transitioning to adult healthcare, partly due to the expectation of increased autonomy [120, 121].

One of the major issues with transition of care based on a survey of adult gastroenterologists was the lack of specific adolescent training [122]. Gastroenterology fellowship programs provide minimal, if any, training in the care of adolescents. The care of young adults in other chronic conditions, such as rheumatologic and cardiac diseases, presents similar concerns [123, 124]. Adult providers will need to be aware of their patients developing independence, differences in the adolescent's style of communication, body image concerns, navigating intimate relationships, and missed school or work [125]. Finally, coordinating insurance coverage as the adolescent transitions off their parents' insurance plan is particularly important because treating IBD often requires expensive biologic drugs, and such advanced preparation may help in avoiding gaps in care.

Some adolescents arrive at the adult gastroenterologist ready to take control of their own health care, while others continue to communicate through their parents. Every adolescent grows at his or her own pace. The first step is for the provider to assess the patient's current level of independence and build from there. Part of fostering independence includes helping adolescents understand what it means to manage IBD. Having IBD often involves frequent lab testing, imaging, and annual screening colonoscopies, procedures that may not have needed to be initiated by their pediatric gastroenterologist.

Fostering independence also includes encouraging adolescents to communicate directly with their physician rather than through their parents. Having this direct connection will help establish trust. Because adolescents often prefer to communicate through email and text, the use of patient portals that allow for electronic communication may be helpful. In gastroenterology, there are many emerging applications (a.k.a. "apps") for disease education and monitoring.

Once communication and trust have been established, there can be an opening to discuss the impact of IBD on body image and sexuality. The diagnosis of IBD is often made in adolescence when body image is forming. Up to two-thirds of adult IBD patients report impaired body image, and one-third blame IBD for negatively affecting their sexual desire and satisfaction [71, 73]. The presence of disfiguring abdominal scars or the presence of an ostomy may lead patients to withdraw from active sexual relationships and have difficulty initiating new ones, especially during the sensitive adolescent period. Patients may want advice on how and when to disclose that they have a chronic illness to their partners. Unfortunately, adequate counseling, especially for women, on sexual health IBD remains low [126]. Not all primary care physicians or gastroenterologists are able to counsel patients. However, they can explain that these important issues are being considered when making medical decisions. For example, if colectomy is required, it is helpful to discuss with patients that an ostomy can be well hidden under clothing and that there are bathing suits that are designed to hide ostomies. PCPs can help advocate for their patients if these sensitive topics are more easily discussed with them than with a gastroenterologist. Whether or not the adolescent seems well adjusted, referral to a psychologist should be offered to all patients to support them while they navigate this sensitive time.

Missed school or work can be difficult for young adults as they attempt to establish themselves in their careers. The indirect costs of missed work and unemployment are estimated at $3.6 billion per year [127]. Physicians can help minimize the disruption to the lives of their patients by being sensitive to the possible need to delay a surgery or start a new medication when conflicts with work, school, weddings, or travel may exist. College students can be advised that they may be eligible for exam extensions or taking a leave from school if necessary. Many pharmaceutical companies offer scholarships to help support patients with IBD. There are also camps for children with Crohn's (Camp Oasis), where an adolescent can provide counsel to younger children navigating their disease and allow them to meet others with similar issues.

As children grow up, they eventually age off of their parent's health insurance. A 2014 survey demonstrated that only up to 24 % of young adults received counseling with respect to obtaining insurance coverage [128]. Interruption in the administration of biological agents can prevent their usefulness in the future. Therefore, notifying patients to be proactive regarding their coverage can be life changing. If possible, access to a social worker would be helpful.

Conclusion

Acknowledging issues that are important to adolescents with IBD when they arrive in an adult practice will establish trust and ultimately lead to better patient outcomes and satisfaction ("Appendix"). It is important to maintain careful coordination of care between the PCP and subspecialist to assure the delivery of comprehensive care to patients with IBD.

Appendix

Inflammatory bowel disease (IBD) fact sheet

Definition	**Inflammatory Bowel Disease (IBD)** is characterized by chronic, relapsing inflammation within the gastrointestinal tract. IBD consists of Crohn's disease (CD) and ulcerative colitis (UC). • UC: affects the mucosal layer of the colon and rectum • CD: affects all layers of the bowel and can occur in any part of the gastrointestinal tract from mouth to anus.
Prevalence	• Affects more than 5 million people worldwide, with more than 1.7 million in the United States • Lifetime risk of development is 1 % • ¼ of patients are diagnosed in childhood or adolescence
Pathophysiology	Inflammation is a result of inappropriate and ongoing activation of the innate immune system of the gut mucosa, driven by the commensal luminal flora in a genetically susceptible host • Unclear as to specific flora responsible for activation • Limited variation in gut bacteria is typically seen in an IBD host
Symptoms	Symptoms can overlap between CD and UC but each has distinctive attributes that can help differentiate: • Abdominal pain, diarrhea • Perianal fistulas (CD) • Weight loss • Anemia, vitamin deficiencies • Bloody stools (higher risk in UC)
Challenges in transition	The transition from pediatric to adult care can be complicated due to the complexity of disease management. • Complications related to the underlying disease and advanced therapies in IBD can be difficult to assess. • Limited scope on routine health maintenance, to include vaccinations and cancer screening (for example, annual colon cancer screening with colonoscopy) • Compliance of medication therapy • Access to therapy and care if college-bound • Discussions in intimacy and pregnancy • Gaining trust in new provider • Dietary management
Helpful resources	• Crohn's and Colitis Foundation of America (resources for patients and family members, may include local chapters in communities throughout the US): http://www.ccfa.org • American College of Gastroenterology Guidelines on Crohn's disease and Ulcerative Colitis management (developed by expert panel): http://gi.org/clinical-guidelines/clinical-guidelines-sortable-list/

References

1. Escher J. Transition from pediatrics to adult health care in inflammatory bowel disease. Dig Dis. 2009;27:382–6.
2. Dabadie A, Troadec F, Heresbach D, Siproudhis L, Pagenault M, Bretagne JF. Transition of patients with inflammatory bowel disease from pediatric to adult care. Gastroenterol Clin Biol. 2008;32(5 Pt 1):451–9.
3. El-Matary W. Transition of children with inflammatory bowel disease: big task, little evidence. World J Gastroenterol. 2009;15(30):3744.
4. Van Assche G, Vermeire S, Ballet V, Gabriels F, Noman M, D'Haens G, et al. Switch to adalimumab in patients with Crohn's disease controlled by maintenance infliximab: prospective randomised switch trial. Gut. 2012;61(2):229–34.
5. Burisch J, Jess T, Martinato M, Lakatos PL. The burden of inflammatory bowel disease in Europe. J Crohns Colitis. 2013;7(4):322–37.

6. Bernstein C, Wajda A, Svenson L, MacKenzie A, Koehoorn M, Jackson M. The epidemiology of inflammatory bowel disease in canada: a population-based study. Am J Gastroenterol. 2006;101:1559–68.
7. Burisch J, Pedersen N, Cukovic-Cavka S, Brinar M, Kaimakliotis I, Duricova D, et al. East-west gradient in the incidence of inflammatory bowel disease in Europe: the ecco-epicom inception cohort. Gut. 2014;63(4):588–97.
8. Sawczenko A, Sandhu BK, Logan RFA, Jenkins H, Taylor CJ, Mian S, et al. Prospective survey of childhood inflammatory bowel disease in the british isles. Lancet. 2001;357(9262):1093–4.
9. Malaty HM, Fan X, Opekun AR, Thibodeaux C, Ferry GD. Rising incidence of inflammatory bowel disease among children: a 12-year study. J Pediatr Gastroenterol Nutr. 2010;50(1):27–31.
10. Loftus CG, Loftus EV Jr, Harmsen WS, Zinsmeister AR, Tremaine WJ, Melton LJ 3rd, et al. Update on the incidence and prevalence of Crohn's disease and ulcerative colitis in olmsted county, minnesota, 1940-2000. Inflamm Bowel Dis. 2007;13(3):254–61.
11. Romberg-Camps MJL, Hesselink-van de Kruijs MAM, Schouten LJ, Dagnelie PC, Limonard CB, Kester AD. Inflammatory bowel disease in South Limburg (the Netherlands) 1991–2002: incidence, diagnostic delay, and seasonal variations in onset of symptoms. J Crohns Colitis. 2009;3:115–24.
12. Trallori G, Palli D, Saieva C, Bardazzi G, Bonanomi A, D'Albasio G. A population-based study of inflammatory bowel disease in florence over 15 years (1978-92). Scand J Gastroenterol. 1996;31:892–9.
13. Robison WW, Bentlif PS, Kelsey JR. Observations on 261 consecutive patients with inflammatory bowel disease seen in the southwest united states. Dig Dis Sci. 1980;25:198–204.
14. Anderson CA, Boucher G, Lees CW, Franke A, D'Amato M, Taylor KD, et al. Meta-analysis identifies 29 additional ulcerative colitis risk loci, increasing the number of confirmed associations to 47. Nat Genet. 2011;43(3):246–52.
15. Franke A, McGovern DP, Barrett JC, Wang K, Radford-Smith GL, Ahmad T, et al. Genome-wide meta-analysis increases to 71 the number of confirmed Crohn's disease susceptibility loci. Nat Genet. 2010;42(12):1118–25.
16. Bellaguarda E, Chang EB. IBD and the gut microbiota–from bench to personalized medicine. Curr Gastroenterol Rep. 2015;17(4):15.
17. Hart AL, Ng SC, Mann E, Al-Hassi HO, Bernardo D, Knight SC. Homing of immune cells: role in homeostasis and intestinal inflammation. Inflamm Bowel Dis. 2010;16(11):1969–77.
18. Hold GL, Smith M, Grange C, Watt ER, El-Omar EM, Mukhopadhya I. Role of the gut microbiota in inflammatory bowel disease pathogenesis: what have we learnt in the past 10 years? World J Gastroenterol. 2014;20(5):1192–210.
19. Monstad I, Hovde O, Solberg IC, Moum BA. Clinical course and prognosis in ulcerative colitis: results from population-based and observational studies. Ann Gastroenterol. 2014;27(2):95–104.
20. Kornbluth A, Sachar DB, Practice Parameters Committee of the American College of G. Ulcerative colitis practice guidelines in adults: American college of gastroenterology, practice parameters committee. Am J Gastroenterol. 2010;105(3):501–23 (quiz 524).
21. Louis E, Collard A, Oger AF, Degroote E, Aboul Nasr El Yafi FA, Belaiche J. Behaviour of Crohn's disease according to the vienna classification: changing pattern over the course of the disease. Gut. 2001;49(6):777–82.
22. Maser EA, Sachar DB, Kruse D, Harpaz N, Ullman T, Bauer JJ. High rates of metachronous colon cancer or dysplasia after segmental resection or subtotal colectomy in Crohn's colitis. Inflamm Bowel Dis. 2013;19(9):1827–32.
23. Hanauer S. Epidemiology, pathogenesis, and treatment of ibd. Inflamm Bowel Dis. 2006;12(1):S3–9.
24. Frank DN, St Amand AL, Feldman RA, Boedeker EC, Harpaz N, Pace NR. Molecular-phylogenetic characterization of microbial community imbalances in human inflammatory bowel diseases. Proc Natl Acad Sci USA. 2007;104(34):13780–5.
25. Manichanh C, Rigottier-Gois L, Bonnaud E, Gloux K, Pelletier E, Frangeul L, et al. Reduced diversity of faecal microbiota in Crohn's disease revealed by a metagenomic approach. Gut. 2006;55(2):205–11.
26. Papadakis KA, Targan SR. Role of cytokines in the pathogenesis of inflammatory bowel disease. Annu Rev Med. 2000;51:289–98.
27. Satsangi J, Jewell D, Bell J. The genetics of inflammatory bowel disease. Gut. 1997;40(5):572.
28. Satsangi J, Morecroft J, Shah N, Nimmo E. Genetics of inflammatory bowel disease: scientific and clinical implications. Best Pract Res Clin Gastroenterol. 2003;17(1):3–18.
29. Khor B, Gardet A, Xavier RJ. Genetics and pathogenesis of inflammatory bowel disease. Nature. 2011;474(7351):307–17.
30. Halme L, Paavola-Sakki P, Turunen U, Lappalainen M, Farkkila M, Kontula K. Family and twin studies in inflammatory bowel disease. World J Gastroenterol. 2006;12(23):3668–72.
31. Yang H, McElree C, Roth M, Shanahan F, Targan S, Rotter J. Familial empirical risks for inflammatory bowel disease: differences between jews and non-jews. Gut. 1993;34(4):517–24.
32. Bouma G, Strober W. The immunological and genetic basis of inflammatory bowel disease. Nat Rev Immunol. 2003;3(7):521–33.
33. Hugot J, Laurent-Puig P, Gower-Rousseau C, Olson J, Lee J, Beaugerie L, et al. Mapping a

susceptibility locus for Crohn's disease on chromosome 16. Nature. 1996;379(6568):821–3.
34. Jostins L, Ripke S, Weersma RK, Duerr RH, McGovern DP, Hui KY, et al. Host-microbe interactions have shaped the genetic architecture of inflammatory bowel disease. Nature. 2012;491 (7422):119–24.
35. Hugot J, Chamaillard M, Zouali H, Lesage S, Cezard J, Belaiche J, et al. Association of nod2 leucine-rich repeat variants with susceptibility to Crohn's disease. Nature. 2001;411(6837):599–603.
36. Ogura Y, Bonen D, Inohara N, Nicolae D, Chen F, Ramos R, et al. A frameshift mutation in nod2 associated with susceptibility to Crohn's disease. Nature. 2001;411(6837):603–6.
37. Strachan D. Hay fever, hygiene, and household size. BMJ. 1989;299(6710):1259–60.
38. Radon K, Windstetter D, Poluda AL, Mueller B, von Mutius E, Koletzko S, et al. Contact with farm animals in early life and juvenile inflammatory bowel disease: a case-control study. Pediatrics. 2007;120(2):354–61.
39. Van Kruiningen H, Joosens M, Vermeire S, Joosens S, Debeugny S, Gower-Rousseau C, et al. Environmental factors in familial Crohn's disease in belgium. Inflamm Bowel Dis. 2005;11(4):360–5.
40. Bager P, Simonsen J, Nielsen NM, Frisch M. Cesarean section and offspring's risk of inflammatory bowel disease: a national cohort study. Inflamm Bowel Dis. 2012;18(5):857–62.
41. Barclay A, Russell R, Wilson M, Gilmour W, Satsangi J, Wilson D. Systematic review: the role of breastfeeding in the development of pediatric inflammatory bowel disease. J Pedatr. 2009;155(3):421–6.
42. Cosnes J, Carbonnel F, Beaugerie L, Le Quintrec Y, Gendre J. Effects of cigarette smoking on the long-term course of Crohn's disease. Gastroenterology. 1996;110(2):424–31.
43. Mahid S, Minor K, Soto R, Hornung C, Galandiuk S. Smoking and inflammatory bowel disease: a meta-analysis. Mayo Clin Proc. 2006;81 (11):1462–71.
44. Higuchi LM, Khalili H, Chan AT, Richter JM, Bousvaros A, Fuchs CS. A prospective study of cigarette smoking and the risk of inflammatory bowel disease in women. Am J Gastroenterol. 2012;107(9):1399–406.
45. Mahid SS, Minor KS, Stromberg AJ, Galandiuk S. Active and passive smoking in childhood is related to the development of inflammatory bowel disease. Inflamm Bowel Dis. 2007;13(4):431–8.
46. Ungaro R, Bernstein CN, Gearry R, Hviid A, Kolho KL, Kronman MP, et al. Antibiotics associated with increased risk of new-onset Crohn's disease but not ulcerative colitis: a meta-analysis. Am J Gastroenterol. 2014;109(11):1728–38.
47. Kronman MP, Zaoutis TE, Haynes K, Feng R, Coffin SE. Antibiotic exposure and ibd development among children: a population-based cohort study. Pediatrics. 2012;130(4):e794–803.
48. Gevers D, Kugathasan S, Denson LA, Vazquez-Baeza Y, Van Treuren W, Ren B, et al. The treatment-naive microbiome in new-onset Crohn's disease. Cell Host Microbe. 2014;15 (3):382–92.
49. Felder J, Korelitz B, Rajapakse R, Schwarz S, Horatagis A, Gleim G. Effects of nonsteroidal antiinflammatory drugs on inflammatory bowel disease: a case-control study. Am J Gastroenterol. 2000;95(8):1949.
50. Kaufmann H, Taubin H. Nonsteroidal anti-inflammatory drugs activate quiescent inflammatory bowel disease. Ann Intern Med. 1987;107 (4):513.
51. Ananthakrishnan A, Higuchi L, Huang E, Khalili H, Richter J, Fuchs C, et al. Aspirin, nonsteroidal anti-inflammatory drug use, and risk for Crohn disease and ulcerative colitis a cohort study. Ann Intern Med. 2012;156(5):350–9.
52. Tanner A, Raghunath A. Colonic inflammation and nonsteroidal anti-inflammatory drug administration: an assessment of the frequency of the problem. Digestion. 1988;41(2):116.
53. Bankar R, Dafe C, Kohnke A, Babu P. Ulcerative colitis probably associated with isotretinoin. Indian J Gastroenterol. 2006;25(3):171–2.
54. Bernstein CN, Nugent Z, Longobardi T, Blanchard JF. Isotretinoin is not associated with inflammatory bowel disease: a population-based case-control study. Am J Gastroenterol. 2009;104 (11):2774–8.
55. Etminan M, Bird ST, Delaney JA, Bressler B, Brophy JM. Isotretinoin and risk for inflammatory bowel disease: a nested case-control study and meta-analysis of published and unpublished data. JAMA Dermatol. 2013;149(2):216–20.
56. Khalili H, Higuchi LM, Ananthakrishnan AN, Manson JE, Feskanich D, Richter JM, et al. Hormone therapy increases risk of ulcerative colitis but not Crohn's disease. Gastroenterology. 2012;143 (5):1199–206.
57. Khalili H, Higuchi LM, Ananthakrishnan AN, Richter JM, Feskanich D, Fuchs CS, et al. Oral contraceptives, reproductive factors and risk of inflammatory bowel disease. Gut. 2013;62(8):1153–9.
58. Ananthakrishnan AN, Khalili H, Pan A, Higuchi LM, de Silva P, Richter JM, et al. Association between depressive symptoms and incidence of Crohn's disease and ulcerative colitis: results from the nurses' health study. Clin Gastroenterol Hepatol. 2013;11(1):57–62.
59. Bitton A, Dobkin PL, Edwardes MD, Sewitch MJ, Meddings JB, Rawal S, et al. Predicting relapse in Crohn's disease: a biopsychosocial model. Gut. 2008;57(10):1386–92.
60. Goodhand JR, Wahed M, Mawdsley JE, Farmer AD, Aziz Q, Rampton DS. Mood disorders in inflammatory bowel disease: relation to diagnosis, disease activity, perceived stress, and other factors. Inflamm Bowel Dis. 2012;18(12):2301–9.

61. Triantafillidis JK, Merikas E, Gikas A. Psychological factors and stress in inflammatory bowel disease. Expert Rev Gastroenterol Hepatol. 2013;7(3):225–38.
62. Chan SS, Luben R, Olsen A, Tjonneland A, Kaaks R, Teucher B, et al. Body mass index and the risk for Crohn's disease and ulcerative colitis: data from a European prospective cohort study (the ibd in epic study). Am J Gastroenterol. 2013;108(4):575–82.
63. Mendall MA, Gunasekera AV, John BJ, Kumar D. Is obesity a risk factor for Crohn's disease? Dig Dis Sci. 2011;56(3):837–44.
64. Desreumaux P, Ernst O, Geboes K, Gambiez L, Berrebi D, Muller-Alouf H, et al. Inflammatory alterations in mesenteic adipose tissue in Crohn's disease. Gastroenterology. 1999;117(1):73–81.
65. Blain A, Cattan S, Beaugerie L, Carbonnel F, Gendre JP, Cosnes J. Crohn's disease clinical course and severity in obese patients. Clin Nutr. 2002;21(1):51–7.
66. Long MD, Crandall WV, Leibowitz IH, Duffy L, del Rosario F, Kim SC, et al. Prevalence and epidemiology of overweight and obesity in children with inflammatory bowel disease. Inflamm Bowel Dis. 2011;17(10):2162–8.
67. Khalili H, Ananthakrishnan AN, Konijeti GG, Liao X, Higuchi LM, Fuchs CS, et al. Physical activity and risk of inflammatory bowel disease: prospective study from the nurses' health study cohorts. BMJ. 2013;347:f6633.
68. Ali T, Madhoun MF, Orr WC, Rubin DT. Assessment of the relationship between quality of sleep and disease activity in inflammatory bowel disease patients. Inflamm Bowel Dis. 2013;19(11):2440–3.
69. Ananthakrishnan AN, Khalili H, Konijeti GG, Higuchi LM, de Silva P, Fuchs CS, et al. Sleep duration affects risk for ulcerative colitis: a prospective cohort study. Clin Gastroenterol Hepatol. 2014;12(11):1879–86.
70. Drossman D, Leserman J, Li Z, Mitchell C, Zagami E, Patrick D. The rating form of ibd patient concerns: a new measure of health status. Psychosom Med. 1991;53(6):701–12.
71. Marin L, Manosa M, Garcia-Planella E, Gordillo J, Zabana Y, Cabre E, et al. Sexual function and patients' perceptions in inflammatory bowel disease: a case-control survey. J Gastroenterol. 2013;48(6):713–20.
72. Timmer A, Bauer A, Dignass A, Rogler G. Sexual function in persons with inflammatory bowel disease: a survey with matched controls. Clin Gastroenterol Hepatol. 2007;5(1):87–94.
73. Muller KR, Prosser R, Bampton P, Mountifield R, Andrews JM. Female gender and surgery impair relationships, body image, and sexuality in inflammatory bowel disease: patient perceptions. Inflamm Bowel Dis. 2010;16(4):657–63.
74. Johnson P, Richard C, Ravid A, Spencer L, Pinto E, Hanna M, et al. Female infertility after ileal pouch-anal anastomosis for ulcerative colitis. Dis Colon Rectum. 2004;47(7):1119–26.
75. Mountifield R, Bampton P, Prosser R, Muller K, Andrews JM. Fear and fertility in inflammatory bowel disease: a mismatch of perception and reality affects family planning decisions. Inflamm Bowel Dis. 2009;15(5):720–5.
76. Tavernier N, Fumery M, Peyrin-Biroulet L, Colombel JF, Gower-Rousseau C. Systematic review: fertility in non-surgically treated inflammatory bowel disease. Aliment Pharmacol Ther. 2013;38(8):847–53.
77. Fonager K, Sorensen H, Olsen J, Dahlerup J, Rasmussen S. Pregnancy outcome for women with Crohn's disease: a follow-up study based on linkage between national registries. Am J Gastroenterol. 1998;93(12):2426–30.
78. Mahadevan U, Sandborn WJ, Li DK, Hakimian S, Kane S, Corley DA. Pregnancy outcomes in women with inflammatory bowel disease: a large community-based study from northern california. Gastroenterology. 2007;133(4):1106–12.
79. Norgard B, Fonager K, Sorensen H, Olsen J. Birth outcomes of women with ulcerative colitis: a nationwide danish cohort study. Am J Gastroenterol. 2000;95(11):3165–70.
80. Katz J. Pregnancy and inflammatory bowel disease. Curr Opin Gastroenterol. 2004;20(4):328–32.
81. Ujihara M, Ando T, Ishiguro K. Appropriate pharmaceutical management is crucial for pregnant women complicated by ulcerative colitis. San Diego, CA: Digestive Disease Week San Diego; 2012. p. 19–22.
82. Bhatia J, Bratcher J, Korelitz B, Vakher K, Mannor S, Shevchuk M, et al. Abnormalities of uterine cervix in women with inflammatory bowel disease. World J Gastroenterol. 2006;12(38):6167–71.
83. Kane S, Khatibi B, Reddy D. Higher incidence of abnormal pap smears in women with inflammatory bowel disease. Am J Gastroenterol. 2008;103(3):631–6.
84. ACOG. ACOG practice bulletin no. 131: screening for cervical cancer. Obstet Gynecol. 2012;120:1222–38.
85. Moscandrew M, Mahadevan U, Kane S. General health maintenance in ibd. Inflamm Bowel Dis. 2009;15(9):1399–409.
86. Peyrin-Biroulet L, Khosrotehrani K, Carrat F, Bouvier AM, Chevaux JB, Simon T, et al. Increased risk for nonmelanoma skin cancers in patients who receive thiopurines for inflammatory bowel disease. Gastroenterology. 2011;141(5):1621–8 (e1621–1625).
87. Nyboe Andersen N, Pasternak B, Basit S, Andersson M, Svanstrom H, Caspersen S, et al. Association between tumor necrosis factor-alpha antagonists and risk of cancer in patients with inflammatory bowel disease. JAMA. 2014;311(23):2406–13.
88. USPTF. Screening for osteoporosis: U.S. Preventative services task force recommendation statement. Ann Intern Med. 2011;154(5):356–64.

89. Long MD, Martin C, Sandler RS, Kappelman MD. Increased risk of pneumonia among patients with inflammatory bowel disease. Am J Gastroenterol. 2013;108(2):240–8.
90. Melmed GY, Ippoliti AF, Papadakis KA, Tran TT, Birt JL, Lee SK, et al. Patients with inflammatory bowel disease are at risk for vaccine-preventable illnesses. Am J Gastroenterol. 2006;101(8):1834–40.
91. Wasan SK, Calderwood AH, Long MD, Kappelman MD, Sandler RS, Farraye FA. Immunization rates and vaccine beliefs among patients with inflammatory bowel disease: an opportunity for improvement. Inflamm Bowel Dis. 2014;20(2):246–50.
92. Dezfoli S, Melmed GY. Vaccination issues in patients with inflammatory bowel disease receiving immunosuppression. Gastroenterol Hepatol (NY). 2012;8(8):504–12.
93. Rubin LG, Levin MJ, Ljungman P, Davies EG, Avery R, Tomblyn M, et al. 2013 idsa clinical practice guideline for vaccination of the immunocompromised host. Clin Infect Dis. 2014;58(3):309–18.
94. Desjardins C, Duling BR. Heparinase treatment suggests a role for the endothelial cell glycocalyx in regulation of capillary hematocrit. Am J Physiol. 1990;258(3 Pt 2):H647–54.
95. Sandhu BK, Fell JM, Beattie RM, Mitton SG, Wilson DC, Jenkins H, et al. Guidelines for the management of inflammatory bowel disease in children in the united kingdom. J Pediatr Gastroenterol Nutr. 2010;50(Suppl 1):S1–13.
96. Borrelli O, Cordischi L, Cirulli M, Paganelli M, Labalestra V, Uccini S, et al. Polymeric diet alone versus corticosteroids in the treatment of active pediatric Crohn's disease: a randomized controlled open-label trial. Clin Gastroenterol Hepatol. 2006;4(6):744–53.
97. Ananthakrishnan AN, Khalili H, Konijeti GG, Higuchi LM, de Silva P, Korzenik JR, et al. A prospective study of long-term intake of dietary fiber and risk of Crohn's disease and ulcerative colitis. Gastroenterology. 2013;145(5):970–7.
98. Hou JK, Abraham B, El-Serag H. Dietary intake and risk of developing inflammatory bowel disease: a systematic review of the literature. Am J Gastroenterol. 2011;106(4):563–73.
99. Weiss G. Iron in the inflammed gut: another pro-inflammatory hit? Gut. 2011;60(3):287–8.
100. Cantorna M, Zhu Y, Froicu M, Wittke A. Vitamin d status, 1,25-dihyroxyvitamin d3, and the immune system. Am J Clin Nutr. 2004;80(6):17175–205.
101. Ford AC, Kane SV, Khan KJ, Achkar JP, Talley NJ, Marshall JK, et al. Efficacy of 5-aminosalicylates in Crohn's disease: systematic review and meta-analysis. Am J Gastroenterol. 2011;106(4):617–29.
102. Gordon GL, Zakko S, Murthy U, Sedghi S, Pruitt R, Barrett AC, et al. Once-daily mesalamine formulation for maintenance of remission in ulcerative colitis: a randomized, placebo-controlled clinical trial. J Clin Gastroenterol. 2016;50(4):318–25.
103. World M, Stevens P, Ashton M, Rainford D. Mesalazine-associated interstitial nephritis. Nephrol Dial Transplant. 1996;11:614–21.
104. Connell W, Kamm M, Ritchie J, Lennard-Jones J. Bone marrow toxicity caused by azathioprine in inflammatory bowel disease: 27 years of experience. Gut. 1993;34:1081–5.
105. Moshkowitz M, Oren R, Tishler M, Konikoff F, Graff E, Brill S, et al. The absorption of low-dose methotrexate in patients with inflammatory bowel disease. Aliment Pharmacol Ther. 1997;11:569–73.
106. Singh JA, Furst DE, Bharat A, Curtis JR, Kavanaugh AF, Kremer JM, et al. 2012 update of the 2008 american college of rheumatology recommendations for the use of disease-modifying antirheumatic drugs and biologic agents in the treatment of rheumatoid arthritis. Arthritis Care Res (Hoboken). 2012;64(5):625–39.
107. Hanauer SB, Feagan BG, Lichtenstein GR, Mayer LF, Schreiber S, Colombel JF, et al. Maintenance infliximab for Crohn's disease: the accent i randomised trial. Lancet. 2002;359(9317):1541–9.
108. Rutgeerts P, Sandborn WJ, Feagan BG, Reinisch W, Olson A, Johanns J, et al. Infliximab for induction and maintenance therapy for ulcerative colitis. N Engl J Med. 2005;353(23):2462–72.
109. Sands BE, Anderson FH, Bernstein CN, Chey WY, Feagan BG, Fedorak RN, et al. Infliximab maintenance therapy for fistulizing Crohn's disease. N Engl J Med. 2004;350(9):876–85.
110. Kotlyar DS, Osterman MT, Diamond RH, Porter D, Blonski WC, Wasik M, et al. A systematic review of factors that contribute to hepatosplenic t-cell lymphoma in patients with inflammatory bowel disease. Clin Gastroenterol Hepatol. 2011;9(1):36–41 e31.
111. Bernstein CN, Blanchard JF, Rawsthorne P, Yu N. The prevalence of extraintestinal diseases in inflammatory bowel disease: a population-based study. Am J Gastroenterol. 2001;96(4):1116–22.
112. Stawarski A, Iwańczak B, Krzesiek E, Iwańczak F. Intestinal complications and extraintestinal manifestations in children with inflammatory bowel disease. Pol Merkur Lekarski. 2006;20(115):22–5.
113. Smale S, Natt RS, Orchard TR, Russell AS, Bjarnason I. Inflammatory bowel disease and spondylarthropathy. Arthritis Rheum. 2001;44(12):2728–36.
114. Felder JB, Korelitz B, Rajapakse R, Schwarz S, Horatagis AP, Gleim G. Effects of nonsteroidal antiinflammatory drugs on inflammatory bowel disease: a case-control study. Am J Gastroenterol. 2000;95(8):1949–54.
115. Vavricka SR, Brun L, Ballabeni P, Pittet V, Prinz Vavricka BM, Zeitz J, et al. Frequency and risk factors for extraintestinal manifestations in the swiss inflammatory bowel disease cohort. Am J Gastroenterol. 2011;106(1):110–9.

116. Requena L, Yus ES. Erythema nodosum. Dermatol Clin. 2008;26(4):425–38 (v).
117. DeFilippis EM, Feldman SR, Huang WW. The genetics of pyoderma gangrenosum and implications for treatment: a systematic review. Br J Dermatol. 2015;172(6):1487–97.
118. Callen JP. Pyoderma gangrenosum. Lancet. 1998;351:581–5.
119. Su CG, Judge TA, Lichtenstein GR. Extraintestinal manifestations of inflammatory bowel disease. Gastroenterol Clin North Am. 2002;31(1):307–27.
120. Annunziato RA, Emre S, Shneider B, Barton C, Dugan CA, Shemesh E. Adherence and medical outcomes in pediatric liver transplant recipients who transition to adult services. Pediatr Transplant. 2007;11(6):608–14.
121. Hersh AO, Pang S, Curran ML, Milojevic DS, von Scheven E. The challenges of transferring chronic illness patients to adult care: reflections from pediatric and adult rheumatology at a us academic center. Pediatr Rheumatol Online J. 2009;7:13.
122. Sebastian S, Jenkins H, McCartney S, Ahmad T, Arnott I, Croft N, et al. The requirements and barriers to successful transition of adolescents with inflammatory bowel disease: differing perceptions from a survey of adult and paediatric gastroenterologists. J Crohns Colitis. 2012;6(8):830–44.
123. Reid GJ, Irvine MJ, McCrindle BW, Sananes R, Ritvo PG, Siu SC, et al. Prevalence and correlates of successful transfer from pediatric to adult health care among a cohort of young adults with complex congenital heart defects. Pediatrics. 2004;113(3):e197–205.
124. McDonagh JE, Southwood TR, Shaw KL, British Paediatric Rheumatology G. Unmet education and training needs of rheumatology health professionals in adolescent health and transitional care. Rheumatology (Oxford). 2004;43(6):737–43.
125. Trivedi I, Keefer L. The emerging adult with inflammatory bowel disease: challenges and recommendations for the adult gastroenterologist. Gastroenterol Res Pract. 2015;2015:260807.
126. Gawron LM, Hammond C, Keefer L. Documentation of reproductive health counseling and contraception in women with inflammatory bowel diseases. Patient Educ Couns. 2014;94(1):134–7.
127. Longobardi T. Work losses related to inflammatory bowel disease in the united states results from the national health interview survey. Am J Gastroenterol. 2003;98(5):1064–72.
128. Sawicki GS, Whitworth R, Gunn L, Butterfield R, Lukens-Bull K, Wood D. Receipt of health care transition counseling in the national survey of adult transition and health. Pediatrics. 2011;128(3):e521–9.

Intellectual Disability

13

Kamala Gullapalli Cotts

Case Presentation

Mr. C.B. is a 52-year-old African American male with a history of diplegic cerebral palsy and intellectual disability. He has lower extremity weakness and has been using a wheelchair since early childhood, has a left hand contracture, and experiences rare urinary tract infections. He is obese with a body mass index (BMI) of 35 kg/m^2. He has severe dysarthria and no decubiti. Family history is significant for hypertension and a myocardial infarction (at age 58) in his father. He moved from the East Coast to live with his brother in Chicago. He had not been to see a physician in almost 3 years as his mother was progressively more ill and was unable to care for him.

Mr. C.B. completed high school at age 18 and has not had further education. He requires help with all activities of daily life including feeding, dressing, and toileting due to his contractures. He is not able to do math but knows how much a plane trip costs and that he can buy 2 airplane tickets with his monthly Social Security income. Although he is not able to call the doctor's office and make an appointment, he is able to converse on the telephone about sporting events and television shows. He had been living with his mother until her recent death. He becomes tearful as he talks about his mother's death. He misses his former neighbors that used to visit frequently. He has difficulty falling asleep at least twice a week, but when he does fall asleep he does not awaken early. He reveals that his wheelchair is nearly 10 years old. Over the course of the next several months, he is diagnosed with and treated for hypertension, diabetes mellitus, and hyperlipidemia. His brother asks about resources to care for his brother while he is at work. On a subsequent visit, his brother states that he has recently had a colonoscopy and asks if Mr. C.B. should have a colonoscopy as well.

Case Discussion

After surviving elderly parents, Mr. C.B. has moved to a different state. Although he is a middle-aged individual, he still requires transitional assessment. Although he is able to participate in the medical decision-making process, he requires help. He is unable to make financial decisions. Information should be provided about the physician certification form and local affordable or volunteer legal services to establish guardianship. Formal neuropsychiatric testing is often performed when an individual is receiving special education under the age of 18 and often updated as one transitions to adulthood. As he has moved here from another state, such

K.G. Cotts (✉)
Department of Internal Medicine, University of Chicago Medicine, 5841 S. Maryland Ave. MC 3051, Lagrange, IL 60525, USA
e-mail: kcotts@medicine.bsd.uchicago.edu

M. Pilapil et al. (eds.), *Care of Adults with Chronic Childhood Conditions*,
DOI 10.1007/978-3-319-43827-6_13

information is not readily available. An office assessment of his intellectual disability and adaptive functioning may be sufficient. The family requires information for local Pre-Admission Screening Agencies (PAS) to obtain information about finding local supports required for his degree of adaptive functioning. Often, these agencies require formal neuropsychological testing in order to establish the need for the services. Referral to a social worker is helpful to provide information on local resources such as the local department of rehabilitation and vocational services as well as homemaker services. Additionally, he requires counseling services and resources within the community.

Mr. C.B. requires subspecialty referral to multiple healthcare providers. He should be evaluated by orthopedic surgery given his chronic contractures as well as physical and occupational therapy assessments and referrals for durable medical equipment needs, including braces and a new wheelchair. In addition to providing general medical care for his newly diagnosed hypertension, diabetes, and hyperlipidemia, his health maintenance needs must be addressed. At subsequent visits, he may require referrals for vision, hearing, and dental evaluation. His vaccinations should be reviewed and updated. Finally, screening procedures such as colonoscopy and bone mineral density assessment, which are recommended by the United States Preventive Services Task Force (USPSTF) guidelines, should be reviewed with Mr. C.B. and his brother.

Background

The term intellectual disability (ID) refers to a condition in which an individual has significant limitations in both cognitive functioning and adaptive behavior. The diagnosis of ID requires formal psychometric testing to assess the intelligence quotient (IQ) and adaptive functioning. ID is initially identified in early childhood [1]. In adulthood, ID impacts the ability to live independently, find employment, and obtain healthcare, and also influences the need for federal and state-based supportive services. Medical care of individuals with ID requires delivering general medical care, treating behavioral symptoms, continuing transitional special education, and providing variable degrees of community-based support. Adults with ID are living longer as a result of improved medical care, environmental conditions, and technology. As these individuals live longer, they require primary care that targets the associated health condition that led to their initial impairment in intellectual functioning, such as cerebral palsy and Down syndrome [2]. In addition, patients with ID often have comorbid medical conditions that are neither caused by nor occur as a result of the ID, such as diabetes and hypertension. Complications of these comorbidities, such as decubitus ulcers and psychiatric disorders, also occur at a higher frequency compared to the general population. Adults with ID require the same considerations for improving quality of life and health screening, particularly for cardiovascular disease and cancer. This chapter reviews the definition and epidemiology of ID, as well as common medical conditions among and health maintenance screening guidelines for individuals with ID.

Definition of Intellectual Disability

The American Association of Intellectual and Developmental Disabilities (AAIDD) defines intellectual disability as a disability acquired prior to the age of 18 years and characterized by significant limitations both in intellectual functioning and in adaptive behavior as expressed in conceptual, social, and practical adaptive skills [1]. The terminology has evolved from idiocy to mental retardation to intellectual disability when the original medical terms lost their neutral meaning and became socially stigmatizing. The term intellectual disability more adequately describes complex individuals with a wide range of abilities, gifts, and supportive needs. Table 13.1 summarizes the diagnostic criteria for intellectual disability [1].

The AAIDD emphasizes several additional considerations. An individual's limitations in

Table 13.1 Diagnostic criteria for intellectual disability

Intellectual disability: significant limitations in both intellectual functioning and in adaptive behavior. Disability originates prior to the age of 18 years.		
Intellectual functioning		
IQ score below the range of 70–75; 2 standard deviations (SD) below the population mean		
Limitations in adaptive skill areas		
Individuals cannot function adequately in their environment, assessed through standardized testing. Scores must fall 2 SD below the mean in one of these areas or on a combined score of all three of the following areas:		
Conceptual deficits	***Social deficits***	***Practical deficits***
Receptive and expressive language, reading, writing, math, reasoning, knowledge and memory	Interpersonal communication skills, friendship, empathy, social judgment skills including gullibility, naiveté, following rules, obeying laws, avoiding victimization	Personal care activities including eating, dressing, bathing, meal preparation, telephone communication, transportation, and occupational skills including organizing school and work activities, money management, job duties

Source The American Association of Intellectual and Developmental Disabilities (AAIDD) [1]

functioning are assessed within the context of the culture and community environment typical of the individual's peers. Assessments consider linguistic and cultural diversity as well as differences in communication, sensory, motor, and behavioral factors. Additionally, the AAIDD recognizes that limitations often coexist with strengths. An essential purpose of identifying limitations is to develop personalized supports that, over a sustained period of time, will improve an individual's level of life functioning.

The Diagnostic and Statistical Manual of Mental Disorders, 5th edition (DSM-V), published in 2013, also agrees that IQ below 70–75 is no longer the only diagnostic criteria. Severity is based on a combination of IQ and adaptive functioning in comparison with population norms. An individual with an IQ score of 75 with significant adaptive disability will be considered to have ID, whereas an individual with no adaptive disability and an IQ score of 65 may not be considered to have intellectual disability [3].

The Individuals with Disabilities Education Act (IDEA) defines intellectual disability as "significantly sub-average general intellectual functioning, existing concurrently with deficits in adaptive behavior and manifested during the developmental period, that adversely affect a child's educational performance." Again, the 2 key components identified within this definition are a student's IQ and his or her capability to function independently, referred to as adaptive behavior. In 2010, the federal government enacted legislation changing the term "mental retardation" to "intellectual disabilities" in all federal law. Most states have made this change in their legislation and documents [4].

An extensive multifaceted evaluation is essential to determine whether an individual has intellectual disability and then tailor individualized support plans. The various levels of severity are defined on the basis of adaptive functioning, not IQ scores, because it is adaptive functioning that determines the level of supports required. Moreover, IQ measures are less valid in the lower end of the IQ range [4, 5]. In situations where it is difficult to assess the degree of ID, clinical judgment must be used to specify the severity. Classification of severity of ID and intensity of required support is shown in Table 13.2 [3, 6, 7].

Etiology of Intellectual Disability

Conditions that result in an impairment of intellectual functioning may be related to a genetic abnormality or a brain injury occurring prenatally, perinatally, or in early childhood. Genetic disorders are the underlying etiology for the majority of individuals with severe ID. More than 500 different genetic defects have been

Table 13.2 Classification of intellectual disability severity

Severity level	Intelligence quotient range	Adaptive functioning	Intensity of supports needed in daily living activities
Mild	55–70 (±5)	• Unskilled job capacity • Income support • Stable relationships • Poor parenting skills • Able to communicate by phone and in writing • Decision-making: able to make some medical, financial, and personal decisions	Intermittent: Support on as-needed basis; episodic or short term
Moderate	40–50 (±5)	• Supported employment • Income support • Residential supervision • Help with shopping • Vocabulary adequate for daily functioning • Decision-making: help with medical decision-making in all areas: personal, medical, and financial	Limited: Consistent over time, but time limited
Severe	25–35 (±5)	• Supervision in residential and day programs • Decision-making: – Unable to make most medical decisions – Not capable of making financial decisions	Extensive: Regular, consistent lifetime support. Regular support in at least 1 aspect such as work, home
Profound	Less than 20–25	• 24-h support and supervision • Nonverbal • Dependent for self-care/hygiene • Does not have decision-making capacity	Pervasive: High intensity, across all environments, lifetime, and potentially life-sustaining

Sources: DSM 2013 [6]; Patel [3]; Edwards [7]

associated with ID. The 2 most common genetic disorders leading to ID are Down syndrome and Fragile X Syndrome. Down syndrome is the most common identified cause of intellectual disability [8]. Nongenetic causes are less commonly the root of ID than genetic causes and are responsible for the majority of cases of mild ID. Brain injuries resulting in impaired brain development include trauma, congenital infections, toxin exposures (i.e., maternal alcohol and polysubstance abuse), pediatric infections such as meningitis or encephalitis, or metabolic abnormalities such as congenital hypothyroidism. Fetal alcohol syndrome is one of the 3 most common congenital causes of ID. Approximately 30 % of cerebral palsy (CP) children will have concomitant intellectual disability. In one-third of individuals with ID, no underlying etiology is identified. Identification of an underlying etiology leads to improved survival and health status of individuals with ID [8]. Table 13.3 shows common etiologies of ID.

Prevalence and Life Span

The increasing need for medical care for adults with intellectual disabilities is due to increased prevalence and increased survival to adulthood. In the United States, the overall prevalence of ID was 1.27 % in 2011–2013 and 1.10 % in 2014, with an anticipated growth rate due to increasing survival rates related to improvements in neonatal care, nutrition, and socioeconomic conditions [9, 10]. The United States prevalence of ID is 11.4 per 1000 in children and 6.6 per 1000 in adults. There is a ninefold variation from state to state [1]. The number of adults with ID at 60 years and

Table 13.3 Intellectual disability of all etiologies

Known causes: 2/3 of individuals with ID	
Genetic causes:	Nongenetic causes
1. Down syndrome	1. Fetal alcohol syndrome
2. Fragile X syndrome	2. Cerebral palsy
3. Rett syndrome	3. Infections: meningitis, rubella, etc.
4. Williams syndrome	4. Teratogenic causes
5. Prader–Willi	5. Traumatic brain injury
6. Phenylketonuria	6. Autism (genetic component as well)
7. Angelman syndrome	7. Seizure Disorder
8. Other genetic causes	
Unknown causes: 1/3 of individuals with ID	

older is projected to nearly double from 641,860 in 2000 to 1.2 million by 2030 [11].

The increasing life expectancy of individuals with ID follows similar trends in the general population. As with the general population, in which the average lifespan has increased from 66 years in 1950 to 78 years of age in 2007, [12] the life expectancy for people with ID has increased from the mid-50s for those with more severe disabilities or Down syndrome, to the early 70s for adults with mild/moderate ID [13, 14]. Although the life expectancy of people with ID is increasing, it still remains lower than that of the general population, with an average age at death of 66.1 years [8, 14]. Because adults with ID are a highly heterogeneous group, differing in degree and cause of impairment as well as their biological, psychological, and social background, life spans of those with ID are highly individualized. Table 13.4 shows the prevalence and life expectancy of common etiologies of ID [8, 15].

Aging starts earlier in persons with ID and medical problems are related to the natural history of the original disability. There is a higher prevalence of some age-related diseases such as hypothyroidism, obesity, epilepsy, sensory deficits, behavioral/mental health problems, frailty, and early onset of dementia [8, 14, 16]. These medical conditions contribute to the higher rates of mortality in adults with ID. Causes of mortality are more easily identifiable if there is an underlying etiology of ID. Dementia seems to be the most important cause of morbidity and mortality in adults with Down syndrome [14]. In a study of older persons with Down syndrome, persons with a severe to profound level of ID had a higher death rate compared to those with mild to moderate ID, and those living in institutions had a higher death rate than those living in the community [17]. In adults with CP, there were higher death rates as a result of aspiration and pneumonia due to dysphagia [18]. Awareness and monitoring of age-related and disease-associated risks provide opportunities to intervene and thus prolong lives of those with ID.

Adults with intellectual disabilities are more likely to live in community-based settings rather than large institutions [19]. More than 75 % of adults with ID live with families, more than 25 % of family care providers are over the age of 60, and 38 % are between 41 and 59 years of age [11, 20]. There is an increasing need for medical care for aging adults with ID and for access to quality supports that address health and social changes [11].

Health Status and Health Disparities in Adults with Intellectual Disabilities

Although there has been progress, adults with intellectual disabilities experience inequities in health status at a disproportionately higher rate than the general population. In 2006, AAIDD declared "there's a marked disparity of health between persons with intellectual and developmental disability and the general population" [21]. The etiology of these differences in health status for individuals with ID is multifactorial. Health disparities can be due to decreased life expectancy, increased morbidity, increases in negative determinants of health such as poverty, and the differences in healthcare access or quality of services (see Box 13.1) [22].

Table 13.4 Prevalence and life expectancy of common causes of intellectual disability (ID)

Etiology of ID	Prevalence in live births[a]	Mean life expectancy (years)[b]
Down syndrome	1/700	82
Cerebral palsy	1.5–4/1000 or 1/323	55
Phenylketonuria	1/10,000	70
Rett syndrome	1/10,000–1/20,000 (females only)	55
Angelman syndrome	1/12,000–1/20,000	72
Williams–Beuren syndrome	1/7500–10,000	55
Prader–Willi syndrome	1/10,000–1/25,000	72
Seizure disorder	10.2/1000 (lifetime prevalence)	decreased
Fetal alcohol syndrome	0.2–1.5/1000	decreased
Fragile X syndrome	1/5000 males	87

[a]From www.cdc.gov [15]
[b]From Coppus et al. 2013 [8]

Box 13.1 Determinants of health disparities in adults with intellectual disabilities

- Genetics
- Social circumstances (i.e., poverty, lack of employment, lack of social networks)
- Environmental conditions
- Health promotion
- Healthcare access

As previously discussed, although life expectancy in adults with ID has increased in recent years, it remains decreased compared to the general population. Individuals with ID are more likely to have certain comorbidities such as epilepsy, psychiatric disorders, sensory impairment, poor dental hygiene, limited mobility, and gastrointestinal problems [23, 24]. Determinants of health include individual behavior, genetics, environmental exposures, social circumstances (i.e., poverty, lack of employment opportunities and social networks, and access to healthcare) [25]. The barriers to accessing quality healthcare include lack of formal training for healthcare providers in the care of adults with ID, communication deficits between providers and patients, complex health care financing systems that limit access to necessary care, and health care providers that lack awareness about steps required to ensure that individuals with ID have access to appropriate, culturally competent care [26]. The medical complexity of adults with ID is itself a crucial barrier [27]. In 2001, "Closing the Gap: A National Blueprint to Improve the Health of Persons with Mental Retardation: report of the Surgeon General's Conference on Health Disparities and Mental Retardation" prioritized increasing sources of healthcare for people with ID [28].

It is important to distinguish 3 distinct types of health conditions experienced by people with ID; these conditions can all contribute to measured health disparities but reflect different points of entry along the cascade of disparities. *Associated health conditions* are medical conditions that are regarded as having led to the impairment in intellectual functioning [2]. For example, cerebral palsy, Down syndrome, fetal alcohol syndrome, and encephalitis are examples of associated health conditions leading to ID. *Secondary conditions* refer to those conditions that a person with a preexisting disability experiences at higher rates than the general population and are generally regarded as preventable [29]. For people with ID, these may include decubitus ulcers, bowel obstruction, and depression. *Comorbid conditions* refer to concomitant but unrelated pathological processes that have an adverse impact on health. Examples of comorbid conditions in individuals with ID are adverse health conditions such as cancer or hypertension. As adults with ID are living longer, all of these conditions must be addressed.

People with ID experience lower rates of preventive care and health promotion practices than the general population [29]. Multiple international studies have documented inequities of preventive services within specific countries and between countries in adults with ID. In addition to hearing and vision evaluations, the literature addresses specific concerns of preventive screening and management of chronic overweight/obesity and has identified disparities based on type of residence [30]. Studies in the United Kingdom showed that being overweight was more common in individual settings than in group homes and more of a problem in the US than in the UK. For example, a 2002 study reported 54 % of its California sample to be overweight or obese, while a subsequent 2003 study reported only 22 % of the UK residential sample as overweight [30, 31]. In the California study, there was a greater risk for obesity for individuals living at home (67 %) or with family or friends (57 %) compared with those living in a group residence (47 %). Those living at home also reported more smoking and drinking. In contrast to those living at home, people living in a group residence were more likely to have current tuberculosis screening tests and influenza vaccination [31].

In order to address equity in healthcare for individuals with disabilities, the United Nations Convention on the rights of persons with disabilities was updated in 2006. Article 25 of the convention outlines that persons with disabilities have the right to the following:

1. The same quality of free or affordable healthcare as the general population
2. Health services that are specific to their disabilities, including early identification and intervention, with services designed to minimize and prevent further disabilities
3. Health services as close as possible to people's own communities
4. Care of the same quality, including ethical considerations of informed consent by raising awareness of the human rights, dignity, autonomy, and needs of persons with disabilities through training
5. The provision of health insurance and life insurance that is permitted by national law and shall be provided in a fair and reasonable manner [27, 32].

In summary, there have been significant efforts to address the health care needs and status of people with intellectual disabilities across their life spans. Adults with ID more fully participate in their communities when they are not constrained by poor health and can access healthcare resources to address conditions affecting their health status [33, 34].

Common Medical Considerations in Providing Care for Adults with Intellectual Disabilities

Medical conditions in individuals with ID differ from those that occur in the general population with regards to prevalence, age of onset, rate of progression, degree of severity, and presentation. Additionally, they are likely to be multiple and complex conditions [35].

Primary care providers (PCPs) are essential for the care of individuals with ID in that they provide continuous healthcare services, interact regularly with caregivers, integrate psychological and social factors, and coordinate subspecialty and interdisciplinary health services. Their role is critical for early detection, disease prevention, and chronic management [36].

Because the definition of ID is broad, the etiology of ID guides management of chronic diseases as well as preventative services. For example, management of mobility issues, urinary tract infections, and dysphagia in patients with CP, or hypothyroidism in those with Down syndrome (for additional information, please see Chaps. 5 and 10). There are many conditions that are common to most people with intellectual disability. The revised Canadian Consensus Guidelines from 2011 summarizes evidenced-based data in providing primary care for adults with intellectual disabilities [36]. Other resources for health maintenance guidelines are the

Massachusetts DDS Health Screening Recommendations and the guidelines provided by AAIDD [1, 37].

Unique Considerations for the Office Visit

It is important to assess the *living situation* of the individual with ID during each visit. Individuals with ID live in a variety of settings with varying degrees of being able to care for themselves. They may live with family members, live independently, or in shared-living situations with supervised help versus structured group homes. Changes in living situation are a common cause of upheaval that may impact on wellbeing and behavior. Some additional social, physical, and behavior barriers to providing medical care for patients with ID are notable.

Communication challenges can make interaction between the provider, caregiver, and patient difficult. It is critically important not to make assumptions about the individual's ability to communicate, even though providers may obtain much of the medical history from caregivers for individuals with limited communication. Directly communicate with the adult with ID unless instructed otherwise. In the case discussed at the beginning of this chapter, Mr. C.B. has dysarthria and is difficult to understand. He reported that when he was seen in an urgent care setting for a urinary tract infection, results of his urinalysis were given to his brother who accompanied him, rather than directly to him. As with patients in the general population, the provider communicating directly with each patient is essential to developing mutual respect and trust. Providers often obtain information from individuals who accompany them to their appointments. However, these individuals may not be the primary caregivers and may not be able to provide essential information. Thus, each provider should know the identity of the caregiver accompanying the patient and know their relationship and depth of interaction. As individuals with ID have medically complex conditions, it is important to communicate with caregivers most familiar with the individual either during the span of a clinic visit or afterward.

Physical challenges can affect both the adults with ID and the providers. For example, individuals who require wheelchairs may have difficulty in accessing a healthcare facility or with gynecological exams. Finally, *behavioral issues* may impact upon the quality of healthcare delivery for those with ID. Prior negative experiences with providers, clinics, and hospitals may engender fear and anxiety. Such emotions may negatively impact the individual's cooperation for exams, tests, or injections. For respect of the patient, a provider must be open to rescheduling or modifying a nonemergent procedure or test when a patient expresses anxiety.

In addition to the aforementioned challenges, barriers from the provider's perspective include lack of formal training in caring for adults with ID, time constraints, reduced reimbursement, and difficulty in obtaining informed consent [38, 39]. Providers may require a longer visit to examine contractures or evaluate for decubitus ulcers. Many patients with ID have insurance plans with reduced reimbursement schedules. In a busy clinical practice where revenue is a consideration, this provides a challenge. Strategies for providers to improve a clinic visit include a chart review prior to the visit and making goals for the visit. Some portions of the exam may need to be deferred to a future visit. Additionally, a short-acting benzodiazepine for anxiety may facilitate obtaining blood work or other testing [38, 39].

Providers should routinely assess the medication regimen. *Polypharmacy* is common for the ID population; many have numerous medications and they often are prescribed by multiple providers. Medication reconciliation at each visit helps to sort out medication use, capacity to follow the medication regimen, and provide assistance required to support medication compliance. A review of *vaccinations* at the initial visit is essential. Adults with ID receive vaccinations at a lower rate than the general population. Individuals in group homes typically have the highest rate of vaccination among adults with ID as they follow state-based regulations. Adults with ID living at home with family have the lowest rates of vaccination [31]. Individuals transitioning from pediatrics typically have extensive records. For individuals who do not have documentation, it is important to check titers and update accordingly [38].

Medical Considerations

Physical inactivity and obesity are common among adults with ID and have been documented in multiple studies [31, 40]. Obesity in adults with ID is associated with adverse outcomes such as cardiovascular disease, diabetes, osteoporosis, constipation, and early mortality [41]. It is crucial for primary care providers to monitor body mass index and to involve caregivers, regional service coordination agencies, and other health professionals to promote a healthy lifestyle [42].

Vision impairments are common in adults with ID. The most common cause of decreased vision in individuals with ID is refractive errors, including hyperopia (farsightedness), myopia (nearsightedness), and astigmatism [43]. Strabismus, cataracts, and keratoconus are also more common in individuals with ID than those without ID [43]. Individuals with ID should have annual vision screening in the office and be referred for vision assessments to detect glaucoma and cataracts every 5 years after the age of 45.

Hearing impairments are also much more prevalent in adults with ID. In adults with severe ID, changes in behavior and adaptive functioning may be clues to a worsening or a new hearing or vision impairment. Cerumen impaction is a common cause of decreased hearing sensation. Assess for cerumen impaction every 6 months. Referral should be made to audiology for hearing assessment if indicated by screening (change in behavior, decreased communication) and for age-related hearing loss every 5 years after the age of 45 [36, 44].

Oral health problems such as dental caries, gingivitis, and periodontal disease are among the top 10 secondary conditions among individuals with ID that cause limitations in their daily activities [23]. Primary care providers should promote dental hygiene practices and referral to a dental professional. Cleaning is recommended every 6 months. Complicated dental procedures may require sedation, and it is important for the primary care provider to identify state-specific Department of Human and Health Services resources for dentists who provide services to adults with intellectual and developmental disabilities [37].

Even in those with the most severe impairment, maintaining *musculoskeletal health* is strongly linked to survival into adulthood [45]. Scoliosis, contractures, and spasticity occur frequently in individuals with ID and can lead to pain, reduced mobility, and adverse health outcomes including decreased quality of life [36, 45]. Additionally, osteoarthritis is becoming more prevalent as adults with ID are living longer and is a common cause of pain leading to behavioral changes [45]. The need for physical or occupational therapy services should be assessed annually and when there's functional decline. The need for durable medical equipment including a new wheelchair, modified seating plans, or orthotic devices should also be periodically assessed.

Seizure disorders are common among individuals with intellectual disability and can increase with the severity of the intellectual disability. Typically, individuals with seizure disorders are under the care of a neurologist. The role of the primary care provider is to monitor the effects of antiepileptic medications. This involves not only checking levels but also monitoring for bone loss/osteoporosis. Phenytoin, a common antiepileptic, can cause significant bone loss over time, at a much higher rate than phenobarbital or carbamazepine. It is important to screen for osteoporosis more frequently among individuals with ID compared to the general population [22].

Cardiac considerations include assessing for congenital heart disease when intellectual disability is associated with certain genetic conditions such as Down syndrome and Williams syndrome. Antibiotic prophylaxis may be required for those individuals who meet criteria [36, 46].

Respiratory disorders are common in adults with ID. These include dysphagia and aspiration. Dysphagia is prevalent in up to 5 % of individuals with ID. Adults with CP have a high death rate as a result of aspiration pneumonia [18]. If the individual with ID has symptoms of coughing and choking with meals, provide a referral for a speech therapy evaluation.

Gastrointestinal and feeding problems are common as well. Adults with intellectual disability have an increased risk of poor nutrition. A retrospective study on individuals with severe to profound ID in the UK showed the importance of nutrition and the improvement in body weight as a result of dietetic referrals. Better nutrition also led to other improvements in medical conditions, including resolution of amenorrhea, improved diarrhea, increased balance and mobility, and improvement in pressure sores [47].

Gastroesophageal reflux disease due to upper gastrointestinal dysmotility is common among individuals with ID. It is more prevalent in individuals with gastrostomy tubes. As it is difficult to identify reflux symptoms in profound ID, providers must evaluate for changes in behavior or adaptive functioning. There is a higher frequency of *Helicobacter pylori* infection in adults with ID than those in the general population [48]. Screening for *H. pylori* infection is recommended in symptomatic or in asymptomatic adults with ID who are in group homes at a frequency of every 3–5 years [48].

Constipation has been reported in up to 40 % of individuals with ID, due to immobility and a lack of exercise. Medications with anticholinergic effects may be contributing as well. An aggressive bowel regimen is important in preventing and treating constipation and has been shown to reduce the incidence of impaction and intestinal obstruction. A necessary strategy is a daily regimen of fiber, increasing fluids, and stool softeners. Frequent laxatives may be necessary and tolerance to stimulant laxatives is less of a concern than the complications of untreated constipation [49].

Hypothyroidism is common in adults with ID and occurs with a much higher frequency in associated conditions such as Down syndrome (see Chap. 10: Down syndrome). It also occurs more frequently in individuals taking lithium or atypical or second-generation antipsychotic medications [36]. For individuals taking these medications, a primary care provider should establish a baseline thyroid screening test and check annually.

Osteoporosis is more prevalent in adults with ID, including in premenopausal women and in men [50, 51]. A review on women with ID highlighted risk factors for osteoporosis including inactivity, long-term anticonvulsant use, CP, and possibly Down syndrome [52]. Low vitamin D level is an additional risk factor [53]. Earlier screening than the general population is recommended; age 40 for individuals who are institutionalized and age 45 for individuals who live in the community [53].

Providers uniformly agree on a variety of reasons to provide *contraception*. Multiple studies described that people with ID are sexually victimized more often than others who do not have a disability [54]. One study reported that 25 % of girls and women with intellectual disability who were referred for birth control had a history of sexual violence [55]. Communication and behavioral disorders contribute to very high levels of risk, and having multiple disabilities (e.g., intellectual disability and behavior disorders) result in even higher risk levels [56]. Another reason for contraception is therapeutic amenorrhea to treat dysmenorrhea/menorrhagia, or in individuals who are frightened or for whom hygiene issues are difficult.

Behavioral and Mental Health Considerations

Aggressive, challenging behavior is frequently reported in adults with intellectual disability. Antipsychotic medications are frequently used, although evidence for their benefit is limited. A 2002 study examined the quality of preventive and psychiatric services of intellectually disabled adults living in California in 1997 [31]. One-third of the individuals in their study received psychotropic medications, but only 24 % of these individuals had received psychiatric consultations. Despite the polypharmacy of psychotropic medications, 36 %

of this group did not have an identifiable diagnosis. A randomized trial comparing risperidone, haloperidol, and placebo in the treatment of aggressive challenging behavior in patients with intellectual disability did not show any clinically significant differences among the 3 study groups [57]. The authors concluded that antipsychotic drugs should no longer be regarded as an acceptable routine treatment for aggressive challenging behavior in people with intellectual disabilities.

The role of primary care providers is to screen for new behavioral issues or worsening of a previously well-controlled behavior disorder at each clinic visit. If new or worsening behavior patterns are identified, the provider pursues an evaluation of underlying medical causes or associated conditions leading to behavioral changes. Pain and distress are common causes of behavioral changes and can be assessed with a caregiver's help as well as pain assessment tools adapted for adults with ID [7]. There are multiple primary care toolkits to assess behavior changes provided by the American Academy of Pediatrics and Got Transition. These assessments include evaluation of physical, environmental, and emotional factors. While not comprehensive, Table 13.5 describes components of a primary care checklist to evaluate behavioral/emotional concerns [7, 58, 59].

The primary care provider should also be routinely monitoring psychotropic medications for side effects such as weight gain and QT prolongation. Phenothiazines such as haloperidol and chlorpromazine are generally accepted to cause QT prolongation with an increased risk for reentrant tachycardias. Other commonly used antipsychotics that can possibly cause QT prolongation include risperidone, quetiapine, and lithium. Periodic electrocardiogram (EKG) monitoring is prudent [60]. Box 13.2 describes considerations during the initial and then subsequent visits for evaluating the individual with intellectual disability.

Box 13.2 Multidisciplinary care at initial visit and then annual updates

- Guardianship assessment
- Residential environment:
  - Home with family
  - Independent living with support
  - Group home
- Medical evaluation:
  - Management of associated, comorbid, and secondary conditions
  - Health screening, vaccines
  - Behavioral evaluation
- Assess for polypharmacy
- Subspecialty evaluation:
  - Orthopedics: musculoskeletal issues such as contractures, scoliosis
  - Neurology: seizure disorders
  - Psychiatry: behavior disorders
- Dental evaluation
- Ophthalmology/hearing evaluation
- Occupational/physical/speech therapy needs
- Durable medical equipment
- Assess for caregiver stress
- Need for respite services
- Social services referral

Table 13.5 Primary care evaluation of agitation/behavioral changes in adults with ID [7]

Physical	Environmental	Emotional
• Medical conditions leading to pain; peptic ulcer disease, dental pain, musculoskeletal disorders, arthritis, spasticity • Infections: e.g., pneumonia, urinary tract infection • Medication adverse effects • Constipation • Sensory discomfort; new clothes, shoes • New hearing/vision impairment • Hypothyroidism	• Reduced supports; loss of staffing • Change in residence • Changes in routines • Lack of adequate communication with family, friends, caregivers • Lack of activities	Depression or anxiety due to: • Addition of a new roommate or sibling • Loss of a parent/caregiver • Social isolation

Health Maintenance/Preventative Health

As individuals transition to adulthood, the American Academy of Pediatrics (AAP), American College of Physicians (ACP), and American Academy of Family Physicians (AAFP) recommend applying the same guidelines for primary and preventive care for all adolescents and young adults, including those with special health care needs. Examples of such guidelines include the American Medical Association's *Guidelines for Adolescent Preventive Services (GAPS)* and the US Public Health Service's Guidelines to Clinical Preventive Services [28, 61].

Several studies have looked at screening tests for individuals with intellectual disabilities. A 2007 study examined screening recommendations for common preventable conditions using the US Preventive Services Task Force guidelines and reviewed the literature about the prevalence of these conditions in adults with intellectual disabilities [62]. Effective health screening requires that a disease must be serious and have important consequences, that early intervention will improve outcomes, that a preclinical phase has a long duration and can be easily identified by a screening test and that the disease is prevalent in the screened population. In adults with ID, the prevalence of various diseases is often not known, and these individuals may have a longer preclinical phase since limitations in cognitive functioning can make it difficult to identify symptoms. Even if early intervention is possible, it may be difficult to implement treatment [63]. Additionally, there are barriers to screening in adults with ID. These include anxiety, lack of understanding of the test, and requiring additional family members or extra staff from residential facilities to accompany individuals for these procedures [39].

Cardiovascular Screening

As previously discussed, there is a higher rate of overweight/obesity among individuals with ID. It is important to provide the same screenings for risk factors for cardiovascular disease including hypertension, hyperlipidemia, and diabetes as recommended by the USPSTF guidelines [37, 64]. Follow blood pressures at each clinic visit and then annually, check lipids at approximately 18 years of age and then every 5 years depending on other risk factors, and follow glycosylated hemoglobin levels every 3 years beginning 45—earlier if at higher risk. As with the general population, encourage smoking cessation [65].

Cervical Cancer Screening

Fewer women with ID are sexually active compared to the general female population [66]. Two large studies of institutionalized women showed low rates of abnormal Pap smears [51, 67]. However, this study was limited in that it did not include community-dwelling women, who are most likely among those with ID to be sexually active. Women with ID may not be able to give a sexual history. There is a high rate of sexual abuse in adults with ID [54]. After obtaining the initial Papanicolaou test, additional screening should be individualized based on a woman's sexual history, rather than her cognitive ability. For those women with ID who are sexually active, providers must counsel and screen for sexually transmitted diseases (STDs). As with the general population, women with ID should also undergo pelvic examinations as appropriate to evaluate symptoms such as menorrhagia, dysmenorrhea, and pelvic pain.

Breast Cancer Screening

Primary care providers should obtain mammograms for women with ID at the same frequency as for the general population. In general, women with ID are less likely to have children and to breastfeed. These factors may increase their risk for breast cancer. Two studies from England and Australia showed that only one-third of eligible women with ID were screened due to low rates of physician referral [68]. As women with ID live longer, the primary care provider should make every effort to obtain mammograms at regular intervals.

Colon Cancer Screening

Constipation is a common problem for adults with ID and this makes the onset of colon cancer symptoms difficult to evaluate. The data for colon cancer prevalence in adults with ID is not clear. In a large international study, colon cancer was more prevalent in adults with ID [67]. In a smaller study, rates of adenomatous polyps in institutionalized adults approximated the general population [69]. The recommendation to pursue colon cancer screening in adults with ID is the same as that for the general population. Some adults with ID may require sedation for the colonoscopy.

Sedation

Some adults with ID may require sedation for health screening procedures. In an ideal setting, primary care providers and subspecialty colleagues can coordinate services to perform multiple procedures such as routine phlebotomy, immunizations, dental examinations, and gynecologic exam while the patient is under sedation. As adults with ID are living longer, it is important to maintain the same screening guidelines to maintain the same quality of life as the general population.

Ethical Considerations

For adults with ID, providers often consider the concept of quality of life when making treatment decisions regarding both management of chronic medical conditions as well as for performing health maintenance procedures. The quality of life (QOL) construct has been examined by several researchers. The key to self-report of quality of life among people with disabilities is accurate modified instrumentation [70]. Studies have shown that individuals with disabilities can accurately assess their quality of life [26, 70]. The public opinion of individuals with disabilities was described in one 2010 study as: "Non-disabled people believe that the quality of life of people who live with disabilities is extremely low… When disabled people report about their own QOL, they rate it as only slightly lower than when non-disabled people self-report their own QOL" [71]. Healthcare professionals' opinion of QOL of people with disabilities is lower than both the opinion of the general public and the disabled individual's own opinion of QOL [71, 72]. Healthcare professionals must be aware of this bias in individuals with intellectual disabilities when discussing treatment options for medical conditions as well as for preventative measures.

The informed consent and decision-making process varies depending on the degree of intellectual disabilities. Individuals with moderate to severe intellectual disabilities typically do not have the decision-making capacity to comply with the principles of informed consent. The substitute decision maker is required to make a decision based on the best interest of the individual with ID. A "bonded" guardian is an individual who has a previous relationship with the patient, such as a parent or caregiver. A nonbonded guardian is typically someone appointed through the courts. Providers typically prefer bonded guardians as they are better able to incorporate a patient's wishes into the healthcare decision-making process [73]. As with the general population, end-of-life issues should be addressed prior to the occurrence of a life-threatening event. ID alone should not be a reason to forgo medical treatments of complicated conditions such as end-stage renal disease requiring dialysis, cancer, or organ transplantation. For those with mild intellectual disability, it is important to remember that although they are not capable of some aspects of decision-making (such as financial management), it does not mean that they are unable to participate in their health care decision-making process. Individuals with ID can still convey their wishes based on a lifetime pattern of expressing their needs to their caregivers, who in turn, can make the best decision for the individual. Providers must take this into consideration when making treatment decisions to improve quality of life by maintaining health and prolonging life [73].

Community Resources

Each state has an office for intellectual/developmental disabilities and adults with ID should be registered with this state-specific office, if they have not already done so. The state agency is an important resource for long-term or short-term services, particularly around residential and vocational/day supports. Each state also has an Aging and Disability Resource Center (ADRC) (https://www.adrc-tae.acl.gov), which is a database of community resources broken down by area. In addition, each state has at least 1 University Center for Excellence in Developmental Disabilities (UCEDDs) (https://www.aucd.org). These centers are a wealth of information for programs, services, advocacy, legislation, and consumer-guidance. Adult providers should use these agencies to find out more about local resources for adults with ID.

Conclusion

Adults with intellectual disabilities have complex medical conditions differing from the general population. Aging starts earlier in persons with ID and medical problems are related to the natural history of the original disability ("Appendix"). It is essential to screen for medical conditions that occur at an equal or higher prevalence than in the general population to avoid morbidity complications and premature death. As adults with intellectual disabilities are living longer due to improved medical care, technology, and environmental conditions, they require the same considerations for improving quality of life, improving access to health care, and health screening as the general population. The goal is to provide the same quality of healthcare for adults with intellectual disability by raising awareness of the human rights, dignity, autonomy, and needs of persons with disabilities through training and implementation of ethical standards for public and private healthcare.

Acknowledgment Special thanks to Cory Nourie who wrote the section on Community Resources.

Appendix

Intellectual disability (ID) condition fact sheet

Definition	**Intellectual disability (ID) is a lifelong neurodevelopmental condition characterized by the following:** IQ score below the range of 70–75; 2 standard deviations (SD) below the mean Limitations in adaptive skill areas; 2 SD below the mean in 1 of these areas or in combination of all 3 areas: • **Conceptual deficits**: receptive and expressive language, reading, writing, math, reasoning, knowledge, and memory • **Social deficits**: interpersonal communication skills, friendship, empathy, social judgment skills including gullibility, naiveté, following rules, obeying laws, avoiding victimization • **Practical deficits:** personal care activities including eating, dressing, bathing, meal preparation, telephone communication, transportation, and occupational skills including organizing school and work activities, money management, job duties These limitations must be present prior to age 18 years
Epidemiology	• Prevalence of ID is estimated at ~1 % of the population in the U.S. and western European countries. • Although the life expectancy of people with ID is increasing, it is still lower than that of the general population, with an average age at death of ~66 years • Many individuals with ID have an underlying etiology; genetic and nongenetic causes • Aging starts earlier in persons with ID and medical problems are related to the natural history of the original disability • More than 75 % of adults with ID live with families • More than 25 % of family care providers are over the age of 60 • Increasing need for medical care for aging adults with ID and their families and for access to quality supports that address health and social changes
Special considerations	**Individuals with intellectual disability have higher prevalence of physical and mental health conditions, including the following:** • Physical inactivity/obesity • Vision impairments: refractive errors, hyperopia, myopia • Hearing impairments • Oral health problems: dental caries, gingivitis, and periodontal disease • musculoskeletal problems • Seizure disorder • Congenital heart disease • Respiratory conditions: dysphagia, aspiration • Gastrointestinal problems: gastroesophageal reflux disease, *H. pylori* infection • Osteoporosis • Anxiety and depression
Recommended preventive screening	• Vision: Annually, glaucoma, and cataract screening every 5 years after age 45 • Hearing exams: age-related reduced hearing every 5 years after age 45 • Cerumen impaction; assess every 6 months • Dental evaluation: cleaning every 6 months • Osteoporosis screening: age 40 in group home, 45 if in community, modify based on condition; e.g., cerebral palsy, anticonvulsant therapy. • Cardiovascular screening: same as USPSTF guidelines Hypertension: BP each visit, annually Diabetes: hemoglobin A1C every 3 years >45, if risk factors, start <45 BMI: counsel regularly Lipids: Initial 18+, then every 5 years • Thyroid function: at initial visit, if on psychotropic medications, annually, modify based on conditions; e.g., Down syndrome **Cancer screening:** • Breast cancer: same as in the USPSTF guidelines • Colon cancer: No modifications from USPSTF guidelines • Cervical cancer: After initial Papanicolaou smear, modify based on sexual history

References

1. Shalock RL, Borthwick-Duffy SA, Bradley VJ, Buntinx WHE, Coulter DL, Craig EM, et al. Intellectual disability: definition, classification, and system of support. 11th ed. Washington, DC: AAIDD; 2010. p. 259.
2. McNeil JM, Binette J. Prevalence of disabilities and associated health conditions among adults: United States. Morbid Mortal Wkly Rep. 2001;50:120–5.
3. Patel D, Merrick J. Intellectual disability. In: Greydanus D, Patel D, Pratt H, Calles JJ, editors. Behavioral pediatrics, vol. 3. New York: Nova Science; 2009.
4. Individuals with Disabilities Education Act (IDEA) [Internet]. American Psychological Association. http://www.apa.org/about/gr/issues/disability/idea.aspx. Accessed 12 Jan 2016.
5. American Psychiatric Association. Diagnostic and statistical manual of mental disorders: DSM-IV-TR. Washington, DC: American Psychiatric Association; 2000.
6. American Psychiatric Association. Diagnostic and statistical manual of mental disorders: DSM-5. Washington, DC: American Psychiatric Association; 2013.
7. Edwards B, Temple V, Dunn L. Adaptive functioning and communication associated with different levels of intellectual and developmental disabilities (IDD) [Internet]. Health care for adults with intellectual and developmental disabilities toolkit for primary care providers. Vanderbilt Kennedy Center for Excellence in Developmental Disabilities. http://vkc.mc.vanderbilt.edu/etoolkit/general-issues/adaptive-functioning-communication/. Accessed 1 April 2016.
8. Coppus AM, Evenhuis HM, Verberne GJ. People with intellectual disability: what do we know about adulthood and life expectancy? Dev Disabil Res Rev. 2013;18(1):6–16.
9. Zablotsky B, Black LI, Maenner MJ, Schieve LA, Blumberg SJ. Estimated prevalence of autism and other developmental disabilities following questionnaire changes in the 2014 National Health Interview Survey. National Health Statistics Reports. Nov 13, 2015; no 87. http://www.cdc.gov/nchs/data/nhsr/nhsr087.pdf Accessed 1 April 2016.
10. Cooper S, Melville C, Morrison J. People with intellectual disabilities. Br Med J. 2004;329:414–5.
11. Heller T, Stafford P, Davis LA, Sedlezky L, Gaylord V, editors. Impact: feature issue on aging and people with intellectual and developmental disabilities, vol. 23(1). Minneapolis: University of Minnesota, Institute on Community Integration; 2010.
12. Miniño AM, Xu J, Kochanek KD, Tejada VB. Death in the United States, 2007. NCHS data brief, no 26. Hyattsville: National Center for Health Statistics; 2009.
13. Bittles A, Petterson B, Sullivan S, Hussain R, Glasson E, Montgomery P. The influence of intellectual disability on life expectancy. J Gerontol A Biol Sci Med Sci. 2002;57(7):M470–2.
14. Janicki MP, Dalton AJ, Henderson CM, Davidson PW. Mortality and morbidity among older adults with intellectual disability: health services considerations. Disabil Rehabil. 1999;21(5–6):284–94.
15. Diseases and Conditions [Internet]. Diseases and conditions. Centers for Disease Control and Prevention. http://www.cdc.gov/nchs/fastats/diseases-and-conditions.htm. Accessed 1 Jan 2016.
16. Evenhuis H, Henderson CM, Beange H, Lennox N, Chicoine B. Healthy aging—adults with intellectual disabilities: physical health issues. J Appl Res Int Dis. 2001;14(3):175–94.
17. Coppus AMW, Evenhuis HM, Verberne G-J, Visser FE, Oostra BA, Eikelenboom P, et al. Survival in elderly persons with Down syndrome. J Am Geriatr Soc. 2008;56(12):2311–6.
18. Strauss D, Cable W, Shavelle R. Causes of excess mortality in cerebral palsy. Dev Med Child Neurol. 1999;41(9):580–5.
19. Luckasson R, Borthwick-Duffy S, Buntinx WHE, Coulter DL, Craig EN, et al. Mental retardation: definition, classification and systems of support. 10th ed. Washington, DC: American Association of Mental Retardation; 2002.
20. Braddock D, Hemp R, Rizzolo MC. State of the States in developmental disabilities. Ment Retard. 2004;42(5):356–70.
21. American Association on Intellectual and Developmental Disabilities. Declaration on health parity for persons with intellectual and developmental disabilities. Washington, DC: American Association on Intellectual and Developmental Disabilities; 2006.
22. Kerr M, Scheepers M, Arvio M, Beavis J, Brandt C, Brown S, et al. Consensus guidelines into the management of epilepsy in adults with an intellectual disability. J Intellect Disabil Res. 2009;53(8):687–94.
23. Traci MA, Seekins T, Szalda-Petree A, Ravesloot C. Assessing secondary conditions among adults with developmental disabilities: a preliminary study. Ment Retard. 2002;40(2):119–31.
24. Scheepers M, Kerr M, O'Hara D, Bainbridge D, Cooper S, Davis R, et al. Reducing health disparity in people with intellectual disabilities: a report from Health Issues Special Interest Research Group of the International Association for the Scientific Study of Intellectual Disabilities. J Policy Pract Intell Disabil. 2005;2(3–4):249–55.
25. McGinnis MJ, Williams-Russo P, Knickman JR. The case for more active policy attention to health promotion: to succeed, we need leadership that informs and motivates, economic incentives that encourage change, and science that moves the frontiers. Health Aff. 2002;21:78–93.
26. Finlay WML, Lyons E. Methodological issues in interviewing and using self-report questionnaires with people with mental retardation. Psychol Assess. 2001;13(3):319–35.

27. Ervin DA, Williams A, Merrick J. Primary care: mental and behavioral health and persons with intellectual and developmental disabilities. Front Public Health. 2014;2:76.
28. US Public Health Service. Closing the gap: a national blueprint for improving the health of individuals with mental retardation. Report of the Surgeon General's Conference on Health Disparities and Mental Retardation. Washington, DC: US Public Health Service; February 2001.
29. Krahn GL, Hammond L, Turner A. A cascade of disparities: health and health care access for people with intellectual disabilities. Ment Retard Dev Disabil Res Rev. 2006;12(1):70–82.
30. Kerr AM, Mcculloch D, Oliver K, Mclean B, Coleman E, Law T, et al. Medical needs of people with intellectual disability require regular reassessment, and the provision of client- and carer-held reports. J Intellect Disabil Res. 2003;47(2):134–45.
31. Lewis MA, Lewis CE, Leake B, King BH, Lindemann R. The quality of health care for adults with developmental disabilities. Public Health Rep. 2002;117:174–84.
32. United Nations Convention on the Rights of Persons with Disabilities [Internet]. United Nations convention on the rights of persons with disabilities. http://www.un.org/disabilities/documents/convention/convention_accessible_pdf. Accessed 1 April 2016.
33. Rubin IL, Crocker AC, editors. Medical care for children and adults with developmental disabilities. 2nd ed. Baltimore: Paul H. Brookes Publishing Co.; 2006. p. 255–71.
34. Marks B, Sisirak J, Heller T. Health matters for people with developmental disabilities: creating a sustainable health promotion program. Baltimore: Paul H. Brookes Pub. Co.; 2010.
35. Haveman MJ, Heller T, Lee LA, Maaskant MA, Shooshtari S, Stydom A. Report of the state of science on health risks and ageing in people with intellectual disabilities. IASSID Special Interest Research Group on Ageing and Intellectual Disabilities/Faculty Rehabilitation Sciences, University of Dortmund; 2009.
36. Sullivan WF, Berg JM, Bradley E, Cheetham T, Denton R, Heng J, et al. Primary care of adults with developmental disabilities: Canadian consensus guidelines. Can Fam Physician. 2011;57:541–53.
37. Massachusetts Department of Developmental Services in partnership with the Center for Developmental Disabilities Evaluation and Research (CDDER)/UMass Medical School. Preventive health recommendations for adults with intellectual disability. Last Revised Oct 2014. http://www.mass.gov/eohhs/docs/dmr/reports/health-screening-brochure.pdf. Accessed 13 June 2016.
38. Messinger-Rapport BJ, Rapport DJ. Primary care for the developmentally disabled adult. J Gen Intern Med. 1997;12(10):629–36.
39. Doostan D, Wilkes M. Treating the developmentally disabled. West J Med. 1999;171(2):92–6.
40. Merrick J, Davidson PW, Morad M, Janicki MP, Wexler O, Henderson CM. Older adults with intellectual disability in residential care centers in Israel: health status and service utilization. Am J Ment Retard. 2004;109:413–20.
41. Rimmer JH, Braddock D, Fujiura G. Prevalence of obesity in adults with mental retardation: implications for health promotion and disease prevention. Ment Retard. 1993;31:105–10.
42. Bhaumik S, Watson JM, Thorp CF, Tyrer F, Mcgrother CW. Body mass index in adults with intellectual disability: distribution, associations and service implications: a population-based prevalence study. J Intellect Disabil Res. 2008;52(4):287–98.
43. Owens PL, Kerker BD, Zigler E, Horwitz SM. Vision and oral health needs of individuals with intellectual disability. Ment Retard Dev Disabil Res Rev. 2006;12(1):28–40.
44. Evenhuis HM, Natzgam LM. IASSID international consensus statement: early identification of hearing and visual impairment in children and adults with an intellectual disability. Leiden: International Association of Scientific Studies on Intellectual Disability, Special Interest Group on Health Issues; 1997.
45. Blair E, Watson L, Badawi N, Stanley FJ. Life expectancy among people with cerebral palsy in Western Australia. Dev Med Child Neurol. 2001;43(08):508.
46. Wilson W, Taubert KA, Gewitz M, Lockhart PB, Baddour LM, Levison M, et al. Prevention of infective endocarditis: guidelines from the American Heart Association: a guideline from the American Heart Association Rheumatic Fever, Endocarditis and Kawasaki Disease Committee, Council on Cardiovascular Disease in the Young, and the Council on Clinical Cardiology, Council on Cardiovascular Surgery and Anesthesia, and the Quality of Care and Outcomes Research Interdisciplinary Working Group. J Am Dent Assoc 2007;138(6):739–45, 747–60.
47. Jolly C, Jamieson JM. The nutritional problems of adults with severe learning disabilities living in the community. J Hum Nutr Diet. 1999;12:29–34.
48. Wallace R, Schluter PJ, Duff M, Ouellette-Kuntz H, Webb PM. A review of the risk factors for, consequences, diagnosis, and management of Helicobacter pylori in adults with intellectual disabilities. J Policy Pract Intell Disabil. 2004;1(3–4):147–63.
49. Kozma A, Mansell J, Beadle-Brown J. Outcomes in different residential settings for people with intellectual disability: a systematic review. Am J Intellect Dev Disabil. 2009;114(3):193–222.
50. Tyler CV, Snyder CW, Zyzanski S. Screening for osteoporosis in community-dwelling adults with mental retardation. Ment Retard. 2000;38:316–21.
51. Jaffe JS, Timell AM, Eisenberg MS, Chambers JT. Low prevalence of abnormal cervical cytology in an

institutionalized population with intellectual disability. J Intell Disabil Res. 2002;46(Pt 7):569–74.
52. Schrager S. Epidemiology of osteoporosis in women with cognitive impairment. Ment Retard. 2006;44: 203–11.
53. Dreyfus D, Lauer E, Wilkinson J. Characteristics associated with bone mineral density screening in adults with intellectual disabilities. J Am Board Fam Med. 2014;27(1):104–14.
54. Furey E. Sexual abuse of adults with mental retardation: who and where. Ment Retard. 1994;32(3):173–80.
55. Sobsey R. Violence and abuse in the lives of people with disabilities: the end of silent acceptance?. Baltimore: P.H. Brooks Pub. Co.; 1994.
56. Sullivan PM, Knutson JF. The relationship between child abuse and neglect and disabilities: Implications for research and practice. Omaha: Boys Town National Research Hospital; 1994.
57. Tyrer P, Oliver-Africano PC, Ahmed Z, Bouras N, Cooray S, Deb S, et al. Risperidone, haloperidol, and placebo in the treatment of aggressive challenging behaviour in patients with intellectual disability: a randomised controlled trial. Lancet. 2008;371 (9606):57–63.
58. Helping Adolescents Transition to Adult Health Care [Internet]. Helping adolescents transition to adult health care. American Academy of Pediatrics. 2011. https://www.aap.org/en-us/about-the-aap/aap-press-room/pages/helping-adolescents-transition-to-adult-health-care.aspx?nfstatus=401. Accessed 1 April 2016.
59. GotTransition. Transitioning to an adult approach to health care without changing providers—introduction. http://www.gottransition.org/providers/staying.cfm. Accessed 1 April 2016.
60. Nielsen J, Graff C, Kanters JK, Toft E, Taylor D, Meyer JM. Assessing QT interval prolongation and its associated risks with antipsychotics. CNS Drugs. 2011;25:473.
61. Department of Adolescent Health. American Medical Association. Guidelines for adolescent preventive services. Chicago: American Medical Association; 1992.
62. Wilkinson JE, Culpepper L, Cerreto M. Screening tests for adults with intellectual disabilities. J Am Board Fam Med. 2007;20(4):399–407.
63. Aschengrau A, Seage GM. Essentials of epidemiology in public health. Sudbury, MA: Jones and Bartlett Publishers; 2003.
64. US Preventive Services Task Force. Home—US preventive services task force. US preventive services task force. 2016. http://www.uspreventiveservicestaskforce.org/. Accessed 1 April 2016.
65. Wallace RA, Schluter P. Audit of cardiovascular disease risk factors among supported adults with intellectual disability attending an ageing clinic. J Intellect Dev Disabil. 2008;33(1):48–58.
66. Wilkinson JE, Cerreto MC. Primary care for women with intellectual disabilities. J Am Board Fam Med. 2008;21(3):215–22.
67. Quint E, Elkins T. Cervical cytology in women with mental retardation. Obstet Gynecol. 1997;89:123–6.
68. Sullivan SG, Hussain R, Threlfall T. Bittles, AH The incidence of cancer in people with intellectual disabilities. Cancer Causes Control. 2004;15 (10):1021–5.
69. Uno Y. Mental retardation and colorectal disease: colonoscopic mass screening to determine whether the risk of adenomatous polyposis screening is increased in the mentally retarded. J Gastroenterol Hepatol. 1996;11:275–8.
70. Cummins RA. Self-rated quality of life scales for people with an intellectual disability: a review. J Appl Res Intellect Disabil. 1997;10(3):199–216.
71. Amundson R. Quality of life, disability, and hedonic psychology. J Theory Soc Behav. 2010;40(4):374–92.
72. Albrecht GL, Devlieger PJ. The disability paradox: high quality of life against all odds. Soc Sci Med. 1999;48(8):977–88.
73. Veatch RM. Limits of guardian treatment refusal: a reasonableness standard. Am J Law Med. 1984;9 (4):427–68.
74. Sullivan SG, Glasson EJ, Hussain R, Petterson BA, Slack-Smith LM, Montgomery PD, Bittles AH. Breast cancer and the uptake of mammography screening services by women with intellectual disabilities. Prev Med. 2013;37(5):507–12.

14 Juvenile Idiopathic Arthritis

Tova Ronis and Patience H. White

Case Presentation

Tina is an 18-year-old female with a history of polyarticular juvenile idiopathic arthritis (JIA). She will be starting college at a university near your practice and presents to the internal medicine office with her parents to establish care. Tina recently graduated high school and will be studying engineering at a local university that is a 4-h drive from her home.

Tina reports that she was diagnosed with arthritis when she was 3 years of age. Her arthritis has involved her knees, ankles, wrist, and temporomandibular joint (TMJ). She has been followed regularly by an ophthalmologist and never had any eye complications. She was treated initially with intra-articular corticosteroid injections of the affected joints as well as naproxen and methotrexate when she was younger and was able to wean off of all her medications by the time she was 9. She then had a flare of wrist arthritis when she was 14 and is currently being treated with methotrexate and adalimumab injections, which she administers independently. She was recently treated with antibiotics for a urinary tract infection and continued her arthritis medications at that time. She has regular menstrual periods. On dietary history, she notes no restrictions but does not like drinking milk. She has no other health problems and her immunizations are up to date. There is no family history of autoimmune disease. Her father and maternal grandfather have coronary artery disease.

On musculoskeletal exam, you notice that Tina has micrognathia and a decreased oral aperture. Wrist range of motion is mildly decreased in both flexion and extension. Otherwise, the remainder of her musculoskeletal and general exam is normal. Gait evaluation reveals a 1.5 cm leg-length discrepancy. She compensates for this by wearing a shoe lift on the shorter side.

Recent labs showed borderline elevated cholesterol and a negative rheumatoid factor (RF) and anti-citrullinated cyclic peptide (CCP).

Tina is excited to be starting university. She graduated from a public high school where she had a 504 plan that provided accommodations for her physical limitations, such as the use of a computer to type notes in class and additional time to take tests if her wrists were in pain. She

T. Ronis (✉)
Department of Pediatrics, Division of Rheumatology, Children's National Health System, 111 Michigan Ave NW, Washington, DC 20010, USA
e-mail: tronis@childrensnational.org

P.H. White
Got Transition: the Center for Health Care Transition Improvement, Department of Medicine and Pediatrics, George Washington University School of Medicine and Health Sciences, 1615 M Street, NW, Suite 290, Washington, DC 20036, USA
e-mail: PWhite@thenationalalliance.org

M. Pilapil et al. (eds.), *Care of Adults with Chronic Childhood Conditions*,
DOI 10.1007/978-3-319-43827-6_14

will be living in campus housing. At this initial appointment, her mother raises concern about her immunocompromised state and the risk of exposure to infections in the school dormitory. She will still be covered under her parents' medical insurance plan. She will be responsible for getting her medications while at college. Additionally, she needs to have screening labs for methotrexate toxicity every 3 months.

Case Discussion

This case demonstrates a typical course of polyarticular RF negative JIA and raises several issues that are faced by patients with JIA as they graduate from high school and enter college. In the United States, the Americans with Disabilities Act (ADA) states that postsecondary schools cannot deny enrollment based on the presence of physical or mental disabilities. The U.S. Department of Education shares that "academic adjustments may include auxiliary aids and modifications to academic requirements as are necessary to ensure equal educational opportunity." [1] (see more at: http://www2.ed.gov/about/offices/list/ocr/transition.html). Applications cannot ask about health conditions and prospective students do not need to disclose a health condition on applying. Most colleges and universities have an office for students with disabilities where students like Tina can register. This office can help provide accommodations now or at any time during the school year such as extra test time and excused absences for doctor's appointments or acute illness. If patients are significantly immunocompromised, this office can also help them find single rooms without a roommate to reduce the exposure to infections. However, this is not always necessary and college life should be normalized as much as possible. Students need to register with this office with documentation from their physician each year and, if not complete, the student can be denied any accommodation due to their condition. (For additional information on education among adults with chronic childhood conditions, please see Chap. 27 of this book).

Because Tina will be living in a dormitory, she may be at higher risk of infection. Immunizations should be reviewed and patients on immunosuppressive medications should not be given live virus vaccines including intranasal flu, measles mumps rubella, varicella, and zoster vaccines. She will need a yearly injectable influenza vaccine and should have received both pneumococcal 13-valent conjugate (PCV13) and pneumococcal polysaccharide (PPSV23) as she is immunocompromised. She should also be given the meningitis MenACWY vaccine as she will be living in campus housing [2].

Often, immunosuppressive therapies will be temporarily held if a patient gets a serious infection such as a urinary tract infection requiring antibiotics. In this case Tina should be counseled to stop her methotrexate and adalimumab if this happens again. Corticosteroids are usually continued despite infection given the risk for adrenal insufficiency if they are stopped abruptly.

A challenge faced by many teenagers and young adults at this phase is adherence. Since Tina will be responsible for getting and administering her own medications, she is at risk of having poor adherence. It is normal for adolescents and young adults to want to appear like their peers at this developmental stage. Patients with no outwardly apparent chronic diseases may not want to disclose to their peers that they have a health condition. If their arthritis has been asymptomatic, they may have some denial about their illness and stop taking their medications. There are web-based tools and applications (apps) to help patients remember to take their medications that may be helpful. (Free apps are available on both the Apple iTunes and Google Play stores).

Additionally, many adolescent and young adult patients do not have experience in managing their own chronic disease if their care has been previously coordinated by their parents. Research has demonstrated that mature decision-making often does not emerge until the middle of the third decade of life [3]. You may need to assess Tina's knowledge of her disease and her skills of managing her health care in the adult care system. An American College of Rheumatology self-care assessment tool is available online for this purpose [4]. If she is accustomed to her parents ordering her medications and taking her to have her regular labs done, this may be difficult for her at first. Logistically, Tina is still covered under her parents' insurance plan but she will be responsible for managing her disease at college. It may be helpful to find a mail order pharmacy that can deliver her medications if there is no pharmacy close to her dormitory. She needs a plan for needle disposal on campus. She will also need to find a location to have her regular labs drawn (see schedule for lab tests for methotrexate screening in Table 14.1) [5]. Sometimes this can be done at a campus student health office, and she should find out where that is located on campus and make arrangements to have the results sent to the office. She should have access to a portable summary of her disease and her current medications at all times, which she can store in her cell phone (e.g., see Medical ID in the Health app on recent models of Apple's iPhone). Young adults are familiar with electronic communication, and Tina should be encouraged to sign up for the office electronic portal, if available. It is also important to have a discussion with Tina about what is the best way to communicate with her about her appointments (e.g., text reminders) and for her to communicate with the office and her primary care physician about her questions. Young adults ages 18–25 years are one of the biggest users of the emergency room under the age of 75 in the US and are poorly connected to primary care.

Now that Tina is 18, her medical information is protected under the Health Insurance Portability and Accountability Act (HIPAA). This includes confidentiality from her parents. If Tina wants her parents to continue to receive her medical information, she should be asked to sign a HIPAA waiver granting them this right. As she is a young adult, she should be interviewed without her parents present for at least part of the visit. Ideally, she has been seen alone for part of her visits to her pediatrician for the past few years so asking her parents to step out during the visit will not be a surprise. Parents are usually willing to step out of the room once their medical concerns about their child have been expressed. Methotrexate is a teratogenic medication with risk of hepatotoxicity, and Tina should be counseled about safe sexual practices and alcohol. Two simultaneous forms of contraception are recommended for patients who are sexually active and taking teratogenic medications (e.g., barrier methods and hormonal birth control). The latter is safe to use in young adults with JIA.

Medically, this case illustrates the deformities that can occur due to arthritis in a growing joint. Some joints such as the knee will grow faster when inflamed, resulting in leg-length discrepancy. Leg lengths should be measured along with a scoliosis assessment. If quadriceps muscle bulk is asymmetric due to disuse of the arthritic knee, physical therapy can assist with strengthening. When the TMJ is involved, this can lead to micrognathia and decreased range of motion of the jaw.

This patient will also need referrals to specialty care. She will need an adult rheumatologist, an

Table 14.1 American College of Rheumatology recommendations for follow-up laboratory monitoring intervals for complete blood count, liver transaminase levels, and serum creatinine levels for patients receiving DMARDs. Modified with permission obtained from [5]

Medication	Monitoring interval based on duration of treatment[a]		
	<3 months[b]	3–6 months	>6 months
Hydroxychloroquine	None after baseline	None	None
Methotrexate (weeks)	2–4	8–12	12
Leflunomide (weeks)	2–4	8–12	12
Sulfasalazine (weeks)	2–4	8–12	12

[a]Patients with comorbidities, abnormal laboratory results, and/or multiple therapies may require more frequent laboratory testing than what is generally recommended
[b]More frequent monitoring is recommended within the first 3 months of therapy or after increasing the dose

ophthalmologist (see later section on "Uveitis"), a dentist, and a gynecologist (if gynecological care is not provided at the primary care provider's office). Tina may also be at higher risk of dyslipidemia and cardiac disease given her history of JIA and family history and this would require special consideration (see later section on "Cardiovascular disease"). Tina's diet may be low in calcium and vitamin D and she is at increased risk of osteoporosis (see "Bone health" section later). She should be counseled to increase her intake of calcium and vitamin D.

Definition

The International League of Associations for Rheumatology (ILAR) classification of JIA (Table 14.2) replaces previous terms juvenile rheumatoid arthritis (JRA) and juvenile chronic arthritis (JCA) [6–8]. JIA is an autoimmune disease defined by arthritis occurring for greater than 6 weeks in a child younger than 16. Even as they enter adulthood, they keep the diagnosis of JIA and their diagnosis does not change to rheumatoid arthritis. There are several subtypes of JIA and the characteristic features of each of these subtypes will be discussed in this section.

Systemic Arthritis

This form of childhood arthritis is analogous to adult-onset Still's disease and accounts for 5–15 % of all children with JIA. Diagnosis requires the presence of arthritis, 2 weeks of daily fevers, plus 1 of the following: classic evanescent rash, generalized lymphadenopathy, hepatomegaly or splenomegaly, or serositis [9]. This type of arthritis can occur at any age and affects males and females equally [10]. Patients can be very ill at the time of diagnosis. Systemic features

Table 14.2 ILAR Classification of JIA

Characteristic	Clinical features
Age at onset	<16 years old
Minimum Duration	$\geq$6 weeks
Subtypes:	
Systemic	Arthritis 2 weeks of daily fever Presence of at least one of: rash, lymphadenopathy, organomegaly, or serositis Risk of macrophage activation syndrome
Oligoarticular	Up to four involved joints in the first 6 months *Persistent*—no more than four joints involved *Extended*—more than four joints involved after first 6 months
Polyarticular	Involves five or more joints in the first 6 months Rheumatoid factor negative or positive
Enthesitis-related arthritis	Arthritis and enthesitis, or arthritis or enthesitis with at least two of the following: Sacroiliac joint tenderness and/or inflammatory back pain HLA-B27 antigen positive Onset of arthritis in a male over 6 years old Acute (symptomatic) anterior uveitis Family history of ankylosing spondylitis or HLA-B27-positive related disease in first-degree relative
Psoriatic arthritis	Arthritis and psoriasis Arthritis and at least two of: Dactylitis Nail pitting or onycholysis Psoriasis in a first-degree relative
Undifferentiated	Arthritis that fulfills none of the above categories or two or more categories

Adapted from [8]

including fevers and elevated inflammatory markers are common early in the course of disease; however, arthritis can predominate later in the course and can affect any number of both large and small joints [7]. This is a diagnosis of exclusion and has a broad differential diagnosis. Malignancy often needs to be excluded. Patients are at risk of developing the possibly fatal complication of macrophage activation syndrome (MAS), characterized by hemophagocytosis in the bone marrow or liver causing fever, fatigue, cytopenias, hyperferritinemia, and hepatic and neurologic abnormalities. Treatment for systemic arthritis depends on severity of disease and may include nonsteroidal anti-inflammatory drugs (NSAIDs); systemic or intra-articular corticosteroids; disease modifying anti-rheumatic agents (DMARDs), such as methotrexate; and biologic agents, particularly blockade of interleukin (IL)-1 (anakinra, canakinumab) or IL-6 (tocilizumab) [7]. Prognosis depends on the response to therapy and the amount of joint involvement. Patients can have long-term morbidity due to protracted use of systemic corticosteroids. The arthritis in this subtype can be destructive and lead to general growth abnormalities. Some patients eventually require joint replacement.

Oligoarthritis

This is a chronic inflammatory arthritis lasting for at least 6 weeks involving 4 or fewer joints. It is called *persistent-oligoarthritis* if no more than four joints are involved throughout the disease course and *extended-oligoarthritis* if more than four joints become affected in the period following the initial 6 months [7]. Oligoarthritis is the most common subtype of childhood arthritis, affecting 50–80 % of all children with chronic arthritis. The peak incidence is between the ages of 1–3 years and is more common in girls [7]. These patients should not have psoriasis or a family history of psoriasis, ankylosing spondylitis, or inflammatory bowel disease are not systemically ill and are rheumatoid factor (RF) negative. Larger joints and joints of the lower extremities are most commonly involved [10]. Patients are at risk for developing asymptomatic uveitis, which can be present at onset and can affect up to 20 % of oligoarthritis patients [7] (see "Uveitis" section). They are at risk for growth abnormalities from persistent inflammation, most commonly leg-length discrepancy from unilateral knee arthritis. Treatment includes NSAIDs, intra-articular corticosteroid injections, and physical therapy. DMARDs and biologic therapies are occasionally required [7]. Patients require regular slit lamp exams for screening for uveitis, and the frequency of recommended eye exams varies based on presence of positive antinuclear antibody (ANA), age at disease onset, and duration of disease [11].

Polyarthritis (Rheumatoid Factor Negative)

Polyarthritis accounts for approximately 20 % of all JIA patients and Tina, the case presented earlier in this chapter, has this form of JIA [7]. This is a chronic arthritis affecting five or more joints within the first 6 months after disease onset [6]. Approximately 85 % of polyarthritis patients test negative for RF. This is defined as a separate entity than those who test positive for RF. There is a biphasic age of onset with 1 peak at age 1–3 and another peak in later childhood and adolescence. It is 4 times more common in females [7]. Articular disease predominates, though some patients also have systemic features such as fatigue, growth failure, and elevated inflammatory markers. The onset is usually insidious and patients have significant morning stiffness and gelling after inactivity. Wrists and ankles are the most commonly affected joints. Small joint involvement of hands and feet may also occur. This subtype of patients is more likely to have TMJ involvement, which can eventually lead to micrognathia. The cervical spine can be involved, leading to loss of neck extension. Up to 15 % of these patients develop uveitis, which, like oligoarticular arthritis, tend to occur in patients with younger age of onset and positive ANA. [7] This is a chronic disease that can last into adulthood. Arthritis can persist into the late 20s and 30s. Substantial functional disability may ensue.

Polyarthritis (Rheumatoid Factor Positive)

This is also a chronic arthritis affecting five or more joints within the first 6 months after disease onset. RF is positive on two occasions at least 3 months apart [6]. This subtype has similar features to adult rheumatoid arthritis [10]. It occurs in approximately 3 % of patients with JIA and is much more common in females. The mean age of onset is 9–11 years of age [7]. Patients often test positive for anti-citrullinated protein (CCP) antibodies [12], and up to 56 % of patients have a positive ANA [13]. This form of arthritis is often symmetric and can involve upper and lower extremities, small joints, as well as the TMJ and cervical spine. Early limitation of the wrist can progress to substantial deformity and debility. Erosive joint disease often occurs. Systemic manifestations include fatigue and weight loss with active disease. Rheumatoid nodules may occur. The presence of CCP antibodies is often associated with more severe disease course [14]. This subtype has a poor articular prognosis and early aggressive medical therapy is indicated [7]. These patients may have increased disability, which has been shown to persist into adulthood [15].

Enthesitis-Related Arthritis

This subtype of arthritis is defined as patients having arthritis and enthesitis (defined as inflammation at the sites of attachment of ligament, tendon, fascia, or capsule to bone). Alternatively, patients can have either arthritis or enthesitis with at least two of the following: sacroiliac joint tenderness and/or inflammatory spine pain; presence of HLA-B27; family history in at least one first- or second-degree relative with HLA-B27 associated disease; anterior uveitis associated with pain, redness, or photophobia; or onset of arthritis in a boy after 6 years of age [7]. This subtype affects the joints of the lower extremities and axial skeleton. There is a strong association with HLA-B27, which is positive in 90 % of patients. Autoantibodies such as ANA and RF are characteristically absent [7]. Peripheral joint disease can precede axial involvement by years. Many patients eventually evolve to resemble adult ankylosing spondylitis (AS), however, the characteristic features of AS are usually absent in childhood. Up to 10 % of patients with JIA have enthesitis-related arthritis. Up to 11 % of patients with adult AS had their disease onset in childhood [16]. Onset typically occurs in late childhood or adolescence and is more common in males with a male-to-female ratio of 7:1 [7]. This form of arthritis may resemble that found in inflammatory bowel disease, which should be included on the differential diagnosis. This disease is often progressive, and symptoms persist into adulthood [17].

Juvenile Psoriatic Arthritis

Clinical features of patients with psoriatic arthritis overlap with those of the other subtypes. The diagnostic criteria include patients with arthritis for 6 weeks associated with either psoriasis or at least two of the following: dactylitis (defined as swelling of a digit that extends beyond the borders of the joints,) nail pitting or onycholysis, or psoriasis in a first-degree relative [6]. Development of psoriasis can lag behind arthritis in about half of children. The proportion of patients with JIA who have psoriatic arthritis is approximately 7 %. The age of onset is biphasic, with a first peak occurring around 2–3 years and a second peak in late childhood. It is more common in females. Clinical manifestations are heterogeneous. Younger children are often females, can have a positive ANA, and are at risk for developing uveitis. Older children have a tendency to develop enthesitis and axial disease. RF is frequently absent. Patients often present with asymmetric monoarticular or oligoarticular disease. The highly destructive arthritis mutilans seen in adults is rare in children [7]. Outcome is not well defined, however, up to 33 % of patients continued to require DMARD therapy at 15 years of follow-up in one study [18].

Undifferentiated Arthritis

Patients who have onset of inflammatory arthritis before the age of 16 which fits multiple categories or no category are classified as undifferentiated JIA [6].

Epidemiology and Outcome

JIA is not rare, but the incidence and prevalence vary around the world. Incidence rates of childhood arthritis range from 1 to 20 per 100,000 in various studies [7]. Prevalence ranges from under 10 to 400 per 100,000 [7]. In reports from North America, Australia, and Europe, there is at least a 2:1 female-to-male ratio. Boys are more often affected in reports from Asia [7]. There are geographic and ethnic differences in rates of subtypes of arthritis. Specific data for the individual JIA subtypes was summarized previously. As discussed previously, a substantial number of JIA patients continue to have active arthritis into adulthood. The disease course can be characterized by periods of remission and flare with accumulation of more joint involvement over time.

Pathophysiology

The etiology of JIA is largely unknown but is believed to be multifactorial with genetic and environmental influences and differs among subtypes. Autoantibodies are common in oligoarthritis (ANA) and in RF-positive polyarthritis (IgM rheumatoid factor and anti-citrullinated protein antibodies), suggesting the role of the humoral immune system in the pathophysiology of JIA. Other subtypes are associated with polymorphisms at the histocompatibility locus, but familial arthritis is rare. Systemic JIA is not associated with antibodies or a strong genetic signal and has been considered an autoinflammatory disease [7]. In all subtypes, T-cells and macrophages are involved in pathogenesis and lead to synovial inflammation.

Clinical Manifestations

Clinical manifestations include pain, stiffness, and joint inflammation with swelling, tenderness, warmth, and limitation. Tenosynovitis is common. Children who are growing also have extra-articular manifestations of JIA such as abnormal growth and physical development due to the direct effect of disease, systemic inflammation, or medications. Localized growth disturbances of affected joints can be striking and lead to limb inequality and micrognathia. Puberty and sexual maturation are often delayed.

Uveitis

Patients with JIA are at risk of developing the ocular complication of uveitis that is more common in patients with a positive ANA who present at a younger age, usually before the age of 7 years. The risk of developing uveitis diminishes over time but it can persist into adulthood. If untreated, uveitis can cause significant visual impairment and blindness. This complication is usually asymptomatic, and therefore patients are screened with slit lamp exams routinely according to generally accepted guidelines, with frequency varying depending on the JIA subtype [11]. Older patients, especially those with enthesitis-related arthritis, tend to have symptomatic uveitis.

Therapy

All forms of JIA require a multifaceted approach to treatment. Mainstays in management include early anti-inflammatory treatment and physical and occupational therapy. Healthy lifestyle, including diet and physical activity, should be promoted. Medical management generally begins with NSAIDs unless contraindicated. In patients with limited number of joints involved, intra-articular corticosteroid injections may be beneficial. Systemic corticosteroids are rarely used other than in systemic arthritis. DMARDs including methotrexate, leflunomide, and sulfasalazine are often required, and many patients have an excellent response. In those who do not, biologic therapies including tumor necrosis factor (TNF)-antagonists and others, have been shown to be very effective. There is little to no role for opiate analgesia, a class of agents that will not address the underlying inflammatory problem and also has an adverse side effect profile as well as risk for dependency and addiction. Novel therapies including JAK inhibitors (tofacitinib) are being developed. Treatment for systemic JIA was previously summarized.

The overall goal of therapy is to achieve disease remission quickly and to maintain remission with medications. There is no consensus to the approach, but if remission occurs, the medications can be tapered. The aim is to prevent flare since every episode of arthritis can cause irreversible joint destruction.

Periodic monitoring labs are indicated. For patients taking daily NSAIDs, complete blood count, serum creatinine, liver enzymes, and urinalysis are recommended approximately twice yearly [19]. American College of Rheumatology (ACR) guidelines for laboratory monitoring frequency in patients taking DMARD therapies from 2015 are summarized in Table 14.1 [5]. Basic labs should be assessed at baseline. Tuberculosis (TB) testing should be performed before starting patients on biologic therapies and tofacitinib [5]. Hepatitis B and C serologies should be assessed before initiating biologic therapies in high-risk populations. For patients taking TNF-antagonists, labs should be checked every 3–6 months [19].

If an adult patient with JIA presents with acute pain, other causes such as trauma or amplified pain syndromes should be excluded. If there is acute onset swelling of a single joint, infection must be considered, including gonococcal arthritis, and medication adherence should be assessed. Arthritis flares may be addressed with local corticosteroid injection, escalation of therapy, or switching medications in conjunction with a rheumatologist.

Most medications used in JIA can be given safely over a long period. Long-term corticosteroids, however, should be avoided due to their multiple side effects. Risks of long-term immunosuppressive therapy include infection. Patients taking chronic corticosteroids have higher incidences of hospitalized bacterial infections [20]. The risk of TB remains a concern in patients taking biologic medications. While patients with JIA may have an increased risk of developing malignancy, this risk seems to be independent of DMARD and biologic therapy [21].

Methotrexate and leflunomide are teratogenic (pregnancy category X), and TNF-antagonist biologics are pregnancy category B drugs. Teratogenic medications should be discontinued in the face of unplanned pregnancy. Patients on leflunomide require cholestyramine washout therapy prior to planning a pregnancy or in the event of an unplanned pregnancy. Methotrexate should be discontinued ≥ 1 ovulatory cycle before planning a pregnancy.

Common Adult Conditions in the JIA Population

Arthritis and Musculoskeletal Abnormalities

The most common adult condition in this population of patients is persistent arthritis in adulthood either due to ongoing disease that is refractory to treatment or flare of previously controlled arthritis. Patients are at risk of developing early secondary osteoarthritis due to joint damage from prior joint inflammation. This can lead to chronic pain and the need for arthroplasty. If present prior to cessation of growth, local growth abnormalities such as leg-length discrepancies, bony fusions, and TMJ involvement can lead to functional difficulties. TMJ arthritis, in particular, can lead to long-term consequences in oral health such as decreased chewing ability, malocclusion (in 66 % of patients), and micrognathia (in 30 % of patients). [22] Treatment of

TMJ arthritis includes local corticosteroid injections and escalation to biologic therapy. Patients who have had cervical spine arthritis may have ankylosis, erosions, and narrowing of cranio-cervical junction [23] and be at risk for atlanto-axial subluxation, which should be noted prior to any surgical procedure requiring anesthesia.

Ocular Complications

Patients who had significant uveitis may have visual morbidity with low vision due to the disease itself or cataract formation as a result of treatment with topical glucocorticoids.

Cardiovascular Disease

As in adult RA, there is evidence that patients with JIA may be at increased risk for premature atherosclerosis or accelerated cardiovascular disease [24, 25]. One study showed increased rates of heart disease in women with JIA [26]. Another study showed no increase in cardiovascular events in patients with JIA 29 years following disease onset when compared to the general population [27]. One study reported that 18 % of patients with JIA were obese. Obesity was not associated with disease activity [28]. Patients with systemic JIA with prolonged exposure to corticosteroids may have dyslipidemia, hypertension, and diabetes. The long-term risk of cardiovascular disease for individuals with JIA remains unclear and there are no guidelines on cholesterol-lowering treatment in JIA patients currently available. Recent publications have shown increased mortality risk among adult RA patients [29], and given the potential for longer disease duration in people with JIA, perhaps mortality risk in this group might be increased, especially if a family history of cardiovascular disease is present. Therefore, one might consider aggressive management of elevated cholesterol in a patient such as the clinical vignette presented previously in this chapter.

Oral Health

There have been rare reports of secondary Sjögren's syndrome occurring years after diagnosis of JIA [30]. Good oral hygiene is important especially for those on immunosuppressive treatment or with Sjögren's symptoms.

Special Issues that Arise in Patients with Juvenile Idiopathic Arthritis

Arthritis Flares

If a patient has an arthritis flare, adherence should be assessed. Monoarthritis is rare in adults and should raise the question of infectious arthritis due to sexually transmitted infections, or Lyme disease in endemic areas.

Macrophage Activation Syndrome

Macrophage activation syndrome (MAS) is a potentially fatal complication most commonly associated with systemic JIA but can also be seen in other forms of autoimmune disease. It is due to hemophagocytosis by macrophages, which can occur in the bone marrow and liver. This can be triggered in the setting of infections such as with mononucleosis. Patients appear unwell and can be febrile. Viral serologies should be checked. Labs show cytopenias, elevated liver enzymes, low erythrocyte sedimentation rate (ESR), hyperferritinemia, elevated triglycerides, elevated D-dimers, and low serum fibrinogen levels. Patients can have hepatic dysfunction, seizures, and can worsen rapidly. MAS is an indication for hospitalization.

Bone Health

Many children with arthritis do not develop adequate bone mineralization. A failure to undergo the normal increase in bone mass during puberty is common and patients are therefore less able to achieve an adequate peak skeletal mass [31]. These patients may then be at an increased risk for fractures in adulthood and for an earlier onset of osteoporosis [32]. There are no recommendations for regular bone densitometry screening exams. The recommended daily allowance (RDA) of calcium for 14–18 years old is 1300 mg/day, decreasing to 1000 mg/day for ages 19–30. RDA for vitamin D is 600 IU/day [33]. It is preferable that this come from dietary intake rather than supplements.

Psychosocial Function

There have been multiple studies investigating the long-term social outcomes of patients with JIA. Young adults with rheumatic diseases reported challenges with job absenteeism, disruptions, and loss of productivity [34]. A meta-analysis found that in general, young adults with a history of JIA were less likely to be employed when compared with healthy peers. This was associated with worse disease, less educational attainment, and female sex [35]. Adults with JIA may have more pain, depression, and anxiety than their peers. A German study found that adults with JIA who completed a health-related quality of life questionnaire were more likely to report depression and anxiety symptoms compared to healthy controls (28 vs 4 %) as well as more pain symptoms (56 vs 28 %) [36].

Reproductive Health

Women with inflammatory arthritis may have lower fertility rates than the general population [37]. Patients with JIA can have normal healthy children. Special issues related to medication toxicity are discussed above (see "Therapy" section). The use of oral contraceptive pills is considered safe in women with rheumatoid arthritis. There is a theoretical concern about increased risk of pelvic infection with intrauterine devices (IUDs), however, this has not been reported in other immunocompromised patients. There is a paucity of data on IUDs and depot medroxyprogesterone acetate in women with inflammatory arthritis [38].

Pain

Some patients may continue to have pain despite clinical improvement of their arthritis. Arthritis pain is typically associated with morning stiffness and improvement with activity. If the history shows increased pain with activity, osteoarthritis, injury, or other mechanical causes should be considered. Pain syndromes are also seen in this population and JIA and fibromyalgia can coexist in the same patient. Pain syndromes should be considered if a patient's reported symptoms are not congruent with their physical exam findings [39]. If a pain syndrome is diagnosed, the mainstays of treatment are physical therapy, psychotherapy, and ensuring adequate sleep [40]. There is limited role for opiate analgesics in the treatment of JIA or pain syndromes and they should be used sparingly given the risk of dependency and addiction.

Immunizations

If patients are taking immunosuppressive medications, then live vaccines (varicella, zoster, MMR, nasal influenza) are contraindicated. Patients should receive a yearly injectable influenza vaccine, pneumococcal vaccines, and routine adult vaccinations [2].

Healthcare Transition

Another challenge in this population is transfer of care to adult rheumatology [41]. Many patients have difficulty making contact with an adult rheumatologist or are lost to follow-up after transfer. This can lead to uncontrolled disease and poor functional outcome [17].

Conclusion

JIA is a chronic autoimmune condition, and arthritis can persist into adulthood. The goal of therapy is to eliminate inflammation to prevent joint destruction. Patients are at risk for long-term consequences of growth disturbance and joint abnormalities. They may suffer from comorbid conditions such as vision loss and chronic pain. They are at risk for associated conditions such as cardiovascular disease and osteoporosis. They may have other concerns related to transition care, employment, and reproductive health. Adult providers need to be aware of the wide range of issues relating to patients with JIA ("Appendix").

Appendix

Juvenile Idiopathic Arthritis (JIA) condition fact sheet

Definition	JIA is an autoimmune disease defined by arthritis occurring for greater than 6 weeks in a child younger than 16 • Subtypes of JIA include: systemic, oligoarticular, polyarticular (rheumatoid factor positive or negative), enthesitis-related arthritis, psoriatic arthritis, and undifferentiated • Each subtype of JIA has a different presentation
Epidemiology	• Prevalence of JIA ranges from 10 to 400 per 100,000 around the world • There is overall a 2:1 female-to-male ratio • Oligoarthritis is the most common subtype of childhood arthritis affecting 50–80 % of all children with chronic arthritis • A substantial number of JIA patients continue to have active arthritis into adulthood
Special considerations	Individuals with JIA are at risk for comorbid physical and mental health conditions, including • Persistent arthritis • Growth abnormalities • Ocular complications • Medication toxicity including infection, teratogenic risk • Anxiety and depression • Macrophage activation syndrome • Chronic pain Individuals are at heightened risk for chronic conditions, including • Uveitis • Atherosclerosis and coronary heart disease • Osteoporosis and fractures • Osteoarthritis • Malignancy • Need for joint replacement surgery • Sjögren's syndrome
Recommended screening	Patients may require lab screening for medication side effects

Suggested Reading List

- Petty RE, Laxer RM, Lindsley CB, Wedderburn L, Cassidy JT (eds). Textbook of pediatric rheumatology, Seventh edition. Philadelphia, PA: Elsevier. 2016
- Espinosa M, Gottlieb BS. Juvenile Idiopathic Arthritis. Pediatr. Rev. 2012;33, 303–313.
- Coulson EJ, Hanson HJM, Foster HE. What does an adult rheumatologist need to know about juvenile idiopathic arthritis? Rheumatol Oxf Engl. 2014 Dec;53(12):2155–66.

Patient/Caregiver/Provider Resources

- Arthritis Foundation: http://www.kidsgetarthritistoo.org
- Getting Accommodations for Juvenile Arthritis at College: https://www.youtube.com/watch?v=ctuj0nXkey0
- Transition and Secondary School Issues Resources: http://www.gottransition.org

References

1. U.S. Department of Education, Office for Civil Rights. Students with disabilities preparing for postsecondary education: know your rights and responsibilities http://www2.ed.gov/about/offices/list/ocr/transition.html. Accessed 13 June 2016.
2. Centers for Disease Control and Prevention. Adult immunization schedules. http://www.cdc.gov/vaccines/schedules/hcp/adult.html Accessed 7 May 2016.
3. Cauffman E, Steinberg L. (Im)maturity of judgment in adolescence: why adolescents may be less culpable than adults. Behav Sci Law. 2000;18(6):741–60.
4. ACP High Value Care JIA. https://www.acponline.org/system/files/documents/clinical_information/high_value_care/clinician_resources/pediatric_adult_care_transitions/rheumatology/jia_transition_tools.pdf. Accessed 7 May 2016.
5. Singh JA, Saag KG, Bridges SL, Akl EA, Bannuru RR, Sullivan MC, et al. American College of Rheumatology guideline for the treatment of rheumatoid arthritis. Arthritis Rheumatol. 2016;68(1):1–26.
6. Petty RE, Southwood TR, Manners P, Baum J, Glass DN, Goldenberg J, et al. International League of Associations for Rheumatology classification of juvenile idiopathic arthritis: second revision, Edmonton, 2001. J Rheumatol. 2004;31(2):390–2.
7. Petty RE, Laxer RM, Lindsley CB, Wedderburn L, Cassidy JT, editors. Textbook of pediatric rheumatology. 7th ed. Philadelphia: Elsevier; 2016.
8. Coulson EJ, Hanson HJM, Foster HE. What does an adult rheumatologist need to know about juvenile idiopathic arthritis? Rheumatol Oxf Engl. 2014;53(12):2155–66.
9. Behrens EM, Beukelman T, Gallo L, Spangler J, Rosenkranz M, Arkachaisri T, et al. Evaluation of the presentation of systemic onset juvenile rheumatoid arthritis: data from the Pennsylvania Systemic Onset Juvenile Arthritis Registry (PASOJAR). J Rheumatol. 2008;35(2):343–8.
10. Ravelli A, Martini A. Juvenile idiopathic arthritis. Lancet Lond Engl. 2007;369(9563):767–78.
11. Heiligenhaus A, Niewerth M, Ganser G, Heinz C, Minden K, German Uveitis in Childhood Study Group. Prevalence and complications of uveitis in juvenile idiopathic arthritis in a population-based nation-wide study in Germany: suggested modification of the current screening guidelines. Rheumatol Oxf Engl. 2007;46(6):1015–9.
12. Tebo AE, Jaskowski T, Davis KW, Whiting A, Clifford B, Zeft A, et al. Profiling anti-cyclic citrullinated peptide antibodies in patients with juvenile idiopathic arthritis. Pediatr Rheumatol Online J. 2012;10(1):29.
13. Saurenmann RK, Rose JB, Tyrrell P, Feldman BM, Laxer RM, Schneider R, et al. Epidemiology of juvenile idiopathic arthritis in a multiethnic cohort: ethnicity as a risk factor. Arthritis Rheum. 2007;56(6):1974–84.
14. Farragher TM, Lunt M, Plant D, Bunn DK, Barton A, Symmons DPM. Benefit of early treatment in inflammatory polyarthritis patients with anti-cyclic citrullinated peptide antibodies versus those without antibodies. Arthritis Care Res. 2010;62(5):664–75.
15. Packham JC, Hall MA. Long-term follow-up of 246 adults with juvenile idiopathic arthritis: functional outcome. Rheumatol Oxf Engl. 2002;41(12):1428–35.
16. Gomez KS, Raza K, Jones SD, Kennedy LG, Calin A. Juvenile onset ankylosing spondylitis—more girls than we thought? J Rheumatol. 1997;24(4):735–7.
17. Hersh A, von Scheven E, Yelin E. Adult outcomes of childhood-onset rheumatic diseases. Nat Rev Rheumatol. 2011;7(5):290–5.
18. Flatø B, Lien G, Smerdel-Ramoya A, Vinje O. Juvenile psoriatic arthritis: longterm outcome and differentiation from other subtypes of juvenile idiopathic arthritis. J Rheumatol. 2009;36(3):642–50.
19. Beukelman T, Patkar NM, Saag KG, Tolleson-Rinehart S, Cron RQ, DeWitt EM, et al. American College of Rheumatology recommendations for the treatment of juvenile idiopathic arthritis: initiation and safety monitoring of therapeutic agents

for the treatment of arthritis and systemic features. Arthritis Care Res. 2011;63(4):465–82.
20. Beukelman T, Xie F, Chen L, Baddley JW, Delzell E, Grijalva CG, et al. Rates of hospitalized bacterial infection associated with juvenile idiopathic arthritis and its treatment. Arthritis Rheum. 2012;64(8):2773–80.
21. Beukelman T, Haynes K, Curtis JR, Xie F, Chen L, Bemrich-Stolz CJ, et al. Rates of malignancy associated with juvenile idiopathic arthritis and its treatment. Arthritis Rheum. 2012;64(4):1263–71.
22. Ringold S, Cron RQ. The temporomandibular joint in juvenile idiopathic arthritis: frequently used and frequently arthritic. Pediatr Rheumatol. 2009;7(1):11.
23. Hospach T, Maier J, Müller-Abt P, Patel A, Horneff G, von Kalle T. Cervical spine involvement in patients with juvenile idiopathic arthritis—MRI follow-up study. Pediatr Rheumatol Online J. 2014;4(12):9.
24. Bohr A-H, Fuhlbrigge RC, Pedersen FK, de Ferranti SD, Müller K. Premature subclinical atherosclerosis in children and young adults with juvenile idiopathic arthritis. A review considering preventive measures. Pediatr Rheumatol Online J. 2016;14. http://www.ncbi.nlm.nih.gov/pmc/articles/PMC4704268/ Accessed 10 May 2016.
25. Coulson EJ, Ng W-F, Goff I, Foster HE. Cardiovascular risk in juvenile idiopathic arthritis. Rheumatology. 2013 Mar 15;ket106.
26. Feldman DE, Vinet É, Bérard A, Duffy C, Hazel B, Meshefedjian G, et al. Heart disease, hypertension, gestational diabetes and pre-eclampsia/eclampsia in mothers with juvenile arthritis: a nested case-control study. Arthritis Care Res. 2016 (Epub ahead of print) PMID: 27111101.
27. Anderson JH, Anderson KR, Aulie HA, Crowson CS, Mason TG, Ardoin SP, et al. Juvenile idiopathic arthritis and future risk for cardiovascular disease: a multicenter study. Scand J Rheumatol. 2016;8:1–5.
28. Pelajo CF, Lopez-Benitez JM, Miller LC. Obesity and disease activity in juvenile idiopathic arthritis. Pediatr Rheumatol Online J. 2012;12(10):3.
29. Pincus T, Gibson KA, Block JA. Premature mortality: a neglected outcome in rheumatic diseases? Arthritis Care Res. 2015;67(8):1043–6.
30. Bouayed K, Alyanakian M-A, Cordonnier C, Caillat-Zucman S, Testelin S, Lambrey G, et al. Sjögren syndrome: an unexpected disease occurring fourteen years after oligoarticular onset juvenile idiopathic arthritis. Rheumatology. 2002;41(10):1190–3.
31. Cassidy JT, Hillman LS. Abnormalities in skeletal growth in children with juvenile rheumatoid arthritis. Rheum Dis Clin N Am. 1997;23(3):499–522.
32. Zak M, Hassager C, Lovell DJ, Nielsen S, Henderson CJ, Pedersen FK. Assessment of bone mineral density in adults with a history of juvenile chronic arthritis: a cross-sectional long-term followup study. Arthritis Rheum. 1999;42(4):790–8.
33. Ross AC, Taylor CL, Yaktine AL, Del Valle HB (eds); Committee to Review Dietary Reference Intakes for Vitamin D and Calcium; Food and Nutrition Board; Institute of Medicine. Dietary reference intakes for calcium and vitamin D. Washington, DC: National Academies Press. 2011. http://www.nap.edu/catalog/13050/dietary-reference-intakes-for-calcium-and-vitamin-d Accessed 10 May 2016.
34. Jetha A, Badley E, Beaton D, Fortin PR, Shiff NJ, Gignac MAM. Unpacking early work experiences of young adults with rheumatic disease: an examination of absenteeism, job disruptions and productivity loss. Arthritis Care Res. 2015;67(9):1246–54.
35. Jetha A. The impact of arthritis on the early employment experiences of young adults: a literature review. Disabil Health J. 2015;8(3):317–24.
36. Barth S, Haas J-P, Schlichtiger J, Molz J, Bisdorff B, Michels H, et al. Long-term health-related quality of life in German patients with juvenile idiopathic arthritis in comparison to German general population. PLoS ONE. 2016;11(4):e0153267.
37. Wallenius M, Skomsvoll JF, Irgens LM, Salvesen KÅ, Nordvåg B-Y, Koldingsnes W, et al. Fertility in women with chronic inflammatory arthritides. Rheumatol Oxf Engl. 2011;50(6):1162–7.
38. Farr SL, Folger SG, Paulen ME, Curtis KM. Safety of contraceptive methods for women with rheumatoid arthritis: a systematic review. Contraception. 2010;82(1):64–71.
39. Schikler KN. Is it juvenile rheumatoid arthritis or fibromyalgia? Med Clin N Am. 2000;84(4):967–82.
40. Anthony KK, Schanberg LE. Pediatric pain syndromes and management of pain in children and adolescents with rheumatic disease. Pediatr Clin N Am. 2005;52(2):611–39, vii.
41. White PH, Ardoin S. Transitioning wisely: improving the connection from pediatric to adult health care. Arthritis Rheumatol. 2016;68(4):789–94.

15 Muscular Dystrophy

Elba Y. Gerena Maldonado

Case Presentation

Luis Antonio is a pleasant 21-year-old male with Duchenne muscular dystrophy (DMD) who presents with his mother to establish care at the primary care clinic. Review of his medical records from his pediatrician and from several specialists at the local children's hospital reveals he was being treated for cardiomyopathy, restrictive lung disease, low bone density, and for his limited functional status given his severe muscle weakness.

One of the main concerns that his mother brings up during the appointment is his recent unplanned weight loss. While obtaining his vitals, the clinic medical assistant was unable to get his current body weight because she could not transfer him off the power wheelchair to the exam table. On examination, the patient has tetraplegia with trace pincer grasp, which he uses to move the joystick of the wheelchair. He is also using a "Sip-n-Puff" machine that is mounted on the back of the power wheelchair. At one point during the appointment the mother states that she misses the multidisciplinary clinics at the children's hospital and states that the family is having a hard time transitioning out of the system into the adult healthcare system.

During the interview process, the patient is able to provide most of his history and is cooperative and agreeable; however, his mother tends to interrupt the patient's answers. While speaking to Luis alone, he reveals that his career goal is to finish a teaching degree in community college and start working. A close friend of Luis, who also had DMD, has recently died and he is wondering about life and death and what measures he should start taking at this moment.

Case Discussion

The story of Luis Antonio is a typical case of a young adult with Duchenne muscular dystrophy, which is a rapidly progressive neuromuscular disease with multi-systemic involvement. For these patients and their families, the transition period from pediatric to adult health care systems is a challenging one. As they are often dealing with numerous changes simultaneously, many of these patients and their families tend to feel overwhelmed and unsupported by the adult healthcare system. Although efforts are being made by most pediatric hospitals to prepare and aid patients and their families in the transition process, it is still a taxing period for all those involved.

E.Y. Gerena Maldonado (✉)
Montana Providence Health and Services, Montana Spine and Pain Center, 500 West Broadway, 3rd Floor, Missoula, MT 59802, USA
e-mail: Elba.GerenaMaldonado@providence.org

M. Pilapil et al. (eds.), *Care of Adults with Chronic Childhood Conditions*,
DOI 10.1007/978-3-319-43827-6_15

A 2012 study conducted in the United Kingdom in which patients with DMD older than 15 years of age and their family members were interviewed, it was self-reported that these patients were more likely to receive fewer healthcare services and were less satisfied with their current health care compared to when they were children [1]. This period of transition to the adult healthcare system has been associated with a decline in health outcomes not only among the muscular dystrophy population but also among patients with many other chronic conditions of childhood [2]. It is for this reason that most experts in Duchenne muscular dystrophy urge that transition not be thought of as a single event but as a continuing process of increased choices and autonomy [3].

For adult primary care providers (PCPs), the initial evaluation of a new patient with multiple comorbidities associated with a rare progressive disease can be an overwhelming process. The focus should be to organize multidisciplinary care, even when the providers are not in the same location. This process can be carried out in the adult healthcare system by having clear and open communication between the cardiologist, pulmonologist, endocrinologist, neuromuscular specialist, and primary care physician. Current guidelines emphasize the need for coordination among all the adult specialists as the key to providing successful care to these patients [4, 5].

This case also illustrates the need to improve the architectural barriers that are still present in most adult practices. There is a growing population of patients that will need proper wheelchair access, special weighing scales that can accommodate wheelchairs or beds with integrated weighing systems, and Hoyer or ceiling lifts for safe transfers. Although these patients are likely going to establish care with an adult cardiologist and pulmonologist, it will be the primary care physician who will likely monitor the patient's weight, skin integrity, and nutrition.

Furthermore, adult healthcare providers need to reinforce the autonomy that these patients have while being respectful to the family dynamics. Among the discussions that should take place include sexual health, advance directives, physician orders for life-sustaining treatment (POLST) forms (if needed), and death and dying. These are important topics for discussion since many patients with DMD are now surviving into their fourth and fifth decade of life [6], and some parents might not have wanted these issues previously addressed with their children. However, given the multiple comorbidities associated with this condition, patients with DMD are at a higher risk for rapid and serious complications from pneumonia, cardiac arrhythmia, and other life-threatening events. Therefore, it is imperative that patients are aware of the POLST forms and resources that might be needed in the future.

Optimal care for patients with DMD should maximize function and quality of life. Early involvement of palliative care specialists as part of the multidisciplinary team is theorized to likely improve the quality of life for these patients. The main goal is to help these young men attain the necessary skills to manage their own personal needs and healthcare. It is important that they become effective self-advocates and be able to pursue their own interests. (For additional information on palliative care for adults with chronic childhood conditions, please see Chap. 24 of this book).

Definition

Muscular dystrophies encompass a diverse group of primarily muscle disorders, all of which fall under the category of orphan (rare) diseases. Most of the muscular dystrophies can be linked back to a genetic mutation, each with its own clinical course and expression [7, 8]. The most common symptom is muscle weakness that worsens with time. Some of these conditions have a rapid progressive course and tend to lead to an early death in childhood, whereas others are not immediately evident and manifest an "adult-onset" phenotype.

Prevalence

Duchenne muscular dystrophy, myotonic dystrophy, and facioscapulohumeral muscular dystrophy are among the most common muscular dystrophies [9–11]. Duchenne muscular dystrophy is an X-linked disease that affects approximately 1 in 4087 males worldwide with a prevalence of 6 in 100,000 males [12]. Myotonic dystrophy type 1 and type 2 have a combined prevalence of 1 in 8000 (12.5/100,000), based on clinical ascertainment [13]. Facioscapulohumeral muscular dystrophy (FSHD) is the third most common form of muscular dystrophy, with a prevalence of approximately 1:15,000–1:20,000 [9, 14].

Pathophysiology

The underlying molecular abnormalities in the muscular dystrophies involve structural proteins. DMD is clinically manifested when there is an absence of dystrophin, a key component of the sarcolemma of the skeletal muscle cell. Dystrophin is involved in the stabilization of the muscle cell membrane during contraction and relaxation and acts as a link between the intracellular cytoskeleton and extracellular matrix [15, 16]. Dystrophin also plays a role in the ability of muscle fibers to differentiate and may play a role in organization of postsynaptic membrane [17]. Loss or abnormal dystrophin destabilizes the sarcolemma, making the muscle fibers susceptible to contraction injury [18]. The repeated process of injury and necrosis eventually leads to replacement of muscles by fat and connective tissue that is clinically manifested as progressive muscle weakness [19]. Dystrophin not only exists in the sarcolemma of skeletal muscle but also exists as a number of other tissue-specific isoforms, some exclusively or predominantly expressed in the brain, heart, and/or in other tissues [20].

The responsible gene, *DMD*, is located on the short arm of the X chromosome at locus Xp21 [21, 22]. Approximately two-thirds of cases are associated with a detectable deletion or duplication of segments within the *DMD* gene [23]. There is a variable phenotypic expression that generally correlates with the type of mutation found on this gene. Milder allelic variants of Duchenne muscular dystrophy include: Becker muscular dystrophy, X-linked dilated cardiomyopathy, and manifesting female carriers. In Becker muscular dystrophy, the abnormal dystrophin preserves enough function to slow down the progression of the illness. Therefore, these patients tend to preserve ambulation well into their late teens or early 20s. However, in Duchenne muscular dystrophy, the absence of the dystrophin is characterized by a progressive muscular weakness that leads to loss of ambulation early in childhood, usually before 12 years of age.

About 10 % of all the female carriers will manifest with some muscle weakness, mostly in cognitive and/or cardiac function [24]. This is thought to be the result of skewed X inactivation.

In patients with DMD, death usually results from either cardiac or respiratory failure. However, the implementation of better respiratory care has improved the mean age of survival in these patients [6, 25].

Management of Comorbidities

Musculoskeletal

The natural history of muscular dystrophy has changed in the last few decades due to the widespread use of corticosteroids as a pharmacological intervention for muscle strength and function [4, 26]. Glucocorticoids, such as prednisone and deflazacort, have been shown to prolong walking by transiently increasing and then slowing the decline in muscle strength [27], and improving pulmonary measures by decreasing the progression of scoliosis [26]. Due to the latter, many experts continue the use of glucocorticoids long after the patient has lost the ability to ambulate. This treatment has to be coupled with a comprehensive physiotherapy program that includes regular stretching exercises for upper and lower limbs with the goal to avoid and/or minimize contractures.

Most often, boys are started on corticosteroids between 5 and 7 years of age, before they start to lose motor milestones. However, some specialists favor starting as early as 3–4 years of age. This has had an impact on the lives of these patients, as they have to deal with the consequences of long-term use of glucocorticoids, including behavioral issues, fracture risk, and obesity. Those patients who are not treated with corticosteroids have about a 90 % chance of developing a progressive scoliosis [28]. Depending on the rate of progression of the scoliosis, the patients might be eligible for spinal fusion surgery. Bone health is an important part of the lifelong care of patients with Duchenne muscular dystrophy, and awareness of potential problems and means to assess these problems are preferably done by the primary care physician in conjunction with bone health specialists. Experts recommend that these patients have their serum vitamin D monitored (at least annually) and undergo an assessment for nutritional intake of calcium and vitamin D, with appropriate supplementation of vitamin D and calcium, if needed. Patients are also encouraged to have physical activity (including standing), exposure to sunshine, and an endocrine consultation should be sought if no pubertal signs are present by 14 years. In regard to imaging studies to aid in the screening process, it is recommended that a baseline lumbar spine dual energy X-ray absorptiometry (DEXA) is obtained at 3 years old or when the patient is started on glucocorticoids and subsequently repeated at 12–24 monthly intervals [29, 30]. If back pain is present, a spine radiograph should be obtained to assess for vertebral fractures [31].

Respiratory

Duchenne muscular dystrophy is associated with progressive loss of respiratory muscle strength and high risk for respiratory complications due to ineffective cough, nocturnal hypoventilation, sleep disordered breathing, and daytime respiratory failure. There have been several published guidelines for respiratory management in DMD [32]. The proactive approach to respiratory management with the use of assisted cough and nocturnal ventilation has been shown to prolong survival [6]. Nevertheless, there has previously been controversy among experts regarding the best method of assisting ventilation, that is, whether to choose noninvasive ventilation or ventilation via tracheostomy. The currently favored method is the use of noninvasive ventilation in almost all clinical situations [33].

Cardiac

Cardiac disease in DMD manifests most often as a dilated cardiomyopathy and/or cardiac arrhythmia [34]. Patients with DMD should be followed by a cardiologist for regular monitoring with electrocardiogram (ECG), Holter monitor, and echocardiography. Published guidelines recommend a baseline assessment of cardiac function should be done at diagnosis or by the age of 6 years, especially if this can be done without sedation [34, 35]. It should be done every 2 years until the age of 10, at which time it should be done annually. Angiotensin-converting enzyme (ACE) inhibitors, beta-blockers, and other cardioprotective agents are currently used to reduce progression and can improve ventricular function [36]. A retrospective cohort study published in 2013 sought to determine the impact of steroid therapy on cardiomyopathy and mortality in patients with DMD. The study found that steroid therapy was associated with a considerably lower all-cause mortality rate, due largely to a significant reduction in heart failure-related deaths. Steroid-treated patients experienced a much lower incidence of new-onset cardiomyopathy [37].

Gastrointestinal

Gastrointestinal and nutritional issues become more prominent in later stages of the disease. Older patients with DMD have progressive pharyngeal weakness that eventually leads to dysphagia, which can result in severe weight loss and the need to consider enteral tube feeding [38]. Other gastrointestinal complications that have been reported include gastric and intestinal dilatation related to air swallowing due to ventilator use and delayed gastric emptying or ileus. For motility issues, stool softeners, laxatives, and stimulants can be used [5]. There is limited published data on recommendations for gastrointestinal issues in the DMD population. Nevertheless, access to a dietitian or nutritionist, a swallowing/speech and language therapist, and a gastroenterologist is of importance as the condition progresses.

Neurologic/Psychiatric

Cognitive involvement is common in patients with Duchenne muscular dystrophy. Of patients with DMD, about 30 % have intellectual disability [39]. A recent large, multicenter, international cohort study reported cognitive function being lower in DMD patients as compared to the general population. It also reported that 21 % of DMD males scored above the threshold for autism spectrum disorder (ASD), 24 % for hyperactivity, and 44 % for inattention. Similarly, 19 % of patients with Duchenne/Becker muscular dystrophies met the criteria for ASD using the Autism Diagnostic Interview—Revised [40].

Duchenne muscular dystrophy is a multisystem disease. As these patients grow up and reach young adulthood, physicians might encounter issues with emotional adjustment and depression. Anxiety might also be an issue and can be exacerbated by the cognitive deficits in mental flexibility and adaptability (i.e., overly rigid thought processes) [40]. Increased rates of depression in parents of children who have DMD underscore the need for assessment and support of the entire family [41]. Recommendations are to have a comprehensive neuropsychological assessment at or near the time of diagnosis and prior to entering formal schooling [4].

Preoperative/Anesthesia

The risks of anesthesia depend on the type of muscular dystrophy. Patients with *DMD* and *RYR1* mutations are at a higher risk of malignant hyperthermia-like reactions and rhabdomyolysis with exposure to inhalational anesthetic agents, such as halothane and isoflurane [42]. For this reason, it is strongly recommended that intravenous anesthetic techniques be used for DMD patients. Other agents, such as depolarizing muscle relaxants, are contraindicated in this population due to the risk of fatal reactions.

In the preoperative setting, it is recommended to have an echocardiogram and electrocardiogram before general and/or local anesthesia. Preoperative training in the use of manual and assisted cough techniques is necessary and the use of noninvasive ventilation is strongly recommended for patients with a baseline forced vital capacity below 50 % of predicted value [43].

Palliative Care

Palliative care is a field with an inherent interdisciplinary nature that is now recognized as a medical subspecialty. The focus of palliative care includes the relief of suffering for patients with life-threatening or serious debilitating illness, as described by the American Academy of Hospice and Palliative Medicine. The intent of palliative care is to neither hasten nor postpone death but instead to offer a support system to help patients live as fully as possible through the integration of medical, psychosocial, and spiritual aspects of patient care [44].

Palliative care services are often provided initially as part of an acute care hospital stay and may be organized around an interdisciplinary consultation service with or without an acute inpatient palliative care ward. However, in the setting of severely progressive neuromuscular diseases, such as Duchenne muscular dystrophy, palliative care services are ideally first introduced as part of the multidisciplinary team that will be involved in the patient's care.

There is still a prevalent underutilization of these services, likely due to the existing misconceptions or lack of knowledge about this specialty by both providers and families alike. A 2011 study of 34 families of patients with DMD demonstrated that most families (85 %) had never heard the term "palliative care," regardless of their socioeconomic status. The same study also reported that there was a low receipt of other important services, such as pastoral care (27 %), respite care (18 %), pain management (12 %), and hospice care (6 %). Only 8 respondents (25 %) reported having any type of directive document in place [45]. All of these services are an integral part of the services provided by the palliative care team.

Unlike hospice, palliative care is applicable earlier in the course of illness, in conjunction with other therapies that may indeed prolong life. The key to effective palliative care is communication. This enables the patient to feel empowered to make informed choices regarding their future care. Progressive conditions such as Duchenne muscular dystrophy pose medical and ethical challenges for the patient, the family, and the health care staff that are involved in their care. These patients often have high symptom burdens and the patients and their families must make complex medical decisions regarding the potential use of life-prolonging therapies, such as mechanical ventilation. A significant portion of the impact may be felt by family-caregivers who are simultaneously struggling with physical, emotional, and financial stressors associated with the disease [46]. Palliative care can provide the support that family-caregivers and primary care providers need to aid in the process of taking care of these medically complex patients.

It is important to remember that optimal care should maximize function and quality of life for patients with muscular dystrophy. Expert multidisciplinary care may improve both quality and length of life of patients with this type of progressive disease. Coordination and partnerships with hospice programs is a major feature in which palliative care can aid as the patient continues across the trajectory of their disease. The depth of support available from each palliative care program varies from institution to institution [47]. Therefore, the primary care providers should reach out to the local palliative care services and agencies and know the resources that are available for them and their patients.

Conclusion

Patients with muscular dystrophies, in particular Duchenne muscular dystrophy, are surviving well into their 30 and 40 s, in part due to early detection and adequate management of their cardiac and pulmonary complications ("Appendix"). Nevertheless, there is still a disparity in regards to the medical care that these patients experience in the pediatric setting compared to the adult healthcare system. It is for this reason that the adult healthcare system needs to continue its efforts in modifying its infrastructure to accommodate the needs of these patients. As part of the team of providers taking care of these patients, the role of the primary care provider is of the utmost importance, as they are at the center of this objective of maintaining adequate continuity of care. The ultimate goal is to be able to let these patients achieve the quality of life they deserve.

Appendix

Muscular dystrophy condition fact sheet

Definition	**Muscular dystrophies are a heterogeneous group of neurodegenerative diseases characterized by:** • Genetic inheritance • Progressive muscle weakness as the primary symptom • Onset of symptoms can be in the pediatric or adult setting
Epidemiology	• In the United States, the most common forms of muscular dystrophy are Duchenne muscular dystrophy (DMD), myotonic dystrophy, and facioscapulohumeral muscular dystrophy (FSHD) • DMD is an X-linked disease, whereas myotonic dystrophy and FSHD are autosomal dominant • Newborn screening for DMD places the incidence closer to 1:5,000 live male births • The worldwide prevalence of myotonic dystrophy lies in the 5–20 per 100,000 range • The myotonic dystrophies afflict mostly people of European heritage, with lesser frequencies in Asia and a virtual absence of disease in sub-Saharan Africa • FSHD has a prevalence of approximately 1:15,000–1:20,000
Special considerations	**Individuals with muscular dystrophies have high rates of co-morbid physical and mental health conditions, including:** • Loss of ambulation • Joint contractures • Cardiomyopathy • Osteopenia/Osteoporosis • Gastrointestinal problems • Dysphagia • Sleep disorders • Autism spectrum disorders • Anxiety and depression • Respiratory Failure
Recommended screening	• **Cardiac:** ECG, echocardiogram annually after the age of 10 years old • **Respiratory:** spirometry every 6 months and polysomnography if presenting with nocturnal hypercapnia • **Dysphagia:** weight and nutritional assessment at every office visit • **Bone health:** serum vitamin D levels at every visit, and DEXA scan every 1–2 years

Suggested Reading List

- Guidelines for diagnosis and management of Duchenne Muscular Dystrophy (Lancet Neurology): http://www.parentprojectmd.org/site/DocServer/120409Lancet_Neuro_online_combo.pdf?docID=8601
- Guidelines for evaluation, diagnosis, and management of facioscapulohumeral muscular dystrophy (American Academy of Neurology and the American Association of Neuromuscular and Electrodiagnostic Medicine): http://www.neurology.org/content/85/4/357.full.pdf+html
- Guidelines for diagnosis and treatment of Limb-Girdle and Distal Muscular Dystrophies (American Academy of Neurology and the American Association of Neuromuscular and Electrodiagnostic Medicine): https://www.aan.com/Guidelines/home/GetGuidelineContent/672

Patient/Caregiver Resources

- Family Guide for the diagnosis and management of Duchenne Muscular Dystrophy: http://www.parentprojectmd.org/site/DocServer/dmd_us_familyguide_june2010.pdf?docID=10781
- Family Guide for the diagnosis and management of Myotonic Muscular Dystrophy: http://www.myotonic.org/what-dm/start-here
- Family Guide for the diagnosis and management of FSHD: https://www.aan.com/Guidelines/Home/GetGuidelineContent/702

References

1. Abbott D, Carpenter J, Bushby K. Transition to adulthood for young men with duchenne muscular dystrophy: research from the UK. Neuromuscul Disord NMD. 2012;22(5):445–6.
2. Goodman DM, Hall M, Levin A, Watson RS, Williams RG, Shah SS, et al. Adults with chronic health conditions originating in childhood: inpatient experience in children's hospitals. Pediatrics. 2011;128(1):5–13.
3. Schrans DG, Abbott D, Peay HL, Pangalila RF, Vroom E, Goemans N, et al. Transition in duchenne muscular dystrophy: an expert meeting report and description of transition needs in an emergent patient population: (parent project muscular dystrophy transition expert meeting 17–18 June 2011, Amsterdam, The Netherlands). Neuromuscul Disord NMD. 2013;23(3):283–6.
4. Bushby K, Finkel R, Birnkrant DJ, Case LE, Clemens PR, Cripe L, et al. Diagnosis and management of duchenne muscular dystrophy, part 1: diagnosis, and pharmacological and psychosocial management. Lancet Neurol. 2010;9(1):77–93.
5. Bushby K, Finkel R, Birnkrant DJ, Case LE, Clemens PR, Cripe L, et al. Diagnosis and management of duchenne muscular dystrophy, part 2: implementation of multidisciplinary care. Lancet Neurol. 2010;9(2):177–89.
6. Eagle M, Baudouin SV, Chandler C, Giddings DR, Bullock R, Bushby K. Survival in duchenne muscular dystrophy: improvements in life expectancy since 1967 and the impact of home nocturnal ventilation. Neuromuscul Diso NMD. 2002;12(10):926–9.
7. Wicklund MP. The muscular dystrophies. Continuum (Minneap Minn). 2013;19(6 Muscle Disease):1535–70.
8. Griggs RC, Amato AA. Muscular dystrophies. Preface. Handb Clin Neurol. 2011;101:9.
9. Flanigan KM, Coffeen CM, Sexton L, Stauffer D, Brunner S, Leppert MF. Genetic characterization of a large, historically significant utah kindred with facioscapulohumeral dystrophy. Neuromuscul Disord NMD. 2001;11(6–7):525–9.
10. Parsons EP, Bradley DM, Clarke AJ. Newborn screening for duchenne muscular dystrophy. Arch Dis Child. 2003;88(1):91–2.
11. Mathieu J, Allard P, Potvin L, Prevost C, Begin P. A 10-year study of mortality in a cohort of patients with myotonic dystrophy. Neurology. 1999;52(8):1658–62.
12. Mendell JR, Shilling C, Leslie ND, Flanigan KM, Al-Dahhak R, Gastier-Foster J, et al. Evidence-based path to newborn screening for duchenne muscular dystrophy. Ann Neurol. 2012;71(3):304–13.
13. Harper PS, van Engelen BG, Eymard B, Rogers M, Wilcox D. 99th ENMC international workshop: myotonic dystrophy: present management, future therapy. 9–11 November 2001, Naarden, The Netherlands. Neuromuscul Disord NMD. 2002;12(6):596–9.
14. Padberg G, Eriksson AW, Volkers WS, Bernini L, Van Loghem E, Meera Khan P, et al. Linkage studies in autosomal dominant facioscapulohumeral muscular dystrophy. J Neurol Sci. 1984;65(3):261–8.
15. Berthier C, Blaineau S. Supramolecular organization of the subsarcolemmal cytoskeleton of adult skeletal muscle fibers. A review. Biol Cell. 1997;89(7):413–34.
16. Koenig M, Kunkel LM. Detailed analysis of the repeat domain of dystrophin reveals four potential hinge segments that may confer flexibility. J Biol Chem. 1990;265(8):4560–6.

17. Cacchiarelli D, Martone J, Girardi E, Cesana M, Incitti T, Morlando M, et al. Micrornas involved in molecular circuitries relevant for the duchenne muscular dystrophy pathogenesis are controlled by the dystrophin/nnos pathway. Cell Metab. 2010;12 (4):341–51.
18. Petrof BJ, Shrager JB, Stedman HH, Kelly AM, Sweeney HL. Dystrophin protects the sarcolemma from stresses developed during muscle contraction. Proc Natl Acad Sci USA. 1993;90(8):3710–4.
19. Blake DJ, Weir A, Newey SE, Davies KE. Function and genetics of dystrophin and dystrophin-related proteins in muscle. Physiol Rev. 2002;82(2):291–329.
20. Muntoni F, Torelli S, Ferlini A. Dystrophin and mutations: one gene, several proteins, multiple phenotypes. Lancet Neurol. 2003;2(12):731–40.
21. Kunkel LM, Beggs AH, Hoffman EP. Molecular genetics of duchenne and becker muscular dystrophy: emphasis on improved diagnosis. Clin Chem. 1989;35(7 Suppl):B21–4.
22. Mandel JL. Dystrophin. The gene and its product. Nature. 1989;339(6226):584–6.
23. Monaco AP, Bertelson CJ, Liechti-Gallati S, Moser H, Kunkel LM. An explanation for the phenotypic differences between patients bearing partial deletions of the DMD locus. Genomics. 1988;2 (1):90–5.
24. Hoffman EP, Arahata K, Minetti C, Bonilla E, Rowland LP. Dystrophinopathy in isolated cases of myopathy in females. Neurology. 1992;42(5):967–75.
25. Passamano L, Taglia A, Palladino A, Viggiano E, D'Ambrosio P, Scutifero M, et al. Improvement of survival in duchenne muscular dystrophy: retrospective analysis of 835 patients. Acta Myol. 2012;31 (2):121–5.
26. Biggar WD, Harris VA, Eliasoph L, Alman B. Long-term benefits of deflazacort treatment for boys with duchenne muscular dystrophy in their second decade. Neuromuscul Disord NMD. 2006;16(4):249–55.
27. King WM, Ruttencutter R, Nagaraja HN, Matkovic V, Landoll J, Hoyle C, et al. Orthopedic outcomes of long-term daily corticosteroid treatment in duchenne muscular dystrophy. Neurology. 2007;68 (19):1607–13.
28. Smith AD, Koreska J, Moseley CF. Progression of scoliosis in duchenne muscular dystrophy. J Bone Joint Surg Am Vol. 1989;71(7):1066–74.
29. Quinlivan R, Shaw N, Bushby K. 170th ENMC international workshop: bone protection for corticosteroid treated duchenne muscular dystrophy. 27–29 November 2009, Naarden, The Netherlands. Neuromuscul Disord NMD. 2010;20(11):761–9.
30. Leung DG, Germain-Lee EL, Denger BE, Wagner KR. Report on the second endocrine aspects of duchenne muscular dystrophy conference December 1–2, 2010, Baltimore, Maryland, USA. Neuromuscul Disord NMD. 2011;21(8):594–601.
31. McDonald DG, Kinali M, Gallagher AC, Mercuri E, Muntoni F, Roper H, et al. Fracture prevalence in duchenne muscular dystrophy. Dev Med Child Neurol. 2002;44(10):695–8.
32. Finder JD, Birnkrant D, Carl J, Farber HJ, Gozal D, Iannaccone ST, et al. Respiratory care of the patient with duchenne muscular dystrophy: ATS consensus statement. Am J Respir Crit Care Med. 2004;170 (4):456–65.
33. Birnkrant DJ, Bushby KM, Amin RS, Bach JR, Benditt JO, Eagle M, et al. The respiratory management of patients with duchenne muscular dystrophy: a DMD care considerations working group specialty article. Pediatr Pulmonol. 2010;45(8):739–48.
34. American Academy of Pediatrics Section on C, Cardiac S. Cardiovascular health supervision for individuals affected by duchenne or becker muscular dystrophy. Pediatrics. 2005;116(6):1569–73.
35. Bushby K, Muntoni F, Bourke JP. 107th ENMC international workshop: the management of cardiac involvement in muscular dystrophy and myotonic dystrophy. 7th–9th June 2002, Naarden, The Netherlands. Neuromuscul Disord NMD. 2003;13(2):166–72.
36. Hunt SA, Abraham WT, Chin MH, Feldman AM, Francis GS, Ganiats TG, et al. Acc/AHA 2005 guideline update for the diagnosis and management of chronic heart failure in the adult: a report of the american college of cardiology/American heart association task force on practice guidelines (writing committee to update the 2001 guidelines for the evaluation and management of heart failure): developed in collaboration with the american college of chest physicians and the international society for heart and lung transplantation: endorsed by the heart rhythm society. Circulation. 2005;112(12):e154–235.
37. Schram G, Fournier A, Leduc H, Dahdah N, Therien J, Vanasse M, et al. All-cause mortality and cardiovascular outcomes with prophylactic steroid therapy in duchenne muscular dystrophy. J Am Coll Cardiol. 2013;61(9):948–54.
38. Jaffe KM, McDonald CM, Ingman E, Haas J. Symptoms of upper gastrointestinal dysfunction in duchenne muscular dystrophy: case-control study. Arch Phys Med Rehabil. 1990;71(10):742–4.
39. Hendriksen JG, Vles JS. Neuropsychiatric disorders in males with duchenne muscular dystrophy: frequency rate of attention-deficit hyperactivity disorder (ADHD), autism spectrum disorder, and obsessive–compulsive disorder. J Child Neurol. 2008;23 (5):477–81.
40. Ricotti V, Mandy WP, Scoto M, Pane M, Deconinck N, Messina S, et al. Neurodevelopmental, emotional, and behavioural problems in duchenne muscular dystrophy in relation to underlying dystrophin gene mutations. Dev Med Child Neurol. 2016;58(1):77–84.
41. Daoud MSA, Dooley JM, Gordon KE. Depression in parents of children with duchenne muscular dystrophy. Pediatr Neurol. 2004;31(1):16–9.
42. Yemen TA, McClain C. Muscular dystrophy, anesthesia and the safety of inhalational agents revisited; again. Paediatr Anaesth. 2006;16(2):105–8.

43. Birnkrant DJ, Panitch HB, Benditt JO, Boitano LJ, Carter ER, Cwik VA, et al. American college of chest physicians consensus statement on the respiratory and related management of patients with duchenne muscular dystrophy undergoing anesthesia or sedation. Chest. 2007;132(6):1977–86.
44. Carter GT, Joyce NC, Abresch AL, Smith AE, VandeKeift GK. Using palliative care in progressive neuromuscular disease to maximize quality of life. Phys Med Rehabil Clin N Am. 2012;23(4):903–9.
45. Arias R, Andrews J, Pandya S, Pettit K, Trout C, Apkon S, et al. Palliative care services in families of males with duchenne muscular dystrophy. Muscle Nerve. 2011;44(1):93–101.
46. Nozoe KT, Moreira GA, Hachul H, Tufik S, Andersen ML. The strength beyond the muscle. J Palliat Med. 2014;17(11):1280–1.
47. Grant M, Elk R, Ferrell B, Morrison RS, von Gunten CF. Current status of palliative care—clinical implementation, education, and research. CA Cancer J Clin. 2009;59(5):327–35.

Sickle Cell Disease

16

Linda S. Overholser, Tiffiny Diers and Kathryn Hassell

Case Presentation

A 20-year-old African American woman presents to an adult medical practice for a new patient appointment. She has just recently started classes at the local community college where she is a freshman living in the dorms. In providing her health history, she reports that she has a diagnosis of hemoglobin SS (HbSS) sickle cell disease (SCD). She is single and lives with a roommate.

At the age of 10, she underwent a transcranial Doppler and has since been receiving regular blood transfusions, which she was told would help reduce the risk of having a stroke. Because of the transfusions, she was also prescribed a medication to help minimize the buildup of iron in her blood, although she reports that it tastes bad and she frequently skips doses. Because of how it has helped her in the past, she would like to continue on transfusion therapy. However, she has concerns about how to arrange for this therapy with her specialist who is now located remotely and whether the local blood supply will be a match for her. She has heard about a medicine called hydroxyurea that might be an option for her now. However, she has also heard that she should not get pregnant while taking this medicine. Though she does not currently desire pregnancy, she would like to be in a relationship and to understand the risks associated with hydroxyurea and sexual activity. Moreover, she would like to know what her options are for contraceptive therapy.

She also confirms that at 3 years of age she had to have her spleen removed. As far back as she can remember, she had frequent hospitalizations, up to 5 times a year, and twice she was told that she had a "chest crisis." This pattern continued until she started her transfusions at age 10, and then things seemed to get better, until she started her menses at around age 13. With her menstrual cycles, she has an increase in her pain, and she also has developed pain in both of her hips that she was told was because of her sickle cell disease. Her pain is bad enough that at times she requires doses of opioid pain medications, and about 3–4 times each year she has to go to the hospital for a brief stay to help control her

L.S. Overholser (✉)
Division of General Internal Medicine, University of Colorado School of Medicine, 12631 E 17th Avenue, Mail Stop B180, 8th Floor, Aurora, CO 80045, USA
e-mail: Linda.Overholser@ucdenver.edu

T. Diers
Department of Internal Medicine, University of Cincinnati Medical Center, 231 Albert B. Sabin Way, Cincinnati, OH 45267-0557, USA
e-mail: dierstl@uc.edu; Tiffiny.diers@uc.edu

K. Hassell
Division of Internal Medicine/Hematology, University of Colorado School of Medicine, 12700 E. 19th Avenue, Room 9122, RC 2/MS B170, Aurora, CO 80045, USA
e-mail: kathryn.hassell@ucdenver.edu

M. Pilapil et al. (eds.), *Care of Adults with Chronic Childhood Conditions*,
DOI 10.1007/978-3-319-43827-6_16

symptoms. She has been told to avoid medications such as ibuprofen because it could be bad for her kidneys. Though the adult medical practice is located in a major metropolitan area and she is excited to be attending college, she has expressed anxiety about the move and her medical care.

Case Discussion

This case highlights a combination of complex yet common medical issues that can be present in young adults affected by sickle cell disease (SCD). Though significant advances have been made in strategies to screen for, diagnose, and treat the complications of SCD, resulting in prolongation of life expectancy in affected individuals, these advances have not yet been sufficient to reduce the cumulative burden of acute and chronic complications in the adult population. Several studies have described that both hospitalization and mortality rates increase in individuals with SCD at or after the time of transition from pediatric-oriented to adult-oriented care [1–4], and there is evidence that beneficial therapies are underutilized in this age group [4]. In order to improve clinical outcomes in transition age youth affected by SCD, strategies to overcome these gaps are needed.

A combination of medical, socioeconomic, and provider-related factors combine to pose unique challenges for adolescents and young adults living with sickle cell disease, but the specific contributors to the increased morbidity and mortality in transition age individuals have not yet been fully clarified. In addition to biological worsening of the disease, patient factors such as multiple concurrent life transitions and provider factors such as a lack of familiarity with SCD in adult non-hematology and even specialty care settings are worth considering. As advances in therapy continue to evolve, it is imperative that the adult health care workforce, and in particular the adult primary care workforce, be adequately prepared to anticipate needs and coordinate care for these individuals. This chapter will focus on major themes that highlight the unique needs for young adults with SCD transitioning into adult care.

This case discussion focuses on a young woman who is furthering her education by attending community college for the first time at age 20. Assuming that she has completed her secondary education, it is notable that she is slightly older than the typical college-age freshman. Children diagnosed with SCD are at risk for frequent acute sickle cell crises requiring intensive medical intervention that may begin in infancy. As they age and schooling begins, these episodes can result in missed days of school that accumulate over time. Additionally, progressive vascular changes in the brain can lead to stroke, estimated to affect up to 10 % of children with sickle cell anemia (HbSS or Sβ[beta]^{0}thalassemia), with onset beginning in the first few years of life [5]. Importantly, however, this underlying process may manifest as silent cerebral infarction, with a clinical presentation that may be subtle but that can affect brain function nonetheless. For individuals who have already had or who are at an increased risk of neurological complications, there is a significant risk of new events, progression, and cumulative cognitive and physical impairment unless long-term treatment to address the underlying SCD pathophysiology is undertaken.

Strategies have now been outlined to help not only identify the risk of strokes but also to reduce the risk of first and recurrent strokes, as will be discussed in more detail in a later section of this chapter. This young woman has received evidence-based strategies including screening with transcranial Doppler to identify an increased risk of stroke and then use of transfusion therapy to reduce this risk. Although transfusion therapy is increasingly initiated in children before they actually develop significant neurological complications, and though most individuals are aware of a history of overt stroke, it is not known from this case study if the patient has sustained any silent neurological injury. As such, neuropsychological testing is indicated to provide insight into specific cognitive abilities and potential confounding psychological factors that affect cognition, such as depression. If she has evidence of cognitive challenges or difficulty adjusting socially given the age difference with her school peers, vocational–educational counseling with specialized educational planning might be helpful. An important challenge in this case is to ensure that the patient can continue to receive transfusion therapy to reduce the risk of further neurologic damage. If resources to continue this locally are unavailable or if she does not want to continue transfusions, then other therapeutic options such as use of hydroxyurea (HU) should be considered. There is no data to support the benefit of using HU together with chronic transfusion therapy, since HU affects only the endogenous red blood cells, which are replaced by transfused red blood cells in an individual receiving chronic transfusion therapy. If transfusion therapy is continued, then the use of medication to reduce iron overload will also need to be addressed, along with the barriers she has identified in medication adherence.

HU therapy in general has been proven to be of significant benefit in individuals with sickle cell anemia (HbSS or Sβ[beta]^{0}thalassemia), reducing pain episodes [6], morbidity and mortality [7, 8]. The National Heart, Lung, and Blood Institute (NHLBI) has recently published guidelines outlining the use of HU therapy for individuals with sickle cell disease [9]. HU therapy is recommended for adults with sickle cell anemia (HbSS disease) who meet any of the following conditions:

- 3 or more acute pain episodes in a year
- pain that is severe enough to impair quality of life or daily functioning
- recurrent severe episodes of acute chest syndrome
- severe anemia

There are no studies to demonstrate whether HU can be safely substituted for transfusion therapy for those individuals who have had a stroke. However, a recent study demonstrated that using HU was as good as transfusion therapy for the prevention of a first stroke in individuals with an abnormal transcranial Doppler, similar to the young woman in this case [10].

There are several practical points when considering HU therapy. It is critical to educate patients who are being considered for HU therapy on the indications for and goals of therapy as well as the need for long-term monitoring for complications of therapy, including low white blood cell (WBC) and platelet counts. Monitoring includes baseline assessment of a complete blood count (CBC) including differential, reticulocyte count, fetal hemoglobin measurement, kidney and liver function assessment, as well as pregnancy testing for women [11], followed by monthly assessments during dose adjustments and every 2–3 month assessments when stable. Dosages may need to be adjusted for renal dysfunction, not uncommon in adults with a history of SCD, and should be titrated to threshold levels of both platelets and neutrophil counts. Therapy can be temporarily held if needed for recovery of abnormally low blood cell parameters, as described in the NHLBI guidelines [11]. A systematic review of adherence of predominately pediatric patients with medications used in the treatment of sickle cell disease, including HU therapy, indicated that HU compliance was much higher in the context of monitoring as a part of a clinical drug trial (74–94 %); adherence in studies that did not include intensive monitoring as part of a clinical trial were much lower (49–85 %) [12]. For young adults, many of whom are on their own for the first time and experiencing other new life changes, adherence may be even more challenging. This may not be the case when treatment is directed at improving symptoms affecting quality of life in the short-term, such as pain. However, among the young adult population, preventing longer term complications of the disease may not seem as compelling of a reason to take medication requiring close monitoring. Despite these challenges, HU therapy can be prescribed and managed in primary care settings, preferably in partnership with an adult hematology specialist. Given the potential risks of HU therapy, collaborative decision-making with SCD patients, especially those of transition age, is critical initially and should be followed by adherence counseling at each office visit. Partnership with pharmacists to assist in this counseling can provide added support.

Another consideration is the impact of HU therapy on reproductive decision-making. Young adults are in a phase of life where entering into intimate relationships and starting families may be high priorities. Men and women are advised against pregnancy when taking HU as it is unclear if there are adverse effects on the fetus. NHLBI guidelines suggest discontinuing HU therapy if women become pregnant or in women who are breastfeeding [9]. The young woman in the case should be counseled about this and other potential risks to her health with pregnancy [12]. Contraceptive options should be offered if she expresses a desire to avoid pregnancy. NHLBI guidelines note that all forms of contraception can be considered, including estrogen-containing contraceptives, as the benefits generally outweigh risks. However, if there is a history of stroke or other thrombosis, this particular form of contraception should be avoided.

If the young woman in this case prefers to continue with transfusion therapy to reduce her risk of stroke, resources to support this therapy should be explored, including collaboration or at least consultation with a sickle cell provider. The NHBLI guidelines provide a consensus protocol for monitoring transfusion therapy, which generally entails transfusion of 1–2 units of packed red blood cells (PRBCs) provided at regular intervals, usually monthly, based on hemoglobin values and intermittent monitoring of HbS levels in the blood. As outlined in the NHLBI guidelines, minor antigen-matched blood is preferred to avoid the development of alloantibodies that could preclude future transfusions. Primary care providers may play a key role in monitoring for evidence of iron overload and for toxicities from iron chelation therapy.

Young adults with chronic conditions often have hesitation at the thought of transferring care from a pediatric specialty setting to primary care, for fear that their primary care provider (PCP) may not be as willing or able to care for them due to a lack of familiarity with the condition. Surveys of providers support there are variable levels of comfort in dealing with sickle cell disease [13]. This may be especially true for individuals with less prevalent and lifelong medical conditions such as SCD, where care is often dependent upon an ongoing relationship with a specialist. Stigmatization related to the pain issues so interwoven with SCD is also a concern. In this case, with the requirement for frequent blood transfusions and a diagnosis of one of the most severe forms of SCD, coordination of care with a hematology specialist is crucial. Likewise, while guidelines now exist for primary care management of HU therapy [9], initiation in most settings still involves coordination with hematology. Over time, coordination may also need to occur with other adult subspecialists as chronic medical conditions arise as described in later sections of this chapter. To capitalize on the gains that have been made in SCD survival, it is prudent for adults with SCD to have a primary care medical home where routine health maintenance and general medical care can be provided and care coordination can occur. Support for accessing primary care and for care coordination within the medical home through community health workers or patient navigators has been helpful in SCD care [14].

Overview of Sickle Cell Disease

Definition and Epidemiology

Though exact numbers are not known, it is estimated that SCD affects anywhere from 70,000 to 140,000 individuals in the United States [11, 14–16]. SCD is a group of blood disorders characterized by the production of hemoglobin S (HbS) due to a point mutation in the hemoglobin β(beta)-globin chain gene. Newborn infants are born producing fetal hemoglobin (HbF), though within 6 months of life this transitions to production of normal adult hemoglobin (HbA). For infants with sickle cell disease, HbS is produced instead of HbA. Individuals with the sickle mutation in both β(beta)-globin genes (HbSS) or those who have 1 gene with the sickle mutation and 1 which does not produce any HbA (HbSβ[beta]^{0}thalassemia) have the most severe forms of the disease—often lumped together and called "sickle cell anemia." [10, 17]. Other individuals have one β(beta)-globin gene with a sickle mutation and the other with a mutation producing another abnormal hemoglobin (e.g., HbC) or underproducing HbA (i.e., β[beta]$^+$thalassemia). The resulting conditions, HbSC and HbS β(beta)$^+$thalassemia, are generally milder with less severe anemia. The presence of 1 sickle gene and 1 normal hemoglobin gene results in sickle cell trait, which does not cause any form of sickle cell disease or hematological manifestations. In this discussion, we will focus on SCD. SCD disproportionately affects individuals of African or Mediterranean descent, but is found in Hispanic populations and less commonly among Caucasians as well. Approximately 1 in 2474 live births in the United States are of children diagnosed with SCD (HbSS and HbSC) [2, 18]. It is important to remember, however, that worldwide population shifts and demographic migration patterns can affect local prevalence.

Throughout much of the twentieth century, SCD was considered a disease of childhood, with high infant mortality rates and few children living into adulthood. However, the average life expectancy of individuals with SCD has increased over the last quarter century. A prospective cohort study across multiple US institutions from 1978 to 1988 indicates that the average life expectancy of those diagnosed with sickle cell anemia was 42 years for males and 48 years for females, 25–30 years shorter than African Americans not affected by SCD [17]. For those diagnosed with HbSC disease, the average life expectancy was 60 years for males and 68 years for females. A prospective cohort study of newborns affected by SCD published in 2010 revealed that almost 94 % of children affected by the most severe forms of SCD (HbSS and HbSβ[beta]^0) lived to 18 years of age, while almost 99 % of those affected by HbSC and HbSβ(beta)$^+$ lived to age 18. The authors note that in this most recent analysis of the cohort, the highest mortality rate now occurs in individuals over the age of 18 years [16]. Cohort data from a 40-year longitudinal study suggest a projected average life expectancy of 53 years for those with HbSS if born after 1975—a 16-year improvement over those born before that date [19], though still significantly shorter than African Americans without SCD.

Pathophysiology and Natural History

The abnormal hemoglobin that is produced in individuals affected by SCD causes reversible deformation of red blood cells ("sickling") due to polymerization of the hemoglobin molecules within the cell after oxygen is released. This phenomenon causes the red blood cells to sustain membrane damage that promotes adhesion to microvascular endothelium, even when unsickled, leading to vasoocclusion, which can in turn lead to disruption or complete blockage of normal blood flow to tissues and organs [2]. Sickled red blood cells are also fragile and may easily hemolyze, severely reducing their lifespan and producing a chronic hemolytic anemia. This ongoing adhesion to vascular endothelium, toxic effects of hemoglobin and iron released from lysed red blood cells, and ischemia created by intermittent vasoocclusion result in a continuous cascade of inflammation, activation of white blood cells, platelets, and endothelial cells through complex biochemical processes, leading to progressive vascular damage. Over time, cumulative vascular and end organ damage can lead to secondary comorbidities and, ultimately, premature death. Relatively abrupt, more extensive vasoocclusion of the microvasculature in a given area can occur episodically, resulting in the characteristic sickle cell "pain crisis" and other acute complications such as acute chest syndrome.

The only known cure for SCD is a bone marrow transplant, though this option is limited by availability of matched donors, and the optimal approach in adults is still under investigation. Advances in diagnosis and therapy have led to an increasing range of options to help prevent complications and reduce morbidity. These advances have also been important factors in increasing survival rates. Important milestones have included the use of prophylactic penicillin in children to reduce morbidity and mortality from life-threatening infections, the introduction of transcranial Doppler ultrasounds to predict stroke risk, the use of blood transfusion as a therapeutic measure, iron chelation therapy to reduce morbidity from iron overload, and the introduction of oral HU therapy to improve outcomes. The NHLBI published guidelines in 2014 that detail the use of most of these therapies, based on a review of available highest level evidence [11].

Common Clinical Issues for Adults with Sickle Cell Disease

SCD is a lifelong medical condition, the clinical manifestations of which begin shortly after birth as protective levels of fetal hemoglobin decline. Infants and young children present with acute complications of SCD in an episodic fashion. However, as individuals age, these episodic presentations lead to cumulative damage to the organ systems most commonly affected by the vascular pathology of SCD, including the brain, lungs, and kidneys. In addition to treating acute complications such as pain crises and acute chest syndrome, chronic organ system disease must be managed just as it would be for those individuals without SCD. Further, strategies to manage the symptoms of acute episodes of pain may need to be altered or adjusted as a result of accumulated chronic organ damage. Because of the advancing complexity of disease over time, a multidisciplinary team approach and involvement of multiple specialists involved in care decisions becomes increasingly important over time. Notably, the role of the adult primary care provider, particularly as pertains to addressing adult preventive care recommendations, is central to the coordination of this care. This section will review several of the most prevalent issues observed among the adolescent and young adult population of individuals living with SCD.

Chronic Pain

Pain is a hallmark of SCD and a symptom that significantly impacts quality of life. It is among the most recognizable symptoms associated with SCD. While certainly acute pain episodes are a classic presentation, pain is listed intentionally here as a common chronic condition to highlight the variety of pain presentations that can be seen in SCD from childhood into adulthood. Specifically, the pain pattern experienced in infants and children can evolve into a chronic pain syndrome by the time an individual reaches adulthood as cumulative organ damage occurs. Complications such as avascular necrosis, arthritis, chronic skin ulceration, peripheral neuropathy, or organ infarction often result in chronic pain conditions that can underlie acute pain episodes. Both frequency and severity of pain have been associated with mortality [17]. Management plans for pain that were established with pediatric medical providers are at risk of being interrupted during the transition period into young adulthood and may require modification throughout adulthood to optimize pain management.

While HU therapy can reduce the frequency of acute complications and hospitalizations, it is not indicated for the treatment of chronic pain. Patients must often rely on opioid pain medications that are administered in an acute care setting and need help in managing their pain regimens upon discharge to an outpatient setting. Use of opioid analgesics can lead to frustration in both patients and providers, with patients too often labeled as drug seeking and providers concerned about addiction and abuse while challenged by the difficulty of accurate pain assessment [20]. It is necessary to acknowledge both perspectives and the important role of trust in a treatment relationship, as reliance on opioids can erode that trust [21]. While opioid pain medications are commonly used, adjunctive therapies such as nonsteroidal anti-inflammatory therapies, neuropathic pain regimens, and other medications and treatment approaches indicated for chronic pain should also be considered. As with other chronic pain syndromes, addressing the emotional toll and distress associated with living with a chronic disease are paramount. This often requires a multidisciplinary team.

Approaches utilized in the management of other chronic pain syndromes should be considered in individuals with SCD. In addition to the aforementioned strategies, these include focusing on functional goals, use of pain treatment agreements, provision of care with a medical home approach to avoid multiple prescribers of pain medications, and considering and addressing causes of pain other than SCD. There has been a growing focus in the literature about the role of supporting self-efficacy and self-management [21–23], although very few interventions have been described or tested to clarify their role in treatment. Much can be learned from patients themselves. For example, 1 study highlighted differences in pain management strategies utilized by those with lower hospital use compared to those with higher hospital use [20]. Specifically, helpful patient strategies included increasing knowledge of the disease process, maintaining a stable provider relationship, engaging in a provider–patient relationship that is viewed as a partnership, documenting evidence of symptoms, use of adjunctive modalities such as heat or massage, improving nutrition and hydration, and exercise.

Pulmonary Issues

Acute chest syndrome is a potentially life-threatening event that occurs when acute vasoocclusion occurs in the microvasculature of the lung, with resulting capillary leak and ischemia. Preexisting asthma can worsen outcomes for pulmonary complications, and asthma has been described itself as being a predictor of mortality [2]. Over time, repeated damage to the pulmonary microvasculature can result in pulmonary hypertension (PH), even in the absence of a history of acute chest syndrome. The prevalence of PH in individuals with SCD has been estimated at around 6–11 % [24]. The American Thoracic Society (ATS) has set forth guidelines to help delineate both the diagnostic approach to and management of PH in sickle cell disease, including the requirement of right heart catheterization to make an accurate diagnosis of PH in individuals with SCD [24]. Key points of the published guidelines include assessment of cardiopulmonary status with careful history taking, physical examination, and testing such as echocardiography. An elevated tricuspid regurgitant jet velocity (TRV) on echocardiogram is associated with an increased risk of early mortality, even in the absence of pulmonary hypertension. The ATS guidelines recommend the initiation of HU therapy for individuals with this finding [25], although there is no direct evidence that this intervention reduces mortality. Echocardiography to assess tricuspid regurgitant jet velocity is recommended, with referral to a PH specialist if TRV > 2.5 m/s is detected. For the primary care provider focused on preventive health, it is critical to assess smoking status, treat nicotine dependence, and ensure that appropriate preventive measures are taken to reduce overlapping pulmonary morbidity from non-SCD causes, such as asthma or infection with influenza virus or pneumococcal infection. The Advisory Committee on Immunization Practices (ACIP) regularly updates recommendations for vaccinations for adults without splenic function, which includes individuals with HbSS/Sβ(beta)^{0}thalassemia [25].

Renal Issues

The kidney is a target organ affected by many vascular diseases including SCD. The kidney is highly metabolically active and the local environment of the kidney may predispose this organ system in particular to red cell adhesion, endothelial activation, intermittent ischemia, and reperfusion injury [26], resulting in a cycle of worsening blood flow to the kidney and glomeruli. This can initially result in hyperfiltration of the kidneys and over time lead to glomerulopathies. Proteinuria in the form of albuminuria is commonly the clinical manifestation of chronic SCD kidney damage, and hypertension can also result. In youth under the age of 21 years, the prevalence of albuminuria has been estimated to be as much as 26 % [26], but in older adults prevalence increases. As with other conditions that cause protein-losing nephropathies, angiotensin-converting enzyme (ACE) inhibitors and angiotensin receptor blockers are recommended when proteinuria is present [26]. Additionally, it is important for hypertension to be appropriately managed, as this can lead to worsening renal function over time. Management principles are similar to the general population with hypertension, though care should be taken to avoid dehydration due to diuretic medications. It is possible the HU therapy may provide renal protective benefits in SCD [26], but data are lacking and further research is needed.

Brain-Related Issues

In the brain, cerebral infarcts may lead not only to clinically symptomatic strokes but small silent infarcts as well. These silent infarcts can lead to progressive cognitive decline and pose educational challenges for children. One of the major therapeutic advances of the last few decades has been the ability to predict risk of strokes in children using transcranial Doppler (TCD) imaging, permitting an opportunity for primary prevention of strokes [27]. It is now recommended that children with sickle cell anemia (HbSS disease) begin screening for stroke using TCD at the age of 2 years and continue annual screening until the age of 16 years [11]. When evidence of abnormally elevated transcranial velocities are found, referral to a specialist for consideration and initiation of red blood cell transfusion therapy should be made [11]. This is largely based on clinical trials that demonstrated significant reductions in stroke risk in individuals receiving regular transfusion therapy compared to no transfusion therapy [27, 28]. For prevention of strokes, chronic red blood cell transfusion therapy, with the goal of reducing the percentage of HbS relative to normal hemoglobin, has become the standard treatment [5]. The introduction of HU therapy, which increases the proportion of fetal hemoglobin in the blood, has been shown to be an alternative strategy to reduce the risk of some SCD complications [6]. The Stroke with Transfusions Changing to Hydroxyurea (SWiTCH) randomized non-inferiority trial evaluated HU as an alternative therapy for recurrent (secondary) stroke prevention. The trial found that while the incidence of recurrent strokes was similar for HU therapy versus chronic transfusion, HU did not confer any advantage in reducing the main complication of chronic RBC transfusion therapy, which is iron overload [29]. However, a primary prevention study comparing continued chronic transfusion therapy to the use of HU for children with an abnormal transcranial Doppler recently demonstrated that HU is non-inferior to chronic transfusion therapy [10]. Thus, HU has now been demonstrated to be an alternative for adults such as our young adult patient who is on transfusion for an abnormal TCD, and it may be an alternative for adults who have a history of overt childhood stroke for whom transfusion therapy may not be possible [11].

Ophthalmologic Complications

The visual manifestations of SCD are varied and depend on the area of the orbital blood supply that is affected. Presentations can range from conjunctival vessel dilation, orbital cellulitis, atrophy or irregularity of the iris, retinal artery occlusion, glaucoma, angioid streaks, and proliferative sickle retinopathy (PSR) [30]. PSR has been well described and characterized [30] and can lead to both vitreous hemorrhage and retinal detachment, which are the primary mechanisms through which visual loss occurs. PSR and other eye diseases associated with SCD can be identified by an eye specialist and treatments are available. Yearly eye exams are recommended.

Immune-Related Concerns

Splenic sequestration of sickled red blood cells results in splenic infarction and functional asplenia within the first 1–2 years of life in children with HbSS/Sβ(beta)^{0}thalassemia, leading to high risk for overwhelming bacterial infections. Death from bacterial sepsis has traditionally been a major cause of mortality in infants and young children with HbSS/ Sβ(beta)^{0}thalassemia, until the use of prophylactic penicillin in early childhood was demonstrated to markedly reduce life-threatening infections [31]. There are no data supporting the use of this prophylaxis into adulthood, however. In patients with HbSC and HbSβ(beta)$^{+}$thalassemia, the spleen is often not infarcted early in childhood. These individuals may have an enlarged spleen and may experience episodes of acute splenic sequestration and infarctions. Chronic subclinical repeated insults to the spleen and splenic sequestration can lead to functional asplenia in these patients. Immunization recommendations in adult patients include coverage with pneumococcal vaccinations, both 23-valent and 13-valent vaccines [11]. Additionally, for individuals that have received or are receiving blood transfusion therapy, screening should occur for hepatitis C.

Pregnancy/Genetic Counseling

Knowledge about the type of sickle cell disease is key for both provider and patient. Young men and women should fully understand their own risk of having offspring with SCD or sickle cell trait. Those affected with sickle cell disease will pass on an abnormal hemoglobin gene. This would be a HbS gene if they have HbSS, or it could be a gene for another abnormal hemoglobin-like HbC if they have HbSC disease. If actively planning a family, they should not assume that they are without risk of having offspring affected by SCD if their partner is not having symptoms of SCD, as they may have sickle cell trait or another abnormal hemoglobin trait (e.g., HbC or β[beta]-thalassemia) that could lead to a form of sickle cell disease. Appropriate testing (complete blood count and hemoglobin electrophoresis) of the partner is needed to be able to provide specific genetic counseling. Women with HbSS/Sβ(beta)^{0}thalassemia have higher rates of pregnancy complications and may experience increased episodes of sickle cell pain [32]. These high-risk pregnancies should be comanaged by obstetrical and specialty providers with knowledge of sickle cell disease.

Special Circumstance: Pain Management in the Young Adult

The management of adolescent and young adult patients with chronic pain presents special challenges for primary care providers. Defined as "pain that recurs or persists over a period of at least three months or more," chronic pain is a common problem affecting 15–25 % of adolescents and young adults [33–35]. Chronic pain in adolescents and young adults increases with age, with females reporting more severe pain and reporting it more frequently than males [36]. Common causes include headaches, abdominal pain, limb pain, and back pain [37], with many adolescents reporting pain at multiple sites [34]. Adolescents report that living with chronic pain affects multiple aspects of life, including school, play, and sleep [37–39]. Parents are also affected, with increased rates of mood disorders and stress of parenting among parents of adolescents with chronic pain [40, 41].

In response to increasing advocacy about management of pain, providers are prescribing controlled substances to adolescents and young adults at a rate that has doubled in the last 14 years. A review of more than 2 million visits between 1994 and 2007 found the rate of prescription of controlled substances for adolescents increasing from 6.4 to 11.2 % and for young adults from 8.3 to 16.1 % [42]. This is concerning given that adolescents and young adults are the age group most likely to abuse controlled substances [43–45]. In fact, the nonmedical use of controlled substances has surpassed the use of all illicit substances other than marijuana [43]. One study found an estimated lifetime medical use of opioids among US high school seniors of 17.6 % and lifetime nonmedical use of 12.9 % [46]. Further complicating management, young adults in particular have decreased use of preventive care services, limiting a proactive, comprehensive management approach [47].

Assessment

A structured approach to chronic pain assessment is recommended by the American Pain Society and American Association of Pain Management's clinical guidelines published in 2009 [48]. Standardized pain assessment instruments such as pain intensity self-report scales, including the visual analog scale [49] and the Faces Pain Scale-Revised [50], as well as pain questionnaires such as the Varni/Thompson Pediatric Pain Questionnaire [51], are well-established and recommended for use in the adolescent age group [52]. Despite the recognition of the negative impact of chronic pain on multiple dimensions of life, however, few structured assessments address domains beyond pain such as functional status or social and educational functioning [53]. One such instrument is the Bath Adolescent Pain Questionnaire [54]. Psychological assessment with instruments validated for use in adolescents and young adults, such as the Beck Depression Inventory [55] or the Center for Epidemiologic Studies-Depression Scale [56], is particularly important due to the high rate of comorbid mental health diagnoses in the chronic pain population, especially among those prescribed opioids [57]. Likewise, assessment of risk for opioid abuse—for example, with the Opioid Risk Tool or Brief Risk Assessment [58, 59]—can help identify patients for whom prescription of controlled substances might be particularly hazardous.

Management

A multimodal treatment strategy that addresses the multiple impacts of chronic pain on the lives of adolescents and young adults is needed. Best results are achieved with an interprofessional (IP) approach [60], although access to IP team members is often limited in primary care settings [61]. Collaborative decision-making with patients and families can improve adherence to treatment plans and self-management. In particular, education and support for behavioral changes in lifestyle habits that affect pain—such as sleep, exercise, diet, and stress management—are critical, but may not be provided at home by parents or in the office by providers. Innovative approaches to self-management incorporating technology and tailored to adolescents and young adults may increase effectiveness [62, 63]. Psychological therapies including cognitive behavioral therapy, relaxation training, and biofeedback have also been found effective in adolescents and young adults [64].

Medication use can be guided by the type of pain being experienced, co-morbid conditions, especially mood disorders, and effectiveness of non-pharmacologic therapies. A challenge in medication use in adolescents and young adults is that most evidence is extrapolated from studies on adults. Some uses for common pain syndromes that have been studied in adolescents and young adults include acetaminophen, ibuprofen, and sumatriptan nasal spray for headache [65, 66] and famotidine, pizotifen, and peppermint oil in recurrent abdominal pain [67]. Opioids specifically have little long-term role in the management of chronic nonmalignant pain in adolescents and young adults [68]. Education on medication safety for adolescents and young adults and their families is needed, as adolescents and young adults have decreased awareness of safe use of over-the-counter medications and increased risk of abuse, diversion, and overdose of controlled substances [42]. Invasive treatments such as injections, nerve blocks, and neurostimulators are rarely used in younger age groups relative to adult practice [68].

Conclusion

Chronic pain in adolescents and young adults benefits from a structured approach with use of standardized assessments and a multimodal treatment plan determined in partnership with adolescents and young adults and their support people. An awareness of the abuse potential of controlled substances is warranted to manage pain without increasing risk. Attention to primary prevention (preventing injuries or overuse that could lead to pain problems) and secondary prevention (minimizing progression of acute to chronic pain through effective treatment and follow up) is also in the realm of primary care ("Appendix").

Appendix

Sickle cell disease (SCD) fact sheet

Definition	Healthy newborn infants are born with fetal hemoglobin (HbF), which transitions to normal adult hemoglobin (HbA) within 6 months of life. **Sickle cell disease (SCD)** is a group of blood disorders characterized by the presence of hemoglobin S (HbS) instead of normal HbA due to a point mutation in the hemoglobin β(beta)-globin chain gene. Disease classification depends upon the specific combinations of abnormal hemoglobin present: • The most severe forms of SCD are HbSS (sickle mutation in both β[beta]-globin genes) and HbSβ(beta)^{0}thalassemia (sickle mutation in one gene and absent production of HbA in the other gene) • These are also referred to as "sickle cell anemia" • Less severe forms of SCD include HbSC (sickle mutation in 1 gene and another mutation causing abnormal hemoglobin in the other gene) and HbSβ(beta)$^+$thalassemia (sickle mutation in 1 gene and underproduction of HbA in the other gene)

Prevalence	SCD disproportionately affects individuals of African or Mediterranean descent, approximately 1 in 2474 live births in US
	  • It can be found, however, in Hispanic and Caucasian populations
	  • Demographic shifts affect local prevalence
	Survival rates into adulthood are increasing

Pathophysiology	Disease manifestations are results of polymerization of abnormal red blood cell (RBC) hemoglobin in low oxygen states
	• Leads to deformation ("sickling") of RBC
	  • Can lead to RBC membrane deformation and vascular wall adhesion even when not sickled
	  • Leads to fragility and decreased RBC lifespan, chronic hemolytic anemia of varying severity
	• Continuous cascade of inflammation, activation of white blood cells, platelets, and endothelial cells through complex biochemical processes affect microvascular blood flow
	  • End organ damage results

Symptoms	**Individuals are at heightened risk for important chronic conditions as they age, including:**
	  • Chronic pain syndromes, acute or chronic pain episodes
	  • Pulmonary hypertension
	  • Chronic renal disease, hypertension, proteinuria
	  • Strokes, silent cerebral infarctions affecting brain function
	  • Proliferative sickle retinopathy, visual loss
	  • Functional asplenia
	  • Iron overload in organs if receiving chronic transfusion therapy

Challenges in transition	The transition from pediatric to adult phase of life is known to be associated with increased SCD complications The use of beneficial therapies to manage SCD complications may also be underutilized in affected adults Many adult health care providers, especially primary care providers, are unfamiliar with the care of those living with SCD. Stigma and lack of trust are key issues when chronic pain is involved
Helpful resources	• Sickle Cell Disease Association of America (resources for patients and family members, may include local chapters in communities throughout the US): http://www.sicklecelldisease.org • Sickle Cell Adult Provider Network (resources for health care providers, includes links to connect with SCD experts): http://www.scapn.net/ohana • National Heart, Lung and Blood Institute Sickle Cell Disease Guidelines (developed by expert panel): http://www.nhlbi.nih.gov/health-pro/guidelines/sickle-cell-disease-guidelines

References

1. Hamideh D, Alvarez O. Sickle cell disease related mortality in the United States (1999–2009). Pediatr Blood Cancer. 2013;60(9):1482–6.
2. Kanter J, Kruse-Jarres R. Management of sickle cell disease from childhood through adulthood. Blood Rev. 2013;27(6):279–87.
3. Hemker BG, Brousseau DC, Yan K, Hoffmann RG, Panepinto JA. When children with sickle-cell disease become adults: lack of outpatient care leads to increased use of the emergency department. Am J Hematol. 2011;86(10):863–5.
4. Blinder MA, Vekeman F, Sasane M, Trahey A, Paley C, Duh MS. Age-related treatment patterns in sickle cell disease patients and the associated sickle cell complications and healthcare costs. Pediatr Blood Cancer. 2013;60(5):828–35.
5. Helton KJ, Adams RJ, Kesler KL, Lockhart A, Aygun B, Driscoll C, et al. Magnetic resonance imaging/angiography and transcranial Doppler velocities in sickle cell anemia: results from the SWiTCH trial. Blood. 2014;124(6):891–8.
6. Charache S, Terrin ML, Moore RD, Dover GJ, Barton FB, Eckert SV, et al. Effect of hydroxyurea on the frequency of painful crises in sickle cell anemia. N Engl J Med. 1995;332(20):1317–22.
7. Steinberg MH, Barton F, Castro O, Pegelow CH, Ballas SK, Kutlar A, et al. Effect of hydroxyurea on mortality and morbidity in adult sickle cell anemia: risks and benefits up to 9 years of treatment. JAMA. 2003;289(13):1645–51.
8. Steinberg MH, McCarthy WF, Castro O, Ballas SK, Armstrong FD, Smith W, et al. The risks and benefits of long-term use of hydroxyurea in sickle cell anemia: a 17.5 year follow-up. Am J Hematol. 2010;85 (6):403–8.
9. Evidence Based Management of Sickle Cell Disease: Expert Report 2014. Expert Panel Report, 2014. US Department of Health and Human Services, National Institutes of Health. National Heart, Lung, and Blood Institute. https://www.nhlbi.nih.gov/sites/www.nhlbi.nih.gov/files/sickle-cell-disease-report.pdf.
10. Ware RE, Davis BR, Schultz WH, Brown RC, Aygun B, Sarnaik S, et al. Hydroxycarbamide versus chronic transfusion for maintenance of transcranial doppler flow velocities in children with sickle cell anaemia—TCD With Transfusions Changing to Hydroxyurea (TWiTCH): a multicentre, open-label, phase 3, non-inferiority trial. Lancet. 2016;387 (10019):661–70. doi:10.1016/S0140-6736(15)01041-7. Epub 2015 Dec 6.
11. Yawn BP, Buchanan GR, Afenyi-Annan AN, Ballas SK, Hassell KL, James AH, et al. Management of sickle cell disease: summary of the 2014 evidence-based report by expert panel members. JAMA. 2014;312(10):1033–48. https://www.nhlbi.nih.gov/health-pro/guidelines/sickle-cell-disease-guidelines.
12. Walsh KE, Cutrona SL, Kavanagh PL, Crosby LE, Malone C, Lobner K, et al. Medication adherence among pediatric patients with sickle cell disease: a systematic review. Pediatrics. 2014;134(6):1175–83.
13. Mainous AG, Tanner RJ, Harle CA, Baker R, Shokar NK, Hulihan MM. Attitudes toward management of sickle cell disease and its complications: a national survey of academic family physicians. Anemia. 2015;2015:853835.
14. National Institute for Children's Health Quality. SCDTDP Congressional Report: Recommendations for improving care for people with sickle cell disease. 2014. http://sicklecell.nichq.org/resources/scdtdp-congressional-report.
15. Brousseau DC, Panepinto AJ, Nimmer M, Hoffmann RG. The number of people with sickle-cell disease in the United States: national and state estimates. Am J Hematol. 2010;85(1):77–8.
16. Hassell KL. Population estimates of sickle cell disease in the U.S. American. J Prevent Med. 2010;38(4, Supplement):S512–21.
17. Platt OS, Brambilla DJ, Rosse WF, Milner PF, Castro O, Steinberg MH, et al. Mortality in sickle cell disease—life expectancy and risk factors for early death. N Engl J Med. 1994;330(23):1639–44.
18. Therrell BLHWH. National evaluation of US newborn screening system components. Ment Retard Dev Disabil Res Rev 2006;12(4):236–45.
19. Powars DR, Chan L, Hiti AL, Ramicone E, Johnson C. Outcome of sickle cell anemia: a 4-decade observational study of 1056 patients. Medicine. 2005;84(6):363–376.
20. Brown S-E, Weisberg DF, Balf-Soran G, Sledge WH. Sickle cell disease patients with and without extremely high hospital use: pain, opioids, and coping. J Pain Symptom Manag. 2015;49(3):539–47.
21. Matthie N, Jenerette C, McMillan S. Role of self-care in sickle cell disease. Pain Manag Nurs. 2015;16 (3):257–66.
22. Molter BL, Abrahamson K. Self-efficacy, transition, and patient outcomes in the sickle cell disease population. Pain Manag Nurs. 2015;16(3):418–24.
23. Crosby L, Quinn C, Kalinyak K. A biopsychosocial model for the management of patients with sickle-cell disease transitioning to adult medical care. Adv Ther. 2015;32(4):293–305.
24. Klings ES, Machado RF, Barst RJ, Morris CR, Mubarak KK, Gordeuk VR, et al. An official american thoracic society clinical practice guideline: diagnosis, risk stratification, and management of pulmonary hypertension of sickle cell disease. Am J Respir Crit Care Med. 2014;189(6):727–40.
25. Centers for Disease Control and Prevention (CDC). Use of 13-valent pneumococcal conjugate vaccine

and 23-valent pneumococcal polysaccharide vaccine for adults with immunocompromising conditions: recommendations of the Advisory Committee on Immunization Practices (ACIP. MMWR Morb Mortal Wkly Rep. 2012;61(40):816–9.
26. Ataga KI, Derebail VK, Archer DR. The glomerulopathy of sickle cell disease. Am J Hematol. 2014;89 (9):907–14.
27. Adams RJ, McKie VC, Hsu L, Files B, Vichinsky E, Pegelow C, et al. Prevention of a first stroke by transfusions in children with sickle cell anemia and abnormal results on transcranial Doppler ultrasonography. N Engl J Med. 1998;339(1):5–11.
28. Lee MT, Piomelli S, Granger S, Miller ST, Harkness S, Brambilla DJ, et al. Stroke Prevention Trial in Sickle Cell Anemia (STOP): extended follow-up and final results. Blood. 2006;108(3):847–52.
29. Ware RE, Helms RW. Stroke with transfusions changing to hydroxyurea (SWiTCH). Blood. 2012;119(17):3925–32.
30. Elagouz M, Jyothi S, Gupta B, Sivaprasad S. Sickle cell disease and the eye: old and new concepts. Surv Ophthalmol. 2010;55(4):359–77.
31. Gaston MH, Verter JI, Woods G, Pegelow C, Kelleher J, Presbury G, et al. prophylaxis with oral penicillin in children with sickle cell anemia. N Engl J Med. 1986;314(25):1593–9.
32. Rogers DT, Molokie R. Sickle cell disease in pregnancy. Obstet Gynecol Clin North Am. 2010;37 (2):223–37.
33. Goodman J, McGrath P. The epidemiology of pain in children and adolescents: a review. Pain. 1991;46 (1758709):247–64.
34. Perquin C, Hazebroek-Kampschreur AA, Hunfeld JA, Bohnen AM, van Suijlekom-Smit LW, Passchier J, et al. Pain in children and adolescents: a common experience. Pain. 2000;87(1):51–8.
35. National Center for Health Statistics. Health, United States, 2006, With chartbook on trends in the health of Americans with special feature on pain. Hyattsville, MD; 2006:68–87.
36. Keogh E, Eccleston C. Sex differences in adolescent chronic pain and pain-related coping. Pain. 2006;123 (3):275–84.
37. Roth-Isigkeit A, Thyen U, Raspe HH, Stöven H, Schmucker P. Reports of pain among German children and adolescents: an epidemiological study. Acta Paediatr. 2004;93(2):258–63.
38. Roth-Isigkeit A, Thyen U, Stöven H, Schwarzenberger J, Schmucker P. Pain among children and adolescents: restrictions in daily living and triggering factors. Pediatrics. 2005;115(4):e152–62.
39. Palermo TM, Kiska R. Subjective sleep disturbances in adolescents with chronic pain: relationship to daily functioning and quality of life. J Pain. 2005;6(3):201–7.
40. Jordan AL, Eccleston C, Osborn M. Being a parent of the adolescent with complex chronic pain: an interpretative phenomenological analysis. Eur J Pain. 2007;11(1):49–56.
41. Eccleston C, Crombez G, Scotford A, Clinch J, Connell H. Adolescent chronic pain: patterns and predictors of emotional distress in adolescents with chronic pain and their parents. Pain. 2004;108 (3):221–9.
42. Fortuna R, Robbins B, Caiola E, Joynt M, Halterman J. Prescribing of controlled medications to adolescents and young adults in the united states. Pediatrics. 2010;126(6):1108–16.
43. Manchikanti L, Singh A. Therapeutic opioids: a ten-year perspective on the complexities and complications of the escalating use, abuse, and nonmedical use of opioids. Pain Phys. 2008;11(2 Suppl):S63–88.
44. Johnston L, O'Malley P, Bachman J, Schulenberg J. Monitoring the future national survey results on drug use, 1975–2008: volume 1, Secondary school students. Bethesda, MD: National Institute on Drug Abuse; 2009.
45. Results from the 2008 National Survey on Drug Use and Health: National Findings. Rockville, MD; 2009: HHS SMA 09-4434.
46. Mccabe S, West B, Teter C, Boyd C. Medical and non-medical uses of prescription opioids among high school seniors in the United States. Arch Pediatr Adolesc Med. 2012;166(9):797–802.
47. Fortuna RJ, Robbins BW, Halterman JS. Ambulatory care among young adults in the United States. Ann Intern Med. 2009;151(6):379–85.
48. Chou R, Fanciullo GJ, Fine PG, Adler JA, Ballantyne JC, Davies P, et al. Clinical guidelines for the use of chronic opioid therapy in chronic noncancer pain. J Pain. 2009;10(2):113–30.e22.
49. Stinson J, Kavanagh T, Yamada J, Gill N, Stevens B. Systematic review of the psychometric properties, interpretability and feasibility of self-report pain intensity measures for use in clinical trials in children and adolescents. Pain. 2006;142:143–57.
50. Hicks CL, von Baeyer CL, Spafford PA, van Korlaar I, Goodenough B. The Faces Pain Scale-Revised: toward a common metric in pediatric pain measurement. Pain. 2001;93(2):173–83.
51. Thompson K, Varni J, Hanson V. Comprehensive assessment of pain in juvenile rheumatoid arthritis: an empirical model. J Pediatr Psychol. 1987;12(2):241–55.
52. Cohen LL, Lemanek K, Blount RL, Dahlquist LM, Lim CS, Palermo TM, et al. Evidence-based assessment of pediatric pain. J Pediatr Psychol. 2008;33(9):939–55.
53. Eccleston C, Jordan AL, Crombez G. The impact of chronic pain on adolescents: a review of previously used measures. J Pediatr Psychol. 2006;31(7):684–97.
54. Eccleston C, Jordan A, McCracken L, Sleed M, Connell H, Clinch J. The Bath Adolescent Pain Questionnaire (BAPQ): development and preliminary psychometric evaluation of an instrument to assess the impact of chronic pain on adolescents. Pain. 2005;118:263–70.
55. Teri L. The use of the Beck Depression inventory with adolescents. J Abnorm Child Psychol. 1982;10 (1):277–84.

56. Roberts R, Andrews J, Lewinsohn P, Hops H. Assessment of depression in adolescents using the Center for Epidemiologic Studies Depression Scale. Psychol Assess. 1990;2(2):122–8.
57. Richardson LP, Russo JE, Katon W, McCarty CA, DeVries A, Edlund MJ, et al. Mental health disorders and long-term opioid use among adolescents and young adults with chronic pain. J Adolesc Health. 2012;50(6):553–8.
58. Webster L, Webster R. Predicting aberrant behaviors in opioid-treated patients: preliminary validation of the Opioid Risk Tool. Pain Med. 2005;6(6):432–42.
59. Jones T, Lookatch S, Moore T. Validation of a new risk assessment tool: the Brief Risk Questionnaire. J Opioid Manag. 2015;11(2):171–83.
60. Eccleston C, Clinch J. Adolescent chronic pain and disability: a review of the current evidence in assessment and treatment. Paediatr Child Health. 2007;12(2):117–20.
61. Bodenheimer T. Transforming practice. N Engl J Med. 2008;359(20):2086–9.
62. Stinson J, Lalloo C, Harris L, Isaac L, Campbell F, Brown S, et al. iCanCope with Pain™: user-centred design of a web- and mobile-based self-management program for youth with chronic pain based on identified health care needs. Pain Res Manag. 2014;19(5):257–65.
63. Stinson JN, Mcgrath PJ, Hodnett ED, Feldman BM, Duffy CM, Huber AM, et al. An Internet-based self-management program with telephone support for adolescents with arthritis: a pilot randomized controlled trial. J Rheumatol. 2010;37(9):1944–52.
64. Palermo T, Eccleston C, Lewandowski A, Williams A, Morley S. Randomized controlled trial of psychological therapies for management of chronic pain in children and adolescents: an updated meta-analytic review. Pain. 2010;148(3):387–97.
65. Hamaleinen M, Hoppu K, Valkeila E, Santavuori P. Ibuprofen or acetaminophen for the acute treatment of migraine in children: a double-blind, randomized, placebo-controlled crossover study. Neurology. 1997;48:103–7.
66. Hamaleinen M, Jones M, Loftus J, Saiers J. Sumatriptan nasal spray for migraine: a review of studies in patients aged 17 years and younger. Int J Clin Pract. 2002;56:704–9.
67. Weydert J, Ball T, Davis M. Systematic review of treatments for recurrent abdominal pain. Pediatrics. 2003;111:1–11.
68. Howard R. Chronic pain problems in children and young people. Contin Educ Anesth Crit Care Pain. 2011;11:219–23.

Solid Organ Transplantation

17

Heather Stewart and Eva Waite

Case Presentation

O.T. is a 21-year-old patient, status post-renal transplantation, presenting for evaluation in the process of transitioning to an adult primary care provider (PCP). Her general pediatrician is located in a nearby suburban practice. The patient does not bring any records with her to the appointment but is accompanied by her mother, who is a single parent with one other child. When the patient is asked what her concerns are, she denies any. When addressed, the patient's mother states that she is concerned about her daughter transitioning to a new doctor and also that her daughter has been missing her periods recently.

O.T.'s history is significant for renal transplantation at the age of 6 years. The primary diagnosis necessitating the transplantation is unknown by the patient and her mother. She has been underweight "since before her transplantation" and has a gastrostomy tube (G-tube) in place for nutritional supplementation. She has hypertension for which she takes amlodipine and labetalol. Additionally, she is taking tacrolimus as her chronic immunosuppressive agent. She also has a history of depression for which she is not currently receiving any treatment. Her review of systems is remarkable for irregular menses for the last several months. Her social history is remarkable for no toxic habits. She does have a boyfriend at college but denies having been sexually active. O.T. is currently in her last year of college, pursuing a degree in graphic art design, though she is not sure what she will do when she graduates. Her family history is negative for hypertension and kidney disease.

Her physical exam is remarkable in that the patient makes limited eye contact and is poorly engaged, having deferred to her mother throughout the entire collection of her medical and social history. Her blood pressure (BP) is 126/72, and body mass index (BMI) is low at 16.8 kg/m^2. Her head, eyes, ears, nose, and throat (HEENT) exam is remarkable for jaw opening that is limited but with no associated discomfort. Cardiopulmonary exam and peripheral pulses are normal. She has an intact G-tube in her left upper quadrant and a palpable pelvic kidney in the right lower quadrant. Her skin exam is normal with a few healed surgical scars

H. Stewart
Division of Pediatric Nephrology and Hypertension, Department of Pediatrics, University of South Carolina School of Medicine - Palmetto Richland Children's Hospital, 9 Medical Park, Suite 270, Columbia, SC 29203, USA

E. Waite
Departments of Internal Medicine and Pediatrics, Mount Sinai Medical Center, 17 East 102 St, Seventh Floor, New York, NY 10029, USA
e-mail: eva.waite@mountsinai.org

H. Stewart (✉)
17 East 102 Street, Box 1087, New York, NY 10029, USA
e-mail: heather.stewart@uscmed.sc.edu

M. Pilapil et al. (eds.), *Care of Adults with Chronic Childhood Conditions*,
DOI 10.1007/978-3-319-43827-6_17

but no abnormal nevi. Her musculoskeletal exam is normal and her neurologic exam is non-focal.

Case Discussion

In caring for a patient with a solid organ transplant, it is critical to monitor for and treat the sequelae of the medications used for immunosuppression. In addition, it is important to monitor for the recurrence of the underlying disease that necessitated transplantation. Initially after the transplant procedure, the greatest concern is for infection due to surgical complications or viral infections. As the patient becomes further removed from the transplant, as in this case, the risk for infection is less of an issue. Though the transplant patient is at risk for the usual bacterial or viral infections typically experienced by the general population, the infections can become more serious due to the immunosuppression. More importantly, the immunosuppressant medications required to maintain the transplanted organ often result in a number of metabolic sequelae. These include an increased risk for diabetes mellitus, hyperlipidemia, hypertension, and gout and, as a result, an increased risk for cardiovascular disease as the patient ages. Patients also often develop chronic kidney disease (CKD) over time due to the effect of calcineurin inhibitors (CNIs) on the kidney. The PCP's goal will be to monitor for these adverse affects in comanagement with the transplant team. Additionally, the PCP typically assumes the primary management of secondary hypertension, diabetes, or gout. Providers should always consider possible drug interactions with the patient's transplant regimen and to avoid medications that can decrease the effectiveness of the immunosuppressant or increase its toxicity to the patient. In addition, the PCP will need to monitor the effects of the immunosuppressant medications on continuing development of bone and reproductive health. Finally, the PCP will be responsible for routine health maintenance with increased vigilance for the special screening recommendations for solid organ transplant patients, such as skin cancer screening.

In this particular case it will be beneficial for the PCP to engage with both the patient and the parent. A primary goal should be to encourage the patient to become a more active participant at future visits. Her limited eye contact may be due to shyness but might also be a sign of underlying developmental delay or depression. Screening with the patient health questionnaire-2 (PHQ-2) would be appropriate at this initial visit. Her irregular menses might be attributable to undernutrition as indicated by her low body mass index, an unplanned pregnancy, or hormonal dysfunction. It would be prudent to evaluate with a pregnancy test at the initial visit, and if negative, discuss appropriate forms of contraception. She would benefit from consultation with a nutritionist to evaluate her feeding regimen and to ensure that she is receiving adequate calories from oral intake and supplementation with her G-tube feeding regimen. Her limited jaw mobility should also be addressed as it could also be limiting her ability to chew and consume adequate calories. Finally, given her nutritional status and irregular menses, it would be appropriate to check serum thyroid, androgen, and prolactin hormone levels.

If O.T. is interested in contraception it will be important to choose the method that is safest for her in the context of her medical conditions. Since O.T. has hypertension, she should probably avoid agents containing estrogen, leaving progesterone-only agents as her lone option for hormonal contraception. Initially, one might consider the use of depot medroxyprogesterone acetate (DMPA), as it is a reliable form of contraception and is associated with weight gain. However, it is associated with osteopenia and should probably be avoided in an undernourished patient with a likely history of metabolic bone disease from kidney dysfunction. For this reason oral progesterone pills alone might be the best option. She could also be counseled on the risks and benefits of an intrauterine device (IUD), since she is more than 2 years post transplant, as well as the appropriate use of barrier methods.

Overview

Prevalence and Epidemiology

The optimal treatment for eligible patients with end-stage kidney disease (ESKD) that offers improved patient survival, reduced morbidity, improved quality of life, and economic savings compared to dialysis is kidney transplantation. Pediatric kidney disease affects children of all ages, and with the various renal replacement therapies available, including dialysis and transplantation, these patients are expected to survive into adulthood. Advances in the medical and surgical care of kidney transplant recipients including the judicious use of antibiotics, the improved understanding of the immunobiology of rejection, and advances in immunomodulatory medications for the treatment of rejection and use in maintenance immunosuppression have undoubtedly played a role in the success of patient and allograft survival.

In the United States, the incidence of ESKD in children has been slowly decreasing. As of 2012, there were 7522 children between the ages of 0 and 19 with prevalent ESKD [1]. Of these children, kidney transplant was the most common modality of renal replacement therapy (5485 [72.9 %]), followed by an essentially equal distribution of hemodialysis (1138 [15.1 %]) and peritoneal dialysis (899 [12.0 %]). The number of pediatric patients living with a kidney transplant has more than doubled since 1988, with 5485 children transplanted in 2012. The first-year deceased- and living-donor transplant outcomes have steadily improved over the last 20 years. In 2011, the most recent reporting year, the first-year mortality rates for both deceased-donor (probability of graft failure 0.05 and death 0.01) and living-donor (probability of graft failure 0.04 and death 0.01) pediatric transplant recipients were the same [1].

Kidney transplantation is not a cure. The Organ Procurement and Transplantation Network (OPTN)/Scientific Registry of Transplant Recipients Annual Data Report notes that the conditional 1 year graft half-life for deceased-donor (DD) kidneys is estimated at 12 years and for living-donor (LD) kidneys it is estimated at 16 years [2]. Overall, the number of pediatric kidney transplants peaked in 2005 at 899 and remained steady at approximately 750 over the subsequent 3 years [2]. Since 2006, the number of DD transplants has exceeded the number of LD transplants; in 2013 there were 474 DD transplants and 279 LD transplants [2]. This is partly due to the implementation of allocation policy known as Share 35. This policy was implemented September 2005 and awarded pediatric priority for donors less than 35 years of age.

Pathophysiology, Risk Factors, and Transplantation Complications

The major indications for kidney transplantation in childhood are congenital abnormalities of the kidney and urinary tract (CAKUT), congenital nephrotic syndrome, polycystic diseases, and neonatal kidney injury/cortical necrosis due to thrombosis.

More than one-third of pediatric patients with ESKD have comorbidities, including cerebral palsy, heart disease, chromosomal abnormalities, a syndromic diagnosis, and developmental delay, which may adversely impact the patient's quality of life and overall prognosis following kidney transplant [1].

Post-transplantation patients are at an increased risk of allograft dysfunction, rejection, infection, bone metabolic problems, cardiovascular disease, dyslipidemia, type II diabetes, growth delay, malignancies, alteration in neurocognitive development, poor adherence to medication, and decreased quality of life. The major cause of graft loss is patient death, mainly due to complications related to cardiovascular disease, infection, and malignancy. The patient's transplant status and long-term immunosuppression can impact routine primary care issues and recommended algorithms.

Conditions Associated with Solid Organ Transplant

Hypertension

Hypertension (HTN) is quite common in kidney transplant recipients and is associated with an increased risk of graft failure. Epidemiologic studies indicate that 50–90 % of kidney transplant patients either have hypertension or are on antihypertensive medications [3]. Most recipients require two or more antihypertensive medications to achieve target BP goals. The major goals of antihypertensive therapy after transplant are to preserve kidney function and to decrease cardiovascular risk. After kidney transplantation, poorly controlled blood pressure has been shown to be an independent risk factor for cardiovascular disease (CVD) and is also associated with an increased risk of graft failure [4].

There is no universal agreement as to the optimal BP goals in kidney transplant recipients. However, the kidney disease outcomes quality initiative (KDOQI) clinical practice guidelines on hypertension and antihypertensive agents in CKD recommend reduction of blood pressure in kidney transplant patients to less than 130/80 mmHg, with lower targets in patients with proteinuria [5]. The kidney disease: improving global outcomes (KDIGO) clinical practice guidelines for the care of the kidney transplant recipient include guidelines for the management of hypertension. These guidelines emphasize that target BPs in kidney transplant recipients should be similar to those provided by "The Seventh Report of the Joint National Committee on Prevention, Detection, Evaluation, and Treatment of High Blood Pressure" [6].

The KDIGO guidelines acknowledge that different targets should be set according to the method of BP readings—home readings versus office versus ambulatory blood pressure monitoring [7]. Home readings are usually 5–10 mmHg lower than office readings; night-time readings often 10 to 15 mmHg lower [7]. Loss of the nocturnal systolic BP dip is associated with higher left ventricular mass index, increased cardiovascular events, lower allograft function, and increased risk of allograft failure after kidney transplantation [8, 9].

Post-transplantation hypertension arises from a variety of factors. Some of these factors may have originated pre-transplant while others are related to immunosuppressive medication effects or post-transplant complications. Pre-transplant factors include increased vascular stiffness and vascular calcification. Dialysis patients have functional and structural alterations in their arterial walls leading to increased vascular stiffness. Vascular calcifications also develop in the ESKD population due to deranged calcium-phosphorus metabolism/secondary renal hyperparathyroidism. Post-transplant factors include delayed or poor allograft function, volume overload, presence of native kidneys, and transplant renal artery stenosis. Delayed graft function (DGF) is a risk factor for post-transplant hypertension. DGF results in the kidney's decreased ability to excrete sodium, which contributes to a lag in daily sodium excretion, salt and water retention, rightward shift of the pressure natriuresis curve, and an increase in blood pressure [10, 11]. Native kidneys induce hypertension via renin secretion or through increased sympathetic nerve activity. The overall prevalence of hypertension associated with native kidneys is unknown. Studies have noted that bilateral native nephrectomies in patients with resistant hypertension can lead to the improvement in BP control in most but not all patients. Native nephrectomies are not commonly performed in the recent decades, likely due to improved antihypertensive drug therapies [10, 11]. Transplant renal artery stenosis (TRAS) increases BP by activation of the renin-angiotensin-aldosterone system (RAAS), leading to systemic vasoconstriction and increase in sodium and water retention. Significant TRAS can be refractory to medical management and can contribute to unexplained worsening of allograft function [10, 11].

The immunosuppressive medications most often used in transplant, especially CNIs and prednisone, can potentiate hypertension. CNIs, the mainstay in the prevention of allograft rejection, cause widespread arterial vasoconstriction, thereby increasing systemic vascular resistance. CNIs also cause vasoconstriction of the afferent arteriole leading to a reduction in glomerular filtration rate (GFR), thereby leading to an increase in tubular sodium reabsorption. Prednisone-induced hypertension has been attributed to the activation of free mineralocorticoid receptor promoting sodium and water retention.

All classes of antihypertensive agents can be used to lower blood pressure in kidney transplant patients. Due to the paucity of data favoring any particular antihypertensive class, both KDOQI and KDIGO guidelines do not specify any individual class of antihypertensive medication for the treatment of post-transplant hypertension. When selecting a particular class of antihypertensive as the initial treatment of post-transplant hypertension, it is practical to consider the presence or absence of proteinuria, diabetes mellitus, allograft dysfunction, volume overload, and risk factors for cardiovascular events. It is also important to become familiar with the interactions between antihypertensive and immunosuppressive agents. While calcium channel blockers are useful, it is important to avoid the non-dihydropyridine group, such as diltiazem and verapamil. These drugs are potent inhibitors of the cytochrome p450 system and increase CNI levels. The dihydropyridine class, nifedipine XL, amlodipine and isradipine, are often used since they do not affect GFR or electrolyte balances. They can, however, potentiate gum hyperplasia. Angiotensin converting enzyme (ACE) inhibitors and angiotensin II receptor blockers (ARBs) are useful if a patient has proteinuria, but renal function and electrolytes must be monitored as they can decrease GFR and cause significant hyperkalemia. Beta blockers such as labetalol and carvediol can be useful in diminishing headaches caused by CNIs. Diuretics are particularly effective in volume-dependent hypertension and can be useful in the setting of hyperkalemia. Alpha blockers are less commonly used due to problems with hypotension. Central agents, such as clonidine, can be used as second-line therapy, especially when compliance may be improved with use of the weekly transdermal patch form [12].

New-Onset Diabetes After Transplant (NODAT)

New-onset diabetes after transplantation (NODAT) refers to the occurrence of diabetes in previously nondiabetic persons after organ transplantation. NODAT occurs in an estimated 30 % of patients within the first 3 years after transplantation. The majority of NODAT cases appear during the first 6 months after transplantation, when patients are treated with high doses of immunosuppression. International Consensus Guidelines on NODAT were published in 2003, recommending that NODAT be diagnosed based on the American Diabetes Association (ADA) criteria for type 2 diabetes [13]. Criteria are namely hemoglobinA1C (HgA1c) $\geq$6.5 %; or fasting plasma glucose of $\geq$ 126 mg/dL; or 2 h plasma glucose level of $\geq$200 mg/dL after an oral load of 75 g of anhydrous glucose; or random plasma glucose level of $\geq$200 mg/dL plus the presence of symptoms.

NODAT is associated with increased morbidity, mortality, and healthcare costs. Besides the traditional risk factors for type 2 diabetes mellitus (age, obesity, family history, and ethnicity), hepatitis C virus infection and the exposure to immunosuppressive agents, specifically CNIs and corticosteroid, increase the risk for NODAT [14]. Recipients that develop NODAT are not only at risk for the complications associated with diabetes itself but they are also at an increased risk for graft-related complications such as rejection, graft loss, infection, and vascular complications [4, 14, 15]. Current immunosuppressive regimens rely heavily on the use of agents that have been identified as being diabetogenic, such as corticosteroids, CNIs, and mammalian target of rapamycin inhibitors (mTOR) [4]. Corticosteroids increase hepatic gluconeogenesis, the development of insulin resistance, and defective insulin secretion. CNIs, which have been shown to be superior to cyclosporine in regards to patient and graft-survival, impose a higher risk of promoting the development of diabetes in solid organ transplant recipients. CNIs reduce glucose-stimulated insulin release in a dose-related and reversible manner, without affecting insulin resistance. Data also suggest that CNIs are directly toxic to the pancreatic β(beta)-cells [16, 17]. It should be noted that mTOR inhibitors are also diabetogenic, especially if combined with CNIs [18]. Although the mechanism is not yet completely understood, the use of mTOR inhibitors leads to hypertriglyceridemia-related peripheral insulin resistance and impaired pancreatic β(beta)-cell response [19]. Based on animal and human data, rapamycin appears to induce an insulin secretion defect and impairs β(beta)-cell survival and proliferation [20].

The management of a transplant recipient with NODAT is best accomplished with a multidisciplinary team approach among the PCP, transplant subspecialist, endocrinologist, and dietician. The targets for treatment are the same as for all diabetic patients with sufficiently intensive treatment to maintain normal or near-normal glycemia with a HgA1c lower than 7.0 %. The choice of glucose-lowering agent should take into account the desired level of glucose control, potential drug–drug interactions, and renal function. It is important to note that the majority of kidney transplant recipients with a well-functioning allograft have some degree of CKD. A stepwise approach to the treatment of NODAT is recommended. In consultation with the transplant subspecialist, consideration should be given to modifying the patient's immunosuppressive regimen to reverse or ameliorate diabetes, after weighing the potential adverse effects including the risk of rejection. It is also critical to address modifiable risk factors including weight control, diet, and exercise. For those patients still not at target after such interventions, it is appropriate to initiate medical therapy: initially monotherapy with an oral hypoglycemic agent taking into account patient-specific factors, renal function, side effects, and potential drug–drug interactions with the patient's immunosuppressive regimen. If monotherapy is insufficient in achieving glucose control, one should proceed to combination therapy, adding another hypoglycemic agent with different mechanisms of action. When oral hypoglycemic medications fail to reach glycemic control targets, insulin therapy should be considered.

When selecting the medications used to treat NODAT, it is always important to take into account the patient's renal and hepatic function and assess for possible drug interactions with the patient's immunosuppressants and other medical therapies. Concern for lactic acidosis has limited the use of metformin in kidney transplant recipients. However, there are recent reports suggesting benefit from metformin therapy in patients with mild to moderate CKD. Caution is recommended in using metformin with appropriate dose adjustment based on the estimated GFR (eGFR) and close laboratory monitoring of renal function and electrolytes. There are various recommendations regarding metformin dosing in renal impairment. The ADA proposes the following: For those patients whose renal function has decreased below an eGFR of 45 mL/min/1.73 m^2, metformin must be avoided and that other classes of oral agents should be considered; for those with an eGFR greater than 45 mL/min/1.73 m^2, metformin can be used but renal function must be monitored closely—the interval depending on the level of renal dysfunction [12, 21]. Of the sulfonylureas, glipizide is the preferred agent in patients with impaired renal function; it is primarily converted to inactive metabolites and less likely to cause hypoglycemia than other sulfonylureas. Other classes such as DDP-4 inhibitors can be used in adjusted doses for patient with eGFR less than 30 mL/min/1.73 m^2. Thiazolidinediones (TZDs) such as pioglitazone and rosiglitazone can be used without need for renal clearance adjustment. However, they must be avoided in patients with heart failure. In addition, TZDs have been linked to decreased bone formation, accelerated bone loss, and increased risk for fractures. They must be used with caution in patients with CKD and metabolic bone disease. Other agents such as α(alpha)-glucosidase inhibitors, amylin analogs, and meglitinides can be used at somewhat lower levels of renal function but have less potent blood sugar lowering effect. Liraglutide is a popular GLP-1 agonist injectable that has been associated with weight loss. It is currently not listed as having recommendations for renal or hepatic adjustment. However, when combined with CNIs it can increase risk of renal toxicity. Finally, one should remember that insulin is the safest of the medications used for transplant-associated diabetes with the fewest drug interactions [12, 22].

Cardiovascular Disease and Dyslipidemia

Atherosclerotic cardiovascular disease is the leading cause of mortality and death-censored graft loss after transplantation. The annual rate of fatal or nonfatal CVD events is 3.5–5.0 % in kidney transplant recipients, a rate 50-fold higher than the general population [7]. Kidney transplantation is known to reduce mortality compared with dialysis; studies suggest that this effect may be due to the reduction in cardiovascular risk associated with the improvement in kidney function. The reason for this observation is unknown. Specific risk factors for post-transplantation CAD include age, male gender, hypertension, cardiovascular event prior to transplantation, longer pre-transplant time on dialysis, post-transplant diabetes mellitus, use of corticosteroids, lower serum albumin post-transplant, and higher triglyceride levels post-transplant [23].

Dyslipidemia is often a complication of the use of immunosuppressive drugs. Patients treated with corticosteroids and CNIs can have adverse lipid profiles with elevated LDL and reduced HDL. Sirolimus can also contribute to moderate-to-severe hypercholesterolemia and hypertriglyceridemia. Dyslipidemia can contribute to the patient's preexisting elevated cardiovascular risk profile. In 2009, the KDIGO Working Group did not find new guidelines or systematic reviews since the KDOQI Dyslipidemia Guidelines were published in 2004 [24]. Therefore, the KDIGO working group recommendations include screening with a serum lipid panel for all adult and adolescent kidney transplant recipients, 2–3 months after transplantation, 2–3 months after change in treatment or onset of other conditions known to cause dyslipidemia, and at least annually thereafter. The working group further recommends treating adults to a goal LDL <100 mg/dL and non-HDL <130 mg/dL and adolescents to a goal LDL <130 mg/dL and non-HDL <160 mg/dL.

HMG-CoA reductase inhibitors (statins) are widely used in kidney transplant recipients given their established benefits in the general population. A 2009 systematic review noted that statins did not decrease all-cause mortality but were associated with a significant reduction in total cholesterol, low-density lipoprotein (LDL) cholesterol, and triglycerides levels [25]. Although there are drug–drug interactions that must be monitored in kidney transplant recipients, the use of statins is generally safe. All statins appear to be effective in lowering LDL and total cholesterol with little evidence to support recommending one agent over another. Atorvastatin, simvastatin, pravastatin, and fluvastatin have all been used in studies of kidney transplant recipients. In the assessment of lescol in renal transplantation (ALERT) study, a large placebo-controlled trial, fluvastatin effectively lowered LDL cholesterol to a goal of <100 mg/dL and also demonstrated a 30 % decreased risk in fatal and nonfatal cardiac events [26].

Certain drug interactions should be taken into consideration when using statins in kidney transplant recipients. The hepatic metabolism of statins is affected by concurrent use of CNIs, which increases the risk of rhabdomyolysis. It is important to remain mindful of additional medications that can increase CNI levels (azole antifungals, macrolides, and diltiazem) and magnify the risk of liver toxicity and rhabdomyolysis. Serum transaminase levels and CNI drug levels should be monitored closely when initiating a statin, and serially monitored once stable drug dosing has been achieved.

Bone Mineral Density and Osteoporosis

While many complications of ESKD may be reversed by transplantation, bone and mineral disturbances may persist. Bone disease is common in transplant recipients with multiple factors involved in its pathogenesis. Rates of bone loss are greatest in the first 6–18 months after kidney transplantation and range from 4–9 % at the spine and 5–8 % at the hip [27, 28]. There are numerous contributing factors, but the main factors include preexisting renal osteodystrophy at the time of renal transplantation, transplant-specific therapies, and reduced GFR. In kidney transplant recipients, osteopenia can also be influenced by long-term hemodialysis, age, heredity, gender, exercise habits, and the presence of diabetes mellitus.

Chronic kidney disease-mineral and bone disorder (CKD-MBD) is the most complex pre-transplant bone disease. One or more types of bone disease may be present including low-turnover bone disease states (osteomalacia or adynamic bone disease), osteitis fibrosa cystica due to secondary hyperparathyroidism, osteoporosis, and mixed bone disease (see Table 17.1) [27].

Bone biopsy studies have revealed that the low-turnover bone conditions osteomalacia and adynamic bone disease are the two most common bone disorders seen in kidney transplant recipients.

The risk for fracture after kidney transplant is approximately 2–3 % per patient per year with 7–10 % of all renal transplant patients suffering 1 or more fractures over their lifetime [29, 30]. Hypercalcemia is also common post-kidney transplant and is considered to result from parathyroid hormone (PTH)-induced osteoclast activation and bone resorption. The dominant clinical adverse bone events following transplantation include bone loss, fractures, osteonecrosis, and bone pain. An analysis of 68,814 patients reported to the United States renal data system (USRDS) revealed that 22.5 % of kidney transplant recipients developed a fracture within 5 years [31]. Given the extent of the problem, various screening tools have been suggested to mitigate risk. Strategies include routine measurement of parathyroid hormone, 25-hydroxy vitamin D, and bone mineral density (BMD) assessment by dual-emission X-ray absorptiometry (DEXA).

BMD screening with DEXA is currently recommended for all women who are older than 65 years of age and postmenopausal women who are younger than 65 years of age with one or more additional risk factors for osteoporosis. Densitometry testing is recommended for transplant recipients on the basis of the assumption

Table 17.1 Different types of bone disease seen in kidney transplant recipients

Type of bone disease	Characteristics
Low turnover	
Adynamic	Reduced bone volume and mineralization is paralleled by a decrease in bone formation Few osteoid seams and few osteoblasts Osteoclasts can be low, normal, or high
Osteomalacia	Accumulation of unmineralized matrix Decrease in mineralization precedes or is more pronounced than the inhibition of collagen deposition
High turnover	
Hyperparathyroid	Marked increase in bone turnover Irregularly shaped trabecules with numerous abnormal remodeling sites Unusually high number of bone cells with irregular arrangement and shape
Mixed renal osteodystrophy	Caused by defective mineralization with or without increased bone formation and increased parathyroid hormone (PTH) activity in bone Bone volume is variable and depends on dominant pathogenic cause Increased numbers of heterogeneous remodeling sites Typically an increase in osteoclasts

that data from the general population are pertinent to this cohort. Fractures resulting from osteoporosis typically involve the lumbar spine or hip. However, fractures in the transplant population frequently include the non-axial skeleton (hips, long bones, ankles, feet), supporting the hypothesis that post-transplant bone disease is not a simple form of osteoporosis.

The kidney disease improving global outcomes (KDIGO) Working Group summarizes key observations about the utility of various screening strategies. KDIGO notes: (1) no randomized clinical trials in kidney transplant recipients have examined bone-specific therapies on patient-level outcomes, including mortality or fractures; (2) low bone mineral density in non-kidney transplant recipients predicts fractures but data are scant for kidney transplant recipients; (3) there are insufficient data to suggest any bone-specific therapies after the first year of transplant; (4) treatment with calcium, calcitriol, or vitamin D analogs and/or bisphosphonates has been suggested to improve bone density in kidney transplant recipients; (5) reports of the use of bisphosphonates indicate therapy is associated with improvements in bone density without being adequately powered to note improvements in patient survival or fracture [7].

A major factor in the pathogenesis of post-transplant bone disease is immunosuppressive therapy. Glucocorticoids are commonly used in most maintenance immunosuppressive regimens and in the event of allograft rejection. The highest glucocorticoid-associated rates of bone loss are in the first 6 months after transplantation. Glucocorticoids reduce bone formation by decreasing osteoblast replication, differentiation, and increasing apoptosis [32]. They also promote osteopenia and calcium loss. Additional mechanisms include reduced gonadal hormone production, decreased calcium absorption from the gut, decreased insulin-like growth factor 1 (IGF-1) production, and diminished PTH sensitivity [32–35]. The CNIs cyclosporine and tacrolimus have also been linked to osteoporosis. Both direct and indirect effects of these medications influence bone resorption. Cyclosporine is thought to cause bone loss through direct effects on osteoclasts and by indirectly acting on T-cell function. Tacrolimus inhibits T-cell activation and proliferation and cytokine gene expression. Though rat studies have demonstrated that tacrolimus leads to bone loss, skeletal effects in humans are not well studied [36]. Less intense bone loss has been noted in patients on tacrolimus, probably due to the fact that tacrolimus allows for lower doses of glucocorticoids to be used.

Therapeutic options for post-transplantation bone disease focus on glucocorticoid avoidance or withdrawal, as well as use of vitamin-D analogs, calcium supplementation, calcimimetics, and bisphosphonates. The rational for minimizing glucocorticoid use relates to its established risks of osteoporosis and avascular necrosis. Studies have noted beneficial effects on BMD after early tapering of prednisolone. A 2012 study analyzed both the USRDS and scientific registry of transplant recipients (SRTR) databases to assess whether early corticosteroid withdrawal after kidney transplant would result in lower fracture risk [37]. With adjustment for multiple covariates, investigators found that corticosteroid withdrawal was associated with 31 % fracture risk reduction while fractures requiring hospitalization were also significantly reduced. For patients with persistent hyperparathyroidism, options include vitamin D analogs, cinacalcet, and surgery. PTH levels usually decline rapidly during the first 3–6 months post-transplantation due to the reduction in functional parathyroid gland mass. Persistently elevated levels of serum PTH can lead to complications such as soft tissue calcification, hypophosphatemia, and hypercalciuria. During the first months following transplantation 1,25-dihydroxy vitamin D levels are low due to the action of glucocorticoids, reducing the 1-alpha-hydroxylase activity. In this case, it is recommended to administer cholecalciferol to replace the substrate to calcitriol. Cinacalcet is a calcimimetic drug licensed for the treatment of secondary hyperparathyroidism in patients with ESKD. It is often used off label in patients with persistent hyperparathyroidism after transplantation. It has been demonstrated that this drug is effective in mitigating high PTH levels post-kidney transplantation with no adverse effects on renal function [38]. In a 2004 blinded study, transplant recipients who received calcium and the vitamin D analog calcitriol were shown to have attenuation of bone loss and an increase BMD when compared to transplant recipients receiving calcium alone [39]. There was also no hypercalcemia or decrease in renal function in either study group, though the study did not evaluate for the beneficial or harmful effects of therapy on fracture rate, hospitalization, or mortality [39]. Numerous studies have shown that bisphosphonates are effective in preventing bone loss when used early after transplantation. They may also help improve bone density when used late in the setting of established bone loss. Despite the positive effect on bone density, there are concerns with the use of bisphosphonates, particularly given the issues regarding renal safety, the unknown effects on fracture rates, and the potential exacerbation or induction of adynamic bone disease. Most transplant nephrologists agree that bisphosphonate therapy should be limited to patients who have a particularly high risk of fracture. Ideally in these kidney transplant patients, adynamic bone disease should be excluded by bone biopsy prior to the administration of bisphosphonate therapy. Several different treatment regimens have been shown to improve bone density, including daily or weekly oral therapy, or even intermittent intravenous administration. An individualized approach is necessary for the prevention of post-transplantation bone loss.

Hyperuricemia and Gout

In the general population, hyperuricemia is defined as >6 mg/dL. The risk of developing gout increases twofold for every incremental increase in serum uric acid of 1 mg/dL. Because of gender differences and the absence of detailed information in kidney transplant recipients, KDIGO defines hyperuricemia as >6 mg/dL in women and >7 mg/dL in men. Monitoring and management of hyperuricemia in kidney transplant patients is important due to the increased incidence of gout in addition to the association with loss of kidney function and cardiovascular disease. Hyperuricemia is a common metabolic problem in kidney transplant recipients and is exacerbated by the use of CNIs that impair renal uric acid secretion, use of diuretics, and impaired renal function. Cyclosporine has been associated with an even greater risk of hyperuricemia and gout than the CNI tacrolimus. The annual incidence of gout is 0.5 % for patients with hyperuricemia (7–8.9 mg/dL) and increases exponentially to 4.9 % for patients with serum uric acid levels of >9 mg/dL [40]. The American College of Rheumatology (ACR) guidelines recommend a target serum uric acid level of <6 mg/dL at a minimum in all patients and <5 mg/dL in more severe or complicated cases [41]. KDIGO guidelines reiterate the recommendation of a treatment threshold of <5 mg/dL in kidney transplant patients. In the general population, there is evidence that modifications that decrease risk include weight loss, low purine diet (reduced meat and alcohol consumption), and avoidance of diuretics. Some antihypertensive drugs such as amlodipine and losartan are reported to have a uricosuric effect.

Treatment of asymptomatic hyperuricemia is not generally recommended in the general population or in kidney transplant recipients. However, it is advocated in patients with recurrent symptomatic episodes of gout, tophi, uric acid stones, or radiographic changes of gout. Several therapeutic classes are available. Xanthine oxidase inhibitors, including allopurinol and febuxostat, reduce the production of uric acid by inhibiting xanthine oxidase. Allopurinol dosing is dependent on renal function and should not be used in conjunction with azathioprine due to the risk of severe myelotoxicity. This potentially life-threatening adverse drug–drug interaction results from an increased concentration of 6-mercaptopurine (the active metabolite of azathioprine), which is metabolized by xanthine oxidase [40]. If used together, azathioprine should be reduced by at least 50 %, and frequent complete blood counts should be used to monitor the interaction. Febuxostat has the same mechanism of action as allopurinol. However, since it is a nonpurine analog, it can be used in patients who have had hypersensitivity reactions to allopurinol [29]. While febuxostat does not require renal dose adjustment, caution is advised when used in the presence of severe renal dysfunction (eGFR < 30 mL/min/1.73 m^2) or hepatic disease. Uricosuric agents, such as probenecid and sulfinpyrazone, are not recommended in transplant recipients due to their ineffectiveness in patients with poor renal function (eGFR < 30 mL/min/1.73 m^2) and reports of drug–drug interactions with cyclosporine and mycophenolate mofetil. They are also contraindicated in patients with a history of renal calculi and low urine volume <1500 mL/day.

The ACR recommends the use of non-steroidal anti-inflammatory drugs (NSAIDs), colchicine, or corticosteroids for acute gout in patients without significant renal impairment [41]. These agents are to be used cautiously in kidney transplant patients. Acute gout flares respond to increased doses of oral steroids and colchicine, NSAIDs, and cyclooxygenase-2 inhibitors, however, high doses of these agents are required for uricosuric effect. At high doses these agents can lead to impaired glomerular perfusion, hyperkalemia, and increased sodium retention contributing to hypertension. In conjunction with CNIs there can be additional escalation in acute kidney injury, hyperkalemia, and hypertension due to vasoconstriction. Colchicine is an effective and rapidly acting anti-inflammatory agent. However, it may be poorly tolerated due to the increased likelihood of diarrhea when used in conjunction with immunosuppressant drugs. Toxic effects on muscle tissue have been reported in patients with decreased renal function <50 mL/min/1.73 m^2. Without dose adjustment, kidney transplant recipients are at high risk of experiencing adverse drug effects of colchicine, including myelotoxic effect and myopathy in patients receiving a combination of cyclosporine and colchicine [40]. Serum levels of colchicine are increased by several drugs such as clarithromycin, voriconazole, fluconazole, diltiazem, verapamil, ritonavir, grapefruit juice, and cyclosporine. Corticosteroids' primary anti-inflammatory mechanism of action is the inhibition of nuclear factor xB (NF-xB) via tumor necrosis factor-α(TNF-alpha) or interleukin 1b (IL-1beta) [40]. Corticosteroids are commonly used in kidney disease and kidney transplant patients for the treatment of acute gout attacks. Issues to consider when using them are exacerbation of hypertension, hyperglycemia, impaired wound healing, and rebound gout attack when tapering dosages to prior maintenance immunosuppressive dose.

In summary, as a result of overproduction and undersecretion of uric acid, hyperuricemia and gout are common conditions in the kidney transplant population. Important considerations in the implementation of treatment are impaired organ function and the numerous drug interactions. It is reasonable to consider implementing treatment for asymptomatic hyperuricemia with a serum uric acid level >9 mg/dL. However, the standard prophylactic regimen recommended by the ACR utilizing NSAIDs and colchicine may not be feasible in kidney transplant recipients. The choice of prophylaxis and treatment regimens should be made in consultation with the patient's transplant nephrologist.

Special Transplant Drug Interactions and Long-Term Adverse Effects

During the first-year post-transplant, a typical drug regimen for a recipient consists of 8–10 medications on average. The necessity for polypharmacy increases the potential for serious drug interactions. Interactions affecting drug metabolism are common and typically involve the cytochrome P-450 system. With the increasing number of new agents on the market, it remains challenging for physicians to recognize potential drug interactions without the assistance of pharmacists. Therefore, the information in this section should by no means be considered all-inclusive. We recommend the provider consider discussing the addition of any new medication in a transplant recipient with the transplant center. A list of commonly used classes of

Table 17.2 Common maintenance immunosuppressive medications in transplantation [4, 12, 13, 42]

Class	Agent	Mechanism of action	Adverse side effects
Calcineurin inhibitors (CNI)	Tacrolimus, cyclosporine	Inhibit calcineurin phosphatase and T-cell activation ***Metabolized by cytochrome P450 IIA (CYP3A)***	Tacrolimus: pancreatic islet cell toxicity, neurotoxicity (insomnia, tremor, delirium), alopecia, hyperkalemia, hypomagnesemia Cyclosporine: gingival hyperplasia, hirsutism, tremor, hypertension, hypercholesterolemia, hyperkalemia, hypomagnesemia, hyperuricemia/gout
Mammalian target of rapamycin (mTOR) inhibitors	Sirolimus, everolimus	Inhibit Interleukin-2 induced T-cell proliferation ***Metabolized by cytochrome P450 IIA (CYP3A)***	Nephrotoxicity when used in combination with CNIs; de novo proteinuria, impaired wound healing and dehiscence, hypertriglyceridemia, mucositis, leukoencephalopathy, embryotoxic and fetotoxic
Antimetabolites	Mycophenolate mofetil (MMF), mycophenolic acid (MPA), azathioprine (AZA)	Prevents proliferation of both T & B cells	MMF and MPA: Diarrhea, Leukopenia, Teratogenic AZA: Myelosuppression, hepatic dysfunction, pancreatitis

immunosuppressive medications used in solid organ transplant patients is found in Table 17.2 [4, 12, 13, 42].

A number of drugs interact with immunosuppressants either pharmacodynamically or pharmacokinetically, potentially altering the efficacy and safety of immunosuppressive drugs (see Table 17.3) [12, 14, 21, 42]. Drugs that induce or compete with the cytochrome P450 enzyme system can dramatically increase or decrease the blood concentrations of immunosuppressants. Such alterations place the transplant recipient at risk of under-immunosuppression and rejection or enhanced side effects due to drug toxicity.

Reproductive Health and Fertility

Most female patients have a rapid recovery of normal menstrual cycles after receiving their solid organ transplant. Thus, it is important to discuss the need for contraception and planning for a healthy pregnancy when the time is right to conceive as well as protection from sexually transmitted infections.

Contraception

When selecting contraceptive methods, one should generally consider the effectiveness of the method, relative contraindications in relation to the timing of patient's transplant, and any other comorbidities, such as hypertension or diabetes [43]. The most effective contraceptives are in the long-acting reversible contraceptives (LARC) group, which consist of intrauterine devices (IUDs) and sub-dermal implants. The second most effective class includes the combined hormonal contraceptives (oral contraceptive pills [OCPs], transdermal patch, or intravaginal ring), and injectable DMPA, followed by the progestin-only pill. The final tier consists of barrier methods such as condoms, diaphragm, cervical caps, fertility awareness, and withdrawal [43].

When discussing the relative safety of a contraceptive method, it should be compared to the risks of an unplanned pregnancy. One can refer to the US Centers for Disease Control (CDC) adaptation of the World Health Organization (WHO) United States medical eligibility criteria (USMEC) for contraceptive use (see Table 17.4).

Table 17.3 Selected medications and their interactions with calcineurin inhibitors and mTOR inhibitors [12, 14, 21, 42]

Class	Agent	Major interactions	Side effects
Calcineurin Inhibitors (CNI)	Tacrolimus, Cyclosporine	Drugs that INCREASE blood levels by inhibition of cytochrome P450: • Antibiotics: clarithromycin, erythromycin, azithromycin[a] • Antifungals: ketoconazole, fluconazole, itraconazole, voriconazole • Antiretrovirals: protease inhibitors, especially ritonavir • Calcium channel blockers: verapamil, diltiazem, nicardipine, nifedipine, Amlodipine[a] • Histamine blockers: ranitidine, cimetidine • Hormones: oral contraceptives, anabolic steroids, testosterone analogs, danazol • Others: amiodarone, allopurinol, bromocriptine, carvedilol, cisapride, conivaptan, HMG-CoA reductase inhibitors, metoclopromide, theophylline • Herbals: grapefruit juice, goldenseal, herbal teas (e.g., camomile), Pomegranate juice, schisandra Drugs that DECREASE blood levels by induction of cytochrome P450: • Antibiotics: cephalosporins, imipenem • Antituberculous drugs: Rifabutin, Rifampin, Oxcarbazepine, Isoniazid • Anticonvulsants: Barbiturates, Carbamazepine, Phenytoin • Others: Bosentan, Cholestyramine, Cinacalcet, Sevelamer, Ticlopidine • Herbals: St. John's Wort	Acute Kidney Injury Hypertension Vasoconstriction Thrombotic microangiopathy (TMA) Sodium retention Edema Hyperkalemia Hypomagnesemia Hyperuricemia Hyperlipidemia New-onset diabetes Alopecia Gingival hyperplasia Rhabdomyolysis/Myotoxicity when used in conjunction with HMG-CoA reductase inhibitors
Mammalian target of Rapamycin (mTOR) Inhibitors	Sirolimus, Everolimus	Use of the following are Contraindicated: Clarithromycin, Ketoconazole, Mifepristone, Rifabutin, Rifampin, Voriconazole Share the same metabolism by CYP450 system as CNIs, therefore mTORs have similar interactions with calcium channel blockers,	Potentiation of CNI nephrotoxic effects De novo proteinuria/Nephrotic syndrome Impaired healing Hypertriglyceridemia Interstitial pneumonia Teratogenic

(continued)

Table 17.3 (continued)

Class	Agent	Major interactions	Side effects
		antifungals, anticonvulsants, antituberculous agents, noted above.	
Antimetabolites	Mycophenolate mofetil (MMF), Mycophenolic acid (MPA)	Major interactions • Hematologic/Myelosuppressive—Azathioprine (hematologic toxicity), Hydroxychloroquine, Acyclovir, Ganciclovir • Increase drug level of MMF and MPA—Amoxicillin • Reduce Absorption of MMF and MPA—Antacids, cholestyramine, sevelamer	Diarrhea Nausea/emesis Leukopenia Progressive multifocal leukoencephalopathy (PML) Congenital malformations
	Azathioprine (AZA)	Major interactions Hematologic/Myelosuppressive—Allopurinol	Myelosuppression Nausea/emesis Hepatic dysfunction Pancreatitis

Cautions This table is not a complete list of potential drug interactions. Interaction data refers to systemic drug forms of immunosuppressants. Refer to drug references and transplant pharmacist for assistance on specific agents and for further details on potential interactions

[a]The interaction with these medications is usually minimal

This was adapted in 2010 and includes recommendations for patients who have been solid organ recipients within the last 2 years, when they are at highest risk for complications [44, 45]. The guidelines were developed in four different categories based on the balance of potential risk of pregnancy and benefits of contraception.

For women with uncomplicated transplants, in the first 2 years following their transplant, every contraceptive method is considered a Category 2, indicating that the benefits of contraception generally outweigh the risks [45]. A complicated transplant, defined as graft failure, graft rejection, or cardiac allograft vasculopathy, places the patient in the higher risk Category 4. For these women, estrogen-containing contraceptives that increase the risk of coagulation and thromboembolism are effectively contraindicated. IUD initiation, in the first 2 years following transplant, is considered a category 3 (risks outweighs benefit but still safer than pregnancy), whereas continuation of an IUD is considered Category 2 and can remain safely in place. Estrogen-containing agents remain contraindicated in conditions such as venous thromboembolic disease, hypertension, or diabetic nephropathy. In these conditions, progesterone-only agents are the safest option. Previous concerns about IUDs being contraindicated in transplant patients have been disproven. In a review of >200 solid organ transplant patients who used an IUD, only two had report of method failure and there were no cases of increased risk of pelvic infection

Table 17.4 United States medical eligibility criteria for contraceptive use

United States medical eligibility criteria for contraceptive use	
Category 1	Condition for which there is no restriction for the use of contraceptive method
Category 2	A condition for which the advantages of using the method generally outweighs theoretical or proven risks
Category 3	A condition for which the theoretical or proven risks usually outweighs the advantages of using the method
Category 4	A condition that represents an unacceptable risk if the contraceptive method is used

or tubal infertility [45]. In addition, concerns about increased risk for infection due to IUD have not been born out with other immunocompromised populations, such as women with human immunodeficiency virus (HIV). Combined OCPs are reasonable contraceptive choices and tend to offer good menstrual cycle control. Several small studies in renal and liver transplant patients have not shown increased risk for rejection, although some women require adjustment to their antihypertensive regimen. The fact that OCPs are easily available and familiar to most women must be weighed with their higher failure rate compared to LARC.

DMPA carries a black box warning concerning the bone effects of this agent with long-term use. When counseling transplant patients regarding DMPA, the benefits of decreased bleeding and efficacy should be balanced with theoretical risk to bone health, especially in women younger than 25 years of age who may still be building bone. Emergency contraception is considered a Category 1 in all medical conditions since it is a 1-time dose of hormonal contraception. The current methods of emergency contraception consist of the progestin levonorgestrel (LGN), the selective progesterone receptor modulator (SPRM) ulipristal, and the urgent placement of a copper IUD.

Pregnancy

The recommended time interval between transplant surgery and conception should be at least 12 months and individualized according to the patient's general health, completion of antiviral prophylaxis, and establishment of stable immunosuppression level and graft function [44]. The patient should not be taking teratogenic medications such as mycophenolate, azathioprine, or other Category D medications. Although transplant pregnancies are generally successful, outcomes differ from the general population in terms of prenatal survival rates, indicating that these pregnancies remain high risk in spite of good allograft function. Pregnancy outcomes after kidney and liver transplantation in the United States show a significant increase in the risk of major obstetrical complications including pre-eclampsia, preterm delivery, and low birth weight. Data from a 2014 study revealed the mean gestational age at birth was 35 weeks in transplant recipients, shorter than the national average of 39 weeks. The mean live birth weight for recipients was less at 2485 grams versus 3358 grams [46]. For lung and cardiac transplant recipients, the risk of pre-eclampsia was 18 % (higher than the 7 % in healthy nulliparous women). Lung transplant patients have a high rate of rejection during and after pregnancy and a 5 year mortality rate of 50 %. A number of associated factors such as age, parity, chronic hypertension, or renal disease determine the risk of pregnancy complications, including miscarriage and gestational diabetes, and are probably more important factors than the type of transplant [46].

Cancer

Solid organ transplant recipients have a twofold to threefold increased risk of developing cancer compared to the general population [47]. The risk of developing cancer is most likely multifactorial due to the type of organ transplanted, the immunosuppressant regimen, exposure to oncogenic viruses—Epstein–Barr virus (EBV), human papillomavirus (HPV), and human herpesvirus-8 (HHV-8)—and environmental factors. There are three proposed oncogenic mechanisms by which immunosuppression can increase cancer risk: direct pro-oncogenic property of the immunosuppressant, increased risk of oncoviral driven malignancy, and impaired immune surveillance of neoplastic cells [47]. Cyclosporine, tacrolimus, and azathioprine exert direct effects on cells that promote cancer while mTOR inhibitors and MMF show anti-proliferative effect and decrease cancer risk [47]. Post-transplant cancers can be arbitrarily divided into de novo, donor-related, and recurrent cancers. De novo cancers include non-melanoma skin cancer, post-transplant lymphoproliferative disorder (PTLD), and anogenital cancers, as they are new tumors that develop away from the transplanted organ. Donor-related cancers may be transmitted by the donor organ or may originate within the transplant graft. Recurrent cancers recur from pre-transplant malignancies such as hepatocellular carcinoma and cholangiocarcinoma [47].

Non-melanoma skin cancer is the most common post-transplant malignancy, with an increased incidence up to 250-fold compared to non-transplanted individuals [47]. Squamous cell carcinoma (SCC) is the most common, followed by basal cell, Merkel cell, and Kaposi sarcoma. Post-transplant SCCs are biologically aggressive and often multicentric with a tendency to recur locally in >10 % of patients and leading to metastatic disease in 5 % of patients. PTLD is the second most common malignancy in adults. It is predominantly B cell in origin, accounting for 85–90 % of cases, with many of these being associated with EBV. The remaining 10–15 % are T cell in origin and are usually EBV negative [47]. The greatest risk is in the first-year post-transplant and is affected by host risk factors such as degree of immunosuppression, viral infections, age of the recipient, and type of allograft. PTLD is highest among individuals receiving intestinal transplants (20 %) and lowest for individuals receiving liver/kidney transplants (1–5 %). The relative risk of non-Hodgkin lymphoma (NHL) is elevated eightfold compared to the general population. It can be divided into early disease (a gift from the donor) or late disease, which occurs beyond the second year of transplant. Use of cyclosporine and azathioprine increases risk for NHL.

Hodgkin lymphoma is raised fourfold in transplant recipients. Both Hodgkin lymphoma and NHL are more aggressive than in immunocompetent patients [48].

The next most common group of cancers are the anogenital cancers, which make up <3 % of cancers but again are 100-fold more common in the immunosuppressed population [47]. They are twice as common in females as male patients and have about a 7 year latency from transplant. HPV-related lesions can arise despite a pre-transplant HPV-negative status. HPV-positive renal transplant recipients have 14-fold higher risk for cervical cancer, 50-fold higher risk for vulvar cancer, and 100-fold greater risk for anal carcinoma [47]. Patients with predisposing chronic conditions are at increased risk for developing cancer. Patients with primary sclerosing cholangitis and ulcerative colitis with liver transplants are at an increased risk for cholangiocarcinoma and colon cancer. Patients with renal, liver, and heart transplants are at greater risk of developing renal cell carcinoma, though they are typically small asymptomatic lesions with a favorable surgical prognosis.

Due to the significant increased risk of skin and anogenital cancers, it is recommended that transplant patients have annual skin examinations. Immunosuppressed females should have annual cervical/pelvic examination and not be liberalized to an every 3 or 5 year pap testing strategy [45].

Except for patients with history of ulcerative colitis, there is no change in the recommendations for screening for breast, colon, or prostate cancer in the transplant population. Although lung cancer is increased from 1.4- to 5.4-fold compared to the general population, there is currently no change in the selection criteria of patients to screen for lung cancer.

Conclusion

Solid organ transplant recipients represent a growing population of medically complex patients for whom outcomes are optimized through a well-coordinated plan of care delivered by a multidisciplinary team ("Appendix"). Though much of this care is directed by transplant subspecialists, PCPs have several critical roles to fulfill. PCPs should be familiar with the diagnosis and treatment goals of common comorbid conditions associated with solid organ transplant as well as commonly used immunosuppressive agents and their associated toxicities and drug–drug interactions. PCPs should also address the sexual and reproductive health of patients and be familiar with cancer screening guidelines for transplant patients. Finally, PCPs should help support young adults with solid organ transplants navigate challenges while transitioning to adult-centered care systems.

Appendix

Solid organ transplant fact sheet

Definition	The replacement of a nonfunctioning solid organ such as kidney, liver, or heart with an organ obtained by donation from another individual. It can be either cadaveric or living donor. The individual must remain on immunosuppressant regimen in order to avoid rejecting the organ
Epidemiology	The number of pediatric patients living with a kidney transplant has more than doubled since 1988 with 5485 children transplanted in 2012. The first-year deceased- and living-donor transplant outcomes have steadily improved over the last 20 years
Pathophysiology	The type of solid organ, and whether it is a first or second transplant, often predicates the intensity of the immunosuppressant regimen used The immunosuppressants are from several classes: • Calcineurin inhibitors (tacrolimus, cyclosporine) • Mtor inhibitors (sirolimus, everolimus) • Steroids (prednisone) • Anti-metabolite (mycophenlic acid, mycophenolate and azathioprine) • Costimualtory blocker (Belatacept)—kidney transplantation only
Sequelae of original disease	Poor growth Metabolic bone disease Association with syndromes affecting other organ systems: • Alagille syndrome • Alport syndrome May have some degree of developmental delay associated with underlying disease or complicated treatment course Recurrence of original disease (systemic lupus erythematosus)
Sequelae of immunosuppressant regimen	Infection Increase risk of metabolic disorders: • Diabetes • Hyperlipidemia • Gout • Osteoporosis Hypertension Increased risk for cardiovascular disease Increased risk for kidney dysfunction Increased risk for cytopenias Increased for malignancies: • Dermatologic • Aerodigestive • Vulvar • Post-transplant lymphoproliferative disorder
Medication interaction	Must always adjust for decreased function of the transplanted organ Always evaluate interaction with immunosuppressant regimen
Challenges in transition	Some centers have reported increased risk of graft rejection and loss when transitioning from pediatric to adult providers Adult providers are less familiar with some of the underlying pediatric syndromes
Helpful Resources	CDC contraception 2010 application (app) download for smartphones

CDC Centers for Disease Control

References

1. US Renal Data System (USRDS). USRDS 2014 Annual Report: Atlas of Chronic Kidney Disease and End Stage Renal Disease in the United States. Bethesda, MD: National Institutes of Health, National Institute of Diabetes and Digestive and Kidney Diseases; 2014.
2. Matas AJ, Smith JM, Skeans MA, Thompson B, Gustafson SK, Stewart DE, et al. OPTN/SRTR 2013 annual data report: kidney. Am J Transplant. 2015;15 (Suppl 2):1–34.
3. Kasiske BL, Anjurn S, Shah R, Skogen J, Kandaswamy C, Danielson B, O'Shaughnessy E, et al. Hypertension after kidney transplantation. Am J Kidney Dis. 2004;43(6):1071–81.
4. Pedraza F, Roth D. Medical management of the kidney transplant recipient. Prim Care Clin Office Pract. 2014;41(4):895–906.
5. K/DOQI clinical practice guidelines on hypertension and antihypertensive agents in chronic kidney disease. Am J Kidney Dis 2004;43:S1–S290.
6. Chobanian AV, Bakris GL, Black HR, Cushman W, Green L, Izzo J, Jones D, et al. The seventh report of the joint national committee on prevention, detection, evaluation, and treatment of high blood pressure: the JNC 7 report. JAMA. 2003;289:2560–72.
7. Kidney Disease: Improving Global Outcomes (KDIGO) Transplant Work Group. KDIGO Clinical Practice Guideline for the Care of Kidney Transplant Recipients. Am J Transplant. 2009;9(Suppl 3):S1–S157.
8. Toprak A, Koc M, Tezcan H, Ozener IC, Oktay A, Akoglu E. Night-time blood pressure load is associated with higher left ventricular mass index in renal transplant recipients. J Hum Hypertens. 2003;17:239–44.
9. Ibernon M, Moreso F, Sarrias X, Grinyo J, Fernandez-Real J, Ricart W, Seron D. Reverse dipper pattern of blood pressure at 3 months is associated with inflammation and outcome after renal transplantation. Nephrol Dial Transplant. 2012;27:2089–95.
10. Lakkis J, Weir MR. Treatment-resistant hypertension in the transplant recipient. Semin Nephrol. 2014;34 (5):560–70.
11. Wadei HM, Textor SC. Hypertension in the kidney transplant recipient. Transplant Rev. 2010;24:105–20.
12. Lexicomp Online®. Hudson, Ohio: Lexi-Comp, Inc.; April 04, 2016.
13. Davidson J, Wilkinson A, Dantal J, Dotta, F, Haller, H, Hernandez, D, Kasiske, B, et al. International Expert Panel. New-onset diabetes after transplantation: 2003 international consensus guidelines. Proceedings of an international expert panel meeting Barcelona, Spain, 19 February 2003. Transplantation 2003;75(10, Suppl):SS3–SS24.
14. Padiyar A, Akoum FH, Hricik DE. Management of the kidney transplant recipient. Prim Care Clin Office Pract. 2008;35(3):433–50.
15. Schaefer HM. Long-term management of the kidney transplant recipient. Blood Purif. 2012;33:205–11.
16. Soleimanpour SA, Crutchlow MF, Ferrari AM, Raum JC, Groff DN, Rankin MM, et al. Calcineurin signaling regulates human islet (beta)-cell survival. J Biol Chem. 2010;285:40050–9.
17. Ajabnoor MA, El-Naggar MM, Elayat AA, Abdulrafee A. Functional and morphological study of cultured pancreatic islets treated with cyclosporine. Life Sci. 2007;80:345–55.
18. Flechner SM, Glyda M, Cockfield S, Grinyó J, Legendre Ch, Russ G, et al. The ORION study: comparison of two sirolimus-based regimens versus tacrolimus and mycophenolate mofetil in renal allograft recipients. Am J Transplant. 2011;11:1633–44.
19. Galindo RJ, Fried M, Breen T, Tamler R. Hyperglycemia management in patients with post-transplantation diabetes. Endocr Pract. 2016;22 (4):454–65.
20. Barlow AD, Nicholson ML, Herbert TP. Evidence for rapamycin toxicity in pancreatic β-cells and a review of the underlying mechanisms. Diabetes. 2013;62:2674–82.
21. Lipska KJ, Bailey CJ, Inzucchi SE. Use of metformin in the setting of mild-to-moderate renal insufficiency. Diabetes Care. 2011;34(6):1431–7.
22. Ghisdal L, Van Laecke S, Abramowicz MJ, VanHolder R, Abramowicz D. New-onset diabetes after renal transplantation: risk assessment and management. Diabetes Care. 2012;35(1):181–8.
23. Vanrenterghem YF, Claes K, Montagnino G, Fieuws S, Maes B, Villa M, et al. Risk factors for cardiovascular events after successful renal transplantation. Transplantation. 2008;85:209–16.
24. Kasiske B, Cosio FG, Beto J, Bolton BM, Chavers R, Grimm R, Levin A, et al. Clinical practice guidelines for managing dyslipidemias in kidney transplant patients: a report from the managing dyslipidemias in chronic kidney disease work group of the national kidney foundation kidney disease outcomes quality initiative. Am J Transplant. 2004;4(Suppl 7):13–53.
25. Navaneethan SD, Perkovic V, Johnson DW, Nigwekar SU, Craig JC, Strippoli GF. HMG CoA reductase inhibitors (statins) for kidney transplant recipients. Cochrane Database Syst Rev. 2009;2: CD005019.
26. Holdaas H, Fellstrom B, Jardine AG, Holme I, Nyberg G, Fauchald P, Gonhagen-Riska C, et al. Effect of fluvastatin on cardiac outcomes in renal transplant recipients: a multicenter, randomized, placebo-controlled trial. Lancet. 2003;361(9374):2024–31.
27. Ebeling PR. Approach to the Patient with Transplantation-Related Bone Loss. J Clin Endocrinol Metab. 2009;94:1483–90.
28. Ebeling PR. Transplantation osteoporosis. Curr Osteoporos Rep. 2007;5:29–37.
29. Nisbeth U, Lindh E, Ljunghall S, Backman U, Fellstrom B. Increased fracture rate in diabetes mellitus and females after renal transplantation. Transplantation. 1999;67(9):1218–22.

30. Abbott KC, Ogelsby RJ, Hypolite IO, Kirk AD, Ko CW, Welch PG, et al. Hospitalizations for fractures after renal transplantation in the United States. Ann Epidemiol. 2001;11(7):450–7.
31. Nikkel LE, Hollenbeak CS, Fox EJ, Uemura T, Ghahramani N. Risk of fractures after renal transplantation in the United States. Transplantation. 2009;87(12):1846–51.
32. Canalis E, Mazziotti G, Giustina A, Bilezikian JP. Glucocorticoid-induced osteoporosis: pathophysiology and therapy. Osteoporos Int. 2007;18(10):1319–28.
33. Kuroki Y, Kaji H, Kawano S, Kanda F, Takai Y, Kajiwaka M, et al. Short-term effects of glucocorticoid therapy on biochemical markers of bone metabolism in Japanese patients: a prospective study. J Bone Miner Metab. 2008;26(3):271–8.
34. Guistani A, Mazziotti G, Canalis E. Growth hormone, insulin-like growth factors, and the skeleton. Endocr Rev. 2008;29(5):535–9.
35. Mazziotti G, Giustina A. Glucocorticoids and the regulation of growth hormone secretion. Nat Rev Endocrinol. 2013;9(15):265–76.
36. Epstein S. Post-transplantation bone disease: the role of immunosuppressive agents and the skeleton. J Bone Miner Res. 1996;11(1):1–7.
37. Nikkel LE, Mohan S, Zhang A, McMahon DJ, Boutroy S, Dube G, et al. Reduced fracture risk with early corticosteroid withdrawal after kidney transplant. Am J Transplant. 2012;12:649–59.
38. Bergua C, Torregrosa JV, Fuster D, Gutierrez-Dalmau A, Oppenheimer F, Campistol JM. Effect of cinacalcet on hypercalcemia and bone mineral density in renal transplanted patients with secondary hyperparathyroidism. Transplantation. 2008;86:413–7.
39. Josephson MA, Schumm LP, Chiu MY, Marshall C, Thistlethwaite JR, Sprague SM. Calcium and calcitriol prophylaxis attenuates post transplant bone loss. Transplantation. 2004;78:1233–6.
40. Sullivan PM, William A, Tichy EM. Hyperuricemia and gout in solid-organ transplant: update in pharmacological management. Prog Transplant. 2015;25(3):263–70.
41. Khanna D, Fitzgerald JD, Khanna PP, Bae S, Singh MK, Neogi T, Pillinger MH, et al. 2012 American College of Rheumatology guidelines for the management of gout. Arthritis Care Res. 2012;64(10):1431–61.
42. Danovitch GM. Handbook of kidney transplantation. 5th ed. Philadelphia: Lippincott Williams & Wilkins; 2010.
43. Krajewski CM, Geetha D, Gomez-Lobo V. Contraceptive options for women with a history of solid-organ transplantation. Transplantation. 2013;95(10):1183–6.
44. Josephson MA, McKay DB. Women and Transplantation: fertility, sexuality, pregnancy, contraception. Adv Chronic Kidney Dis. 2013;20(5):433–40.
45. Krajewski C, Sucato G. Reproductive health care after transplantation. Best Pract Res Clin Obstet Gynaecol. 2014;28:1222–34.
46. Brosens I, Brosens J, Benagiano G. The risk of obstetrical syndromes and solid organ transplantation. Best Pract Res Clin Obstet Gynaecol. 2014;28:1211–21.
47. Katabathina V, Menias CO, Pickhardt P, Lubner M, Prasad S. Complications of immunosuppressive therapy in solid organ transplantation. Radiol Clin N Am. 2016;54:303–19.
48. Grulich AE, Vajdic CM. The epidemiology of cancers in human immunodeficiency virus infection and after organ transplantation. Semin Oncology. 2015;42(2):247–57.

Spina Bifida

18

Ellen Fremion, Jonathan Tolentino, Rose Khavari and Julie N. Stewart

Case Presentation

Roxanne is a 19-year-old Latina female with mid-lumbar spina bifida (SB), a ventriculoperitoneal (VP) shunt, and neurogenic bowel and bladder who presents to establish primary adult care. She uses a manual wheelchair in the community and crawls at home. She was previously cared for by a pediatric SB multisubspecialty clinic and general pediatrician. For neurogenic bladder care, her mother performs clean intermittent catheterization (CIC) through the urethra. Roxanne lacks dexterity to catheterize independently. Despite CIC every 4 h, she has urinary incontinence. She was hospitalized for a urinary tract infection (UTI), elevated blood pressure, and acute kidney injury (AKI) 6 months prior. Her bowel regimen is to have timed bowel movements on the toilet every 2–3 days. Her stools are hard and she has fecal incontinence 1–2 times per week. Roxanne graduated from high school but is not attending college or working. During high school, her grades were borderline passing, and she had particular difficulty with math. She has undergone adult disability determination and receives supplemental social security income and Medicaid. She dresses and bathes independently, but she needs help with cooking, household chores, money management, and transportation. She is often anxious and worries about discrimination in future job environments because she has difficulty with her bowel and bladder management and uses a wheelchair. She has never dated or been sexually active, but she would like to be married, have children, and live independently.

Case Discussion

Roxanne's elevated blood pressure and recent AKI are concerning. Individuals with SB have a higher prevalence of prehypertension and

E. Fremion (✉)
Department of Internal Medicine and Pediatrics, Baylor College of Medicine, 6620 Main St Suite 1250, Houston, TX 77030, USA
e-mail: Ellen.Fremion@bcm.edu

J. Tolentino
Department of Pediatrics, Stony Brook University, HSC Level 11, Room 040, 101 Nicolls Road, Stony Brook, NY 11794-8111, USA
e-mail: Jonathan.Tolentino@stonybrookmedicine.edu

R. Khavari · J.N. Stewart
Department of Urology and Restorative Pelvic Medicine, Department of Internal Medicine, Houston Methodist Hospital, 6560 Fannin St. Suite 2100, Houston, TX 77030, USA
e-mail: rkhavari@houstonmethodist.org

J.N. Stewart
e-mail: jnstewart2@houstonmethodist.org

M. Pilapil et al. (eds.), *Care of Adults with Chronic Childhood Conditions*,
DOI 10.1007/978-3-319-43827-6_18

hypertension than the general population due to renal scarring, obstructive uropathy, and obesity [1–3]. Thus, patients with SB presenting with hypertension should have: (1) review of their bladder management including medications and catheterization regimens, (2) chemistry and renal function labs, (3) a renal/bladder ultrasound to evaluate the renal size as well as monitor for hydronephrosis and nephrolithiasis, and (4) a urology evaluation including urodynamics to measure bladder pressure and evaluate for vesicoureteral reflux.

Upon review of Roxanne's labs (see Box 18.1), she has a high normal potassium level and an elevation in her creatinine from baseline. These lab findings along with the finding of hydronephrosis and decreased size of the left kidney are concerning for acute or chronic obstructive uropathy leading to renal damage. Because urodynamics showed small volume, high pressure bladder, and severe ureter reflux, bladder augmentation is indicated (see urology section). Given her difficulty with catheterizing due to dexterity and mobility impairment, a catheterizable abdominal channel for bladder management and Malone antegrade colonic enema (MACE) procedure would be good options to increase her independence.

Box 18.1

Labs Na 138, K 5.0, Cl 110, CO2 18, BUN 13, Cr. 0.9 (previous baseline 0.5 a year ago)

Renal/Bladder US left kidney length 7.8 cm, with decreased echogenicity and hydronephrosis.

The right kidney is 9.8 cm with normal echogenicity. The bladder was small sized with a thickened wall. Debris and possible stone were seen in the bladder.

Video urodynamics small bladder capacity 100 ml (typical adult is 400–500 ml), detrusor overactivity, high bladder pressures >40, stress urinary incontinence, and severe reflux to the left kidney.

In regard to her mental health and social concerns, depression and anxiety are common and often undertreated in SB [4, 5]. Roxanne's frustration that she was not able to do more things independently is a common concern among SB patients. She felt nervous around new people because she had often been bullied at school about her physical impairments and incontinence. Roxanne should be referred to counseling and occupational therapy to help her gain confidence and independent living skills. Once Roxanne's acute medical needs are addressed, she will be better able to manage her bowel and bladder regimens. Referral to vocational rehabilitation to assess her vocational abilities and help with job placement would be highly beneficial to Roxanne. This would enable her to learn about her rights as a person with a disability in the workplace from the Americans with Disabilities Act, including her right to have wheelchair accessible facilities and the necessary modifications to do her self-care at work. She would have the opportunity to practice how to communicate her needs with her employer and coworkers with a family and vocational coach. (For additional information regarding disability rights, please see Chap. 28.)

Overview

SB is the most common neural tube defect (NTD) and is due to failure of the spinal neural tube to close at 25–28 days postconception [6]. An estimated 1500–2000 babies with SB are born in the United States annually with the highest incidence in the Latino population [7, 8]. Approximately 166,000 people in the United States have SB, with the majority being adults [9]. There are 3 SB types: (1) *occulta*, in which there is a cleft in the vertebral bodies with closed skin; (2) *meningocele*, where the meninges protrude through the vertebral cleft with no neural elements; and (3) *myelomeningocele* (MMC), in which the spinal cord and neural elements are exposed through the vertebral cleft. Spina bifida occulta requires no repair and rarely has associated neuromuscular deficits. Meningoceles often can be repaired without neurologic complications. MMCs are the most common lesion and most often referred to as "spina bifida." MMCs are repaired a few days after birth, though some pediatric centers also offer prenatal repairs [10]. Approximately 65–85 % of infants with MMC have hydrocephalus and require a ventricular shunt placement [11, 12]. The majority of individuals with SB have gait impairment and bladder and bowel dysfunction. Neurocognitive ability ranges from no impairment to severe/profound intellectual disability. The degree of impairment usually correlates with MMC level and especially with the presence of hydrocephalus [13]. Other spinal dysraphisms with similar sequelae that are often followed by SB specialists include: caudal regression, lipomyelomeningoceles, lipomyeloceles, and congenital tethered cord. SB is classified by functional level: *thoracic* (flaccid lower extremities), *high lumbar* (hip flexion present), *mid lumbar* (knee extension present), *low lumbar* (dorsiflexion present), and *sacral* (foot plantar flexion present) [11]. The level of function guides expectations for neurocognitive, motor, and organ system comorbidities [14]. About 75–94 % of people with SB survive to adulthood [15]. Common causes of death for adults with SB include sepsis, renal failure, cardiopulmonary failure, and shunt complications [14, 16–18].

Etiology

The etiology of SB, as with all NTDs, is multifactorial, having both genetic and environmental components. Defects in genes regulating neuropore closing, the folic acid metabolic pathway and nucleotide synthesis, and deoxyribonucleic acid (DNA) repair are thought to be responsible for NTDs, but the exact mechanism is not known [6]. Environmental risk factors include maternal hyperthermia, environmental contaminants (pesticides, contaminated water, hazardous waste), and nutritional factors (folic acid deficiency and high intake of high-glucose foods) [19, 20]. Maternal obesity and folic acid deficiency have emerged as consistent risk factors for NTD [13]. A daily dose of 400 mcg of folic acid, a multivitamin, and a healthy, folate-rich diet are recommended for all women of reproductive age as primary prevention [16, 21, 22]. Women who are at high risk for NTDs (those who have a NTD, have had a child with NTD, or have a family history of NTD) are recommended to take at least 4 mg of folic acid 2–3 months prior to conception, during pregnancy, and for 4–6 weeks postpartum or while breastfeeding [23].

Transition from Pediatric to Adult Care

A multisubspecialty clinic associated with an urban academic hospital is the most common model of care for pediatric patients with SB, but adult clinics that specialize in SB care are rare [24, 25]. Research regarding best practices for adults with SB is limited. Young adults with SB need: (1) adult providers who are welcoming and familiar with the management of their condition; (2) care coordination to ensure insurance coverage, subspecialty care, supplies, and equipment; (3) support for self-management and community engagement (education, employment, transportation, independent living, and day activities); (4) general adult health care; and (5) chronic SB management [26–28]. To facilitate these care needs, patients may require the following adult providers: neurosurgery (may only need to follow for acute concerns), pulmonology (for sleep apnea or restrictive lung disease evaluation), urology (for neurogenic bladder management, preferably a neurourologist), physiatry (for equipment selection, spasticity, pain, and mobility management), orthopedics (for scoliosis and limb deformity), obstetrics and gynecology (for pelvic floor health and well woman care), and social work (for community, funding, and vocational resources). Other care needs include equipment (for wheelchairs, orthotics, crutches, lifts, and shower chairs) and supplies (such as catheters, bowel management equipment, and protective undergarments).

Office Visit Considerations

Given the various degrees of ambulation among people with SB, it is important to standardize height, weight, and body mass index (BMI) measurement. For those patients who are ambulatory, height should be measured with a standiometer with shoes/braces off. For nonambulatory individuals, arm length should be measured using a meter/yard stick from middle finger tip to middle finger tip across the laryngeal prominence (Adam's apple). An estimate of patient height can then be made using arm span-to-height ratio formulas: multiply the arm span length (cm) by 0.95 for individuals with mid-lumbar SB and 0.90 for those with high lumbar/thoracic SB [29]. If the patient is able to stand unsupported, weight should be measured without orthotics on a regular scale. Patients who are wheelchair-dependent should be weighed in the wheelchair on a wheelchair accessible scale and then subtract the wheelchair weight. As many people with SB are allergic to latex, latex-free exam gloves should be used. A large exam room and an exam table that can lower to the ground are helpful for patients who use wheelchairs. Extra pillows for the exam table can help make positioning more comfortable, especially if severe scoliosis is present. Patients should be asked for both permission and guidance on how to assist them before assiting with their wheelchair, exam table positioning, transfers, and clothing adjustments.

Specific Care Considerations for Adults with Spina Bifida by Organ System

Adults with SB should have general adult screenings for: (1) reproductive function and sexually transmitted infections, (2) metabolic syndrome (including hypertension, elevated blood sugar, obesity, abnormal cholesterol), (3) mental health, and (4) cancer based on age and risk factors [30]. In addition to these general health needs, patients with SB have condition-specific care needs as will be reviewed in this section.

Neurocognitive Concerns

There is significant variance in the neurocognitive ability of people with SB. Socioeconomic, demographic, and central nervous system (CNS) structural impairments contribute to the neurocognitive profile. Namely, individuals with shunted hydrocephalus, higher MMC lesions, and Latino ethnicity tend to have more difficulty with reading and math, lower intelligence quotient (IQ), and lower adaptive skills [31]. Relative strengths for the population include language fluency and carrying out established routines. Relative weaknesses are inferencing, learning new routines, problem solving, and fine motor skills [32, 33]. Language fluency may mask deficits in comprehension. Knowing the neurocognitive tendencies for people with SB can help providers develop strategies for patient self-management and care plans. Simple written instructions, phone alarm reminders, follow-up calls, patient teaching by nursing and/or home health providers, and frequent follow-up appointments can facilitate engagement in care and plan implementation. Intellectual ability, adaptive function, and executive function testing can help direct educational, employment, and independent living. Adult insurances may not cover neurocognitive testing, but vocational rehabilitation programs may be able to provide testing or results of previous testing may be obtained from high school records.

Neurological Concerns

Unique neurological comorbidities for SB include ventricular shunts, tethered cord, Chiari II malformations (CM II), and syringomyelia/hydromyelia.

Ventricular Shunts

Ventriculoperitoneal shunts drain cerebral spinal fluid (CSF) into the peritoneal cavity. More rarely, ventricular shunts may drain into the pleural space or right ventricle. Programmable shunts control the flow of CSF. If a patient has a programmable shunt, then neurosurgery must be consulted to manage the shunt before and after magnetic resonance imaging (MRI) is performed. Patients who have a shunt should receive pneumococcal 13-valent conjugate (PCV-13) and pneumococcal 23-valent polysaccharide (PPSV23) vaccines in accordance with Centers for Disease Control (CDC) guidelines for patients who have a CSF leak [34]. Shunt revisions are more common during childhood, and some adults may no longer be shunt-dependent [35]. Nevertheless, shunt failure and infections can occur in adulthood, which may result in catastrophic complications if not emergently managed [36]. Symptoms of shunt malfunction include severe headache, fever, vomiting, visual changes, and lethargy [36, 37]. More subtle findings include decreased concentration, decreased work or school performance, and changes in lower extremity or urologic function [37]. If there is a concern for shunt malfunction, an emergent head computed tomography (CT) scan without contrast and shunt series X-ray should be performed. If dilated ventricles are found, immediate neurosurgery evaluation is required. Some individuals with shunt malfunctions may have no change in ventricular size [38]. If symptoms are not otherwise explained, a neurosurgeon familiar with shunt management should be consulted.

Tethered Cord

Clinically significant cord tethering is less common in adulthood but can occur. Tethered cord is due to scar tissue or lipomeningocele causing tension on the spinal cord, usually at the level of the myelomeningocele repair. Triggers for tethered cord include trauma, heavy lifting, and vaginal childbirth [36, 39]. Signs of tethered cord include severe back pain, worsening lower extremity weakness and/or decreased sensation, worsening neurogenic bladder symptoms with resultant urodynamic changes, and rapidly progressive scoliosis or foot deformity [36, 39, 40]. If these clinical findings are present, an MRI (with and without contrast) should be ordered and neurosurgery consulted. The progression, acuity, and severity of symptoms should guide urgency of evaluation. Untethering can help restore neurologic function in symptomatic patients, but surgical complications can occur, including CSF leak, infection, worsening bowel/bladder or neurological function, and decreased mobility [41]. If tethered cord is seen on imaging but the patient is asymptomatic, watchful monitoring is an accepted approach, but neurosurgical evaluation can be considered [41].

Chiari II Malformation

CM II is the downward displacement of cerebellar and brainstem structures into the foramen magnum. Varying degrees of CM II are almost universally present in patients with MMC, but many may be asymptomatic [42, 43]. CM II compression symptoms include occipital headache, neck pain, diplopia, nystagmus, dysphagia/aspiration, dysphonia, stridor, apnea, upper limb paresis and hypertonia, loss of dexterity, and gait instability [43, 44]. The onset can be a rapid deterioration over a couple of days or an insidious decline. Patients can have recurrent symptoms after cervical decompression due to abnormal hindbrain brain development [43]. Other diagnoses can present with CM II symptoms such as shunt malfunction, hydromyelia, syringomyelia, and tethered cord [43]. MRI is the best study to evaluate CM II, but if MRI is not possible, high-resolution CT scan with sagittal reconstructions can be used [45].

Syringomelia and Hydromyelia

Syringomelia (cystic cavitation in the spinal cord parenchyma) and hydromyelia (enlargement of the central spinal canal) occur in 25–45 % of patients with SB, and of these, 60 % may be symptomatic [46]. Syringomelia/hydromyelia symptoms are similar to tethered cord and can coexist with tethered cord. Syringobulbia is a cavity in the cervicomedullary junction and can present with symptoms similar to CM II. If clinical suspicion exists, it is recommended to obtain an MRI spine for evaluation and correlate imaging with clinical findings [46]. Symptomatic patients should be promptly referred to neurosurgery.

Ophthalmologic Concerns

Eye findings associated with SB include strabismus, nystagmus, and optic atrophy [47]. These abnormalities are predominately seen in individuals with hydrocephalus, higher MMC lesions, and multiple shunt revisions [48]. Annual dilated eye exams and assessment of strabismus are recommended. New onset strabismus or nystagmus are concerning for shunt malfunction and hydrocephalus or CM II compression. In these instances, imaging of the brain should be performed.

Cardiopulmonary Concerns

Congenital heart defects are not associated with SB, but many adults have risk factors for cardiovascular disease (CVD) including hypertension, obesity, and metabolic syndrome [2, 49, 50]. Prehypertension and hypertension are associated with diabetes, previous bladder procedures, and renal dysfunction [2]. It is important for primary care providers (PCPs) to regularly monitor blood pressure and weight, screen for hyperlipidemia and diabetes, and counsel on a healthy diet and exercise. General adult guidelines for screening and management of CVD risk factors should be followed.

Pulmonary complications associated with SB are likely under described. Decreased pulmonary function and respiratory muscle weakness are associated with higher SB lesions and more severe scoliosis. Even with reduced vital capacity, many individuals may be functionally asymptomatic [50]. The incidence of sleep-disordered breathing (SDB) is likely under recognized. Individuals with SB are at risk for central or obstructive sleep apnea as well as central hypoventilation syndrome due to CM II, diminished respiratory muscle function, kyphoscoliosis, and obesity [51]. SDB symptoms such as breathing difficulties and apnea may be more common than snoring or daytime sleepiness [52]. Positive pressure therapy can improve central and obstructive apnea and hypopnea [52]. Patients with significant central apnea may warrant CM II decompression. Patients with SB are more likely to have respiratory complications, pneumonia, respiratory insufficiency, prolonged mechanical ventilation, and pulmonary embolism postoperatively [53]. Patients should be screened for SDB and restrictive lung symptoms. Sleep studies and pulmonary function tests for patients with severe CM II, thoracic SB, and severe kyphoscoliosis should be considered, especially preoperatively. Caution should be taken with sleep aids, benzodiazepines, and pain medications that may suppress respiratory function.

Gastrointestinal Concerns

Neurogenic bowel concerns include: (1) constipation due to impaired peristalsis and infrequent voiding, (2) difficulty evacuating stool due to impaired rectal reflex, and (3) incontinence due to impaired anal sphincter tone and voluntary control. Fecal incontinence is a major barrier to quality of life and socialization [54, 55]. With regimen compliance, 70–90 % of patients have bowel accidents less than once per month, (see Table 18.1) [56–58]. Most bowel regimens start with oral laxatives, fiber, and/or a rectal stimulating agent with timed toileting. Secondly, retrograde colonic enema (RCE) using a cone enema or anal irrigation system (Peristeen®, Coloplast Corp., Minneapolis, MN) may be used. A cone enema is a plastic cone tip attached with tubing to a bag of fluid with approximately 20 mL/kg of water or saline (maximum amount is 500 mL). The cone is held in the rectum and while the fluid fills the colon. The cone is then removed, allowing the patient to evacuate into the toilet. Patients with thoracic or high lumbar lesions may have difficulty holding the cone in place and balancing on the toilet. Anal irrigation system (Peristeen®) may offer patients more independence and continence, as it has a balloon

Table 18.1 Neurogenic bowel assessment and management for individuals with SB

Assessment	Rationale	Treatment options
Stool amount	Approximately 12–18″ of stool per day is needed for adequate emptying	Use stool softener, ± motility agent, abdominal massage, and/or rectal stimulating agent (suppository, mini-enema, digital stimulation)
Stool consistency Goal = Bristol 4	Hard balls (Bristol 1) = slow motility	• Bowel prep cleanout may be needed prior to starting regimen if inadequate bowel movement (BM) for >5 days. • Increase water intake, fruits and vegetables, fiber (15–30 g/day), and/or add stool softener (polyethylene glycol, lactulose, docusate, milk of magnesia) • May also need a motility agent like bisacodyl or senna (effective in 6–8 h)
	Oatmeal (Bristol 5–6) = increased motility and/or need for bulking	• Consider bulking agent such as fiber (methylcellulose may cause less gas than other agents) Decrease foods that increase motility: greasy, spicy, some fruit/vegetables, and beans
Anal sphincter tone	If good tone, likely to respond to rectal stimulating agent	• Docusate mini-enema can help to initiate BM in 10–20 min, though some patients may prefer suppository or rectal colonic enema (RCE)
	If poor tone, may be difficult to attain fecal continence without 1–2 BMs daily. May be difficult use RCE	• Schedule toileting 1–2 times daily with mini-enema • If failure to achieve continence refer for Malone antegrade colonic enema (MACE)
Bowel timing	Timed BMs decrease accidents, improve compliance with regimen. Ideal regimen duration is 30–45 min	• Toilet timing 15–30 min postprandial maximizes gastrocolonic reflex • Schedule toileting in relationship to routine activities such as showering • Bowel motility and rectal stimulating agents may shorten duration
Mobility	Review ability to enter bathroom, transfer, and balance on the toilet	• Consider ordering a bedside commode, bath chair to put around toilet, or recommending installing handles around toilet
Goals for bowel regimen	1. Bowel movement every 1–2 days, of adequate amount 2. Maximize independence and compliance 3. Goal regimen time 30–45 min or less 4. No unpredictable accidents	• Start with stool softener ± motility agent with timed toileting • May need to start with rectal medication to initiate BMs • If not at goal with titrating oral and rectal medications and timing, consider RCE or referral for MACE

Adapted from [58]

that inflates around a catheter inserted into the rectum, similar to the cone enema [59]. If the rectal vault is dilated, patients may not be able to use an RCE due to difficulty forming a seal around the cone or balloon, in which case surgical options may be pursued. Surgical options include creation of a stoma for Malone antegrade continence enema (MACE) or colostomy. A MACE offers 90 % continence and independence [59]. For a MACE, a neurourologist or colorectal surgeon creates a continent channel from the terminal ileum or the appendix that connects the cecum and abdominal wall. To perform the MACE evacuation, a catheter attached to a 1000 mL kangaroo bag with water or saline (approximately 20 mL/kg, up to approximately 500 mL) is inserted in the stoma while the individual sits on the toilet. The bowel is flushed from the cecum to the rectum, a process that takes approximately 30–45 min and needs to be repeated every 1–2 days in order to achieve continence.

Bladder and Pelvic Floor Concerns

Neurologic lesions associated with SB bladder innervation can impact bladder storage and emptying. Urologic problems in SB include: (1) UTIs, (2) urinary retention, (3) urolithiasis, (4) urinary incontinence, (5) deterioration of renal function, (6) pelvic organ prolapse, and (7) sexual dysfunction. Preservation of renal function, sexual function, continence, infection prevention, and independent management are the goals of urologic care.

Monitoring and Evaluation

Neurogenic bladder monitoring for SB remains controversial [60]. Most neurourologists recommend annual serum creatinine assessment and renal/bladder ultrasound to monitor for hydronephrosis, urolithiasis, and upper urinary tract concerns. Urodynamic evaluations (preferably a videourodynamic study to also assess for vesicoureteral reflux) are recommended every 2–5 years, or if new hydronephrosis, increased UTIs, or worsening incontinence is present [61]. Urodynamic studies evaluate for: (1) bladder compliance and capacity, (2) detrusor overactivity, (3) bladder neck competence, and (5) bladder emptying issues. Patients with poor bladder compliance and/or detrusor pressures more than 40 cm H_2O without leakage during bladder filling are at risk for vesicoureteral reflux and upper tract deterioration [61].

Medical Management of Neurogenic Bladder

Neurogenic bladder management often involves clean intermittent catheterization (CIC) and anticholinergic medication. CIC allows for timely bladder emptying, decreased incontinence, prevention of urinary tract infections and urolithiasis, lower bladder storage volumes, and safer pressures to protect renal function [60–65]. CIC complications (urethral injury, epididymitis, and meatitis) occur in less than 30 % [66]. However, asymptomatic bacteriuria occurs in 70 % [66]. If anticholinergics fail to increase bladder capacity and decrease pressure, intravesical botulinum toxin A injections can help decrease incontinence, increase capacity, decrease filling pressures, and increase quality of life for a mean duration of 6–7 months [67, 68].

Surgical Management of Neurogenic Bladder

When maximal medical management fails to prevent urinary upper tract deterioration or improve urinary incontinence, surgical reconstruction is recommended. Surgery may include bladder augmentation, creation of a continent catheterizable channel, and/or a bladder neck procedure. Ileocecoplasty (reconfigured portion of terminal ileum attached to the bladder) is the most common augmentation and improves compliance and capacity, preserves renal function, and minimizes incontinence. A continent catheterizable channel allows for easier access to the bladder and more CIC independence. A channel is constructed from the appendix (Mitrofanoff appendicovesicostomy procedure) [69], a transverse ileal tube (Yang-Monti) [70, 71], tapered ileum implant [72], or ileocecal valve (ileocecocystoplasty) [73, 74]. Complications are not common but may include stomal leakage or stenosis. Patients with augmentation may have a slightly higher risk for bladder cancer long term [75]. Some neurourologists recommend regular cystoscopy surveillance starting at 10 years postaugmentation, but this recommendation may lead to overmonitoring. It is reasonable to obtain a cystoscopy evaluation for patients with persistent hematuria and/or chronic UTIs [75]. Lastly, bladder outlet procedures (bladder slings, formal bladder neck closures, or artificial urinary sphincter devices) treat refractory stress urinary incontinence or urethral tract strictures and fistulae.

Pelvic Organ Prolapse

Pelvic organ prolapse (POP) is a prevalent problem in women with SB [76]. POP is the symptomatic descent of the vaginal walls, the apex (cervix/uterus) and/or vaginal vault and is staged from stage 0 (normal) to stage IV (complete prolapse) [77]. POP affects functional status, continence, and sexual function [78]. Women with SB may present with POP at a younger age (mean age 25 years), with more severe prolapse, and with symptoms including vaginal bulge, difficult intercourse, and difficult catheterization [79]. Management options include observation, pessary device, sacrocolpopexy, uterosacral ligament suspension, or sacrospineous suspension.

PCPs should monitor chronic bladder management, including catheterization regimens and incontinence; identify and initiate work up for complications such as difficulty performing catheterization and UTIs; and coordinate care with urology, including visits and supplies. Patients should see urology annually and if complications arise, including recurrent UTIs (three or more per year), difficulty performing catheterization, increased incontinence, urolithiasis, new/worsening hydronephrosis, and/or POP.

Sexual/Reproductive Issues

An estimated 24–68 % of adolescent and young adults with SB (AYASB) are sexually active [80–99]. Many report having had some sex education from school or parents, but physician-directed sex education is uncommon [85, 91, 92]. Most adolescents and young adults with SB report inadequate reproductive and sexual knowledge as issues of physical impairment, fertility, and heredity of SB are rarely addressed [93, 94]. Many AYASB desire sexual relationships and plan to get married [83, 93]. About 50 % of sexually active AYASB report being satisfied with their sexual relationships. Wheelchair dependence and incontinence are barriers to satisfactory sexual relationships [85–88, 91, 93]. Individuals with lesions at or above the lumbar 2 (L2) level are more likely to have decreased genital sensation and decreased likelihood of engaging in sexual activity, but those with lower lumbar and sacral lesions can also have sexual dysfunction [95, 96]. Routine well care for adolescents and young adults with SB should include evaluation of sexual function and individualized sex education.

Men's Health

Sexual dysfunction and infertility concerns for men with SB include difficulties with ejaculation, low sperm counts, and erectile dysfunction (ED) and are more common in high lumbar or thoracic MMC [82, 84, 87, 95–97]. Most men can achieve ejaculation and orgasm, but sometimes ejaculate may be minimal and not associated with orgasm [85]. If the internal urethral sphincter fails to contract during ejaculation, men may have retrograde ejaculation (where semen enters the bladder instead of the urethra) or bladder incontinence with ejaculation. These concerns require urological evaluation. Failure of spermatogenesis may be due to prostatitis, increased testicular temperatures, cryptorchidism, or medications such as chronic antibiotics and tricyclic antidepressants [96]. ED has been reported in up to 70–75 % of men with SB, especially for lesions above the thoracic 10 level (T10), and contributes to a lack of confidence, poor body image and difficulty maintaining intimate relationships [82, 84, 87, 95–98]. ED treatments include touch stimulation, phosphodiesterase type 5 inhibitors (long acting forms maybe more effective), penile rings, self-injection with paperverine or prostagladin E1, a vacuum constriction device, and prostheses [98, 99]. Neurourology or urologists who specialize in male sexual function can help with management.

Women's Health

Gynecologic concerns for women with SB include early menarche (on average 10–11 years); congenital reproductive tract anomalies; orthopedic abnormalities of the pelvis, spine and lower limbs; and POP [100]. Women with SB are recommended to take folic acid 4 mg 2–3 months before and during pregnancy to reduce the risk of having a baby with a NTD, although dose-related outcomes have not been studied [101]. Genetic counseling should be offered, and early management by a high-risk obstetrician can yield the best outcomes [102, 103]. Live births occur in 70–80 % of pregnancies in women with SB. Nevertheless, pregnancy complications occur including shunt problems, UTIs, problems with bowel and bladder conduits, incontinence, and constipation (see Table 18.2) [100, 102–108]. Cesarean

Table 18.2 Complications in pregnancy with spina bifida

Concern	Management	Notes
Bladder incontinence	Oral anti-cholinergics	Pregnancy category B. No evidence of impacts on fertility or fetotoxicity
Recurrent urinary tract infections (UTIs)	Increase frequency of clean intermittent catheterization (CIC) Consider prophylactic antibiotics [108]	Management of recurrent UTIs can assist in preventing miscarriage, prematurity, and low birth weight
Neurogenic bowel dysfunction	Increase fiber, fluids, and exercise Emollient laxatives (mineral oil, glycerin) Osmotic laxatives for refractory cases	Transanal irrigation is not recommended

deliveries are common due to small pelvis, hip bone abnormalities, contractures, severe kyphosis, and vertebral anomalies. Ambulatory women have had more successful vaginal deliveries compared to nonambulatory patients [107, 108].

Osteoporosis

Fracture prevalence in the pediatric population of SB is estimated around 30 %, but studies in adults are limited [109–112]. Medical comorbidities (urinary diversion, kidney disease, and use of anti-epileptics), higher MMC lesions, wheelchair use, hypercalciuria, high body fat levels, contractures, and previous fractures are significant osteoporosis risk factors [109, 110, 112–114]. The distal femur is the most common fracture site [109, 112, 113]. Concluding from sparse studies, a baseline dual energy X-ray absorptiometry (DEXA) with serum and urine calcium, 25-hydroxy vitamin D, phosphorus, and parathyroid hormone levels may be considered in patients with a previous fracture or risk factors. Limitations to using DEXA in this population include positioning due to scoliosis and/or contractures and the use of DEXA software that measures bone density of the wrists, lumbar spine, and hips when the most vulnerable sites among this population are the long bones [109, 112]. Treatment for osteoporosis in SB has not been studied, and bisphosphonate treatment remains controversial [115]. PCPs should encourage patients to take 1000 mg of calcium daily and 800 units of vitamin D daily (more may be required for deficiencies), and engage in physical activity to promote bone health [115].

Skin/Soft Tissue Concerns

Impaired ambulation, decreased sensation, and skeletal abnormalities increase the risk of pressure ulcers in individuals with SB [116–121]. Risk factors are listed in Box 18.2, with the highest risks being wheelchair use and thoracic lesion level [116, 119, 120]. The most common sites for pressure ulcers are the foot, ankle, and buttocks [119, 120]. Infected decubitus ulcers are common reasons for emergency room visits and hospital admissions [121, 122].

Box 18.2 Patients at highest risk for pressure ulcers [116, 119, 120]

- Higher lesion level
- Wheelchair Use
- Improper wheelchair seating
- Urinary incontinence
- Shunt presence
- Arnold Chiari malformation
- Above the knee orthopedic surgery
- Recent surgery
- Male sex
- Prior ulcerations
- Poorly fitting orthotics
- Obesity
- Inadequate nutrition
- Difficulty with transfers

The PCP should assess for risk factors, regularly examine high-risk areas of decreased sensation, and refer to wound care practitioners for early stage ulcers. Patients and/or families should regularly check skin for pressure changes and sores especially on the buttocks, back, lower extremities, angulation areas, and skin folds [117, 118]. Ulcers should be staged based upon the European Pressure Ulcer Grading System [123]. Management considerations are listed in Table 18.3 [123].

Infected decubitus ulcers increase the risk for osteomyelitis. Symptoms often include increased warmth, tenderness, fever, and bone pain. However, many patients with SB may not have or recognize symptoms due to decreased sensation. If concern for osteomyelitis is present, erythrocyte sedimentation rate, C-reactive protein, white blood count, and blood cultures should be obtained. X-ray imaging may show bony changes consistent with osteomyelitis, but MRI is more sensitive. If osteomyelitis is present on imaging, it is necessary to consult surgery for bone cultures and infectious disease for antibiotic plans.

Musculoskeletal Issues

General Mobility and the Use of Assistive Devices

Wheelchair and assistive device use is associated with lower activity participation, decreased quality of life, and decreased independence [124–126]. Overall, 57–60 % of individuals with SB use a wheelchair. Individuals with lesions above L2, hydrocephalus, and/or hip dislocation are likely to be wheelchair-dependent [127–130]. In individuals with lower lumbar and sacral lesions, approximately 35 % require braces and 23 % require walking aides such as walkers, forearm crutches, or canes [124]. While most adults with SB already use assistive devices, functionality may continue to deteriorate with age due to obesity, fractures, and other long-term non-musculoskeletal consequences [130, 131]. Physiatrists, physical therapists, and wheelchair clinics can help determine which assistive technology best suits a patient's mobility needs (see Box 18.3) [125, 130–132].

Box 18.3
The following information is often needed for supply orders
- Equipment needed and date of last new supplies
- Insurance coverage or other funding sources to cover equipment
- Patient's Functional Goals for home, education, employment, and community
- Physical and Functional assessment by physical therapist and/or physiatrist
- Documentation and diagnoses association needed (contact equipment company to clarify)

Table 18.3 Management of pressure ulcers

Preventative measures
- Appropriately fitting orthotics, wheelchairs, and wheelchair cushions
- Regular skin checks by patients and family of high-risk areas
- Regular PCP exams of high-risk areas
- Proper nutrition and healthy weight
- Early evaluation and management by wound care practitioners

Common treatment modalities [123]
- *Stage I or Stage II Ulcers* PCP can manage with hydrocolloid or hydrogel dressing
- *Exuding Stage II, Stage III, or Stage IV Ulcers* Co-management with wound practitioner and/or plastic surgery management. Aliginate dressing, foam dressings, honey impregnated dressing, cadexomer dressing, collagen matrix are often used
- *Recalcitrant ulcers* Comanagement with wound care and/or plastic surgeon. Treatments may include electrostimulation and negative pressure therapy
- *Infected ulcers* Comanagement with wound care and/or plastic surgeon. May use antibiotics and/or silver impregnated dressing. Consider evaluation for osteomyelitis

PCP primary care physician

Shoulder and Upper Extremity Pain

Roughly 30–33 % of adults with SB have shoulder pain, which increases in intensity and incidence with age [133]. Risk factors include manual wheelchair use and obesity [134, 135]. Non-steroidal anti-inflammatories, physical therapy, and equipment adjustment are initial therapies [135]. Rotator cuff disorders should be considered if initial therapy fails [136]. Wheelchair users can also develop wrist pain, nerve entrapment, and median nerve injury [134, 137, 138]. Initial management includes rest, ice, wrist splints, and non-steroidal anti-inflammatories [135]. Intracarpal injections and surgical decompression should be considered in more severe cases.

Hip, Knee, and Foot Deformities

Individuals with lumbar 4 (L4) level or higher lesions and severe scoliosis often have hip dislocation, which can cause chronic pain and limited mobility [139, 140]. Hip reduction surgery is often not effective and may lead to stiffness, contractures, hyperlordosis, and decreased function [141]. Foot deformities are associated with lesion level: thoracic with equinus foot (87 %), mid-lumbar with club foot (55 %), and sacral with calcaneal foot (34 %) [142]. Charcot's arthropathy (joint swelling and pain at the foot, knee, or hip) can lead to deformity, dislocation, and functional decline [143, 144]. Skeletal deformities may contribute to chronic pain, decreased mobility, and wounds. Therapies can include bracing and possibly orthopedic surgery [141].

Chronic Pain

Chronic pain from joint contractures or dislocation or secondary to assistive devices are common. The shoulder, back, wrist, hands, knees, ankle, and feet are the most common sites [145]. General chronic pain management should be followed including non-narcotic medications, physical therapy, bracing, and appropriate wheelchair sizing and mechanics. Amitriptyline, gabapentin, and pregabalin are options for neuropathic pain [146, 147].

Scoliosis

Scoliosis is present in the majority of individuals with SB especially in high lumbar and thoracic lesions [148]. Scoliosis rarely progresses in adulthood, but individuals may have had prior spinal fusion to maximize height and mobility, decrease pain, and improve forced vital lung capacity [149–154]. Nonoperative care—including trunk balance exercises, upper extremity manipulation, and orthotics—may improve or maintain function [152]. Surgery can be considered for scoliosis more than 50°, curvature with pain, or restrictive lung disease, but risks such as wound infections and nonunion of the spinal fusion should be discussed [152].

Obesity

Up to 35–50 % of adolescents and young adults with SB are obese [155]. These patients tend to have lower aerobic fitness, eat less healthy diets, and are more sedentary than their peers, putting them at greater risk for obesity, metabolic syndrome, cardiovascular disease, chronic wounds, and lymphedema [155–164]. Exercise regimens and physical therapy reduce pain, increase efficiency in wheelchair propulsion, and improve physical activity and balance [161]. Barriers to physical activity need to be addressed, including lack of motivation and time, fatigue, body image concerns, lack of knowledge about adaptive exercise, lack of facilities and programs, and weather/environmental limitations [160]. Motivation to stay healthy, improving physical appearance, maintaining physical skills, and social support promote engagement in physical activity [162].

Quality of Life

People with SB have lower quality of life (QOL) scores than the general population in physical functioning, general health, vitality, pain, and social functioning [165]. The presence of a shunt, level of spinal lesion, and decreased IQ correlate with decreased QOL [166–168]. Using a wheelchair full time, difficulty with math and reading, lower executive function skills, and pain are also associated with reduced QOL for people with SB [165–171]. On the other hand, succeeding at college, participating in recreation and sport activities, higher communication efficacy, lower stress, social support, lower parental overprotectiveness, and satisfaction with family positively correlate with QOL [171, 172]. Self-efficacy, personal hope and coping skills, parental hope, psychological stress, and role disability have been found to more strongly correlate with QOL than physical deficits [172, 173]. Thus, QOL for people with SB can be best supported by: (1) engaging them in emerging adult activities (education, employment, recreation, and relationships); (2) supporting them in adaptive skills; (3) promoting self-efficacy and a positive outlook; and (4) addressing pain, mental health, and role concerns.

Conclusion

With more than three-fourths of children born with SB surviving into adulthood, chronic condition management and preventive care for adults with SB will increasingly need to be facilitated by the adult PCP. Adult providers must be prepared to manage the psychosocial as well as medical needs of adults with SB. Adult practices planning to manage this population should prepare for facility accessibility; care coordination with adult subspecialists such as neurosurgeons, physiatrists, physical therapists, wound care, and urologists familiar with the comorbidities associated with SB; healthcare funding support; and community resources to support adaptive living ("Appendix"). The adult PCP should be comfortable recognizing shunt complications; managing and preventing basic complications of neurogenic bowel, bladder, and skin; adapting general health guidelines to individual with SB; and facilitating care coordination and self-management to optimize health and promote quality of life for adults with SB.

Appendix

Spina bifida (SB) condition fact sheet

Definition	• SB is the most common neural tube defect (NTD) and is due to failure of the spinal neural tube to close at 25–28 days postconception • SB is classified by functional level: *thoracic* (flaccid lower extremities), *high lumbar* (hip flexion present), *mid lumbar* (knee extension present), *low lumbar* (dorsiflexion present), and *sacral* (foot plantar flexion present)
Epidemiology	• An estimated 1500–2000 babies with SB are born in the United States annually, with the highest incidence in the Latino population • Approximately 166,000 people in the United States have SB, with the majority being adults • Primary prevention for SB is 4 mcg folic acid for women without SB and no family history of SB, and 4 mg for women with SB or who have a family history of SB
Special considerations	Adults with SB may have the following comorbidities • Shunted hydrocephalus • Neurocognitive impairment • Neurogenic bladder • Pelvic organ prolapse • Neurogenic bowel • Skin ulcers • Musculoskeletal concerns: scoliosis, varying levels of paralysis, contractures, foot deformities, pain • Disuse Osteoporosis • Latex allergy Adults with SB have increased risk of • Obesity • Hypertension • Anxiety/Depression • Impairment of sexual function
Recommended screening and prevention	• Annual chemistry, blood urea nitrogen/creatinine, renal/bladder ultrasound • At least annual urology visit • Regular skin exams • Evaluation of bowel and bladder regimens • Evaluation of mobility impairment and adaptive equipment need • Evaluation of adaptive supports for vocation and independent living • If shunt, administration of pneumococcal vaccines at least 1 time (Pneumococcal 13-valent conjugate vaccine followed at least 8 weeks later by pneumococcal 23-valent polysaccharide vaccine)

Parent/Caregiver Resources

- Spina Bifida Association: http://spinabifidaassociation.org/adults/
- Center for Disease Control – Spina Bifida: http://www.cdc.gov/ncbddd/spinabifida/adult.html
- International Federation for Spina Bifida and Hydrocephalus: http://www.ifglobal.org/en/
- National Institute of Neurological Disorders and Stroke/NIH: http://www.ninds.nih.gov/disorders/spina_bifida/detail_spina_bifida.htm

Suggested Reading List

- Dicianno et al. [106]
- Webb [130]

References

1. Mazur L, Lacy B, Wilsford L. The prevalence of hypertension in children with spina bifida. Acta Paediatr. 2011;100(8):e80–3.
2. Stepanczuk BC, Dicianno BE, Webb TS. Young adults with spina bifida may have higher occurrence of prehypertension and hypertension. Am J Phys Med Rehabil. 2014;93(3):200–6.
3. Veenboer PW, Hobbelink MG, Ruud Bosch JL, Dik P, van Asbeck FW, Beek FJ, de Kort LM. Diagnostic accuracy of Tc-99 m DMSA scintigraphy and renal ultrasonography for detecting renal scarring and relative function in patients with spinal dysraphism. Neurourol Urodyn. 2015;34(6):513–8.
4. Dicianno BE, Kinback N, Bellin MH, Chaikind L, Buhari AM, Holmbeck GN, et al. Depressive symptoms in adults with spina bifida. Rehabil Psychol. 2015;60(3):246–53.
5. Kabra AT, Feustel PJ, Kogan BA. Screening for depression and anxiety in childhood neurogenic bladder dysfunction. J Pediatr Urol. 2015;11(2):75.e1–7.
6. Sadler TW. Embryology for neural tube development. Am J Med Fenetic C Semin Med Genet. 2005;135C(1):2–8.
7. Parker SE, Mai CT, Canfield MA, Rickard R, Wang Y, Meyer RE, et al. Updated national birth prevalence estimates for selected birth defects in the United States, 2004–2006. Birth Defects Res A Clin Mol Teratol. 2010;88(12):1008–16.
8. Spina Bifida Fact Sheet [Internet]. Bethesda: NIH Publication; c2013. http://www.ninds.nih.gov/disorders/spina_bifida/detail_spina_bifida.htm.
9. Centers for Disease Control and Prevention (CDC). Racial/ethnic differences in the birth prevalence of spina bifida - United States, 1995–2005. MMWR Morb Mortal Wkly Rep. 2009;57(53):1409–13.
10. Adzick NS, Thom EA, Spong CY, Brock JW 3rd, Burrows PK, Johnson MP, et al. A randomized trial of prenatal versus postnatal repair of myelomeningocele. N Engl J Med. 2011;364(11):993–1004.
11. Sawin KJ, Liu T, Ward E, Thibadeau J, Schechter MS, Soe MM, et al. The National Spina Bifida Patient Registry: profile of a large cohort of participants from the first 10 clinics. J Pediatr. 2015;166(2):444–50.
12. Hunt GM. Non-selective intervention in newborn babies with open spina bifida: the outcome 30 years on for the complete cohort. Eur J Pediatr Surg. 1999;9:S5–8.
13. Barf HA, Verhoef M, Jennekens-Schinkel A, Post MW, Gooskens RH, Prevo AJ. Cognitive status of young adults with spina bifida. Dev Med Child Neurol. 2003;45(12):813–20.
14. Brei T, Kelly L. Level of Function. Washington, DC: Spina Bifida Association. http://spinabifidaassociation.org/wp-content/uploads/2015/07/HOW-SB-LESIONS-IMPACT-DAILY-FUNCTION1.pdf. Accessed November 16, 2015.
15. Liptak G, Garver K, Dosa NP. Spina bifida grown up. J Dev Behav Pediatr. 2013;34(3):206–15.
16. Dicianno BE, Wilson R. Hospitalizations of adults with SB and congenital spinal cord anomalies. Arch Phys Med Rehabil. 2010;91(4):529–35.
17. Oakeshott P, Hunt GM. Long-term outcome in open spina bifida. Br J Gen Pract. 2003;53:632–6.
18. Werhagen L, Gabrielsson H, Westgren N, Borg L. Medical complication in adults with spina bifida. Clin Neurol Neurosurg. 2013;115(8):1226–9.
19. Green N, Copp A. Neuroal tube defects. Annu Rev Neurosci. 2014;37:221–42.
20. Mitchell LE. Epidemiology of neural tube defects. Am J Med Genet C Semin Med Genet. 2005;135C(1):88–94.
21. Centers for Disease Control and Prevention (CDC). Spina bifida and anencephaly before and after folic acid mandate–United States, 1995–1996 and 1999–2000. MMWR Morb Mortal Wkly Rep. 2004;53(17):362–5.
22. Williams J, Mai CT, Mulinare J, Isenburg J, Flood TJ, Ethen M, et al. Updated estimates of neural tube defects prevented by mandatory folic acid fortification—United States, 1995–2011. Centers Dis Control Prev. 2015; 64(01):1–5. http://www.cdc.gov/mmwr/preview/mmwrhtml/mm6401a2.htm.
23. Wilson RD, Committee Genetics, Wilson RD, Audibert F, Brock JA, Carroll J, Cartier L, Gagnon A, et al. Pre-conception folic acid and multivitamin supplementation for the primary and secondary prevention of neural tube defects and other folic acid-sensitive congenital anomalies. J Obstet Gynaecol Can. 2015;37(6):534–52.

24. Clinics. Arlington, VA: Spina Bifida Association. http://spinabifidaassociation.org/clinics/. Accessed 16 Nov 2015.
25. Brei TJ. The future of the multidisciplinary clinic. ScientificWorldJournal. 2007;7:1752–6.
26. Binks JA, Barden WS, Burke TA, Young NL. What do we really know about the transition to adult-centered health care? A focus on cerebral palsy and spina bifida. Arch Phys Med Rehabil. 2007;88(8):1064–73.
27. Dicianno BE. 21st century challenges to the provision of health care to adults with spina bifida: a rehabilitation approach. Arch Phys Med Rehabil. 2014;95(9):1601–2.
28. Sawin KJ, Betz CL, Linroth R. Gaps and opportunities: an agenda for further research, services, and program development in spina bifida. Pediatr Clin North Am. 2010;57(4):1041–57.
29. Dosa NP, Foley HT, Eckrich M, Woddall-Ruff D, Liptak GS. Obesity across the lifespan among persons with spina bifida. Disabil Rehabil. 2009;21 (11):914–20.
30. USPSTF A and B Recommendations. U.S. Preventive Services Task Force; April 2016. http://www.uspreventiveservicestaskforce.org/Page/Name/uspstf-a-and-b-recommendations. Accessed 3 June 2016.
31. Fletcher JM, Copeland K, Frederick JA, Blaser SE, Kramer LA, Northrup H, et al. Spinal lesion level in spina bifida: a source of neural and cognitive heterogeneity. J Neurosurg. 2005;102(3 Suppl):268–79.
32. Dennis M, Landry SH, Barnes M, Fletcher JM. A model of neurocognitive function in spina bifida over the life span. J Int Neuropsychol Soc. 2006;12 (2):285–96.
33. Dennis M, Jewell D, Drake J, Misakyan T, Spiegler B, Hetherington R, et al. Prospective, declarative, and nondeclarative memory in young adults with spina bifida. J Int Neuropsychol Soc. 2007;13(2):312–23.
34. Centers for Disease Control and Prevention. Recommended adult immunization schedule for adults aged 19 years or older, by vaccine and age group. http://www.cdc.gov/vaccines/schedules/hcp/imz/adult.html. Accessed 3 June 2016.
35. Bowman RM, McLone DG, Grant JA, Tomita T, Ito JA. Spina bifida outcome: a 25-year prospective. Pediatr Neurosurg. 2001;34(3):114–20.
36. Piatt JH. Treatment for myelomeningocele: a review of outcomes and continuing neurosurgical considerations among adults. J Neurosurg Pediatr. 2010;6:515–25.
37. Edwards RJ, Witchell C, Pople IK. Chronic headaches in adults with spina bifida and associated hydrocephalus. Eur J Pediatr Surg. 2003;13:S13–7.
38. Rocque BG, Lapsiwala S, Iskandar BJ. Ventricular shunt tap as a predictor of proximal shunt malfunction in children: a prospective study. J Neurosurg Pediatr. 2008;1(6):439.
39. Drake JM. Occult tethered cord syndrome: not an indication for surgery. J Neurosurg. 2006;104(5 Suppl):305–8.
40. Proctor MR, Bauer SB, Scott RM. The effect of surgery for split spinal cord malformation on neurologic and urologic function. Pediatr Neurosurg. 2000;32(1):13.
41. Cardoso M, Keating RF. Neurosurgical management of spinal dysraphism and neurogenic scoliosis. Spine. 2009;34(17):1775–82.
42. McLone DG. Continuing concepts in the management of spina bifida. Pediatr Neurosurg. 1992; 18:254–6.
43. Stevenson K. Chiari Type II malformation: past, present, and future. Neurosurg Focus. 2004;16920:E5.
44. Rahman M, Perkins L, Pincus D. Aggressive surgical management of patients with Chiari II malformation and brainstem dysfunction. Pediatr Neurosurg. 2009;45:337–44.
45. Gundry CR, Heithoff KB. Imaging evaluation of patients with spinal deformity. Orthop Clin North Am. 1994;25(2):247–64.
46. Tsitouras V, Sgouros S. Syringomyelia and tethered cord in children. Childs Nerv Syst. 2013;29: 1625–34.
47. Gaston H. Ophthalmic complications of spina bifida and hydrocephalus. Eye. 1991;5:279–90.
48. Anderson HA, Stuebing KK, Buncic R, Mazow M, Fletcher JM. Factors associated with strabismus in spina bifida myelomeningocele. J Pediatr Ophthalmol Strabismus. 2012;49(5):284–9.
49. Nelson MD, Widman LM, Abresch RT, Stanhope K, Havel PJ, Styne DM, McDonald CM. Metabolic syndrome in adolescents with spinal cord dysfunction. J Spinal Cord Med. 2007;7:S127–39.
50. Sherman MS, Kapalan JM, Effgen S, Campbell D, Dold F. Pulmonary dysfunction and reduced exercise capacity in patients with myelomeningocele. J Pediatr. 1997;131:413–8.
51. Kirk VG, Morielli A, Brouillette RT. Sleep-disordered breathing in patients with myelomeningocele: the missed diagnosis. Dev Med Child Neurol. 1999;41(1):40–3.
52. Patel DM, Rocque BG, Hopson B, Arynchyna A, Bishop ER, Lozano D, Blount JP. Sleep disordered breathing in patients with myelomeningocele. J Neurosurg Pediatr. 2015;16(1):30–5.
53. Wang HH, Wiener JS, Ferrandino MN, Lipkin ME, Routh JC. Complications of surgical management of upper tract calculi in spina bifida patients: analysis of nationwide data. J Urol. 2015;193(4):1270–4.
54. Krogh K, Lie HR, Bilenberg N, Laurberg S. Bowel function in Danish children with myelomeningocele. APMIS Suppl. 2003;109:81–5.
55. Verhoef M, Lurvink M, Barf HA, Post MW, van Asbeck FW, Gooskens RH, et al. High prevalence of incontinence among young adults with spina bifida: description, prediction and problem perception. Spinal Cord. 2005;43(6):331–40.

56. Velde SV, Biervliet SV, Bruyne RD, Winckel MV. A systematic review on bowel management and the success rate of the various treatment modalities in spina bifida patients. Spinal Cord. 2013;51(12): 873–81.
57. Imai K, Shiroyanagi Y, Kim WJ, Ichiroku T, Yamazaki Y. Satisfaction after the Malone antegrade continence enema procedure in patients with spina bifida. Spinal Cord. 2014;52(1):54–7.
58. Leibold S. Achieving continence with a neurogenic bowel. Pediatr Clin N Am. 2010;57:1013–25.
59. Märzheuser S, Karsten K, Rothe K. Improvements in incontinence with self-management in patients with anorectal malformations. Eur J Pediatr Surg. 2016;26(2):186–91.
60. McGuire EJ, Woodside JR, Borden TA, Weiss RM. The prognostic value of urodynamic testing in myelodysplastic patients. J Urol. 1981;126:205–9.
61. Snow-Lisy DC, Yerkes EB, Cheng EY. Update on urological management of spina bifida from prenatal diagnosis to adulthood. J Urol. 2015;194:288–96.
62. Edelstein RA, Bauer SB, Kelly MD, Darbey MM, Peters CA, Atala A, et al. The long-term urologic response of neonates with myelodysplasia treated proactively with intermittent catheterization and anticholinergic therapy. J Urol. 1995;154:1500–4.
63. Teichman JMH, Scherz HC, Kim KD, Cho DH, Packer MG, Kaplan GW. An alternative approach to myelodysplasia management: aggressive observation and prompt intervention. J Urol. 1994;152: 807–11.
64. Wu H-Y, Baskin LS, Kogan BA. Neurogenic bladder dysfunction due to myelomeningocele: neonates versus childhood treatment. J Urol. 1997;157:2295–7.
65. Kasabian NG, Bauer SB, Dyro FM, Colodny AH, Mandell J, Retik AB. The prophylactic value of clean intermittent catheterization and anticholinergic medication in newborns and infants with myelodysplasia at risk of developing urinary tract deterioration. Am J Dis Child. 1992;146:840–3.
66. Schlager TA, Clark M, Anderson S. Effect of a single-use sterile catheter for each void on the frequency of bacteriuria in children with neurogenic bladder on intermittent catheterization for bladder emptying. Pediatrics. 2001;108:E71.
67. Cruz F, Herschorn S, Aliotta P, Brin M, Thompson C, Lam W, et al. Efficacy and safety of onabotulinumtoxinA in patients with urinary incontinence due to neurogenic detrusor overactivity: a randomized, double-blind, placebo-controlled trial. Eur Urol. 2011;60:742–50.
68. Ginsberg D, Gousse A, Keppenne V, Sievert KD, Thompson C, Lam W, et al. Phase 3 efficacy and tolerability study of onabotulinumtoxinA for urinary incontinence from neurogenic detrusor overactivity. J Urol. 2012;187:2131–9.
69. Mitrofanoff P. Trans-appendicular continent cystostomy in the management of the neurogenic bladder. Chir Pediatr. 1980;21:297–305.
70. Monti PR, Lara RC, Dutra MA, de Carvalho JR. New techniques for construction of efferent conduits based on the Mitrofanoff principle. Urology. 1997; 49:112–5.
71. Yang WH. Yang needle tunneling technique in creating antireflux and continent mechanisms. J Urol. 1993;150:830–4.
72. Abol-Enein H, Ghoneim MA. Serous lined extramural ileal valve: a new continent urinary outlet. J Urol. 1999;161:786–91.
73. Sarosdy MF. Continent urinary diversion using cutaneous ileocecocystoplasty. Urology. 1992;40: 102–6.
74. Sutton MA, Hinson JL, Nickell KG, Boone TB. Continent ileocecal augmentation cystoplasty. Spinal Cord. 1998;36:246–51.
75. Veenboer PW, de Kort LM, Chrzan RJ, de Jong TP. Urinary considerations for adult patients with spinal dysraphism. Nat Rev Urol. 2015;12 (6):331–9.
76. Hendrix SL, Clark A, Nygaard I, Aragaki A, Barnabei V, McTiernan A. Pelvic organ prolapse in the Women's Health Initiative: gravity and gravidity. Am J Obstet Gynecol. 2002;186:1160–6.
77. Abrams P, Andersson KE, Brubaker L, Cardozo L, Cottenden A, Denis L, et al. 3rd International Consultation on Incontinence. Recommendations of the International Scientific Committee: evaluation and treatment of urinary incontinence, pelvic organ prolapse and fecal incontinence. Monaco;2005.
78. Edenfield AL, Levin PJ, Dieter AA, Amundsen CL, Siddiqui NY. Sexual activity and vaginal topography in women with symptomatic pelvic floor disorders. J Sex Med. 2015;12:416–23.
79. Khavari R, Tokaz MC, Stewart JN, Boone TB. Pelvic organ prolapse in female patients presenting to transitional urology care clinic. J Uro. 2015;194 (6):1654–8.
80. Shurtleff DB, Hayden PW, Chapman WH, Broy AB, Hill ML. Myelodysplasia. Problems of long-term survival and social function. West J Med. 1975;122 (3):199–205.
81. Vroege JA, Zeijlemaker BY, Scheers MM. Sexual functioning of adult patients born with meningomyelocele. A pilot study. Eur Urol. 1998; 34(1):25–9.
82. Hirayama A, Yamada K, Tanaka Y, Hirata N, Yamamoto M, Suemori T, et al. Evaluation of sexual function in adults with myelomeningocele. Hinyokika Kiyo. 1995;41(12):985–9.
83. Cromer BA, Enrile B, McCoy K, Gerhardstein MJ, Fitzpatrick M, Judis J. Knowledge, attitudes and behavior related to sexuality in adolescents with chronic disability. Dev Med Child Neurol. 1990;32 (7):602–10.
84. Decter RM, Furness PD 3rd, Nguyen TA, McGowan M, Laudermilch C, Telenko A. Reproductive understanding, sexual functioning and testosterone levels in men with spina bifida. J Urol. 1997;157(4):1466–8.

85. Cardenas DD, Topolski TD, White CJ, McLaughlin JF, Walker WO. Sexual functioning in adolescents and young adults with spina bifida. Arch Phys Med Rehabil. 2008;89(1):31–5.
86. von Linstow ME, Biering-Sørensen I, Liebach A, Lind M, Seitzberg A, Hansen RB, et al. Spina bifida and sexuality. J Rehabil Med. 2014;46(9):891–7.
87. Gamé X, Moscovici J, Gamé L, Sarramon JP, Rischmann P, Malavaud B. Evaluation of sexual function in young men with spina bifida and myelomeningocele using the International Index of Erectile Function. Urology. 2006;67(3):566–70.
88. Lassmann J, Garibay Gonzalez F, Melchionni JB, Pasquariello PS Jr, Snyder HM 3rd. Sexual function in adult patients with spina bifida and its impact on quality of life. J Urol. 2007;178(4 Pt 2):1611–4.
89. Cass AS, Bloom BA, Luxenberg M. Sexual function in adults with myelomeningocele. J Urol. 1986;136 (2):425–6.
90. Gavin L, MacKay AP, Brown K, Harrier S, Ventura SJ, Kann L, et al. Centers for Disease Control and Prevention (CDC). Sexual and reproductive health of persons aged 10-24 years—United States, 2002–2007. MMWR Surveill Summ. 2009;58(6): 1–58.
91. Verhoef M, Barf HA, Vroege JA, Post MW, Van Asbeck FW, Gooskens RH, et al. Sex education, relationships, and sexuality in young adults with spina bifida. Arch Phys Med Rehabil. 2005;86 (5):979–87.
92. Gatti C, Del Rossi C, Ferrari A, Casolari E, Casadio G, Scire G. Predictors of successful sexual partnering of adults with spina bifida. J Urol. 2009;182(4 Suppl):1911–6.
93. Sawyer SM, Roberts KV. Sexual and reproductive health in young people with spina bifida. Dev Med Child Neurol. 1999;41(10):671–5.
94. Dorner S. Sexual interest and activity in adolescents with spina bifida. J Child Psychol Psychiatry. 1977;18(3):229–37.
95. Lee NG, Andrews E, Rosoklija I, Logvinenko T, Johnson EK, Oates RD, et al. The effect of spinal cord level on sexual function in the spina bifida population. J Pediatr Urol. 2015;11(3):142 e1–6.
96. Diamond DA, Rickwood AM, Thomas DG. Penile erections in myelomeningocele patients. Br J Urol. 1986;58(4):434–5.
97. Sandler AD, Worley G, Leroy EC, Stanley SD, Kalman S. Sexual function and erection capability among young men with spina bifida. Dev Med Child Neurol. 1996;38(9):823–9.
98. Palmer JS, Kaplan WE, Firlit CF. Erectile dysfunction in patients with spina bifida is a treatable condition. J Urol. 2000;164(3 Pt 2):958–61.
99. Jackson AB, Mott PK. Reproductive health care for women with spina bifida. ScientificWorldJournal. 2007;7:1875–83.
100. De-Regil LM, Peña-Rosas JP, Fernández-Gaxiola AC, Rayco-Solon P. Effects and safety of periconceptional oral folate supplementation for preventing birth defects. Cochrane Database Syst Rev. 2015;12: CD007950.
101. Finnell RH, Shaw GM, Lammer EJ, Volcik KA. Does prenatal screening for 5,10-methylenetetrahydrofolate reductase (MTHFR) mutations in high-risk neural tube defect pregnancies make sense? Genet Test. 2002;6 (1):47–52.
102. Liakos AM, Bradley NK, Magram G, Muszynski C. Hydrocephalus and the reproductive health of women: the medical implications of maternal shunt dependency in 70 women and 138 pregnancies. Neurol Res. 2000;22(1):69–88.
103. Reitberg CCT, Lindhout D. Adult patients with spina bifida cystica: genetic counseling, pregnancy and delivery. Eur J Obstet Gynecol. 1993;52:63–70.
104. Visconti D, Noia G, Triarico S, Quattrocchi T, Pellegrino M, Carducci B, et al. Sexuality, pre-conception counseling and urological management of pregnancy for young women with spina bifida. Eur J Obstet Gynecol Reprod Biol. 2012;163 (2):129–33.
105. Cameron M, Moran P. Prenatal screening and diagnosis of neural tube defects. Prenat Diagn. 2009;29(4):402–11.
106. Dicianno BE, Kurowski BG, Yang JM, Chancellor MB, Bejjani GK, Fairman AD, et al. Rehabilitation and medical management of the adult with spina bifida. Am J Phys Med Rehabil. 2008;87 (12):1027–50.
107. Arata M, Grover S, Dunne K, Bryan D. Pregnancy outcome and complications in women with spina bifida. J Reprod Med. 2000;45(9):743–8.
108. Salomon J, Schnitzler A, Ville Y, Laffont I, Perronne C, Denys P, et al. Prevention of urinary tract infection in six spinal cord-injured pregnant women who gave birth to seven children under a weekly oral cyclic antibiotic program. Int J Infect Dis. 2009;13(3):399–402.
109. Marreiros H, Loff C, Calado E. Osteoporosis in paediatric patients with spina bifida. J Spinal Cord Med. 2012;35(1):9–21.
110. Marreiros H, Monteiro L, Loff C, Calado E. Fractures in children and adolescents with spina bifida: the experience of a Portuguese tertiary-care hospital. Dev Med Child Neurol. 2010;52(8):754–9.
111. Okurowska-Zawada B, Konstantynowicz J, Kułak W, Kaczmarski M, Piotrowska-Jastrzebska J, Sienkiewicz D, et al. Assessment of risk factors for osteoporosis and fractures in children with meningomyelocele. Adv Med Sci. 2009;54(2): 247–52.
112. Valtonen KM, Goksör LA, Jonsson O, Mellström D, Alaranta HT, Viikari-Juntura ER. Osteoporosis in adults with meningomyelocele: an unrecognized

problem at rehabilitation clinics. Arch Phys Med Rehabil. 2006;87(3):376–82.
113. Alexandre C, Vico L. Pathophysiology of bone loss in disuse osteoporosis. Joint Bone Spine. 2011;78(6):572–6.
114. Jiang SD, Jiang LS, Dai LY. Mechanisms of osteoporosis in spinal cord injury. Clin Endocrinol (Oxf). 2006;65(5):555–65.
115. Boyce AM, Tosi LL, Paul SM. Bisphosphonate treatment for children with disabling conditions. PM&R. 2014;6(5):427–36.
116. Okamoto GA, Lamers JV, Shurtleff DB. Skin breakdown in patients with myelomeningocele. Arch Phys Med Rehabil. 1983;64(1):20–3.
117. Plaum PE, Riemer G, Froslie KF. Risk factors for pressure sores in adult patients with myelomeningocele—a questionnaire-based study. Cerebrospinal Fluid Res. 2006;3:14.
118. Sawin KJ, Liu T, Ward E, Thibadeau J, Schechter MS, Soe MM, et al. NSBPR Coordinating Committee. The National Spina Bifida Patient Registry: profile of a large cohort of participants from the first 10 clinics. J Pediatr. 2015;166(2):444–50.
119. Ottolini K, Harris AB, Amling JK, Kennelly AM, Phillips LA, Tosi LL. Wound care challenges in children and adults with spina bifida: an open-cohort study. J Pediatr Rehabil Med. 2013;6(1):1–10.
120. Kim S, Ward E, Dicianno BE, Clayton GH, Sawin KJ, Beierwaltes P, et al. National Spina Bifida Patient Registry. Factors associated with pressure ulcers in individuals with spina bifida. Arch Phys Med Rehabil. 2015;96(8):1435–41.
121. Caterino JM, Scheatzle MD, D'Antonio JA. Descriptive analysis of 258 emergency department visits by spina bifida patients. J Emerg Med. 2006;31(1):17–22.
122. Kinsman SL, Doehring MC. The cost of preventable conditions in adults with spina bifida. Eur J Pediatr Surg. 1996;6(Suppl 1):17–20.
123. Haesler E, editor. National Pressure Ulcer Advisory Panel, E.P.U.A.P.a.P.P. and P.I. Alliance, Prevention and Treatment of Pressure Ulcers: quick reference guide. Perth: Cambridge Media; 2014.
124. Dicianno BE, Bellin MH, Zabel AT. Spina bifida and mobility in the transition years. Am J Phys Med Rehabil. 2009;88(12):1002–6.
125. Johnson KL, Dudgeon B, Kuehn C, Walker W. Assistive technology use among adolescents and young adults with spina bifida. Am J Public Health. 2007;97(2):330–6.
126. Dicianno BE, Gaines A, Collins DM, Lee S. Mobility, assistive technology use, and social integration among adults with spina bifida. Am J Phys Med Rehabil. 2009;88(7):533–41.
127. Verhoef M, Barf HA, Post MW, van Asbeck FW, Gooskens RH, Prevo AJ. Functional independence among young adults with spina bifida, in relation to hydrocephalus and level of lesion. Dev Med Child Neurol. 2006;48(2):114–9.
128. Williams EN, Broughton NS, Menelaus MB. Age-related walking in children with spina bifida. Dev Med Child Neurol. 1999;41(7):446–9.
129. Danielsson AJ, Bartonek A, Levey E, McHale K, Sponseller P, Saraste H. Associations between orthopaedic findings, ambulation and health-related quality of life in children with myelomeningocele. J Child Orthop. 2008;2(1):45–54.
130. Webb TS. Optimizing health care for adults with spina bifida. Dev Disabil Res Rev. 2010;16(1):76–81.
131. Mazur JM, Shurtleff D, Menelaus M, Colliver J. Orthopaedic management of high-level spina bifida. Early walking compared with early use of a wheelchair. J Bone Joint Surg Am. 1989;71(1):56–61.
132. Minkel JL. Seating and mobility considerations for people with spinal cord injury. Phys Ther. 2000;80(7):701–9.
133. Roehrig S, Like G. Factors affecting shoulder pain in adolescents and young adults with spina bifida. Pediatr Phys Ther. 2008;20(3):224–32.
134. Ferrero G, Mijno E, Actis MV, Zampa A, Ratto N, Arpaia A, Massè A. Risk factors for shoulder pain in patients with spinal cord injury: a multicenter study. Musculoskelet Surg. 2015;99(Suppl 1):53–6.
135. Sawatzky BJ, Slobogean GP, Reilly CW, Chambers CT, Hol AT. Prevalence of shoulder pain in adult-versus childhood-onset wheelchair users: a pilot study. J Rehabil Res Dev. 2005;42(3 Suppl 1):1–8.
136. Escobedo EM, Hunter JC, Hollister MC, Patten RM, Goldstein B. MR imaging of rotator cuff tears in individuals with paraplegia. AJR Am J Roentgenol. 1997;168(4):919–23.
137. Boninger ML, Cooper RA, Baldwin MA, Shimada SD, Koontz A. Wheelchair pushrim kinetics: body weight and median nerve function. Arch Phys Med Rehabil. 1999;80(8):910–5.
138. Schroer W, Lacey S, Frost FS, Keith MW. Carpal instability in the weight-bearing upper extremity. J Bone Joint Surg Am. 1996;78(12):1838–43.
139. Crandall RC, Birkebak RC, Winter RB. The role of hip location and dislocation in the functional status of the myelodysplastic patient. A review of 100 patients. Orthopedics. 1989;12(5):675–84.
140. Roach JW, Short BF, Saltzman HM. Adult consequences of spina bifida: a cohort study. Clin Orthop Relat Res. 2011;469(5):1246–52.
141. Glard Y, Launay F, Viehweger E, Guillaume JM, Jouve JL, Bollini G. Hip flexion contracture and lumbar spine lordosis in myelomeningocele. J Pediatr Orthop. 2005;25(4):476–8.
142. Frischhut B, Stöckl B, Landauer F, Krismer M, Menardi G. Foot deformities in adolescents and young adults with spina bifida. J Pediatr Orthop B. 2000;9(3):161–9.
143. Nagarkatti DG, Banta JV, Thomson JD. Charcot arthropathy in spina bifida. J Pediatr Orthop. 2000;20(1):82–7.

144. Yalcin S, Kocaoglu B, Berker N, Erol B. Conservative treatment of Charcot artroparthy in a series of spina bifida patients: the experience of one center and review of the literature. J Pediatr Orthop B. 2007;16(5):373–9.
145. Clancy CA, McGrath PJ, Oddson BE. Pain in children and adolescents with spina bifida. Dev Med Child Neurol. 2005;47(1):27–34.
146. Rintala DH, Holmes SA, Courtade D, Fiess RN, Tastard LV, Loubser PG. Comparison of the effectiveness of amitriptyline and gabapentin on chronic neuropathic pain in persons with spinal cord injury. Arch Phys Med Rehabil. 2007;88(12): 1547–60.
147. Tzellos TG, Papazisis G, Amaniti E, Kouvelas D. Efficacy of pregabalin and gabapentin for neuropathic pain in spinal-cord injury: an evidence-based evaluation of the literature. Eur J Clin Pharmacol. 2008;64(9):851–8.
148. Thomson JD, Segal LS. Orthopedic management of spina bifida. Dev Disabil Res Rev. 2010;16(1): 96–103.
149. Patel J, Walker JL, Talwalkar VR, Iwinski HJ, Milbrandt TA. Correlation of spine deformity, lung function, and seat pressure in spina bifida. Clin Orthop Relat Res. 2011;469(5):1302–7.
150. Trivedi J, Thomson JD, Slakey JB, Banta JV, Jones PW. Clinical and radiographic predictors of scoliosis in patients with myelomeningocele. J Bone Joint Surg Am. 2002;84-A(8):1389–94.
151. Mercado E, Alman B, Wright JG. Does spinal fusion influence quality of life in neuromuscular scoliosis? Spine (Phila Pa 1976). 2007;32(19 Suppl):S120–5.
152. Wai EK, Young NL, Feldman BM, Badley EM, Wright JG. The relationship between function, self-perception, and spinal deformity: implications for treatment of scoliosis in children with spina bifida. J Pediatr Orthop. 2005;25(1):64–9.
153. Berven S, Bradford DS. Neuromuscular scoliosis: causes of deformity and principles for evaluation and management. Semin Neurol. 2002;22(2): 167–78.
154. Buffart LM, van den Berg-Emons RJ, Burdorf A, Janssen WG, Stam HJ, Roebroeck ME. Cardiovascular disease risk factors and the relationships with physical activity, aerobic fitness, and body fat in adolescents and young adults with myelomeningocele. Arch Phys Med Rehabil. 2008;89(11): 2167–73.
155. Dosa NP, Foley JT, Eckrich M, Woodall-Ruff D, Liptak GS. Obesity across the lifespan among persons with spina bifida. Disabil Rehabil. 2009;31 (11):914–20.
156. McPherson AC, Swift JA, Yung E, Lyons J, Church P. The assessment of weight status in children and young people attending a spina bifida outpatient clinic: a retrospective medical record review. Disabil Rehabil. 2013;35(25):2123–31.
157. McPherson AC, Leo J, Church P, Lyons J, Chen L, Swift J. An environmental scan of weight assessment and management practices in paediatric spina bifida clinics across Canada. J Pediatr Rehabil Med. 2014;7(3):207–17.
158. Shurtleff DB, Walker WO, Duguay S, Peterson D, Cardenas D. Obesity and myelomeningocele: anthropometric measures. J Spinal Cord Med. 2010;33(4):410–9.
159. Nelson MD, Widman LM, Abresch RT, Stanhope K, Havel PJ, Styne DM, et al. Metabolic syndrome in adolescents with spinal cord dysfunction. J Spinal Cord Med. 2007;30(Suppl 1):S127–39.
160. Buffart LM, Roebroeck ME, Rol M, Stam HJ, van den Berg-Emons RJ. Transition Research Group South-West Netherlands. Triad of physical activity, aerobic fitness and obesity in adolescents and young adults with myelomeningocele. J Rehabil Med. 2008;40(1):70–5.
161. van den Berg-Emons HJ, Bussmann JB, Meyerink HJ, Roebroeck ME, Stam HJ. Body fat, fitness and level of everyday physical activity in adolescents and young adults with meningomyelocele. J Rehabil Med. 2003;35(6):271–5.
162. Buffart LM, van den Berg-Emons RJ, van Mechelen W, van Meeteren J, van der Slot W, Stam HJ, et al. Promoting physical activity in an adolescent and a young adult with physical disabilities. Disabil Health J. 2010;3(2):86–92.
163. Davis G, Plyley MJ, Shephard RJ. Gains of cardiorespiratory fitness with arm-crank training in spinally disabled men. Can J Sport Sci. 1991;16 (1):64–72.
164. Miyano G, Kalra M, Inge TH. Adolescent paraplegia, morbid obesity, and pickwickian syndrome: outcome of gastric bypass surgery. J Pediatr Surg. 2009;44(3):e41–4.
165. Rofail D, Maguire L, Kissner M, Colligs A, Abetz-Webb L. Health-related quality of life is compromised in individuals with spina bifida: results from qualitative and quantitative studies. Eur J Obstet Gynecol Reprod Biol. 2014;181C: 214–22.
166. Cope H, McMahon K, Heise E, Eubanks S, Garrett M, Gregory S, Ashley-Koch A. Outcome and life satisfaction of adults with myelomeningocele. Disabil Health J. 2013;6(3):236–43.
167. Barf HA, Post MW, Verhoef M, Gooskens RHJM, Prevo AJH. Is cognitive functioning associated with subjective quality of life in young adults with spina bifida and hydrocephalus? J Rehabil Med. 2010;42 (1):56–9.
168. Sawin KJ, Brei TJ, Bura CF, Fastenau PS. Factors associated with quality of life in adolescents with spina bifida. J Holist Nurs. 2002;20:279–304.
169. Dicianno BE, Bellin MH, Zabel AT. Spina bifida and mobility in the transition years. Am J Phys Med Rehabil. 2009;88(12):1002–6.

170. Bellin MH, Dicianno BE, Osteen P, Dosa N, Aparicio E, Braun P, Zabel TA. Family satisfaction, pain, and quality-of-life in emerging adults with spina bifida: a longitudinal analysis. Am J Phys Med Rehabil. 2013;92(1):641–55.
171. Leger RR. Severity of illness, functional status, and HRQOL in youth with spina bifida. Rehabil Nurs. 2005;30(5):180–7.
172. Kirpalani HM, Parkin PC, Willan AR, Fehlings DL, Rosenbaum PL, King D, Van Nie AJ. Quality of life in spina bifida: importance of parental hope. Arch Dis Child. 2000;83(4):293–7.
173. Padua L, Rendeli C, Rabini A, Girardi E, Tonali P, Salvaggio E. Health-related quality of life and disability in young patients with spina bifida. Arch Phys Med Rehabil. 2002;83(10):1384–8.

Part IV

Other Clinical Considerations in the Care of Adults with Chronic Childhood Conditions

19 Respiratory Care of Adults with Chronic Pulmonary Disease

Tara Lynn Barto

Introduction

The last 30 years has seen a shift in the care of chronic pulmonary disease owing in large part to the advancements in medicine and technology. Comprehensive chronic disease management, as demonstrated in cystic fibrosis (CF) and muscular dystrophy (MD), has led to improved survival and quality of life for children diagnosed with previously fatal conditions, such that now these patients are living well into adulthood. The care of patients with chronic respiratory failure (CRF) has followed suit with this changing landscape of chronic disease management. CRF is defined as a condition persisting for greater than one month and requiring mechanical ventilation for part (at least 6 h) or all of the day to provide adequate ventilation [1]. Previously, children with CRF would be confined to a hospital with personnel trained in respiratory care and ventilator management, with patients and their families choosing home only for palliative or hospice care. Today, patients are offered multiple options for management of respiratory failure at home, albeit requiring significant education, family commitment, and medical community support.

T.L. Barto (✉)
Division of Pulmonary, Sleep and Critical Care Medicine, Baylor College of Medicine, 6620 Main Street, Houston, TX 77030, USA
e-mail: Tara.Barto@bcm.edu

Like many changes in medicine, the initial impetus to move toward home care for patients with (CRF) was financial in origin. However, what seems to have grown out of this movement is a paradigm for managing complex medical patients safely while improving survival and quality of life. Integral to these improvements has been the development of programs supporting the care of chronically ventilated patients with CRF at home as well as multidisciplinary teams knowledgeable in the care of these patients. In addition to these changes, the trends in parental expectations of long-term survival in children with chronic respiratory failure has led to more parents initially taking on the long-term responsibility for these patients.

Chronic Respiratory Failure

CRF can be divided into three categories, each with different expectations of progression and need for lifelong mechanical ventilation. The first is CRF related to ventilatory muscle weakness, for example, neuromuscular diseases such as Duchenne's muscular dystrophy or quadriplegia. As home care for CRF was gaining popularity, these patients comprised more than 50 % of patients offered home mechanical ventilation (HMV), although reports reviewing the trends in HMV have shown that patients with other categories of CRF are being offered home care options more often [2]. Because these conditions

M. Pilapil et al. (eds.), *Care of Adults with Chronic Childhood Conditions*,
DOI 10.1007/978-3-319-43827-6_19

are typically chronic and progressive, it is unlikely once a patient requires mechanical ventilatory support that they would be able to be successfully weaned from such support.

The second category of CRF is related to disorders of the lung parenchyma and airways, which in turn cause an increase in work of breathing. Examples include patients with bronchopulmonary dysplasia, interstitial lung disease, or chest wall deformities. As children with such conditions age and grow, their respiratory mechanics may improve, allowing them to be potentially weaned from ventilation.

The final category of CRF is related to disorders that cause a failure of neurologic control of breathing, for example, postencephalitis, brain trauma, or rarer conditions such as congenital central hypoventilation syndrome (CCHS). These conditions typically require lifelong ventilation, although in certain conditions, such as CCHS, ventilation may only be required at night.

Mechanical Ventilation

Home mechanical ventilation (HMV) can be described in different ways: positive versus negative pressure ventilation, invasive versus noninvasive ventilation (NIV), and mode of ventilation, to name a few. As a primary care provider (PCP), it is most important to understand the difference between invasive and the noninvasive mechanical ventilation and possible complications of each. Initiation of HMV should be accomplished in coordination with a specialist in pulmonary disease. Further, the ventilator settings, regardless of whether invasive or noninvasive ventilation is being employed, should first be established with inpatient titration and monitoring, typically during a sleep study. Optimal ventilation is achieved once the partial pressure of carbon dioxide ($PaCO_2$) normalizes. If a patient remains hypoxemic at this point, then oxygen supplementation is added. Oxygen should not be used until adequate ventilation is maintained, as it can mask cyanosis, worsen hypercapnea, and delay the initiation of ventilatory support [3]. Chronic management of mechanically ventilated patients employs monitoring carbon dioxide levels, typically with venous blood gases and intermittent sleep studies to ensure appropriate ventilation. Such monitoring may be required more frequently in children, as they tend to grow and require more frequent changes in their settings than do adults.

The goals of initiating HMV are to improve quality of life, improve mobility and rehabilitation potential, and to improve growth and development. Qualitative data on patients' experiences before and after initiation of mechanical ventilation are limited but suggest that patients' improvement in dyspnea directly impacts their quality of life. Though a minority of patients report negative social impacts and low self-esteem, these outcomes do not negate the reported improvement in quality of life due to relief of dyspnea [4]. The standard outcome measure of quality of life in children has been the patient's ability to reintegrate into the school system [5–7]. In order to accomplish these goals of HMV, ventilators must be small, lightweight, portable, durable, and able to be powered by a battery. As technology is advancing, these devices are becoming more portable and user friendly [8].

Noninvasive ventilation (NIV) employs a simpler device and is accomplished using a mask or nasal pillows, making this device less cumbersome. The success of NIV is highly dependent on the patient's ability to tolerate the masks. These devices exert a pressure on the face to maintain the seal and reduce air leak potential, leading to a risk of midface hypoplasia in children or pressure ulcers in adults. Regular monitoring of the site of contact of the mask on the face is important. Additionally, NIV cannot meet high-flow demands of certain patients, causing dyssynchrony between the patient and the ventilator, which the patient would perceive as dyspnea. As such, certain patients may not be comfortably ventilated with this type of ventilator.

Invasive mechanical ventilation is accomplished with a traditional home ventilator through a tracheostomy. This type of ventilator is a more cumbersome machine but can provide more sophisticated modes of ventilation, allowing for improved patient comfort. Despite placement of a tracheostomy, most patients will still be able to vocalize.

The decision to use invasive or noninvasive ventilation should be made only after discussion among the patient, family, pulmonologist, and, if desired, the PCP. Traditionally if a patient requires mechanical ventilation for 24 h per day, then the invasive modality is recommended. However, in children, even those requiring ventilation for 24 h per day, noninvasive ventilation is often initiated until there is failure to adequately ventilate, failure to tolerate the mask, high risk of ongoing aspiration due to changes in bulbar function, or ineffective management of airway secretions [3, 5, 9].

Tracheostomy

A tracheostomy tube is a tube surgically placed in the neck extending into the trachea to allow for adequate ventilation, both assisted and non-assisted. These tubes require special attention and care to ensure proper cleaning and use. Typically, tracheostomy care is coordinated with an otolaryngologist (ENT)—a surgeon who most commonly places these devices. Once the decision is made to pursue invasive mechanical ventilation a tracheostomy tube is placed. The choice of the type of tube to use is made based on many factors. The two most common types of tracheostomies are plastic and metal. Plastic tubes are more flexible and typically smaller in nature. They are comprised of an outer cannula and an inner removable or disposable cannula. They come in standard sizes, although custom tubes can be made if a patient needs to have a longer portion entering the trachea, for example, in individuals with significant redundant neck tissue. Metal tubes are less flexible but more easily cleaned and therefore are used when patients have thick tenacious secretions or if they frequently obstruct their plastic tube. Tubes can also be uncuffed or cuffed, meaning there is a cuff on the distal intratracheal limb that is used to prevent air leaks in patients requiring mechanical ventilation. It is important to know that cuffs, if not managed properly, can cause damage as high pressure over extended periods of time can cause tracheal scarring. Tracheostomy tube cuffs are designed to be a high-volume, low-pressure system, but cuffs should only be inflated enough to prevent air leaks during mechanical ventilation, as overinflation can cause tracheal damage over time. Tracheostomy cuff tubes should not be inflated above a maximum pressure of 20 cm of water (cmH_2O).

Patients and caregivers will need training in tracheostomy care, which should be performed once a day. This typically involves changing the dressings and tracheostomy ties as well as cleaning the inner cannula. Plastic tubes must also be removed and new ones placed periodically. The ENT physician changes the tube the first time, typically 1–2 weeks after placement. There are no well-established guidelines on how often chronic tracheostomy tubes need to be changed thereafter, but recommendations range from every 2 weeks to every 3–4 months. This decision is best made in consultation with the ENT physician [10].

Complications of tracheostomy tubes are categorized into early and late. Early complications are those complications most commonly occurring up until the first tube change. They can be directly related to placement; for example, development of a false tract or pneumothorax, or local complications including infection, bleeding, or obstruction. The tracheostomy tube is sutured in place until the first change, so decannulation is uncommon. Late complications also include infection, obstruction, and bleeding, the most concerning of which would be an innominate artery fistula, typically occurring in the first 3 weeks after placement. Chronic tracheostomy tube placement can result in other complications over time including recurrent tracheitis, granulation tissue formation, which would lead to recurrent obstruction, and permanent tracheocutaneous fistula. Routine monitoring for development of these complications is mandatory. Some patients will develop chronic or recurrent tracheitis, as such they should routinely have tracheal cultures performed to determine the nature of the bacterial flora in their airway in the event of an infection or an exacerbation.

Airway Clearance and Humidification

Patients with CRF due to any number of reasons often have difficulty managing respiratory secretions. For example, muscle weakness in patients with MD, increased secretion production in individuals with CF, and loss of cough reflex in those with central neurologic conditions can all pose challenges in the handling of respiratory secretions. To assist patients in managing these secretions, additional respiratory therapies should be administered 2–4 times daily. These therapies include inhaled airway hydration, mechanical airway clearance techniques, and frequent suctioning. There a multiple forms of airway clearance techniques including chest physiotherapy (CPT), high-frequency chest wall compression (HFCWC), and intrapulmonary percussive ventilation, all of which can be used with both invasive and noninvasive mechanical ventilation. Consultation with the pulmonologist should be sought to determine if the patient would benefit from these therapies.

Heated humidification is the delivery of air, with or without supplemental oxygen, that has been heated and passed over sterile water to increase the humidity. Heated humidification is mandatory for all patients who use invasive mechanical ventilation. Its benefits include prevention of tracheal mucosa dryness, preventing infection, prevention of inspissated secretions by increasing hydration, decreasing the risk of hypothermia, and increasing patient comfort. Care must be taken to ensure proper cleaning of the humidifier and use of sterile water.

Emergency Action Plans

Emergency action plans should be devised early in the planning of mechanical ventilation with input from the pulmonologist, ENT, and PCP. Key topics to include would be which physician should be contacted for an acute illness or particular issue and who is responsible for ordering specific equipment and supplies. Families should be provided with the appropriate equipment in the event of an emergency. For example, they should have equipment and training to perform manual ventilation in the event of power outages and extra tracheostomy tubes for placement in the event of an accidental decannulation.

Weaning from Ventilation

Patients will ask if weaning off of the ventilator is an option. This often is not possible if the condition requiring mechanical ventilation is a chronic progressive condition. However, for children who are placed on mechanical ventilation due to bronchopulmonary dysplasia or tracheobronchomalacia, it is possible that, as they grow, their respiratory mechanics may improve such that HMV is no longer required. If weaning is a potential option, after consultation with the pulmonologist, patients are usually liberated from the ventilator for progressively longer periods of time rather than adjusting ventilator settings. Careful monitoring of vital signs and assessment of patient tolerance of being off the ventilator are critical. The final steps of weaning from a ventilator at night should be done in a monitored setting, such as an inpatient stay or during sleep study.

Caregivers

Caregivers are the most integral part of the care of a ventilated patient. It has been suggested that it is not the education level of the caregiver that predicts success but rather the commitment and dedication to appropriate home care [8]. It is a very time-consuming, physically and mentally rigorous undertaking to be a caregiver for a patient requiring mechanical ventilation. The role of home health care services is to provide the caregiver a reprieve to allow them to rest and care for themselves as well as to provide support for certain patient activities such as bathing,

Table 19.1 Caregiver Education Checklist. Adapted with permission from Preutthipan [8]

General	Understanding of underlying disease Concerning signs and symptoms Inhaled therapies/airway clearance techniques Emergency care/CPR Emergency call number Medical history document
Oxygen therapy	Understand why it is necessary Oxygen source Care/maintenance of equipment Flow rate of oxygen Complications of oxygen therapy
Tracheostomy care	Understand why it is necessary Safe activities of daily living Communication and speech Cleaning and sterilization of equipment Suctioning techniques and equipment Tube and ties change Accidental decannulation plan In-home safety Transportation safety
Ventilator care	How the ventilator works Understanding alarms/complications Problem-solving ventilator malfunction Check ventilator and humidifier Mask/tracheostomy tube interface Cleaning and sterilization of equipment In-home safety Battery and power supply Manual bag mask ventilation

CPR cardiopulmonary resuscitation

respiratory treatments, and tracheostomy care. Prior to a mechanically ventilated patient being discharged to home, the caregivers must go through extensive education to learn tracheostomy care, understand the ventilator, coordinate emergency action plans, and be instructed in basic life support, among many other things [8] (see Table 19.1).

Conclusion

Over the last decades, improvements in clinical care and technology have afforded patients with CRF increases in survival and improvements in quality of life. Encompassed in these changes is the involvement of multidisciplinary team of family and caregivers as well as pulmonary and primary care physicians. Successful home mechanical ventilation is now an option for these individuals and experience has shown that, with a multidisciplinary approach to care and dedicated family and caregivers, HMV can improve both quality of life and survival among individuals with CRF. Multiple support systems have been established to assist in these endeavors.

References

1. Adams AB, Whitman J, Marcy T. Surveys of long term ventilatory support in Minnesota: 1986 and 1992. Chest. 1993;103(5):1463–9.
2. Chatwin M, Tan HL, Bush A, Rosenthal M, Simonds AK. Long term non-invasive ventilation in children: impact on survival and transition to adult care. PLoS ONE. 2015;10(5):e0125839.
3. Hull J, Aniapravan R, Chan E, Chatwin M, Forton J, Gallagher J, et al. British thoracic society guideline for respiratory management of children with neuromuscular weakness. Thorax. 2012;67:i1–40.

4. Noyes J. Health and quality of life of ventilator-dependent children. J Adv Nurs. 2006;56 (4):392–403.
5. Amin R, Fitton C. Tracheostomy and home ventilation in children. Semin Neonatol. 2003;8:127–35.
6. Gilgoff IS, Kahlstrom E, Maclaughlin E, Keens TG. Long-term ventilatory support in spinal muscular atrophy. J Pediatr. 1989;115(6):904–9.
7. Marcus CL, Jansen MT, Poulson MK, Keens SE, Nield TA, Lipsker LE, et al. Medical and psychosocial outcome of children with congenital central hypoventilation syndrome. J Pediatr. 1991;119 (6):888–95.
8. Preutthipan A. Home mechanical ventilation in children. Indian J Pediatr. 2015;82(9):852–9.
9. Nixon GM, Edwards EA, Cooper D, Fitzgerald DA, Harris M, Martin J, et al. Ventilatory support at home for children. A consensus statement from the Australian Paediatric Respiratory Group. February 2008. APRG Working. https://www.thoracic.org.au/journal-publishing/command/download_file/id/10/filename/Ventilatory_Support_at_Home_for_Children._A_Consensus_Statement_from_the_Australasian_Paediatric_Respiratory_Group.pdf. Accessed 6 June 2016.
10. White AC, Kher S, O'Connor H. When to change a tracheostomy tube. Respir Care. 2010;55(8):1069–75.

Nutritional Support

20

Susan Hunt and Deonna Monnahan

Introduction

As children move into adolescence and young adulthood, their nutritional goals transition from weight gain and linear growth to weight maintenance. For young adults with chronic childhood conditions (YACCC), this transition may be complicated by changes in caloric needs over time as severity of illness or functional ability change and thus requires special attention from their adult providers. Some YACCC may already be receiving nutrition support while others may need to have these issues addressed anew. Assessment of ongoing needs in both groups is needed to prevent malnutrition or overweight and obesity. Involvement of a dietitian may be advisable in complex situations, but medical providers should have a working understanding of potential nutritional issues such as malnutrition and overnutrition as well as types of nutritional support and their potential complications.

S. Hunt (✉)
Departments of General Internal Medicine and Pediatric Medicine, University of Washington Medical Center and Seattle Children's Hospital, 1959 NE Pacific St, Box 356429, Seattle, WA 98195-6429, USA
e-mail: hunts1@uw.edu

D. Monnahan
Department of Nutrition, Seattle Children's Hospital, 4800 Sand Point Way NE, Seattle, WA 98105, USA

Malnutrition

Malnutrition is common in YACCC. Although the diversity of conditions makes general estimates impossible, children with cerebral palsy, as one example, may have rates of 29–46 %, with prevalence increasing with age [1]. Malnutrition is associated with increased morbidity and mortality, more frequent hospital admissions and longer length of stay, and decreased quality of life [2]. Nutritional deficits may be multifactorial in origin and type depending on the young adult's underlying medical condition. For example, in cystic fibrosis (CF), patients may have calorie deficit, fatty acid deficiency, and vitamin deficiency as a result of the multisystem effects of their underlying disorder [3, 4]. Causes of caloric and nutrient deficits in CF further demonstrates the major categories of malnutrition in transition patients:

1. normal nutritional intake but increased needs due to medical condition,
2. inadequate nutritional intake due to oral feeding difficulties or restrictions, and
3. malabsorption, feeding intolerance, and other gastrointestinal (GI) issues that cause nutritional losses.

Increased caloric needs are hypothesized as a common cause of undernutrition in chronic illness, but this is often difficult to quantify due to complexity of measuring resting energy expenditure (REE) and total energy expenditure in real-life situations. CF provides a well-studied

M. Pilapil et al. (eds.), *Care of Adults with Chronic Childhood Conditions*,
DOI 10.1007/978-3-319-43827-6_20

example of this issue. While initial speculation suggested the underlying genetic defect of CF as the source of increased requirements, studies in children with CF show that REE does not differ from that of healthy controls [5]. In adults with preserved lung function, REE is also unchanged. However, as lung function declines, exacerbations become more frequent and secondary complications such as diabetes and liver disease manifest, resulting in an increase in REE, placing patients at risk of caloric deficiency [4]. Cerebral palsy, is another condition where increased REE has been noted in the subset of patients who have athetosis, continuous involuntary movements [6, 7].

Inadequate oral intake, regardless of REE, is the most frequent cause of undernutrition in YACCC. In CF, for example, appetite may decrease due to nausea associated with recurrent pulmonary exacerbations or gastroparesis resulting from CF-related diabetes. Selective eating patterns can also lead to inadequate intake and are common in patients with developmental disability, with some studies indicating prevalence of up to 80 % in children, although rates may show some improvement with age [8]. In children with autism, for example, approximately 60 % have "strong food preferences," often related to texture (up to 70 % of preferences) or restricted food choices, placing them at increased nutritional risk [9]. Finally, dysphagia can be a factor in multiple disorders including central neurologic disorders such as hypoxic-ischemic injury with resultant cerebral palsy, degenerative muscular disorders such as Duchenne muscular dystrophy (DMD), or genetic anomalies with physical variations causing poor oropharyngeal coordination, such as Pierre Robin sequence [10–12].

A subset of underlying conditions impairs adequate absorption from the gastrointestinal tract or leads to increased losses. CF patients may have both insufficient absorption of fats and vitamins, even when symptoms of pancreatic insufficiency are clinically well controlled, as well as sugar loss due to glycosuria from CF-related diabetes [3]. Conditions such as inflammatory bowel disease (IBD) and celiac disease can cause poor absorption during disease flares. Children with Crohn's disease, for example, have high rates of growth failure, up to 56 % in some studies [13]. Young adults with prior intestinal resections, such as those with a history of necrotizing enterocolitis or IBD, may have decreased absorptive intestine or ostomies, which further complicate nutritional status.

Overnutrition

In addition to conditions predisposing to undernutrition, YACCC, like the general population, can also suffer from overnutrition, overweight, and obesity. In cerebral palsy and spina bifida, for example, energy needs are significantly linked to physical activity, and patients who have progressive loss of ambulatory ability due to worsening contractures or weakness may have decreased energy requirements, placing them at risk of weight gain and obesity if feeding is not adjusted [7, 14]. Genetic conditions may predispose to obesity, such as Prader-Willi syndrome, with associated hyperphagia, and trisomy 21 (Down syndrome), due to poor impulse management and carryover dietary habits from childhood [12]. Obesity can have short-term morbidity costs, such as decreased ambulatory ability and caregiver difficulty lifting and transferring nonambulatory patients, as well as the typical long-term costs associated with obesity in adult populations, such as metabolic syndrome and cardiovascular disease.

Types of Nutrition Support

For YACCC whose complex condition includes malnutrition, nutrition support may be indicated [15]. Some transitioning young adults will already have nutrition support in place, with adult practitioners assuming supervising responsibility from their pediatric colleagues. Primary management of nutrition support in pediatric-centered care is often the responsibility of subspecialty medical homes. Conversely, in adult care systems, the primary care provider often assumes this role with support from subspecialists and dietitians. Modes of nutritional support include oral supplementation, enteral nutrition, and parenteral nutrition. Each method has risks and benefits and should be weighed carefully based on the underlying condition and patient and family needs.

Assessing Nutritional Status in YACCC

This section covers basic nutritional concepts and common situations that a primary care provider (PCP) may encounter when caring for YACCC. These include the assessment of weight goals, accurate diagnosis of nutritional status, and gathering a dietary history from a patient with intellectual or developmental disability. Familiarity with these fundamentals will allow PCPs to adequately address the basic nutritional health of most YACCC. In certain instances, though, consultation with a dietitian may be necessary.

Consultation with a Dietitian

For those patients not meeting their nutritional goals after assessment and intervention by the PCP, consideration should be given to involving a registered dietitian, who can complete a thorough evaluation of the patient's nutritional intake and status and help the patient set nutrition goals based on specialized medical needs and lifestyle. A dietitian should be involved in most decisions about initiation or adjustment of enteral and parenteral nutrition. Additional specific conditions may require a dietitian analysis of specific nutrients; for example, a patient with chronic kidney disease (CKD) who struggles to decrease their potassium or phosphorus levels, or a patient with a very low caloric intake who may be at risk for nutrient deficiencies. Some common instances of these conditions and appropriate use of a dietitian's services are highlighted throughout the following sections, although a comprehensive list is beyond the scope of this text.

Assessing Weight Goals

Identifying appropriate caloric intake and weight goals is a foundational step of nutritional assessment. Adult providers are likely to be familiar with the body mass index (BMI) as an indicator of total body fat, with 18.5–24.9 kg/m^2 considered a healthy range for men and women. BMI < 18.5 kg/m^2 indicates underweight, >25 kg/m^2 overweight, and >30 kg/m^2 obese [16]. There are many equations that can be used to calculate ideal body weight but little research to support their validity. A BMI of 22 kg/m^2 is associated with the lowest rate of mortality for those 30–59 years of age and so may be an appropriate goal for healthy adults [17].

When assessing YACCC, weight goals should be individualized with weight history, body type, and degree of muscle mass taken into consideration. For example, in patients with lower muscle mass, a BMI at the low end of normal may be appropriate, such as those who are nonambulatory, with hypotonic cerebral palsy, or Down syndrome. In addition, BMI is only useful if the weight and height are accurately measured, and obtaining an accurate height can be difficult in patients with contractures or who are unable to stand. For wheelchair users, recumbent length gives the most accurate measurement [18]. For those who are unable to safely transfer to a flat table or have contractures, the next best approache is the knee height method or self-report [18].

Diagnosis of Nutritional Status

Correctly diagnosing malnutrition is important for heightened focus on the nutritional status of the patient as well as for accurate coding, billing, and research purposes. Clinical indicators of malnutrition can be identified by a thorough medical history, assessment of nutritional intake, physical signs of nutrient deficiencies, anthropometrics, and possibly hand grip strength (see Table 20.1) [2]. Additional elements that can elucidate increased risk for malnutrition include lab results, in particular markers of inflammation,

Table 20.1 Diagnosing malnutrition

Clinical characteristic	Acute illness or injury		Chronic illness (≥ 3 months)		Social or environmental circumstances	
	Moderate malnutrition	Severe malnutrition	Moderate malnutrition	Severe malnutrition	Moderate malnutrition	Severe malnutrition
Energy intake	<75 % estimated energy requirement for >7 days	≤ 50 % estimated energy requirement for ≥ 5 days	<75 % estimated energy requirement for ≥ 1 month	<75 % estimated energy requirement for ≥ 1 month	<75 % estimated energy requirement for ≥ 3 months	≤ 50 % estimated energy requirement for ≥ 1 month
Weight loss	1–2 % in 1 week, 5 % in 1 month, or 7.5 % in 3 months	>2 % in 1 week, >5 % in 1 month, or >7.5 % in 3 months	5 % in 1 month, 7.5 % in 3 months, 10 % in 6 months, 20 % in 1 year	> 5 % in 1 month, >7.5 % in 3 months, >10 % in 6 months, >20 % in 1 year	5 % in 1 month, 7.5 % in 3 months, 10 % in 6 months, 20 % in 1 year	> 5 % in 1 month, >7.5 % in 3 months, >10 % in 6 months, >20 % in 1 year
Body fat loss	Mild	Moderate	Mild	Severe	Mild	Severe
Muscle loss	Mild	Moderate	Mild	Severe	Mild	Severe
Fluid accumulation	Mild	Moderate to Severe	Mild	Severe	Mild	Severe
Reduced grip strength	N/A	Reduced	N/A	Reduced	N/A	Reduced

At least two characteristics are recommended for diagnosis of moderate or severe malnutrition. Table modified from [2]
There is inadequate evidence to define mild malnutrition [2]

mental health history, and psychosocial factors [2]. When malnutrition is confirmed, the primary care provider should address the etiology/etiologies of the malnutrition, develop an intervention with the patient or caregiver, and confirm a plan for routine monitoring and adjusting of the intervention until the malnutrition is resolved. Basic interventions for malnutrition typically include encouraging consumption of high-calorie, high-protein foods and addressing barriers to doing so, starting a multivitamin and mineral supplement, and any additional supplements indicated by lab abnormalities. For malnourished patients, an appropriate rate of weight gain is 1–2 lb per week toward ideal body weight. Further information on how to support patients who are unable to increase their oral intake to meet their needs will be discussed in subsequent sections of this chapter.

Clinical assessment for overweight and obese patients includes the same factors as for malnutrition. For overweight patients, an appropriate weight loss goal is 0.5–1 lb per week toward achieving 10 % body weight loss over a 6-month period [19]. Regular follow-up is essential to support healthy weight loss, and dietitian support should be considered if patient weight goals are unclear, goals are not being met, or patient and/or caregivers would benefit from additional counseling.

Gathering a Diet History from a Patient with Intellectual or Developmental Disability

The high prevalence of underweight and overweight among adults with intellectual or developmental disabilities makes nutritional evaluation a valuable part of their clinical assessment [20]. Adults with intellectual or developmental disabilities may not be able to provide an accurate diet history, and unfortunately there currently is no validated approach to completing a dietary intake assessment for this population [20]. A proxy reporter may be able to provide accurate information if they are consistently with the patient during eating opportunities [20]. There are many strategies to assessing dietary intake, such as retrospective food record, 24-h recall, food frequency questionnaire, food checklists, and direct observation. There is no evidence to support prospective methods being more accurate than retrospective or vice versa, and no gold standard method using patient report has been established [21]. Underreporting intake is a common reporter bias [21]. Of the various methods, the 24-h recall can be the fastest approach to assessing a patient's intake. This method requires the patient to report all the foods and beverages consumed the day prior, and if time allows including portion sizes. Patients are often more accurate in their reporting if they are prompted to recall the previous day in a sequential order. These principles can be applied to caregiver histories as well. Other comorbidities affecting intake should be noted in the initial nutritional history, such as dysphagia, GI problems, and sensory issues that limit food choices. This information will also help inform a dietary consult, if your history does not reveal causes for weight imbalance.

Common Nutritional Considerations

Bone Health

Growth and bone health are a major focus of medical nutrition therapy for children with chronic disease. Patients will no longer be growing in height by the time they transition to adult care, so this focus should shift to maintaining bone health. Young adults with intellectual or developmental disabilities are at higher risk for poor bone health compared to those who are typically developed [20]. Patients who are nonambulatory are at greater risk for lower bone density [22].

Adequate calcium and phosphorus intake are crucial for bone health, as they make up 80–90 % of bone mineral content. Vitamin D, given its role in promoting calcium absorption and decreased bone turnover, is also a critical nutrient [23]. Dietary phosphorus is typically less of a focus when counseling patients, likely because national surveys have shown that calcium intake is low whereas phosphorus intake is greater than recommended among adults in the United States [23].

At 19 years of age, the recommended dietary allowance (RDA) for calcium decreases from 1300 mg to 1000 mg elemental calcium daily [24]. The National Osteoporosis Foundation has a guide to quickly assess your patient's calcium intake (http://nof.org/articles/542) [25]. Notably, multivitamins and mineral supplements typically do not contain significant amounts of calcium, so separate supplementation is often warranted.

The RDA for vitamin D intake remains 600 IU daily in adulthood, although higher intake is necessary for those with preexisting vitamin D deficiency or insufficiency [24]. Vitamin D deficiency is common among young adults, with the primary causes being inadequate exposure to sunlight and very few foods rich in vitamin D [26, 27]. Screening for vitamin D deficiency should be considered in YACCC, particularly those at high risk such as patients on anticonvulsant therapy and those with dark skin, due to lower rates of synthesis in response to the sun [28, 29]. The Endocrine Society recommends adults on anticonvulsant medications, glucocorticoids, antifungals, and medications used to treat human immunodeficiency virus (HIV) infection/acquired immunodeficiency syndrome (AIDS) receive 2–3 times the RDA for vitamin D, since these medications increase the catabolism of vitamin D [28].

Additional nutrients essential for bone health include protein, magnesium, zinc, copper, iron, fluoride, and vitamins A, C, and K [23].

Drug–Nutrient/Food Interactions

Drug–nutrient and drug–food interactions can have significant impact on patient health and must be evaluated as a part of medication review. Some medications can alter the patient's nutritional status or lead to nutrient deficiencies, and conversely some foods can alter the drug effect [30]. Table 20.2 outlines common drug–nutrient/food interactions that may be seen with YACCC.

Additionally, some medications may affect appetite, such as certain psychiatric medications including antidepressants, antipsychotics, as well as stimulants for attention disorders, and their potential contribution should be assessed in patients with weight management issues.

Nutrition for Wound Healing

Patients with malnutrition and unintentional weight loss are at risk for delayed wound healing and infection [31]. Losing more than 15 % lean body mass will delay wound healing, and losing more than 30 % will actually promote the development of wounds [32]. Ideally all patients with pressure ulcers or who are at risk for pressure ulcers, such as malnourished young adults with immobility from spina bifida or cerebral palsy, should have a formal nutrition assessment by a dietitian [33]. Wounds create a catabolic state that significantly increases calorie and protein requirements. Therefore, PCPs should encourage their patients with a wound to increase their calorie and protein intake [32].

Oral nutrition supplements and a multivitamin and mineral supplement are recommended for those with abnormal weight status or poor nutritional intake [31]. Enteral nutrition support is indicated for those unable to maintain adequate oral intake, either temporarily or chronically. Patients who are underweight or overweight can have micronutrient deficiencies that further impede healing. Vitamin C and zinc deficiencies are associated with poorly healing wounds, and patients with deficiencies benefit from supplementation and repeat labs every 2 weeks until

Table 20.2 Drug–nutrient, drug–food interactions

Anticonvulsants	Can increase need for vitamins D, K, C, B12, folate, and calcium with long-term use associated with low carnitine levels
Corticosteroids	Decreased bone mineral density; ensure adequate intake of calcium and vitamin D
Diuretics	Increased losses of sodium, potassium, chloride, calcium, magnesium, zinc
Immunosuppressants	Grapefruit can increase drug concentration Increased losses of magnesium and potassium Special attention to food safety to avoid food-borne illness
Statins	Grapefruit can increase drug concentration May decrease absorption of fat soluble vitamins (A, D, E, and K), vitamin B12, folic acid, and calcium
Anticoagulants	Vitamin K decreases anticoagulation effect (keep vitamin K intake consistent for best results). Licorice, vitamin E, fish oil, mango, and grapefruit may increase anticoagulation effect
Monoamine oxidase inhibitors	Interaction with tyramine in food can cause severe hypertension
Proton pump inhibitors	May impair absorption of calcium, magnesium, iron, zinc, folic acid, B12 May increase risk of bone fractures; ensure adequate intake of calcium and vitamin D
Calcium channel blockers	Grapefruit can increase drug concentration Large amounts of natural licorice can increase blood pressure
Beta blockers	Large amounts of natural licorice can increase blood pressure

replete [31]. Research has shown no benefit to supplementation when there is no evidence of a vitamin C or zinc deficiency [31].

Oral Supplementation

Formula Supplements

Commercial oral nutrition supplements can be of significant value for patients who are struggling to meet their nutrition needs with traditional foods. Some young adults rely on oral supplements as an exclusive source of nutrition; for example, the patient with autism who has severe food selectivity, or the patient with cerebral palsy who has inadequate muscle tone to coordinate solids but can take liquids safely by mouth. If a patient is taking all or the majority of his or her nutrition from an oral supplement, the PCP must ensure that it is nutritionally complete to prevent nutrient deficiencies (i.e., not missing any essential vitamins or minerals.). Manufacturers use wording such as "sole-source nutrition" or "appropriate for tube feeding" in their descriptions to indicate nutritionally complete formulations. However, when in doubt, the PCP should consult with a dietitian to review the appropriateness of the oral supplement for the patient.

Insurance coverage for oral supplements typically changes as young adults reach transition age, raising concerns for patients using them as a main source of nutrition. The Department of Health and Human Services (DSHS) will cover the oral formula cost for children and adolescents through a home health company after prior authorization, though this coverage may end at age 21 years [34]. Continued insurance coverage, if possible, may require prior authorization and medical justification by the provider, but this varies by state. Addressing this issue prior to reaching the limiting age is recommended to avoid possible gaps in care.

Paying out of pocket for oral supplements can be quite costly. Therefore, for those patients who cannot obtain insurance coverage, a dietitian can explore other options such as homemade high-calorie shakes and smoothies, though these options may not be a realistic or feasible substitute for caregivers.

Vitamin and Mineral Supplements (VMS)

Patients who are malnourished or lacking well-rounded nutrition intake may benefit from a multivitamin and mineral supplement (VMS). For example, a VMS may be indicated for the patient who is tube fed and receives less than 1400 calories per day, since this amount of formula may not meet their protein, vitamin, and mineral requirement. Over-the-counter supplements can vary from incomplete to excessive dosing with the risk for toxicity and should therefore be reviewed carefully. Some supplements contain herbs that could have drug interactions or pose other health risks to the chronically ill, further highlighting the importance of reviewing ingredients with the patient. VMS are commonly recommended supplements, however, their use in YACCC requires special consideration. As noted previously in the section on "Bone Health," VMS do not contain significant amounts of calcium or phosphorus. YACCC with swallowing difficulty, intellectual disability, or those who are tube fed may use alternative forms of VMS, such as liquid or gummy formulations. Liquid VMS are typically not nutritionally complete and specifically often do not contain folic acid, vitamin K, calcium, phosphorus, magnesium, and selenium. Gummy VMS do not contain iron, thus requiring separate supplementation in patients with iron deficiency. VMS may contain higher than recommended doses of some vitamins and minerals posing risk in certain populations, including those with chronic liver or renal disease.

Enteral Nutrition Support

Enteral nutrition (EN) support typically refers to nutrition delivered via feeding tube, and is appropriate for patients unable to take adequate PO intake, as highlighted previously. Though comanagement of EN typically occurs with the support of gastroenterologists and dietitians, PCPs should be familiar with commonly used enteral access devices and their maintenance, available enteral formulas, and the presentation and management of the complications of EN.

Enteral Access Devices

While short-term EN via the nasal route is common in inpatient and acute care settings, young adults with chronic feeding difficulties typically require long-term EN and have more permanent enteral access. Basic knowledge of long-term enteral tube options, placement methods, management, and potential complications are important for clinicians caring for these complex patients. Distinctions between tube types include terminus location (prepyloric versus postpyloric), placement method (endoscopic, radiology guided, or laproscopic/open surgical procedure), and external extension type (standard versus low-profile "button").

The most clinically significant distinction between tube types is prepyloric (gastric) versus postpyloric (jejeunal) terminus location (see Fig. 20.1a, b). In general, prepyloric tubes are preferred because of increased ease of placement, decreased risk of reprocedure (for tube repositioning and replacement), and because they allow more physiologic feeding regimens (bolus feeding). Postpyloric tubes may be indicated in patients with severe gastroesophageal reflux disease (GERD) or recurrent vomiting, gastric dysmotility or outlet obstruction and gastric anomalies (congenital or postsurgical) [35]. Postpyloric tubes are also often recommended for patients with feeding-related aspiration, although aspiration pneumonias from oral secretions can still occur [36]. Postpyloric tubes can be placed through an existing gastrostomy site, known as a percutaneous endoscopic gastrostomy with jejunal extension (PEG-J) tube, or directly into the jejunum, referred to as a direct percutaneous endoscopic jejunostomy (DPEJ) tube [36]. Patients with postpyloric tubes often also have a gastric port, which is used to drain gastric contents, termed "venting." Drawbacks of jejunal tubes include requirement for continuous tube feeding, which may limit patient lifestyle, frequent retrograde dislodgements requiring replacement and increased risk for tube clogging due to smaller caliber of tube [35, 36].

Initial placement of a long-term enteral access device may be percutaneous, laparoscopic, or surgical. Complication rates between these approaches in pediatric patients are comparable, with slightly decreased complications in adults with nonsurgical techniques [37]. Tubes are secured by an internal bolster, typically a balloon or bumper, and an external bolster. Following initial placement, tract maturation takes approximately 4 weeks, after which replacement can be accomplished either at the bedside (in clinic or at home) or by interventional radiology (IR), depending on the type of bolster and tube, with J-tubes typically requirinq IR. Following tract maturation some patients opt for transition to a low-profile "button" connection, which lies flush with the skin and is less visible under clothing but requires a connector for feeding (see Fig. 20.2a, b).

Frequency of tube exchange varies by tube type and use. Prepyloric tubes have the longest life, with routinely used PEG tubes lasting up to 2 years [36]. Low-profile "button" tubes have a shorter lifetime, typically requiring exchange every 6 months, though exchanges can often be done by patient or caregiver at home. Postpyloric tubes usually need to be exchanged more often due to frequency of retrograde dislodgement and obstruction or mechanical failure related to the small caliber of the tube. Mean functional use of postpyloric tubes is around 55 days in adults, with the possibility of shorter duration [37]. Typically, IR recommends exchange every 3–4 months for these postpyloric tubes.

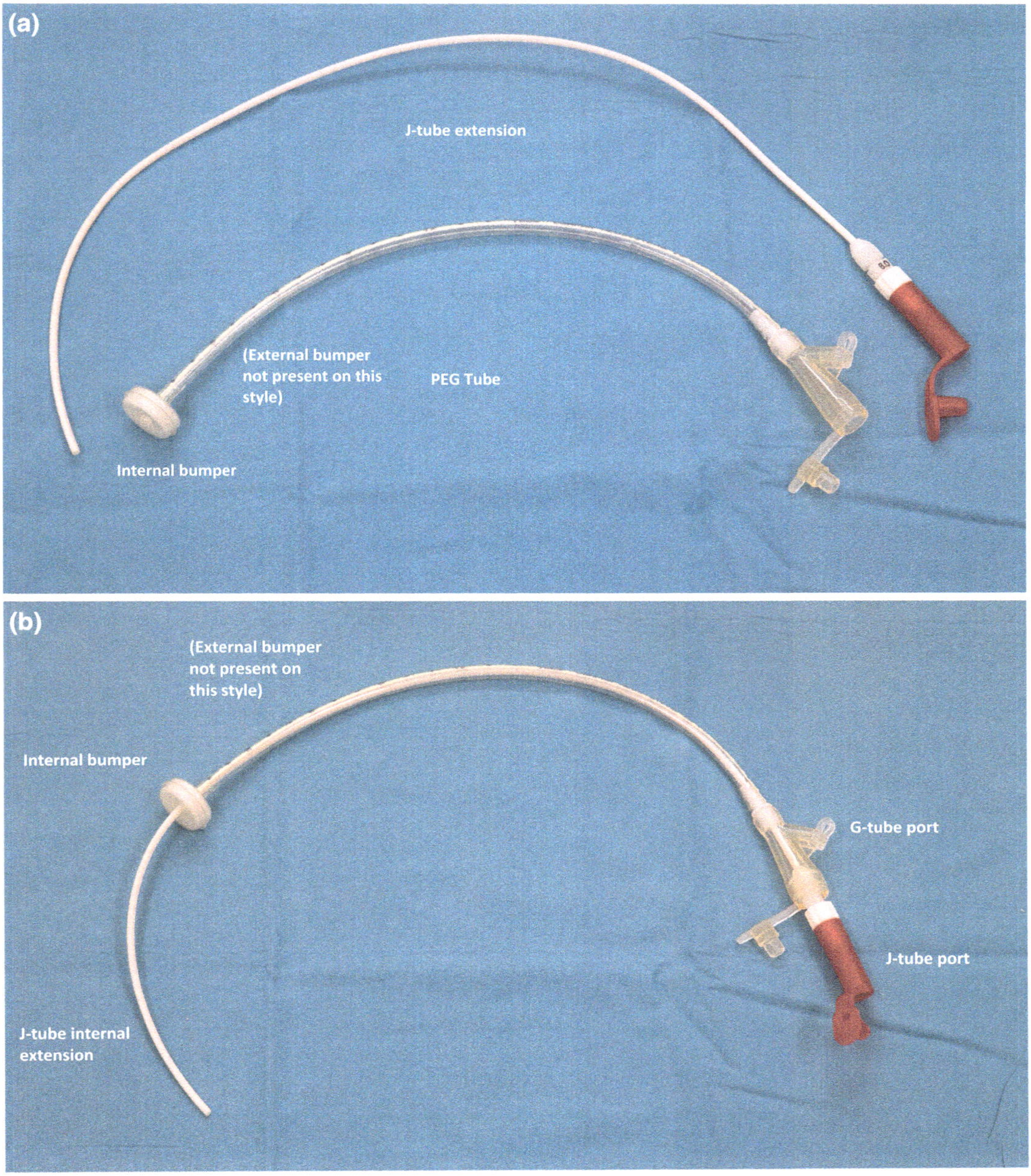

Fig. 20.1 **a** PEG tube length compared with J-tube extension length. This tube style does not have a built-in external bumper, text indicates where this item would be located. **b** PEG tube with J-tube extension in place

Important information to document about the patient's enteral access device includes type, length, frequency of recommended replacement, and method of replacement (bedside by clinician or IR-guided). Patients should have an extra tube at home in case of dislodgement, either for home replacement or to bring with them to the office or emergency department to speed replacement. In absence of an appropriate tube, a Foley catheter with a balloon can typically be placed in the short term to maintain the tract while awaiting definitive tube replacement.

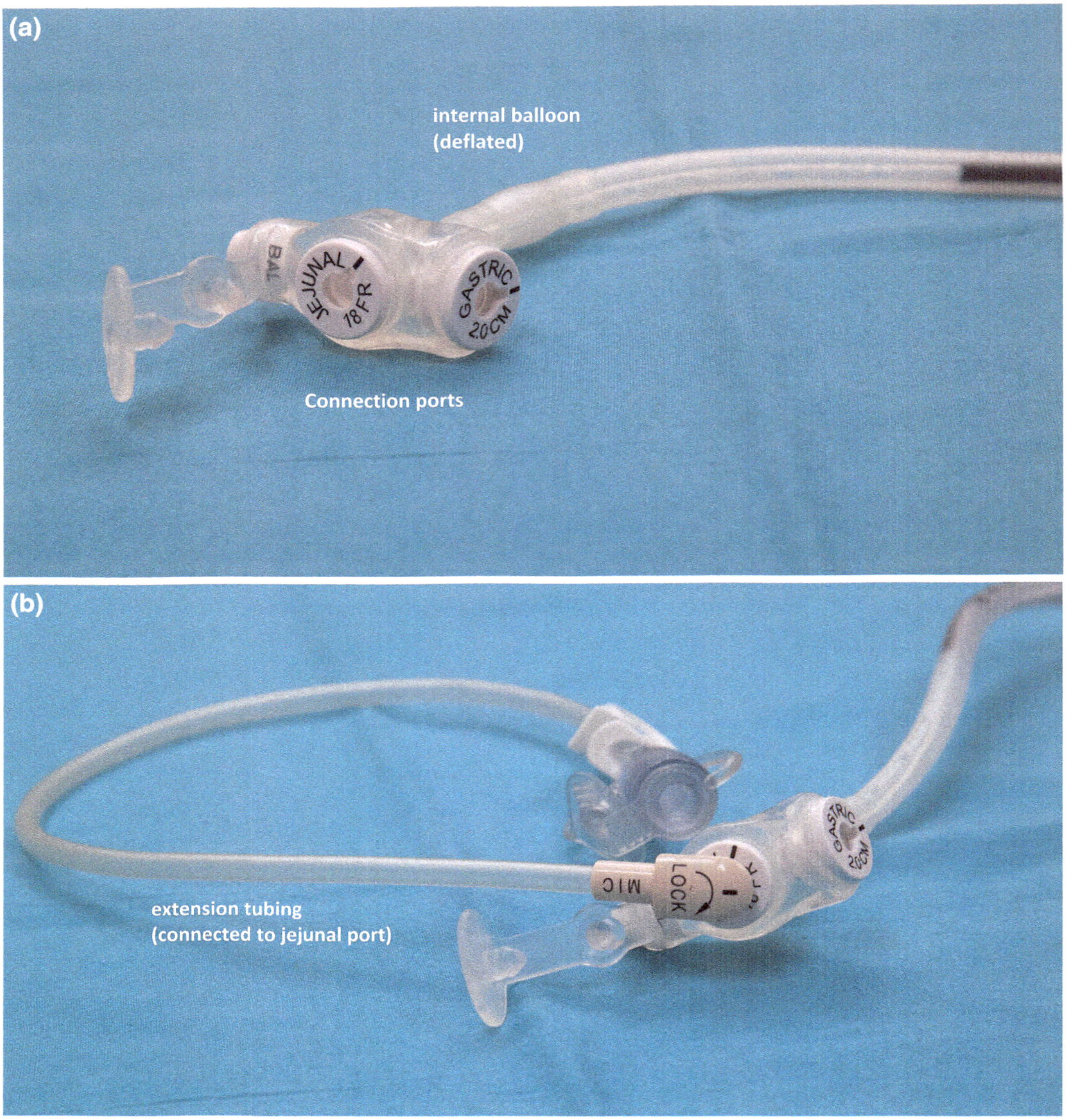

Fig. 20.2 **a** A low-profile tube set up. **b** A low-profile tube with connected extension tubing

Acute complications of long-term enteric tube devices should be addressed with the team who initially placed the tube. PCPs should, however, be familiar with the common complications seen in chronic enteric access and their management, summarized in Table 20.3 [36–38]. Additional less common but severe complications of enteric tubes include fistulous tracts, which are typically related to procedure complications or occur in patients with prior abdominal surgery. Work-up and treatment of fistulae should involve consultation with gastroenterology and surgical colleagues.

Table 20.3 Common complications associated with chronic enteric tube access. Compiled from [36–38]

Complication	Incidence	Symptoms	Risk factors	Prevention	Treatment
Peristomal wound infection	4–30 %	Erythema Swelling Fever Pain	Immunosuppression Diabetes Obesity or malnutrition	Avoid excessive traction on tube Pre-procedure antibiotics	Antibiotics
Clogged tube	23–35 % (higher occurrence among those with postpyloric tubes)	Inability to flush Inability to aspirate	Small caliber tube Crushed medications Use of bulking agents	Avoid gastric residual aspiration Dissolve all medications Frequent water flushes	Pancreatic enzymes mixed with bicarbonate Mechanical clearing Tube replacement
Dislodged tube	1.6–4.4 % (likely higher in practice)	Removed tube	Developmental disability	Low-profile tube Abdominal binder/cover	Replacement with Foley to maintain tract New tube placement by parent, provider or in IR
Peristomal leakage	1–2 % reported (likely higher in practice)	Formula leakage Gastric content leakage Skin irritation	Infection Gastric hypersecretion Traction on tube site	PPI for hypersecretion	Barrier cream Consider replacement or convert to G-J tube Do NOT upsize tube
Buried bumper syndrome (internal bolster migrates)	2–6 % (usually late complication)	Immobile tube Increased resistance to flushes Tube leakage Tube occlusion Abdominal pain	Excessive traction between bumpers	Allow 1.5 cm between skin and external bolster Mobilize PEG every other day	Consult IR regarding removal and new tube placement
Bleeding (delayed)		Anemia Gastroccult positive	Buried bumper GERD (esophagitis is most common cause)	PPI	PPI Consider endoscopic evaluation

IR interventional radiology, *PPI* proton pump inhibitor, *PEG* percutaneous endoscopic gastrostomy, *GERD* gastroesophageal reflux disease

Enteral Formulas

The four major categories of enteral formulas are polymeric (standard), partially hydrolyzed/semi-elemental, elemental, and blended food, summarized in Table 20.4. The formula types can vary in protein, fat, and carbohydrate composition, and PCPs should have a basic understanding of these differences as well as available special formulas and transitioning from pediatric to adult formulas.

Polymeric and blended food formulas contain complete proteins, while in partially hydrolyzed

Table 20.4 Categories of enteral formulas

	Polymeric/standard	Partially hydrolyzed/semi-elemental	Elemental	Blended food
Ingredients	Complete cow's milk protein and/or soy protein, corn syrup/maltodextrin/sugar, MCT, and LCT (oral supplements do not contain MCT), vitamins and minerals With or without fiber	Hydrolyzed whey and/or casein, maltodextrin/sugar, MCT, and LCT With or without fiber	Amino acids, maltodextrin/modified cornstarch, MCT, and LCT	Highly varies Food contains fiber
Indications	Standard formula for normal GI function	Feeding intolerance, GI dysfunction, short bowel syndrome, malabsorption, pancreatic insufficiency	Same indications as partially hydrolyzed formula and severe food allergies	Commercially sterile and convenient alternative for homemade blenderized tube feeding
Examples	Boost, Ensure, Nutren, Jevity, Osmolite	Peptamen, Vital	Vivonex (low fat), Tolerex (very low fat, not for long-term use)	Compleat, liquid hope, real food blends

MCT medium-chain triglycerides, *LCT* long-chain triglycerides, *GI* gastrointestinal

formulas the protein is enzymatically hydrolyzed to small peptides and amino acids. Partially hydrolyzed formulas are typically used with treatment of feeding intolerance, GI dysfunction, short bowel syndrome, malabsorption, pancreatic insufficiency, and intractable diarrhea—although there is conflicting evidence on whether these formulas improve diarrhea [39]. Due to limited evidence supporting the use of hydrolyzed formulas, the American Society of Parenteral and Enteral Nutrition (ASPEN) and the European Society of Parenteral and Enteral Nutrition make no recommendations on the use of these formulas [39]. Elemental formulas contain proteins that are completely broken down into amino acids. These formulas are indicated for severe food allergies as well as all of the same indications as partially hydrolyzed formulas. Drawbacks of elemental formulas include increased cost, more time spent preparing feeds since elemental formulas are powder based, and higher risk of contamination since powdered formulas are not sterile. Therefore, elemental formula is typically reserved for those situations when partially hydrolyzed formulas are not tolerated.

The majority of enteral formulas contain fats in the form of medium-chain triglycerides (MCTs), which do not require pancreatic enzymes or bile to be absorbed and which bypass the lymph system directly into portal circulation. MCTs are essential to promote fat absorption for patients with cholestasis or bile salt malabsorption such as with short gut syndrome. Formulas also contain some long-chain triglycerides (LCTs) because MCTs do not provide essential fatty acids.

Carbohydrate source varies by formula but all pediatric and adult formulas are lactose free. Standard caloric concentration is 30 calories per ounce, but many formulas are also available in 36 and 45 calories per ounce preparations. Other variations include those with high protein concentrations, with or without fiber, and with prebiotics. Prebiotics are a form of fiber that is fermented in the ileum and colon by bacteria, thereby stimulating growth and/or activity of gut microbiota [39].

Commercially-prepared blended food formulas are growing in popularity due to a desire to provide whole foods. Some blended food

Table 20.5 Comparison of bolus and continuous feeding methods

Feeding type	Bolus feeding	Continuous feeding
What	Periodic, moderate volume	Continuous slow infusion
Frequency	Up to 6 times per day	12–24 h/day
How	By syringe, gravity, or over a pump	Pump
Benefits	Physiologic "meals" Ample disconnected time	Improved tolerance for those with poor GI motility May reduce aspiration risk [40, 41]
Drawbacks	Sometimes requires tolerance to large bolus volumes Not possible with postpyloric tubes	Requires pump Prolonged connected time

formulas are nutritionally complete with added vitamins and minerals, and some contain only a few foods per packet with no vitamin, mineral, or electrolyte supplementation. Some caregivers will prepare their own home-blended tube feeding, which requires a very powerful and typically expensive blender, although some blender companies will give discounts if the device will be used to prepare tube feeding. Home-blended diets should be monitored by a dietitian to ensure adequate fluid and nutrient intake as well as food safety.

Explanation of the wide variety of disease-specific formulas is beyond the scope of this chapter, but the PCP should know that specialized options exist for ketogenic diets; for conditions such as renal failure, liver failure, diabetes mellitus, pancreatitis, and specific pulmonary diagnoses; for patients requiring immune-modulating therapy or critical care; and for patients with chylous effusions or who have undergone bariatric surgery.

Some transitioning patients who are tube fed may still be receiving a pediatric formula when they reach adult care. Compared to pediatric formulas, adult formulas typically have more protein, more fiber, less calcium and phosphorus, and a variable content of other vitamins and minerals. An adult patient receiving all or the majority of his or her nutrition from a pediatric formula may be receiving an inadequate or, in some cases, an excess amount of certain nutrients, in particular calcium. Poor feeding tolerance with other formula trials may lead to ongoing use of pediatric formulas, and an adequate history and possible consultation with prior providers should be considered prior to suggesting changes. For those patients who would benefit from a detailed nutrient analysis or change in formula, consultation with a dietitian is appropriate.

Adjusting Enteral Nutrition

Determination of an appropriate feeding schedule is patient-specific and depends on multiple factors, including the type of tube, amount of formula and fluid needed, and patient lifestyle factors. A general comparison of the two methods is outlined in Table 20.5 [40, 41]. Prepyloric tubes allow either feeding type, whereas postpyloric tubes require continuous feeding due to inability to handle volume required for boluses.

In active patients without gastrointestinal contraindications, bolus feeding is usually preferred due to value of intermittent schedule. In patients who still take some nutrition orally, bolus feeding or overnight continuous feeding with disconnection during the day can facilitate hunger cues. In patients with high aspiration risk, continuous feeding is often recommended due to presumed decreased aspiration risk, although most studies demonstrating this decreased risk were conducted in critically ill patients [40, 41]. With continuous feeding, caution must be exercised about overnight feeding as risk of aspiration may be increased with sleep. Proper positioning and prevention of tube dislodgement are important factors to consider.

When assessing a patient's tube feeding regimen, nutrition and fluid needs should be assessed separately, as volume of formula intake may not match fluid requirement. For example, patients with chronic constipation may benefit from a formula that contains fiber and a fluid intake above their maintenance fluids requirement to promote regularity. Additionally, acute illnesses can change fluid needs, particularly if the illness involves vomiting, diarrhea, or increased sweating, requiring temporary increase in fluid intake.

When a patient who is tube fed has chronic unintentional weight loss or gain, a conservative first step is to modify their caloric intake by 10–15 %, keeping in mind weight goals noted earlier in this chapter. If the patient is having rapid weight gain or loss, a more aggressive approach may be necessary with a 20–30 % change in caloric intake. When reducing formula intake, one needs to consider whether the volume should be replaced with water to meet their fluid requirement and whether the decreased formula intake will still meet their protein, vitamin, and mineral requirement. Patients receiving less than 1400 calories per day are at increased risk of inadequate nutrient intake, as noted previously. When uncertainty exists, a dietitian should be consulted for a thorough nutrient analysis. Interval assessments of weight with tube feeding adjustments should be considered every 2–3 weeks to monitor changes and tolerance issues.

Enteral Nutrition Complications and Feeding Intolerance

EN is often associated with changes in gastrointestinal function, with the most common being diarrhea, followed by nausea and constipation [36]. Evaluation of feeding intolerance symptoms by the PCP should follow a stepwise approach.

Normal stool consistency in exclusively tube fed individuals should be soft to mushy, and 2–3 bowel movements per day may be normal. Watery stools or higher frequency may constitute diarrhea. Initial assessment should include review of formula type, any recent changes in formula or medications, evidence of malabsorption, and risk assessment for intestinal infections. In-patients receiving enteral tube feeding have been shown to have a ninefold increased risk of developing *Clostridium difficile* infections [36]. Whether this risk extends to chronic EN is unclear, but the onset of diarrhea in a patient receiving long-term EN should prompt increased clinical suspicion.

Treatment of noninfectious enteral feeding-related diarrhea can include adjustment of formula type or addition of fiber [42]. Such changes may be guided by a dietitian. In theory, fiber may decrease diarrhea due to soluble fiber increasing fluid absorption and insoluble fiber slowing transit time. However, there has been conflicting evidence on whether adding fiber to tube feeding decreases diarrhea [39]. Adding probiotics may be of some help in slowing diarrhea, with minimal risk in otherwise stable patients [43]. Use of antidiarrheal medications such as loperamide should be reserved for refractory cases.

While overall less common than diarrhea in this population, constipation may be more prevalent in patients on long-term EN [36]. In addition, in YACCC, constipation may be compounded by the underlying condition that resulted in need for nutritional support, such as neurogenic bowel in patients with cerebral palsy or spina bifida. Treatment and prevention of constipation is frequently managed with a stable bowel regimen that may include stool softeners, such as colace, and promotility agents, such as senna and miralax. Addition of fiber has not shown consistent benefit for enterally fed patients and is not recommended as first-line therapy [36].

In addition to diarrhea and constipation, feeding intolerance may present as nausea, vomiting, abdominal distention, or discomfort. As with constipation and diarrhea, the patient's clinical status and whether medications, infection, inflammation, or constipation could be causing intolerance should be assessed. When these variables have been addressed or eliminated from consideration, one should look to overfeeding, rapid infusion time, rapid infusion of very cold formula, any recent changes in formula type or fiber intake, or bacterial contamination of enteral feeds as potential causes of the feeding intolerance [39].

If infusion rate is a concern and the patient is receiving gravity bolus feeds, the rate can be decreased by lowering the height of the syringe or feeding bag or by controlling the rate with a feeding pump. High-osmolality formulas rarely cause diarrhea, but this can occur if these formulas are infused too quickly [39]. Osmolality increases with formula caloric density, and elemental and low-fat formulas have a higher osmolality than polymeric formulas.

If infusion rate is ruled out as causative, one might consider a change in formula, such as a trial of partially hydrolyzed formula for the patient not tolerating a polymeric formula or adjustment of fiber content, either with a modified formula or powdered supplement.

Parenteral Nutrition Support

Parenteral nutrition (PN) is most commonly used in the acute care setting for patients who are unable to tolerate EN [44]. Adult providers are likely most familiar with its use in this short-term setting. However, in rare cases, young adults may receive chronic PN support. Clinical conditions in young adults that may warrant PN include short gut syndrome (due to resections from necrotizing enterocolitis, inflammatory bowel disease, or recurrent bowel obstructions), malabsorption syndromes (such as severe inflammatory bowel syndrome or celiac disease), high-output gastric fistulas or severe intestinal dysmotility with inability to tolerate EN [15].

Monitoring and prescribing PN requires the close involvement of a dietitian and pharmacist who work with a home infusion company. The PCP is typically responsible for ordering laboratory testing and communicating with the dietitian and infusion company for periodic adjustment of PN orders, typically on a monthly basis. As young adult nutrition goals shift from growth to maintenance, adjustments are usually less dramatic than in childhood.

PN has multiple risks including those associated with the long-term central intravenous access (IV) required for administration and the nutrition itself. Young adults with long-term central IV access are at risk for line malfunction and catheter-related blood stream infections, a risk that is amplified in the setting of daily access for PN [15]. PN can also cause liver dysfunction, termed parenteral nutrition-associated liver disease (PNALD), which is typically cholestatic and can range from mild to severe liver failure. PNALD risk is also associated with an increased frequency of line infections [45].

In addition to increased medical risks, PN is significantly more expensive than enteral options. Insurance companies typically require strict documentation of the clinical indication for PN in order to provide coverage of PN. This documentation typically needs to be resubmitted periodically to ensure ongoing coverage [15].

Conclusion

YACCC are at increased nutritional risk, and management of nutrition needs is an essential part of primary care for this population. Assessment of nutritional status includes determining caloric and weight goals as well as vitamin and mineral needs. Nutritional needs may vary based on underlying condition, disease progression, and medications, requiring periodic assessment by the PCP. A PCP should have a basic understanding of nutritional support options, including oral, enteral, or parenteral support with additional aid of a dietician in complex cases.

References

1. Marchand V, Motil KJ, NASPGHAN Committee on Nutrition. Nutrition support for neurologically impaired children: a clinical report of the North American society for pediatric gastroenterology, hepatology, and nutrition. J Pediatr Gastroenterol Nutr. 2006;43(1):123–35.

2. White JV, Guenter P, Jensen G, Malone A, Schofield M, Academy of Nutrition and Dietetics Malnutrition Work Group; A.S.P.E.N. Malnutrition Task Force; A.S.P.E.N. Board of Directors. Consensus statement of the academy of nutrition and dietetics/American society for parenteral and enteral nutrition: characteristics recommended for the identification and documentation of adult malnutrition (undernutrition). J Acad Nutr Diet. 2012;112(5):730–8.
3. Sinaasappel M, Stern M, Littlewood J, Wolfe S, Steinkamp G, Heijerman HGM, et al. Nutrition in patients with cystic fibrosis: a European consensus. J Cyst Fibros. 2002;1(2):51–75.
4. Pencharz PB, Durie PR. Pathogenesis of malnutrition in cystic fibrosis. Clin Nutr. 2000;19(6):387–94.
5. Marin VB, Velandia S, Hunter B, Gattas V, Fielbaum O, Herrera O, et al. Energy expenditure, nutrition status, and body composition in children with cystic fibrosis. Nutrition. 2004;20:181–6.
6. Johnson RK, Goran MI, Ferrara MS, Poehlman ET. Athetosis increased resting metabolic rate in adults with cerebral palsy. J Am Diet Assoc. 1996;96:145–8.
7. Johnson RK, Hildreth HG, Contompasis SH, Goran MI. Total energy expenditure in adults with cerebral palsy as assessed by doubly labeled water. J Am Diet Assoc. 1997;97:966–70.
8. Mari-Bauset S, Zazpe I, Mari-Sanchis A, Llopis-Gonzalez A, Morales-Suarez-Varela M. Food selectivity in autism spectrum disorders: a systematic review. J Autism Dev Disord. 2014;29(11):1554–61.
9. Kerwin ML, Eicher PS, Gelsinger J. Parental report of eating problems and gastrointestinal symptoms in children with pervasive developmental disorders. Child Health Care. 2005;34:217–34.
10. Fung EB, Samson-Fang L, Stallings VA, Conaway M, Liptak G, Henderson RC, et al. Feeding dysfunction is associated with poor growth and health status in children with cerebral palsy. J Am Diet Assoc. 2002;102(261–368):373.
11. van den Engel-Hoek L, Erasmus CE, Hendriks JC, Geurts AC, Klein WM, Pillen S, et al. Oral muscles are progressively affectedin Duchenne muscular dystrophy: implications for dysphagia treatment. J Neurol. 2013;260(5):1295–303.
12. Cooper-Brown L, Copeland S, Dailey S, Downey D, Peterson MC, Stimson C, et al. Feeding and swallowing dysfunction in genetic syndromes. Dev Disabil Res Rev. 2008;14:147–57.
13. Abraham BP, Mehta S, El-Serag HB. Natural history of pediatric-onset inflammatory bowel disease: a systematic review. J Clin Gastroenterol. 2012;46 (7):581–9.
14. Bell KL, Samson-Fang L. Nutritional management of children with cerebral palsy. Eur JClin Nutr. 2013;67 (suppl 2):S13–6.
15. ASPEN board of directors and the clinical guidelines task force. Guidelines for the use of parenteral and enteral nutrition in adult and pediatric patients. J Parenter Enteral Nutr. 2002;26(1 Suppl):1SA–138SA.
16. Centers for Disease Control and Prevention. About Adult BMI. 2015. http://www.cdc.gov/healthyweight/assessing/bmi/adult_bmi/index.html.
17. Tokunaga K, Matsuzawa Y, Kotani K, Keno Y, Kobatake T, Fujioka S, et al. Ideal body weight estimated from the body mass index with the lowest morbidity. Int J Obes. 1991;15(1):1–5.
18. Froehlich-Grobe K, Nary DE, Van Sciver A, Lee J, Little TD. Measuring height without a stadiometer: empirical investigation of four height estimates among wheelchair users. Am J Phys Med Rehabil. 2011;90(8):658–66.
19. [no authors listed] NHLBI Obesity Education Initiative Expert Panel. Clinical guidelines on the identification, evaluation, and treatment of overweight and obesity in adults. Obes Res. 1998;6(Suppl 2):51S–209S.
20. Humphries K, Traci MA, Seekins T. Nutrition and adults with intellectual or developmental disabilities: systematic literature review results. Intellect Dev Disabil. 2009;47(3):163–85.
21. Trabulsi J, Schoeller DA. Evaluation of dietary assessment instruments against doubly labeled water, a biomarker of habitual energy intake. Am J Physiol Endocrinol Metab. 2001;281(5):E891–9.
22. Chad KE, McKay HA, Zello GA, Bailey DA, Faulkner RA, Snyder RE. Body composition in nutritionally adequate ambulatory and non-ambulatory children with cerebral palsy and a healthy reference group. Dev Med Child Neurol. 2000;42(5):334–9.
23. Ilich JZ, Kerstetter JE. Nutrition in bone health revisited: a story beyond calcium. J Am Coll Nutr. 2000;19(6):715–37.
24. Institute of Medicine of the National Academies. Report Brief November 2010. Dietary Reference Intakes for Calcium and Vitamin D. http://iom.nationalacademies.org/~/media/Files/Report%20Files/2010/Dietary-Reference-Intakes-for-Calcium-and-Vitamin-D/Vitamin%20D%20and%20Calcium%202010%20Report%20Brief.pdf.
25. National Osteoporosis Foundation. Steps to Estimate Your Calcium Intake. http://nof.org/articles/542.
26. Tangpricha V, Pearce EN, Chen TC, Holick MF. Vitamin D insufficiency among free-living healthy young adults. Am J Med. 2002;112(8):659–62.
27. Holick MF, Chen TC. Vitamin D deficiency: a worldwide problem with health consequences. Am J Clin Nutr. 2008;87(4):1080S–6S.
28. Holick MF, Binkley NC, Bischoff-Ferrari HA, Gordon CM, Hanley DA, Heaney RP, et al. Endocrine society. Evaluation, treatment, and prevention of vitamin D deficiency: an endocrine society clinical practice guideline. J Clin Endocrinol Metab. 2011;96 (7):1911–30.
29. Clemens TL, Adams JS, Henderson SL, Holick MF. Increased skin pigment reduces the capacity of skin to synthesise vitamin D3. Lancet. 1982;1(8263):74–6.
30. Boullata JI, Hudson LM. Drug–nutrient interactions: a broad view with implications for practice. J Acad Nutr Diet. 2012;112(4):506–17.

31. Thompson KL, Leu MG, Drummond KL, Popalisky J, Spencer SM, Lenssen PM. Nutrition interventions to optimize pediatric wound healing an evidence-based clinical pathway. Nutr Clin Pract. 2014;29(4):473–82.
32. Demling RH. Nutrition, anabolism, and the wound healing process: an overview. Eplasty. 2009;9:e9.
33. Dorner B, Posthauer ME, Thomas D, National Pressure Ulcer Advisory Panel. The role of nutrition in pressure ulcer prevention and treatment: national pressure ulcer advisory panel white paper. Adv Skin Wound Care. 2009;22(5):212–21.
34. Washington State Department of Social and Health Services. Medicare Purchasing Administration (MPA). Enteral Nutrition Billing instructions. Chapter 388-554 WAC. 2010. http://www.hca.wa.gov/medicaid/billing/documents/guides/enteral_nutrition_biasof063011.pdf.
35. Gopalan S, Khanna S. Enteral nutrition delivery technique. Curr Opin Clin Nutr Metab Care. 2003;6:313–7.
36. Blumenstein I, Shastir YM, Stein J. Gastroenteric tube feeding: techniques, problems and solutions. World J Gastroenterol. 2014;20(26):8505–24.
37. ASGE Technolgy Committee, Kwon RS, Banerjee S, Desilets D, Diehl DL, Farraye FA, Kaul V, et al. Enteral nutrition access devices. Gastrointest Endosc. 2010;72(2):236–48.
38. Lynch CR, Fang JC. Prevention and management of complications of percutaneous endoscopic gastrostomy (PEG) tubes. Practical Gastroenterol. 2004;28:66–76.
39. The ASPEN Adult Nutrition Support Core Curriculum, 2nd edn. Silver Spring, MD: American Society for Parenteral and Enteral Nutrition; 2012.
40. Alkhawaja S, Martin C, Butler RJ, Gwadry-Sridhar F. Post-pyloric versus gastric tube feeding for preventing pneumonia and improving nutritional outcomes in critically ill adults. Cochrane Database Syst Rev. 2015;8:CD008875.
Wang D, Zheng SQ, Chen XC, Jiang SW, Chen HB. Comparisons between small intestinal and gastric feeding in severe traumatic brain injury: a systematic review and meta-analysis of randomized controlled trials. J Neurosurg. 2015;123:1194–201.
42. Whelan K, Schneider SM. Mechanisms, prevention, and management of diarrhea in enteral nutrition. Curr Opin Gastroenterol. 2011;27:152–9.
43. Whelan K, Myers CE. Safety of probiotics in patients receiving nutritional support: a systematic review of case reports randomized controlled trials, and non-randomized trials. Am J Clin Nutr. 2010;91:687–703.
44. Zaloga GP. Parenteral nutrition in adult inpatients with functioning gastrointestinal tracts: assessment of outcomes. Lancet. 2006;367:1101–11.
45. Wales PW, Allen N, Worthington P, George D, Compher C, American Society for Parenteral and Enteral Nutrition, Teitelbaum D. A.S.P.E.N. Clinical guidelines: support of pediatric patients with intestinal failure at risk of parenteral nutrition-associated liver disease. J Parenter Enteral Nutr. 2014;38(5):538–57.

21 Technology Dependence of the Nervous System

Devesh Upadhya and Cynthia Peacock

Introduction

Multiple childhood medical conditions affect the nervous system, including intracranial hemorrhage, cerebral palsy, spina bifida, and intractable epilepsy. Implantable devices used in these patients can improve quality and duration of life. While the devices are often managed by neurosurgeons or neurologists, a basic understanding of their function allows the primary care physician to recognize and assist in early management of device complications including failure.

Intrathecal Baclofen Therapy

Intrathecal baclofen is an increasingly utilized tool for the management of spasticity. It may be used in the treatment of spasticity associated with cerebral palsy, multiple sclerosis, and other conditions. Intrathecal delivery of baclofen decreases systemic side effects and improves response to therapy. This allows better control of tone and spasm, reducing pain, and improving functional capabilities of patients.

D. Upadhya · C. Peacock (✉)
Department of Internal Medicine and Pediatrics, Baylor College of Medicine, 1 Baylor Plaza – BCM 620, Houston, TX 77030, USA
e-mail: cpeacock@bcm.edu

D. Upadhya
e-mail: upadhya@bcm.edu

Device

The primary device available for delivery of baclofen is the Medtronic Synchromed II [1]. The pump is placed underneath the anterior abdominal skin, typically on the right, with the catheter tunneled laterally to the spine. The device is a 3-in. diameter, 1-in. thickness disc with a peripheral catheter access port and a central port allowing access to the drug reservoir. The device is easily palpated subcutaneously on examination of the lower abdomen. Specific precautions following baclofen pump placement are available from the manufacturer but include the possibility of baclofen overdose and withdrawal (see Complications section below) [1]. Important issues to review at routine visits include regular pump refills, additional sedative medications, and pump alarms. The Synchromed II has a 1-tone alarm that sounds when the pump has a problem or needs to be refilled or replaced. There is a separate, two-tone alarm to indicate discontinuation of baclofen infusion. Two-tone alarming is considered an urgent issue. In addition, pump function should be confirmed following exposure to magnetic resonance imagining (MRI). Routine MRIs can be safely performed, though the physician managing the pump should be contacted before the imaging procedure is done.

M. Pilapil et al. (eds.), *Care of Adults with Chronic Childhood Conditions*,
DOI 10.1007/978-3-319-43827-6_21

Complications

Complications of baclofen pump therapy are managed in concert with the prescribing physical medicine and rehabilitation physician but may also require the involvement of a neurosurgeon. Device complications typically present as baclofen withdrawal or baclofen overdose.

Baclofen overdose is frequently iatrogenic or associated with pump refilling; less frequently, it is associated with pump malfunction. Patients may present with hypotension, hypotonia, flaccid paralysis, somnolence, delirium, respiratory depression, seizures, and cardiac abnormalities. There is no specific antidote for intrathecal baclofen overdose. Instead, supportive care involves resuscitation and mechanical ventilation when necessary. The physician managing the pump should be contacted to assist with urgent discontinuation of drug infusion. If necessary, there is an access port on the pump that can be aspirated to empty baclofen from the reservoir, and lumbar puncture can be used to drain baclofen from the intrathecal space [2].

Baclofen withdrawal is a potential medical emergency. It may be associated with delay in refilling the reservoir, catheter problems such as kinking or line disruption, device problems, or intentional discontinuation of the device by the treating physician. Patients present with recurrence of initial spasticity symptoms, tachycardia, hyperthermia, itching, or seizures. Less frequently, patients may exhibit neuropsychiatric symptoms, malignant hyperthermia, autonomic instability, rhabdomyolysis, disseminated intravascular coagulation, or multi-organ failure. Initial management includes use of various sedative medications, including propofol, benzodiazepenes, or, with more limited efficacy, high-dose oral baclofen. Many patients will have oral baclofen available for emergency administration. Externalized intrathecal catheters have also been used for temporizing therapy. Definitive management requires device interrogation and assessment of catheter continuity and flow [2].

Other complications can be related to device placement or other components of the system [3–5]. Infection of overlying skin or the central nervous system (CNS) has been reported in 5–17 % of patients. Catheter damage, tip migration, kinking, or blockage is seen in 15–20 % of patients, and cerebrospinal fluid (CSF) leak is seen in 22 % of patients. Standard abdominal radiographs, anterior-posterior (AP), and lateral lumbar spine radiographs, and AP thoracic spine radiographs can help identify catheter problems. In the absence of visible catheter disruption, more advanced fluoroscopic and nuclear medicine techniques can aid in the diagnosis of catheter dysfunction [6]. Additional online resources are available for both providers as well as patients [7].

Ventricular Shunts

Ventriculoperitoneal (VP) shunts are extensively used for the treatment of symptomatic hydrocephalus. They consist of an intraventricular portion, typically placed in the right lateral ventricle, a valve that regulates outflow of CSF based on intracranial pressure, and shunt tubing that travels along the lateral neck, across the clavicle and ribs, and into the peritoneum. The shunt is usually palpable subcutaneously via the right parietal scalp and down the lateral neck on physical exam. Although the preferred distal site for shunt placement is the peritoneal space, less commonly used are the ventriculoatrial (VA) shunt, which has CSF flowing from the cerebral ventricular system to the atrium of the heart, or the ventriculopleural shunt, with CSF flowing to the pleural space. There can be many reasons to select these alternative sites, and these options should be discussed by neurosurgeons with patients and their families. This remainder of the discussion in this section will focus on the more commonly used VP shunts.

Complications of VP shunts should be managed in concert with a neurosurgeon. Complications can include infection, obstruction, mechanical failure, over-drainage, loculations within the ventricular system, and abdominal pathology. The type of complication is often associated with the timing since shunt placement. Shunt failure occurs in most patients at some point and can occur years after initial placement, including into adulthood [8, 9].

Infection is most common in the period immediately after shunt placement, but risk persists throughout the lifetime of the shunt. In one retrospective analysis of adults with VP shunt infections, the most frequent presenting symptoms were fever (78 %), neck stiffness (45 %), and local signs of infection such as erythema over shunt tubing (49 %) [10]. In this study, CSF leukocyte count was elevated in 80 % of patients, and cultures were positive in 66 % of patients; yield was highest when the specimen was obtained by valve puncture. Peripheral white blood cell count was not a reliable indicator of infection. Intracranial imaging was of limited value, but intra-abdominal imaging was frequently abnormal when the intra-abdominal portion of the shunt was infected. Computed tomography (CT) scan was more useful than ultrasound in this regard, and findings associated with infection included inflamed fat or muscle around the shunt, thickened gut wall, intra-abdominal abscess, and peritoneal cyst. Common etiologic agents are coagulase-negative staphylococci (CoNS), *Staphylococcous aureus*, and *Propionibacterium acnes*. Notably, infection with CoNS tends to be less symptomatic [11].

A variety of noninfectious shunt complications can occur. Shunt obstruction or mechanical failure can occur anywhere along the system. It usually manifests with signs of elevated intracranial pressure, including nausea, vomiting, headache, lethargy, irritability, decline in academic performance, change in vision, increase in seizure frequency, and ataxia [12]. A shunt series using plain radiographs can assist in diagnosis of mechanical shunt failure, as may occur with cracks in shunt tubing or recession of the shunt tip out of the peritoneum. However, the majority of shunt failure happens in the absence of apparent mechanical failure on plain films. At times, even cross-sectional imaging may not provide definitive diagnosis, and in these cases either further imaging (i.e., radionucleotide injection into the shunt reservoir) or surgery based on clinical suspicion may be undertaken [13]. Over-drainage of CSF can result in the slit ventricle syndrome, with CT findings of very small, "slit-like" ventricles. This condition presents with symptoms similar to shunt obstruction, although symptoms are often worse with the patient in the upright position. Within the abdomen, shunts can become obstructed by pseudocyst formation around the catheter tip. In this situation, patients typically present with abdominal distention. Rarely, distal shunt components can cause perforation of the bladder or intestines [14].

Additional online information is available for providers and patients [15].

Vagal Nerve Stimulator (VNS)

Vagal nerve stimulation is an evolving therapeutic modality. Initially utilized for intractable epilepsy, it is now also indicated for treatment-resistant depression [16]. Notably, in the population of patients with chronic childhood conditions, it has also been observed to have a beneficial effect on disruptive behavior and obesity [16]. The VNS device is usually implanted on the left to avoid interference with sinoatrial node innervation. The electrode is placed adjacent to the vagus nerve in the neck, within the neurovascular bundle containing the common carotid and internal jugular veins. The lead is tunneled subcutaneously to a pocket in the lateral chest. Complete seizure freedom with the use of a VNS is not typical, and most people will still require medications while using the VNS.

Several of the complications associated with VNS placement are procedure-related [17, 18]. The procedure is associated with a 3–6 % infection rate. Injury to the adjacent structures can also result in vocal cord palsy, swallowing difficulty, and neck pain [17, 18].

Other side effects are related to stimulation of the vagus nerve, and adjustment of device settings or postural changes can result in relief. Hoarseness is the most common of these [19]. Others include throat pain, cough, and dyspnea. Respiratory effects, including both obstructive and central sleep apneas, have also been reported, though their clinical significance is unclear [20]. Aspiration may occur in some patients, and causation can be investigated with manipulation of device settings [21]. Symptoms tend to wane with time, and use of an external magnet with a programmable VNS allows individual testing for correlation of symptoms [19].

Use of MRI is limited in patients with VNS due to concerns for heating the tip of the device lead; however, it has been safely performed with modified protocols [22].

Additional online information is available for providers and patients [23–25].

Conclusion

The use of implantable devices to treat neurological conditions continues to evolve and promises significant improvement in life expectancy and quality of life. As use of these applications expands in adult populations, primary care physicians should build the knowledge base to guide patients through the consideration, implantation, and ongoing management of these devices.

References

1. Medtronic. Medtronic for healthcare professionals: intrathecal baclofen therapy. http://professional.medtronic.com/pt/neuro/itb/index.htm#.Vv2w8pwrJhE. Accessed 16 May 2016.
2. Watve SV, Sivan M, Raza WA, Jamil FF. Management of acute overdose or withdrawal state in intrathecal baclofen therapy. Spinal Cord. 2012;50(2):107–11.
3. Motta F, Antonello CE. Analysis of complications in 430 consecutive pediatric patients treated with intrathecal baclofen therapy: 14-year experience. J Neurosurg Pediatr. 2014;13(3):301–6.
4. Dickey MP, Rice M, Kinnett DG, Lambert R, Donauer S, Gerber MA, et al. Infectious complications of intrathecal baclofen pump devices in a pediatric population. Pediatr Infect Dis J. 2013;32(7):715–22.
5. Overgard TM, Kjaersgaard-Hansen L, Soe M, Illum NO. Positive experience with intrathecal baclofen treatment in children with severe cerebral palsy. Dan Med J. 2015;62(1):A4999. Epub 2015/01/06.
6. Miracle AC, Fox MA, Ayyangar RN, Vyas A, Mukherji SK, Quint DJ. Imaging evaluation of intrathecal baclofen pump-catheter systems. AJNR Am J Neuroradiol. 2011;32(7):1158–64.
7. Medtronic. Baclofen pump for ITB therapy. www.baclofenpump.com. Accessed 16 May 2016.
8. Reddy GK, Bollam P, Caldito G, Guthikonda B, Nanda A. Ventriculoperitoneal shunt surgery outcome in adult transition patients with pediatric-onset hydrocephalus. Neurosurgery. 2012;70(2):380–8 (discussion 8–9).
9. Stone JJ, Walker CT, Jacobson M, Phillips V, Silberstein HJ. Revision rate of pediatric ventriculoperitoneal shunts after 15 years. J Neurosurg Pediatr. 2013;11(1):15–9.
10. Conen A, Walti LN, Merlo A, Fluckiger U, Battegay M, Trampuz A. Characteristics and treatment outcome of cerebrospinal fluid shunt-associated infections in adults: a retrospective analysis over an 11-year period. Clin Infect Dis. 2008;47(1):73–82.
11. Prusseit J, Simon M, von der Brelie C, Heep A, Molitor E, Volz S, et al. Epidemiology, prevention and management of ventriculoperitoneal shunt infections in children. Pediatr Neurosurg. 2009;45(5):325–36.
12. Browd SR, Ragel BT, Gottfried ON, Kestle JR. Failure of cerebrospinal fluid shunts: part I: obstruction and mechanical failure. Pediatr Neurol. 2006;34(2):83–92.
13. O'Brien DF, Taylor M, Park TS, Ojemann JG. A critical analysis of 'normal' radionucleotide shuntograms in patients subsequently requiring surgery. Childs Nerv Syst. 2003;19(5–6):337–41.
14. Browd SR, Gottfried ON, Ragel BT, Kestle JR. Failure of cerebrospinal fluid shunts: part II: overdrainage, loculation, and abdominal complications. Pediatr Neurol. 2006;34(3):171–6.
15. Association H. Shunt systems. http://www.hydroassoc.org/shunt-systems/. Accessed 16 May 2016.
16. Ogbonnaya S, Kaliaperumal C. Vagal nerve stimulator: evolving trends. J Nat Sci Biol Med. 2013;4(1):8–13.
17. Kabir SM, Rajaraman C, Rittey C, Zaki HS, Kemeny AA, McMullan J. Vagus nerve stimulation in children with intractable epilepsy: indications, complications and outcome. Childs Nerv Syst. 2009;25(9):1097–100.
18. Kahlow H, Olivecrona M. Complications of vagal nerve stimulation for drug-resistant epilepsy: a single center longitudinal study of 143 patients. Seizure. 2013;22(10):827–33.
19. Ghanem T, Early SV. Vagal nerve stimulator implantation: an otolaryngologist's perspective. Otolaryngol Head Neck Surg. 2006;135(1):46–51.
20. Parhizgar F, Nugent K, Raj R. Obstructive sleep apnea and respiratory complications associated with vagus nerve stimulators. J Clin Sleep Med. 2011;7(4):401–7.

21. Lundgren J, Ekberg O, Olsson R. Aspiration: a potential complication to vagus nerve stimulation. Epilepsia. 1998;39(9):998–1000.
22. Rösch J, Hamer HM, Mennecke A, Kasper B, Engelhorn T, Doerfler A, et al. 3T-MRI in patients with pharmacoresistant epilepsy and a vagus nerve stimulator: a pilot study. Epilepsy Rev. 2015;110:62–70.
23. LivaNova. VNS therapy. http://us.livanova.cyberonics.com/vns-therapy. Accessed 16 May 2016.
24. Foundation E. Vagal nerve stimulation (VNS). http://www.epilepsy.com/learn/treating-seizures-and-epilepsy/devices/vagus-nerve-stimulation-vns. Accessed 16 May 2016.
25. Surgeons AAoN. Vagus nerve stimulation. http://www.aans.org/patient%20information/conditions%20and%20treatments/vagus%20nerve%20stimulation.aspx. Accessed 16 May 2016.

22 Mobility Impairment

Jenny M. Lieberman and Miguel X. Escalon

Patient Factors to Consider in Wheelchair Assessments

Many factors should be considered when evaluating patients for mobility devices as concerns for both functionality for the user as well as prevention of long-term complications. This section will review the most common patient variables that should be addressed when making a mobility device assessment.

Supine Versus Seated Positioning

The effect of gravity on posture and functional mobility is an important consideration. The gravitational pull on a person changes when he or she is seated as opposed to being in the supine position. These forces can impact posture, tone, and skin integrity. For patients requiring mobility assistance, posture should be physically assessed when the patient is supine as well as seated to determine the asymmetrical pull of muscles from gravity, weakness, and spasticity.

Pelvic and Spine Alignment

The pelvis is the base of support when an individual is seated, and in persons with disability it serves as a stabilizing force on the spine. Pelvic asymmetry can thus lead to improper seating and mechanics thereby resulting in long-term adverse outcomes such as skin breakdown and scoliosis. Pelvic asymmetry may be caused directly by the seating system or may be inherent to the individual and not accounted for in the seating system. If the former is true and the asymmetry is flexible, it can be corrected in order to improve postural stability when the patient is seated. This is best confirmed by demonstrating that the patient's collapsed trunk can be straightened. Furthermore, pelvic asymmetry can be a result of spinal position with the pelvis achieving a more neutral position when the spinal asymmetry is encouraged and vice versa. This is an important consideration for function. Forward reach is more difficult when positioned with a posterior pelvic tilt and collapsed trunk and self-propulsion is more difficult when lateral flexion is encouraged.

J.M. Lieberman
Department of Rehabilitation Medicine, The Mount Sinai Hospital, 17 East 102nd Street, 2 East, New York, NY 10029, USA
e-mail: jenny.lieberman@mountsinai.org

J.M. Lieberman
New York, NY 10003, USA

M.X. Escalon (✉)
Department of Rehabilitation Medicine, Icahn School of Medicine at Mount Sinai, 5 East 98th Street, Box 1240B, New York, NY 10029, USA
e-mail: miguel.escalon@mountsinai.org

M. Pilapil et al. (eds.), *Care of Adults with Chronic Childhood Conditions*,
DOI 10.1007/978-3-319-43827-6_22

Upper and Lower Extremity Range of Motion

Lower extremity positioning is extremely important when considering the seated position in a wheelchair. Tight hamstrings and hip extensors are the most common extremity derangement causing impaired skin integrity, and these conditions require unique seating considerations. For example, use of elevating legrests with tight hamstrings often results in the user sliding out of the seat, which can in turn lead to shear forces and increased pressure on the sacrum and bilateral ischial tuberosities. Likewise, forcing an individual to sit more upright than his or her hip extensors will allow results in the user sliding out of the seat, again encouraging negative shear forces. A common deformity in the lower extremities in those individuals with asymmetrical muscle pull is a windswept deformity in which both legs shift to a particular side. This position can sometimes extend into the trunk as well and thus impact overall required seat width. Considerations for upper extremity range relate primarily to propulsion and joystick control. Adults with childhood disabilities have often developed contractures in their upper extremities, impacting wheel access and joystick control. Adjustments can be made in order to allow them better access to wheels and joystick controls, and referral to a specialized therapist to assist in the evaluation is essential.

Muscle Tone and Reflexes

Spasticity, low tone, and abnormal reflexes are all very important considerations with this patient population, as each can directly impact posture and function. For example, some patients require spasticity (hyperreflexia) in order to maintain a seated posture, whereas for others spasticity may be a hindrance to proper seating. Individuals with hypotonia face similar issues.

Mobility Devices

Though a formal assessment of patients who require the assistance of a mobility device is typically done in consultation with a licensed clinical specialist, adult healthcare providers should be familiar with the various types of available devices.

This section will provide an overview of the indications for and limitations of the mobility devices most commonly utilized in clinical practice for young adults with child-onset conditions.

Walkers and Canes

Though not as frequently used by the young adult population, walking devices are a consideration for some individuals. There are various types of devices, determined by the number of supports that are used. Quad canes provide increased stability as compared to a standard cane. Some walkers have wheels while others must be lifted for forward movement. The devices that will best meet the individual's needs should be determined by a physical therapy assessment. For example, individuals with decreased balance from impaired motor control, such as in spastic diplegic cerebral palsy, would benefit from a device with a wider base of support and with wheels so they do not have to lift it when walking. However, individuals with less controlled movements would not benefit from a wheeled walking device as they could more easily lose control of this.

Scooters

Due to their inability to provide postural support, a scooter is not a common mobility device used by young adults with mobility concerns. However, for individuals with slowly progressing debility and without significant neuromuscular impairment, such as those with emphysema or morbid obesity, a scooter can be an effective mobility device.

Manual Wheelchairs

Wheelchairs are classified by categories, with their delineation dependent on axle position. A standard wheelchair and lightweight wheelchair do not have an adjustable axle. These should not be used as long-term mobility devices as they do not allow for an adequate hand-to-wheel ratio, potentially leading to chronic shoulder and upper extremity issues. Ultra-lightweight wheelchairs do allow for an adjustment in the rear wheel position, allowing for movement of the wheel forward and for a discrepancy between front and rear wheel position (as seen in Fig. 22.1). They also allow for camber, which is where the base of the wheel is wider than the top (as seen in Fig. 22.2). These adjustments create a healthy environment for upper extremity propulsion.

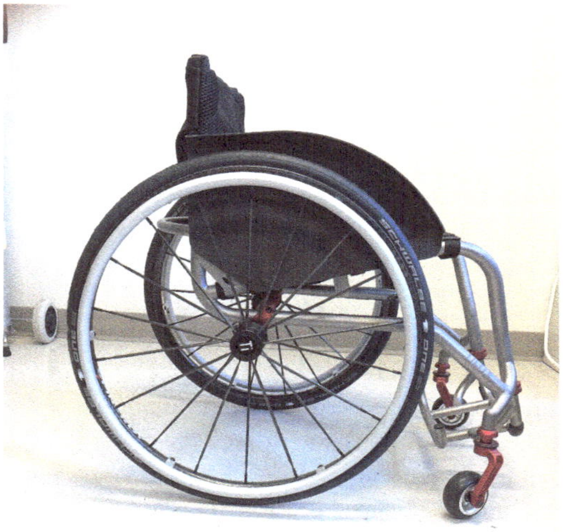

Fig. 22.1 Ultra-lightweight wheelchair that allows adjustment of rear wheel position

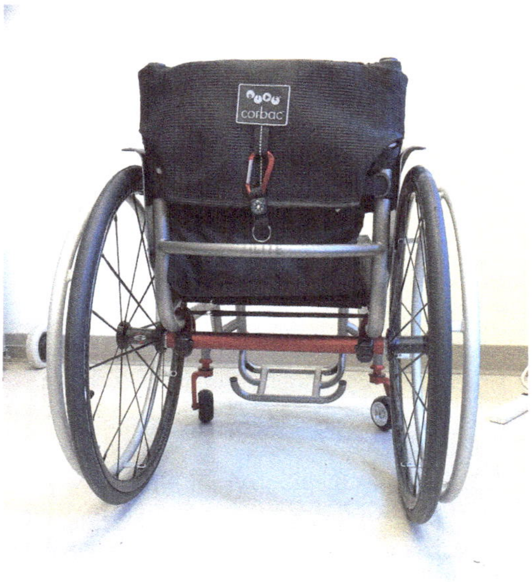

Fig. 22.2 Ultra-lightweight wheelchair showing camber, where the distance between the base of the wheels is wider than the top

Another consideration when evaluating a patient for a manual wheelchair is foot propulsion. Some adults with cerebral palsy, for example, prefer propulsion with their feet in a manual wheelchair. This results in the need for a wheelchair that allows for a lower seat-to-floor height. The ideal, long-term manual wheelchair for this population is customized and requires referral to a proper seating clinic or therapist.

Reclining wheelchairs should not be used as full-time mobility devices since they encourage shear. Transitioning from a reclined to seated position results in sliding of the user down the seat, with shear created along the bony prominence of the pelvis and spine. As a short-term solution—for example, after a lower extremity orthopedic surgery—a reclining wheelchair is an effective mobility device. However, for patients who are dependent long term for mobility, the most appropriate device is a manual tilt-in-space wheelchair. This allows for proper position while allowing for removal of gravity to promote good skin integrity and encourage improved alignment. A manual wheelchair is a dependent mobility device as it requires that someone else help propel the patient. There is also the option for a Power Tilt adds on to a manual base for those who cannot mobilize themselves but would be able to shift their weight with assistance.

Power Wheelchairs

Standard power wheelchairs can either include van seating or rehabilitation seating. The type of seat chosen is dependent upon the postural needs of the individual. Power wheelchairs allow for very basic adjustments to position and electronics, which is necessary for those with impaired upper extremity function.

Adults with childhood-onset conditions often require external assistance for positional change. Power wheelchairs allow for the addition of power tilt, recline, elevating leg rests, and an elevating seat. Though not as frequently used, alternative options are lateral tilt, precline, and anterior tilt. These complex wheelchairs also allow for alternative drive configurations. This makes it possible for those with impaired hand function to use alternative body parts to control the wheelchair; for example, the head, chin, foot, and elbow.

Wheelchair Seating Support Surfaces

Cushions are defined by their supportive and pressure-relieving capabilities. Full-time wheelchair users should avoid general-use standard cushions as they lack the ability to support postural asymmetry and do not promote good skin integrity. There are two principles of pressure relief to consider when selecting a seating support surface: immersion and suspension. Immersion refers to the amount of pressure and is equal to force over area. The better the immersion, the less force there is over the area (as the force or pressure is dispersed throughout the cushion) and the greater the pressure-relieving capabilities. For some individuals, no contact (suspension) is preferred over full contact to facilitate wound healing. This occurs with suspension of the bony prominence by weight bearing through larger support area surfaces.

The most common material used to fabricate cushions is foam. Viscosity determines the stability versus pressure-relieving capabilities. Some pressure-relieving cushions have a rigid foam base to provide stability, whereas others have softer conforming foam on top for pressure relief.

Gel cushions, are a combination of chemicals that allow for a fluid substance that is a cross between water and gel. These cushions have fair to good immersion. This design requires maintenance with fluid moved back into the center of the cushion after each time the patient gets into or transfers out of the chair.

Air is considered the best support surface for skin integrity due to its ability to fully conform to the surface area. Air allows for one to sink into the cushion, often with the lowest pressure gradient achieved. These cushions also require maintenance for proper inflation. Over-inflating or under-inflating these cushions will negatively impact skin integrity. To assess proper inflation, one must place their hand underneath the lowest bony prominence of the pelvis (usually the ischial tuberosity) and feel for the bottom of the cushion. There should only be a palms width of space. For a demonstration, please refer to www.roho.com.

Back Supports for wheelchairs can either be off-the-shelf or custom-molded types. Off-the-shelf back supports are distinguished by the extent of their lateral curve. The more aggressive the support needed, the deeper the lateral wall.

For individuals with custom needs, the only option is custom-molded seating. For example, individuals with scoliosis and rotational spine deformities where there is greater risk for increased pressure or for those with trunk weakness making it impossible to sit unassisted against gravity. This is very common with adults aging with a childhood disability. There are three different styles of custom-molded seat backs: subtle contour, thick aggressive support, and orthotic style. The seat back most appropriate for the individual should be assessed by the licensed specialist. The determining factor of one option over the other is due to several factors, including carryover by caretakers and mobility needs. Orthotic style systems require better carryover to ensure proper positioning and due to their narrower profile are better options for those attempting to propel or easily access a joystick in proximal position. The thicker options are better if there is need for support that is more highly padded as these consist of thicker foam.

Consequences of Long-Term Use of a Mobility Device

Long-term wheelchair use is associated with several adverse health outcomes. Adult healthcare providers should be familiar with the prevention, identification, and management of the more common of these conditions.

Decreased Bone Mineral Density

Prolonged wheelchair use has been shown to impact bone density. Individuals who use wheelchairs as their primary mode of mobilization do not weight bear often. Research has shown that bone density dramatically decreases the longer the period of non-weight bearing [1].

Skin Integrity

Prolonged sitting without pressure relief places wheelchair users at high risk for impairment in skin integrity. Impairment in skin integrity results from pressure, shear, and force. For some individuals, decreased sensation and incontinence can further contribute to skin breakdown.

Peak pressures prevent blood from flowing to the area, resulting in tissue death. This situation arises when direct pressure is applied into one localized area and when bony prominences are not properly supported. Frequent weight shifts help to ensure that there are no prolonged, unsafe pressures. Research has identified that pressure reliefs need to be at least 3 min in order to reduce oxygen tension into tissues [2]. Research has also distinguished proper angles for weight shift, which is only able to be achieved with dynamic seating. The optimal positions are 35° of tilt and 100 of recline, or 15–25° of tilt and 120° of recline, with greater angles providing even greater pressure relief [3–5]. Therefore, weight shifts or change of position in chair, usually by a tilt backwards or lean, should occur every 30 min for a duration of at least 3 min per weight shift.

Shear is a mechanical force that acts on an area of skin in a direction parallel to the body's surface. Shear is affected by the amount of pressure exerted, the coefficient of friction between the materials contacting each other, and the extent to which the body makes contact with the support surface [6]. Shearing forces are a result of pulling or sliding of a person while the skin stays in place, leading to tearing of and lateral damage to tissue. Deeper tissues, such as muscles, are particularly susceptible to shearing. Two common examples of shearing forces are (1) when a patient slides out of his or her seat and is then slid back into the seat and (2) when a patient slides along the tire of a wheelchair during transfers. Shearing ulcers are often difficult to heal due to the mechanism of injury and the fact that deep tissues are affected.

Force is a concept that is used to describe the effect on an object by an external influence. Force has a direction and a magnitude. Perpendicular forces cause pressure. The pressure at the junction between the skin and a support surface is often called "interface pressure." Pressure is defined as the amount of force applied perpendicular to a surface per unit area of application [7]. Force has been found to play a large role in impairment in skin integrity with the intensity of thrust into tissue resulting in greater deforming effects.

To assist in the prevention and identification of impairment in skin integrity, routine health care visits should include skin integrity assessments for individuals who rely on a wheelchair for most of their mobility needs.

Pelvic and Spinal Asymmetry

Prolonged sitting against gravity can lead to spinal and pelvic asymmetry, as mentioned previously. Dynamic seating is essential for positional change for the adult with childhood-onset conditions to provide gravity-assisted positioning [8–10]. Long-term wheelchair users are at very high risk of impairment of the joints of the upper extremities, either from propulsion or from the push-up style weight shift [11, 12]. For this reason, weight shifts and pressure reliefs are best performed by leaning forward or changing dynamic position of the chair.

Pain

Many adults with childhood-onset conditions experience pain, either from immobility, contracture, deformity, or impairment in skin integrity [13]. Many individuals who experience pain and who use power wheelchairs can benefit from proper device, seating, and cushion to decrease their complaints of pain [13]. An increase or change in pain patterns may be related to immobility issues and can require a referral to physical therapy for evaluation of the wheelchair fit.

Considerations for Specific Populations

Though a comprehensive discussion of all conditions that may necessitate use of a mobility device is beyond the scope of this chapter, this section will review several of the more common childhood-onset conditions that may warrant specific modifications to the mobility device.

Cerebral Palsy

Individuals with cerebral palsy (CP) often have abnormal reflexes that might aid in their mobility such that seating that has deep lateral contours may be contraindicated. For example, some patients with CP utilize their abnormal tonic reflex pattern to access the joystick of a power wheelchair for independent mobility. Asymmetrical tonicity can result in dramatic deformity necessitating custom rehabilitation seating. An additional consideration for individuals with CP is foot propulsion versus powered mobility. Foot propellers generally propel backwards. However, the increased exertion required by foot propellers can increase the onset of spasticity worsening overall alignment. For those individuals in which self-propulsion is contraindicated and for whom there are no cognitive generated safety concerns, powered mobility is essential for increased function and participation in daily activities.

Spina Bifida

Though upper spinal levels can be affected in individuals with spina bifida, the most common presentation resembles that of a low-level paraplegic. There are several considerations with this population. First, height is stunted in this population, predominantly due to scoliosis and poor bone growth. When considering seating with this population, trunk length is very important for good postural support. For individuals with a gibbus (short-segment structural thoracolumbar kyphosis), the extent of the gibbus determines the need for customization. More often than not, these individuals will require custom-molded seating to offload the gibbus.

Osteogenesis Imperfecta

Due to the frequency of fracture with individuals with osteogenesis imperfecta, seating needs to be adjustable, allowing for both standard foot support as well as elevating leg rests in the event of fracture. A well-padded seating system can provide some additional protection to decrease risk of fracture.

Arthrogryposis Multiplex

There are several considerations with patients who have arthrogryposis multiplex, including stature, contracture, and limitations in range of motion. Custom seating is necessary as the patient ages to support the spine and encourage elongation.

Muscular Dystrophy

For patients with muscular dystrophy (MD), the subtype of MD determines mobility needs and type of equipment. Considerations should include respiratory function and the need for a ventilator, as well as spinal deformity and hand function. Custom seating is often required due to dramatic asymmetries that may be present. Alternative joystick access (head, finger, elbow, etc.) or joystick accessible to a caregiver may be necessary to power the wheelchair dependent on the individual's hand function. Multiple power seat functions are necessary for continuous mobility to manage discomfort and pain.

Additional Considerations

Referral to a Wheelchair Seating Clinic

Because many young adults with chronic childhood-onset conditions must use a mobility device full time, they should not be provided with basic equipment. This population should be referred to a wheelchair seating clinic for evaluation of their mobility needs whenever possible. A list of clinicians able to complete these assessments can be found at the Rehabilitation Engineering and Assistive Technology Society of America (RESNA) site, found in Section "Helpful Resources" at the end of this chapter.

Insurance Reimbursement

Medicare has specific requirements for documentation of wheelchair needs (refer to the information in Section "Helpful Resources"). Many insurance policies, including private and managed Medicare and Medicaid plans, follow Medicare guidelines. Requirements for insurance reimbursement of a wheelchair are that the individual must have a mobility limitation that significantly impairs his or her function in the "customary locations in the home." Additionally, the mobility limitation must prevent the individual from accomplishing his or her Mobility-Related Activities of Daily Living (MRADL), including toileting, feeding, dressing, grooming, and bathing. Finally, the mobility limitation must place the client at risk of morbidity or mortality when attempting to perform his or her MRADL or must prevent the client from completing his or her MRADL within a reasonable time frame.

If the individual is being considered for a standard K0001 wheelchair, a lightweight K0003 wheelchair, or a K0004 active duty lightweight wheelchair, then the individual must be unable to walk at all and requires a manual wheelchair to access the rooms in their home. To be considered for a K0005 ultra-lightweight wheelchair, the weight of the wheelchair must affect the individual's ability to propel the wheelchair, the individual's medical condition, and position of the rim in relation to the arm position (hand-to-wheel ratio) must be integral to the ability to self-propel the wheelchair, and the individual must have the cognitive ability to independently function in the lightweight wheelchair. Additionally the individual's medical condition requires a frame with multiple adjustments that cannot be achieved with a less costly wheelchair.

To qualify for a tilt-in-space wheelchair, the individual must be dependent for transfers, and there must be in place a plan of care that identifies the need for frequent positional changes for medical reasons. To qualify for a powered wheelchair, an individual must not be able to safely or independently propel a manual wheelchair and/or scooter in his or her home for completion of his or her MRADLs.

In order to qualify for specialized mobility devices, a face-to-face visit between the patient and the provider is usually in order. If the individual is in the hospital, the doctor still needs to document a face-to-face evaluation in the medical record. The physician must clearly state the limitations the patient faces depending on the device selected. For example, in order to qualify for a power wheelchair one must state that the client cannot walk and is unable to propel a manual wheelchair or control a scooter to complete his or her MRADLs. The physician must also document the patient's diagnostic history, physical exam, and functional assessment as well as the individual's willingness to utilize the equipment and cognitive and physical ability to safely and independently control the device. Many equipment companies are familiar with the documentation needed for the different wheelchair requirements and can help the physician understand these requirements.

Conclusion

Many childhood-onset conditions are associated with mobility impairments. With advances in medicine, an increasing number of individuals with these conditions are surviving well into adulthood and being cared for in adult medical practices. In co-management with a licensed clinical specialist, such as occupational therapist or physical therapist, adult healthcare providers should be familiar with the indications for and limitations of the various available mobility devices. Additionally, providers should recognize appropriate prevention, screening, diagnosis, and management strategies for the most common adverse outcomes associated with long-term dependence on mobility devices. The information presented in this chapter is more of an overview and is meant only to serve as a guide. Additional information about wheelchairs and other mobility devices can be found in Section "Helpful Resources" included at the end of this chapter.

Helpful Resources

A list of clinicians able to complete assessments can be found on the Rehabilitation Engineering and Assistive Technology Society of North America (RESNA) site:

- http://www.resna.org/member-directory/individual

Information sheet for physicians on insurance requirements:

- https://www.cms.gov/Outreach-and-Education/Medicare-Learning-Network-MLN/MLNProducts/downloads/pmd_DocCvg_FactSheet_ICN905063.pdf

Consumer support organizations:

- United Cerebral Palsy: www.cerebralpalsy.org
- Muscular Dystrophy Association: www.mda.org
- Spina Bifida: www.spinabifidaassociation.org
- Osteogenesis imperfecta foundation: www.oif.org
- Arthrogryposis Multiplex Congenita: www.amcsupport.org

References

1. King W, Levin R, Schmidt R, Oestrich A, Heubi J. Prevalence of reduced bone mass in children and adults with spastic quadriplegia. Dev Med Child Neurol. 2003;45(1):12–6.
2. Jan YK, Liao F, Jones M, Rice LA, Tisdell T. Effect of durations of wheelchair tilt-in-space and recline on skin perfusion over the ischial tuberosity in people with spinal cord injury. Arch Phys Med. 2012;94(4):667–72.
3. Jan YK, Crane BA, Liao F, Woods JA, Ennis WJ. Comparison of muscle and skin perfusion over the ischial tuberosities in response to wheelchair tilt-in-space and recline angles in people with spinal cord injury. Arch Phys Med. 2013;94(10):1990–6.
4. Chen Y, Wang J, Liu L, Li S. Comparative effects of different posterior tilt sitting postures on buttock pressure in children. In: Paper presented at the 2010 3rd international conference on biomedical engineering and informatics (BMEI). 2010.
5. Sprigle S, Maurer C, Sorenblum SE. Load redistribution in variable position wheelchairs in people with spinal cord injury. J Spinal Cord Med. 2010;33(4):58–64.
6. Bergstrom N, Allman RM, Alvarez OM, Bennett MA, Carlson CE, Frantz RA, et al. Treatment of pressure ulcers guideline panel. Treatment of pressure ulcers. AHCPR clinical practice guidelines, No. 15. AHCPR publication No. 95-0652. Rockville, MD: Agency for Health Care Policy and Research (AHCPR). 1994.
7. International Review. Pressure ulcer prevention: pressure, shear, friction and microclimate in context. A consensus document. London, UK: Wounds International. 2010. http://www.woundsinternational.com/media/issues/300/files/content_8925.pdf. Accessed 19 May 2016.
8. Bushby K, Finkel R, Birnkrant DJ, Case LE, Clemens PR, Cripe L, et al. Diagnosis and management of Duchenne muscular dystrophy, part 2: implementation of multidisciplinary care. Lancet Neurol. 2010;9(2):177–89.
9. Calhoun CL, Schottler J, Vogel LC. Recommendations for mobility in children with spinal cord injury. Top Spinal Cord Inj Rehabil. 2013;19(2):142–51.

10. Mcnamara L, Casey J. Seat inclinations affect the function of children with cerebral palsy: a review of the effect of different seat inclines. Disabil Rehabil Assist Technol. 2007;2(6):309–18.
11. Paralyzed Veterans of America. Consortium for Spinal Cord Medicine. Pressure ulcer prevention and treatment following spinal cord injury: a clinical practice guideline for health-care professionals. 2000. http://www.pva.org/atf/cf/%7BCA2A0FFB-6859-4BC1-BC96-6B57F57F0391%7D/cpg_pressure%20ulcers.pdf. Accessed 19 May 2016.
12. Reyes ML, Gronley JK, Newsam CJ, Mulroy SJ, Perry J. Electromyographic analysis of shoulder muscles of men with low-level paraplegia during weight relief raise. Arch Phys Med Rehabil. 1995;76:433–9.
13. Frank AO, De Souza LH, Frank JL, Neophytou C. The pain experiences of powered wheelchair users. Dis Rehabil. 2012;34:770–8.

Sexual and Reproductive Health 23

Jennifer M. LeComte

Introduction

Reproductive health needs should be incorporated into routine care for patients across their lifespan. Physicians should include education about sexuality, preventative health including immunizations and screening, contraception, and fertility as appropriate for each individual. Unfortunately, reproductive health needs for individuals with physical, intellectual, and developmental disabilities and complex chronic conditions have been largely neglected. Adult medicine providers have an opportunity to provide comprehensive care to this vulnerable population in order to optimize their general health. This chapter will address the needs of this complex population by offering insight to the problems of limited sexuality education, understanding the risk of abuse, addressing alternative approaches to ensuring access to preventative sexual health and routine screenings, and maximizing the opportunities for healthy relationships.

J.M. LeComte (✉)
Transition Care and Pediatric Practices, Christiana Care Health System, 501 W. 14th Street, Wilmington, DE 19801, USA
e-mail: JLecomte@Christianacare.org

Sexuality and Education

Sexuality is a broad topic that incorporates both physical and emotional health with underlying tones of personal and societal values and expectations. The Position Statement published by The Arc, a national community-based organization advocating for and serving people with intellectual and developmental disabilities and their families, and the American Academy for Intellectual and Developmental Disabilities (AAIDD) in 2008 articulated well the issues concerning people with intellectual and/or developmental disabilities and sexuality. It states:

> For decades, people with intellectual and/or developmental disabilities have been thought to be asexual, having no need for loving and fulfilling relationships with others. Individual rights to sexuality, which is essential to human health and well-being, have been denied. This loss has negatively affected people with intellectual disability in gender identity, friendships, self-esteem, body image and awareness, emotional growth, and social behavior. People with intellectual or developmental disabilities frequently lack access to appropriate sex education in schools and other settings. At the same time, some individuals may engage in sexual activity as a result of poor options, manipulation, loneliness or physical force rather than as an expression of their sexuality [1].

As children age and mature, physicians routinely provide them and their families with anticipatory guidance about the next stages of development. Just before the adolescent stage, physicians begin to use various tools to address

M. Pilapil et al. (eds.), *Care of Adults with Chronic Childhood Conditions*,
DOI 10.1007/978-3-319-43827-6_23

the impending changes with the onset of puberty and the social challenges that accompany those changes. Bright Futures from the American Academy of Pediatrics provides guidance on addressing adolescent development. Some tools for screening include **H**ome, **E**ducation/Employment/Eating, **A**ctivities, **D**rugs, **S**uicide/Depression, **S**exuality, **S**afety, **S**pirituality (HEADSSS), **S**trengths/Interests, **S**chool, **H**ome, **A**ctivities, **D**rugs/Substance Abuse, **E**motions/Depression, **S**exuality, **S**afety (SSHADES), and **P**artners, **P**revention of Pregnancy, **P**rotection from sexually transmitted infections, **P**ractices, and **P**ast History (5 P's). Unfortunately, for patients with special health care needs, including those with chronic conditions and physical and cognitive disabilities, the standard of care is often delayed or avoided completely. Education about sexuality should be comprehensive for all. The concept of sexuality should include education about relationship building, developing friendships, social skills, grooming, manners, safety, and privacy in order to promote respect, informed consent, and healthy emotional and physical relationships [2].

There are many barriers that result in physicians and families not addressing sexuality or providing appropriate education and preventative care to patients with disabilities and chronic conditions. Some providers believe that the chronic condition or disability is the paramount focus and therefore discussions of social and physical development can be delayed. Perceptions of the sexuality of people with disabilities spans from asexual to inappropriately sexual. For example, some view a person with a disability as childlike and believe that the person does not need information and training on sexuality. Terri Couwenhoven, a certified sexuality educator for people with disabilities and a mother of a self-advocate with Down syndrome, disagrees. She reflected that she needed to be purposeful about thinking of her daughter in her chronological age rather than her developmental age because many of her daughter's stages of development around sexuality were on track with her typical peers [3]. The challenge is helping patients with intellectual and developmental disabilities understand and respond appropriately to the changes, challenges, and feelings that they encounter. Physicians should encourage families and others to provide education and opportunities to develop confidence and self-esteem and build healthy relationships.

On the other end of the spectrum, some people with intellectual and developmental disabilities are believed to be hypersexual. Every behavior is subject to review and potentially is misinterpreted as having sexual intent requiring constant supervision. Ironically, many people with disabilities have experienced acquaintances or strangers who pinch cheeks or give hugs without regard to their personal space. This invasion of privacy and personal space happens often to people with disabilities of all ages, as they are often perceived as being affectionate or requiring more affection than their typical peers [4]. Understanding appropriate touch and expressions of affection can be very confusing when persons with intellectual and developmental disabilities have their boundaries repeatedly violated regardless of intention. It is understandable that they may begin to violate the space of others and misunderstand what is appropriate behavior.

There are other examples when the privacy of patients with physical and intellectual disabilities leads to confusion about personal boundaries. For people with a disability or chronic condition, limited privacy and a high degree of physical intrusion seems to be routine. If a patient uses attendant services, lives in a group home, or is not able to maintain personal care independently, privacy is viewed very differently. Intrusion is tolerated. Respect for privacy during any physical examination is essential at every age. Physicians and caregivers need to be cognizant when providing personal care and need to ask for permission to examine or assist in personal care and promote modesty. Teaching about private parts is taught early but needs to be reiterated throughout adolescence and beyond. Given the limited opportunities for patients to practice self-advocacy, physicians need to reinforce modesty skills in the office.

Regardless of perceptions, people with intellectual, developmental, and physical disabilities have the desire and the right to develop and express their sexuality. Some studies have shown that the level of sexual activity is not significantly related to the severity of disability [5]. All are capable of having relationships and "enjoying the sensation that comes from being respected and loved" [6]. They have the right to be emotionally and physically involved with an appropriate partner. Issues involving informed consent and guardianship need to be addressed when supporting patients with developmental and intellectual disabilities. When partners mutually agree to pursue a more intimate relationship, they should expect those around them to facilitate that by offering as much privacy as needed when asked. In addition, people with disabilities often need to plan for romantic physical experiences as they may need to alter their bowel or bladder regimens or modify medication to reduce spasticity prior to the activity. While this decreases the ability to be spontaneous, it does not reduce the need for privacy and intimacy. When limits or restrictions are placed on private sexual expression, sexual activity can move into inappropriate settings. Research conducted by the Center for Research on Women with Disabilities (CROWD) through the National Study of Women with Physical Disabilities found that 41 % of the women with disabilities believed that they did not have adequate information about how their disability affects their sexual functioning [5]. Sexual functioning and behavior should be addressed not just to prevent pregnancy and sexually transmitted infections (STIs) but to reassure individuals that they can be sexually active [7].

Looking again at the position paper on sexuality from

> The Arc and AAIDDM, it highlights the rights of patients with respect to sexuality stating individuals have a right to:
> Sexual expression and education, reflective of their own cultural, religious, and moral values and of social responsibility;
> Individualized education and information to encourage informed decision-making, including education about such issues as reproduction, marriage and family life, abstinence, safe sexual practices, sexual orientation, sexual abuse, and sexually transmitted diseases; and
> Protection from sexual harassment and from physical, sexual, and emotional abuse.
> Individuals also have a responsibility to consider the values, rights, and feelings of others [1].

Risk of Exploitation

There is evidence that people with a physical or intellectual disability or chronic condition are at increased risk of being abused. A 2008 study done in British Columbia surveyed high school students and showed that students who reported having a limiting health condition or a disability were two times more likely than their peers to report being physically abused (31 vs. 15 %) or sexually abused (19 vs. 7 %) and were three times more likely to have experienced both physical and sexual abuse (12 vs. 4 %) [8]. The US Department of Justice reports that 68–83 % of women with developmental disabilities will be sexually assaulted in their lifetimes and less than half of them will seek assistance from legal or treatment services [6].

Risk of abuse is due to many factors including limited education and decision-making, dependence on others for basic care including care that often results in public exposure, increased exposure to a large number of caregivers and settings, inappropriate social skills, poor judgment, inability to seek help or report abuse, and lack of strategies to defend themselves against abuse [9]. The realization of such vulnerability may lead parents to increase protection of their children, both young and old, from unsupervised social contacts and even from knowledge about sex. In order to protect and prevent abuse, physicians and caregivers need to be aware of the problem of abuse and report any concerns or signs of abuse. More importantly, they need to provide education and opportunities to promote and enhance self-determination and self-preservation [10].

Screening for Abuse

The Abuse Assessment Screen-Disability (AAS-D) form, which was developed by McFarlane in 2001 and is available on the American College of Obstetrics and Gynecology (ACOG) Website, uses the following questions [11]:

1. Within the last year, have you been hit, slapped, kicked, pushed, shoved, or otherwise physically hurt by someone?
2. Within the last year, has anyone forced you to have sexual activities?
3. Within the last year, has anyone prevented you from using a wheelchair, cane, respirator, or other assistive devices?
4. Within the last year, has anyone you depend on refused to help you with an important personal need, such as taking your medicine, getting to the bathroom, getting out of bed, bathing, getting dressed, or getting food or drink?

If yes to any of the questions above, who? Intimate Partner, Care Provider, Health Professional, Family Member, other (e.g., stranger, clergy)?

Women's Health Exams

Simply stated in *A Provider's Guide for the Care of Women with Physical Disabilities and Chronic Health Conditions*: "Viewing the woman with a disability as a woman first, who happens to have physical differences, will give a better understanding of how her disability affects her health and how her health affects her disability. Recognizing that she is the person most knowledgeable about her own disability will foster effective provider-patient relationships and more active participation in self-care and health promotion" [12].

The need for women's health assessments and preventative care is equal for all women. Health care providers should offer women with disabilities and chronic conditions education, counseling, and exams at the same intervals as all women. Unfortunately, women with disabilities are often discouraged from scheduling exams because the office may not be accessible or they have had a prior negative experience with physicians and other healthcare providers not knowing how to handle disability-related symptoms during the exam such as spasticity, imbalance, and autonomic dysreflexia. Physicians who assume women with disabilities are not sexually active may not screen for STIs or educate them about safe sex practices. Women with disabilities may not detect signs and symptoms of STIs, or they may mistake the symptoms for other common complications of their chronic conditions, such as urinary tract infections. In a patient with a disability, STIs may present differently such as with fatigue or increased spasticity. For these reasons and more, women with disabilities need to have access to women's health exams. ACOG has an interactive site for clinicians serving women with disabilities. The site includes a recorded slide program, *Reproductive Health Care for Women with Disabilities,* to guide physicians to provide the preventative care that all women need while addressing the unique approaches one might need to accommodate women with physical, developmental, and cognitive disabilities [13].

Pap Smears

Pap tests when performed at recommended intervals can prevent at least 70 % of cervical cancers. Women 21 years and older should have a Pap test every 3 years. This is true for all women, including lesbian and bisexual women and women who have never had sexual intercourse. Women with disabilities are just as likely to get cervical cancer as the general population. Women with a disability, however, in one study were less likely than those without a disability to report receiving a Pap test during the past 3 years (78.9 vs. 83.4 %; $p < 0.001$) [14]. As stated previously, physicians need to be aware of accommodations and possible complications when performing pelvic exams, but these factors should not preclude doing the exam. For those rare circumstances for when an exam cannot be performed—for example, when congenital strictures in the vaginal opening prevent the ability to safely perform a speculum exam—human papillomavirus (HPV) testing and/or pelvic ultrasound may be considered as alternatives.

Women with mobility issues may need accommodations in order to perform a women's health exam. They may require adjustable exam tables or need assistance in getting into a comfortable position. The typical pelvic exam position may increase spasticity for some women with mobility disabilities. Variations for the pelvic exam includes the knee-chest position, which is good for women who need to lie on their side (Fig. 23.1a), and the diamond-shaped position (Fig. 23.1b) and V-shaped position where women lie on their backs and the speculum is inserted with handle up [15]. Physicians can also use the OB stirrup position to provide increased support.

If accommodations for positioning and the performance of the pelvic exam are not discussed ahead of time, women with a spinal cord injury or other neurologic impairments may be at the increased risk for experiencing autonomic dysreflexia. Autonomic dysreflexia is a response to painful stimuli below the spinal cord lesion. The patient is not able to feel pain, but the body recognizes it as painful. Signs and symptoms of autonomic dysreflexia include headache, sweating, and piloerection above the level of the lesion, nasal stuffiness, facial flushing, papillary dilatation, rapid heart rate, arrhythmias, and labile hypertension that could be life threatening. The Center for Research on Women with Disabilities (CROWD) has information [16] for providers to be prepared when examining patients at risk for autonomic dysreflexia.

For some women with mobility impairments there is an increased need to monitor for organ prolapse because it can occur at a younger age. Some women may require a referral for genetic counseling depending on their chronic condition. In general, it may take additional accommodations and more time to obtain a history and examine a woman with physical or intellectual/developmental disabilities, but anticipating the patient's needs should improve the experience for all involved.

Mammograms

Breast cancer is the most common cancer in women and does not vary when accounting for women with a disability. In the United States in a study done in 2008, women with a disability aged 50–74 years reported a lower rate of mammography use than women without a disability of the same age (78.1 vs. 82.6 %) [17]. According to data from the Office on Disability of the US Department of Health and Human Services, 68 % of women older than 40 years without disabilities have had a mammogram, as compared to only

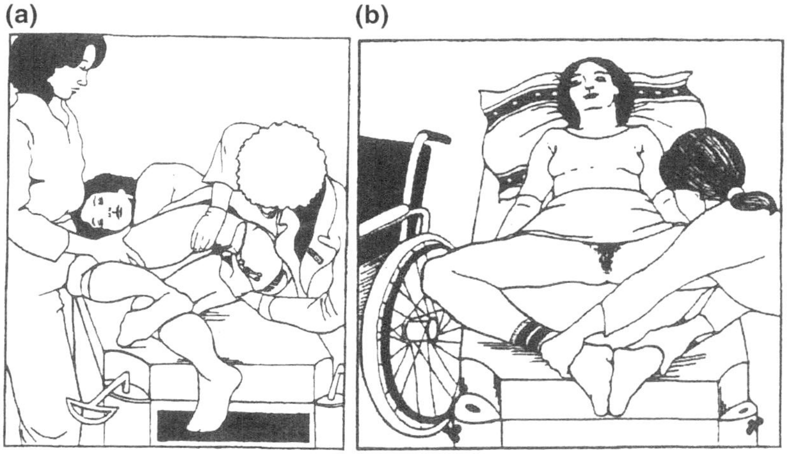

Fig. 23.1 Pelvic exam positions. (**a**) Knee-chest position. (**b**) Diamond-shaped position. Reprinted with permission from Simpson [15]

54 % of women in that age group with a disability [18]. Studies also show higher rates of death related to breast cancer among women with a disability, even when diagnosed at the same stage as women without a disability. Women with disabilities had higher breast cancer mortality rates and were less likely to undergo standard therapy after breast-conserving surgery than other women. Differences in treatment did not explain the differences in breast cancer mortality rates [19]. Additionally, women with intellectual disabilities frequently experience nulliparity, a factor associated with as great as a fourfold increase in risk of developing breast cancer.

The Centers for Disease Control and Prevention (CDC) identified some of the barriers to breast cancer screening for women who have physical disabilities. Barriers included: lack of perceived susceptibility to cancer, preoccupation with other health issues, not knowing where to go for accessible screening, difficulty with positioning, inaccessible facilities and equipment, and provider knowledge and attitudes [20]. The American Association on Health and Disability developed a handout for women to be prepared for a mammogram including how to advocate for accommodations for specific disabilities [21]. The CDC also led a campaign called "Breast Cancer Screening: *The Right to Know*," which offers women stories and resources to promote higher rates of screening among women with disabilities [22].

Menstruation

A discussion about menstruation should happen prior to onset of menses for all women. For women with intellectual and physical disabilities and their families, there can be significant anxiety about the impact menstruation will have on daily functioning. Consideration of menstrual management techniques may come into question for multiple reasons including hygiene, protection from pregnancy, seizure disorder, behavior and mood, and treatment of symptoms including dysmenorrhea and abnormal uterine bleeding. Dr. Quint compiled an overview of menstrual management for teenagers with Special Needs that included benefits and effects on disability (see Table 23.1) [23].

When pursuing a treatment for menstrual management, there are several scenarios to consider. Medication interactions can impact choice. Some anticonvulsants decrease the efficacy of oral contraceptives including barbiturates, carbamazepine and oxcarbazepine, phenytoin, topiramate, and vigabatrin. Some antiepileptic medications induce hepatic enzyme activity and decrease the effectiveness of oral and implanted contraceptives. Combination with other medications, such as antibiotics, can increase the metabolism of oral contraception therapy making the oral contraceptive therapy less effective.

Depo-Medroxyprogesterone acetate (DPMA) injectable is easy to use and can achieve high rates of amenorrhea but can result in bone density loss in healthy adolescent females, which may not reverse completely after discontinuation of the medication. Because of the risk to bone health, patients with mobility impairments should be evaluated with a dual energy X-ray absorptiometry (DEXA) scan and consider supplementation with calcium and vitamin D. Given the high prevalence of obesity across the disability population, the risk of weight gain on DPMA should also play a role in the decision as to whether to use this agent.

Contraception

The medical, social, and psychological issues related to pregnancy and a disability or chronic condition should be assessed prior to conception. All women of reproductive age, including those with disabilities, should receive counseling about the potential effects of their chronic medical conditions, any medications, and their emotional/mental health may have on pregnancy-related outcomes. Discussion about options to alter dosages or switch to safer medications prior to conception and optimizing health conditions are essential before embarking on a pregnancy.

The choice and safety of effective contraception varies from person to person. As discussed earlier, women with disabilities are sexually

Table 23.1 Overview of menstrual management methods for teenagers with special needs

Treatment	Specific benefits	Disability concerns
NSAIDS	Decreases flow and pain	GI issues
Combined oral contraceptives	Can use extended regimen	If immobile: risk for VTE Daily reminders Interfere with certain EI-AED
Contraceptive patch	Weekly application Can use extended regimen	If immobile: risk for VTE Patient can remove from skin Interfere with certain EI-AED
Contraceptive ring	Monthly Can use extended regimen	If immobile: risk for VTE Placement by others (privacy) Interfere with certain EI-AED
Oral progestin	Decreased flow	BTB Daily reminders Interfere with certain EI-AED
Depo Medroxyprogesterone acetate	Every 3 months	Weight gain in obese teens BMD loss with long-term use
Progesterone implant	Every 3 years	BTB Insertion might be challenging
LNG-IUD	Every 3 to 5 years	Insertion might need anesthesia Initial BTB
Surgical methods: endometrial ablation		Variable amenorrhea rates No data on use in adolescents Legal and ethical implications
Surgical methods: hysterectomy	Complete amenorrhea	Major surgery Legal and ethical implications

Reprinted with permission from Quint [23]

BMD bone mineral density, *BTB* breakthrough bleeding, *EI-AED* enzyme inducing antiepileptic drugs, *GI* gastrointestinal, *LNG-IUD* levonorgestrel intrauterine device, *NSAIDS* nonsteroidal anti-inflammatory drugs, *VTE* venous thromboembolism

active and need to be offered contraception keeping in mind their unique needs. The World Health Organization (WHO) created the medical eligibility criteria to offer guidance on the safety of various contraceptive methods for use in specific health conditions to improve the quality of care in family planning [24]. The CROWD Website also offers education about choice of contraceptive methods [25].

The condom is the only contraceptive method proven to be highly effective protection against both pregnancy and STIs. Barrier contraception requires intact balance, physical dexterity, and hand coordination or the willingness of the woman's sexual partner to assume responsibility for its use. Women at risk for latex allergies, such as women with spina bifida, need to be cautioned to select products accordingly. The diaphragm increases the frequency of urinary tract infections, so women who have bladder concerns may require an alternative method.

As discussed previously, medications may decrease the effectiveness of oral contraception, and some medications used for seizures may make implantable methods less effective. Women with mobility impairments may be at increased risk for blood clots with any of the estrogen-containing contraceptive agents.

Some women with spinal cord injuries or chronic conditions that effect sensation should consider avoiding the use of intrauterine devices (IUDs) because of decreased ability to detect movement of the device away from its appropriate location in the uterus and autonomic dysreflexia. IUDs may increase menstrual flow. Spasticity of the lower extremities can increase the difficulty of insertion of an IUD. Women or their partners or caregivers must be able to assess the presence of the IUD string weekly. Women with cardiac valvular disease need to be aware that IUD insertion is associated with transient, minimal bacteremia [26].

Women with multiple disabilities experienced a higher risk of undergoing a hysterectomy than women with no disability (hazard ratio 1.3), and this heightened risk was concentrated at younger ages [27]. Ethical issues surrounding this method of contraception should also be considered.

Men's Health Exams

An important part of the male exam is screening for testicular cancer. It is the most common cancer among men aged 20–34, although men of any age can develop testicular cancer. Testicular cancer can be treated very successfully when it is found early. Planned Parenthood has good resources on how patients can perform a testicular exam [28].

Special Populations

Down Syndrome

Approximately 50 % of women with Down syndrome are fertile and may use any method of contraception without added medical risk. Men with Down syndrome have a significantly lower overall fertility rate than that of other men of comparable ages. The National Down Syndrome Society Website has additional resources [29].

Spina Bifida

Physicians should consider all patients with spina bifida to be at high risk for an allergic reaction to latex. The allergy to latex has to be taken into consideration in the equipment choice when performing Pap smears and when discussing barrier methods for birth control.

Fertility is generally preserved in women but reduced in men with spina bifida. Pre-pregnancy counseling should include informing women with spina bifida of the 5 in 100 risk of bearing children with neural tube defects, the protective effect of folate supplementation, and the potential complications associated with pregnancy. Women with spina bifida are able to receive epidural anesthesia but may need ultrasound guidance for correct placement given alterations in anatomy [30].

The same nerves that control urinary function also control sexual function and can be a concern if a patient with spina bifida has poor sensation. Communicating with a partner about the possibility of urine or stool leakages during sex can alleviate some anxiety. Encouraging patients to start with an empty bladder and bowels prior to sexual activity could decrease the risk of leakage.

In men with spina bifida, one important consideration is erectile dysfunction due to poor sensation or blood supply in the penis. The Spina Bifida Association has additional resources [31].

Muscular Dystrophy

Use of chronic steroids in Duchenne Muscular Dystrophy (DMD) can delay onset of puberty. Though patients with DMD on chronic steroids appear younger, physicians need to be mindful to treat patients appropriate to their chronological age [32].

Sickle Cell Disease

Young men with sickle cell disease should be educated about priapism, as most will have experienced the complication of a prolonged, painful, unwanted erection by the age of 20. Priapism can be seen as young as age 12 and is a medical emergency. Young men need to be educated so that they are not embarrassed and seek care.

Women and men who are taking hydroxyurea should use contraception or discontinue the drug if they plan to conceive a child, since hydroxyurea has been shown to be teratogenic in animal models. Generally, all forms of contraception are reasonable choices for women with sickle cell disease.

There can be several complications seen during pregnancy. One study found that among women with sickle cell disease, the most common complication during pregnancy was hypertension. A high percentage of the pregnancies resulted in preterm deliveries and infants that were small for gestational age [33].

Childhood Cancer Survivors

Surveillance

Several studies have shown that women treated with radiation to the chest for cancer during childhood have an increased risk of developing breast cancer compared to women of the same age in the general population. The risk is related to the dose of radiation and begins to increase between 5 and 9 years following radiation therapy and continues to rise. For women who received a dose of 20 Gy or higher, yearly mammograms should begin starting at age 25 or 8 years after the last dose of radiation [34].

Fertility

The Children's Oncology Group Long-Term Follow-Up Guidelines for Survivors of Childhood, Adolescent, and Young Adult Cancers (COG LTFU Guidelines) are a resource for healthcare professionals who provide ongoing care to survivors of pediatric malignancies. Chemotherapy and radiation may have effects on male and female reproductive function, but this depends on many variables related to the cancer and its treatment. The Children's Oncology Group has guidelines to assess individual risk [35].

Women who had radiation to the whole abdomen, pelvis, lower spine, or total body may have an increased risk of miscarriage, premature delivery, or problems during labor. Also women who received anthracycline chemotherapy and women who received radiation to the upper abdomen or chest may be at risk for heart problems that can worsen with pregnancy and labor. Additional information can be found at LIVESTRONG Fertility, a Website dedicated to providing educational information and access to resources that support cancer patients and survivors whose cancer and its treatment present risks to their fertility [36].

Cystic Fibrosis

Men with cystic fibrosis (CF) are azoospermic due to anatomic abnormalities and are functionally sterile. Women have normal reproductive anatomy.

All pregnancies for a woman with CF should be considered high-risk, especially if the woman has advanced disease, malnutrition, or diabetes [37].

Conclusion

As the population of patients with complex chronic conditions and physical, intellectual and developmental disabilities ages, attention to their longitudinal health care needs will need to be addressed, including their reproductive healthcare needs. Access to care with sensitivity to the unique needs of this vulnerable population will optimize the mental health, safety, and general health outcomes across the spectrum. As adult medicine providers become more educated about the needs of this complex population, they will also be able to partner with appropriate specialists to provide comprehensive care ("Appendix").

Appendix

Resources

- ACOG: http://www.acog.org/About_ACOG/ACOG_Departments/Women_with_Disabilities.
- Baylor College of Medicine—Center for Research on Women with Disabilities (CROWD): https://www.bcm.edu/research/centers/research-on-women-with-disabilities.

- Centers for Disease Control and Prevention: http://www.cdc.gov/ncbddd/disabilityandhealth/women.html.
- Massachusetts Department of Public Health—Healthy Relationships, Sexuality and Disability Resource Guide: http://www.mass.gov/eohhs/docs/dph/com-health/prevention/hrhs-sexuality-and-disability-resource-guide.pdf.
- A Provider's Guide for the Care of Women with Physical Disabilities and Chronic Health Conditions: http://fpg.unc.edu/sites/fpg.unc.edu/files/resources/other-resources/NCODH_ProvidersGuide.pdf.
- Sexuality Resource Center for Parents (SRCP):
  - http://www.srcp.org/for_some_parents/physical_disabilities/generalPD.html
  - http://www.srcp.org/for_some_parents/developmental_disabilities/additional_resources/index.html.
- Sexuality and Disability: A Guide for Parents: http://www.srcp.org/pdf_versions/Alberta.pdf.
- University of Michigan—*YourChild* is a Website especially for parents about kids' development and behavior. Sexuality Education for Youth with Disability or Chronic Illness—A Resource List: http://www.med.umich.edu/yourchild/topics/disabsex.htm.
- Villanova NP guide to disability: https://www1.villanova.edu/villanova/nursing/community/npsknowdisabilitycare.html.

References

1. The Arc Position Statement: Sexuality. Washington, DC. Adopted 2008. http://www.thearc.org/who-we-are/position-statements/life-in-the-community/sexuality. Accessed 24 Apr 2016.
2. Schwier KM, Hingsburger D. Sexuality: your sons and daughters with intellectual disabilities. Baltimore: Paul H. Brookes Publishing; 2000.
3. Fager S, Hancox D, Ely C, Stenhjem P, Gaylord V (eds). Impact: feature issue on sexuality and people with intellectual, developmental and other disabilities. Minneapolis: University of Minnesota, Institute on Community Integration; 2010. https://ici.umn.edu/products/impact/232/8.html. Accessed 24 Apr 2016.
4. Couwenhoven T. Sexuality education: building a foundation for healthy attitudes. [Internet] Lake Oswego: Disability Solutions. 2001;4(5). http://downsyndromenutrition.com/images/stories/dsolnsvol4/4-5.pdf. Accessed 24 Apr 2016.
5. Nosek MA, Howland CA, Rintala DH, Young ME, Chanpong GF. National study of women with physical disabilities: final report. Sex Disabil. 2001;19(1):5–39. https://www.bcm.edu/research/centers/research-on-women-with-disabilities/topics/sexuality-and-reproductive-health/national-study-executive-summary. Accessed 24 Apr 2016.
6. Murphy NA, Elias ER. Sexuality of children and adolescents with developmental disabilities. Pediatrics. 2006;118:398–403. http://www.pediatrics.org/cgi/content/full/118/1/398.
7. Tulloch T, Kaufman M. Adolescent sexuality. Pediatr Rev. 2013;34(1):29–38. http://pedsinreview.aappublications.org/content/34/1/29.
8. Kaufman M. Canadian Paediatric Society Adolescent Health Committee Position Statement: the sexual abuse of young people with a disability or chronic health condition. Posted 2011 reaffirmed 2016. http://www.cps.ca/documents/position/sexual-abuse-youth-disability-chronic-condition. Accessed 24 Apr 2016.
9. Couwenhoven T. Sexuality education: building a foundation for healthy attitudes. Lake Oswego: Disability Solutions; 2001;4(5). http://downsyndromenutrition.com/images/stories/dsolnsvol4/4-5.pdf. Accessed 24 Apr 2016.
10. Davis LA. People with intellectual disabilities and sexual violence. Rev 2011. Washington. http://www.thearc.org/what-we-do/resources/fact-sheets/sexual-violence. Accessed 24 Apr 2016.
11. McFarlane J. Abuse Assessment Screen-Disability (AAS-D): measuring frequency, type, and perpetrator of abuse toward women with physical disabilities. J Women's Health Gend Med. 2001;10(9):861–866. http://www.acog.org/About-ACOG/ACOG-Departments/Women-with-Disabilities/Abuse-Assessment-Screen. Accessed 24 Apr 2016.
12. Smeltzer SC, Sharts-Hopko NC. A provider's guide for the care of women with physical disabilities and chronic health conditions. North Carolina Office on Disability and Health in collaboration with Villanova University College of Nursing. 2005. http://fpg.unc.edu/sites/fpg.unc.edu/files/resources/other-resources/NCODH_ProvidersGuide.pdf. Accessed 24 Apr 2016.
13. Cox RL, Caroline Signore C, Quint E. Reproductive health care for women with disabilities. http://www.acog.org/About-ACOG/ACOG-Departments/Women-with-Disabilities/Interactive-site-for-clinicians-serving-women-with-disabilities. Accessed 24 Apr 2016.
14. Armour BS, Thierry JM, Wolf LA. State-level differences in breast and cervical cancer, 2008. Women's Health Issues. 2009;19(6):406–14.

15. Simpson KM (ed). Table manners and beyond: the gynecological exam for women with developmental disabilities and other functional limitations. Oakland: Women's Wellness Project; 2001. http://lurie.brandeis.edu/pdfs/TableMannersandBeyond.pdf. Accessed 24 Apr 2016.
16. Spinal Cord Injury Model System. Autonomic dysreflexia. 2015. https://media.bcm.edu/documents/2016/58/sci-autonomic-dysreflexia.pdf. Accessed 24 Apr 2016.
17. Centers for Disease Control and Prevention. Behavioral risk factor surveillance system survey data. Atlanta: U.S. Department of Health and Human Services, CDC; 2008. http://www.cdc.gov/brfss/.
18. US Department of Health and Human Services, Office on Disability. Access to quality health services and disability—a companion to chapter 1 of Healthy People; 2010. http://hhs.gov/od/about/fact_sheets/healthypeople2010.html.
19. McCarthy EP, Ngo LH, Roetzheim RG, Chirikos TN, Donglin L, Drews RE, et al. Disparities in breast cancer treatment and survival for women with disabilities. Ann Intern Med. 2006;145(9):637–45.
20. Centers for Disease Control and Prevention. The right to know health promotion campaign. 2008. http://www.cdc.gov/ncbddd/disabilityandhealth/righttoknow/documents/new/234117_rtkdisseminationguide_v5_508_v1.pdf. Accessed 24 Apr 2016.
21. Delaware Breast Cancer Coalition. Tips for Women with Disabilities (WWD): getting your mammogram. 2014. http://debreastcancer.org/index.php/information/mammography_sites_wwd/. Accessed 24 Apr 2016.
22. Centers for Disease Control and Prevention. The right to know health campaign. 2008 http://www.cdc.gov/ncbddd/disabilityandhealth/righttoknow/documents/tipsheetseng.pdf. Accessed 24 Apr 2016.
23. Quint EH. Adolescents with special needs: clinical challenges in reproductive health care. J Pediatr Adolesc Gynecol. 2016;29(1):2–6.
24. World Health Organization. Medical eligibility criteria for contraceptive use, 5th ed. 2015. http://apps.who.int/iris/bitstream/10665/181468/1/9789241549158_eng.pdf?ua=1. Accessed 24 Apr 2016.
25. Center for Research on Women with Disabilities (CROWD). Contraception. https://www.bcm.edu/research/centers/research-on-women-with-disabilities/topics/sexuality-and-reproductive-health/pelvic-health/women-with-disabilities/reproductive-health/contraception. Accessed 24 Apr 2016.
26. Welner S. A provider's guide for the care of women with physical disabilities & chronic medical conditions. Chapel Hill: North Carolina Office on Disability & Health; 1999.
27. Rivera Drew JA. Hysterectomy and disability among U.S. women. Perspect Sex Reprod Health. 2013;45(3):157–63.
28. Planned Parenthood. Testicular Cancer. 2016. https://www.plannedparenthood.org/learn/men/testicular-cancer. Accessed 24 Apr 2016.
29. National Down Syndrome Society (ndss). Sexuality & down syndrome. www.ndss.org/Resources/Wellness/Sexuality/Sexuality-and-Down-Syndrome. Accessed 24 Apr 2016.
30. Spina Bifida Association. Health care for women. 2015. http://spinabifidaassociation.org/project/health-care-for-women/. Accessed 24 Apr 2016.
31. Spina Bifida Association. http://spinabifidaassociation.org. Accessed 24 Apr 2016.
32. Parent Project Muscular Dystrophy. Delayed puberty in duchenne muscular dystrophy. http://www.parentprojectmd.org/site/DocServer/Delayed_Puberty_Parent.pdf?docID=13125. Accessed 24 Apr 2016.
33. National Institutes of Health. National Heart, Lung, and Blood Institute. Division of Blood Diseases and Resources NIH Publication NO. 02-2117. The Management of Sickle Cell Disease. Originally printed 1984 previously revised 1989, 1995 reprinted June 1999 revised June 2002, 4h ed. http://www.nhlbi.nih.gov/files/docs/guidelines/sc_mngt.pdf. Accessed 24 Apr 2016.
34. Children's Oncology Group. Long-term follow-up guidelines for survivors of childhood, adolescent, and young adult cancers. 2013. www.survivorship-guidelines.org. Accessed 24 Apr 2016.
35. Children's Oncology Group. Long-term follow-up guidelines for survivors of childhood, adolescent, and young adult cancers. Version 4. 2013. http://www.survivorshipguidelines.org/pdf/LTFUGuidelines_40.pdf. Accessed 24 Apr 2016.
36. Livestrong. Comprehensive guide for fertility & family planning. http://www.livestrong.org/we-can-help/fertility-services/. Accessed 24 Apr 2016.
37. Yankanskas JR, Marshall BC, Sifian B, Simon RH, Rodman D. Cystic fibrosis adult care. Chest. 2004;125:1S–39S.

Palliative Care

24

Jill Ann Jarrell

Basics of Palliative Care

Definitions

Palliative care is an approach to caring for patients and families of patients with life-threatening illnesses that focuses on improving quality of life.

The word *palliate* comes from the Latin word *palliare*, which means "to cloak" and thus palliative care is often associated with pain and other symptom mitigation. However, palliative care attempts to address and assist with facets of the patient and family's illness experience that may not only be physical, but also emotional, psychosocial, and spiritual.

In this particular population, adults with chronic childhood conditions, it is important to consider aspects of pediatrics in implementing palliative care. The patient's physiology and psychosocial health as well as pertinent legal and ethical issues may be more pediatric in nature than what one is accustomed to in adult medicine or may be unique to this population, all together. The World Health Organization has similar but distinct definitions of adult and pediatric palliative care (Table 24.1) [1].

Who Should Receive Palliative Care?

"Palliative care is for patients of any age, and at any stage of illness, whether that illness is curable, chronic, or life threatening" [2]. Patients do not have to be actively dying or near the end of life to receive palliative care.

Over recent years, there has been a conceptual shift away from identifying diagnoses appropriate for palliative care toward identifying patients with *unmet palliative care needs*. For example, the patient may have complex or refractory pain or other symptoms such as anxiety, depression, insomnia, dyspnea, secretions, or fatigue. Additionally, there may be difficult aspects of the patient's care due to prognostic uncertainly, complex medical decision-making, need for care coordination or transitional services, psychosocial stressors, or spiritual concerns.

When to Implement Palliative Care

Studies have shown that earlier implementation of palliative care can not only improve patient's symptom control and decrease healthcare

J.A. Jarrell (✉)
Section of Palliative Care and Academic General Pediatrics, Texas Children's Hospital, Clinical Care Center, Baylor College of Medicine, 6701 Fannin Street, Suite 1540, Houston, TX 77030, USA
e-mail: jajarrel@texaschildrens.org

M. Pilapil et al. (eds.), *Care of Adults with Chronic Childhood Conditions*,
DOI 10.1007/978-3-319-43827-6_24

Table 24.1 World Health Organization definitions of palliative care for adults and pediatrics

WHO definition of palliative care
Palliative care is an approach to caring for patients and families facing life-threatening illnesses that improves the quality of life through the prevention and relief of suffering by means of early identification and impeccable assessment and treatment of pain and other problems that are physical, psychosocial, emotional and spiritual. Palliative care: • Provides relief from pain and other distressing symptoms; • Affirms life and regards dying as a normal process; • Intends neither to hasten nor postpone death; • Integrates the psychological and spiritual aspects of patient care; • Offers a support system to help patients live as actively as possible until death; • Offers a support system to help the patient and family cope during the illness and in bereavement; • Uses a team approach to address the needs of patients and their families, including bereavement counseling; • Will enhance quality of life, and may also positively influence the course of illness; • Is applicable early in the course of illness and may be used in conjunction with other therapies that are intended to prolong life
WHO definition of palliative care for children
Palliative care for children is the active total care of the child's body, mind and spirit, and also involves giving support to the family; • It begins when illness is diagnosed, and continues regardless of whether or not a child receives treatment directed at the disease; • Health providers must evaluate and alleviate a child's physical, psychological, and social distress; • Effective palliative care requires a broad multidisciplinary approach that includes the family and makes use of available community resources; it can be successfully implemented even if resources are limited; • It can be provided in tertiary care facilities, in community health centers and even in children's homes

Reprinted with permission from World Health Organization. WHO definition of palliative care and WHO Definition of Palliative Care for Children. www.who.int/cancer/palliative/definition/en/

utilization, but early implementation of palliative care can actually prolong life [3, 4].

The components of palliative care should be offered at the time of diagnosis of a life-threatening condition and continued throughout the course of the illness, whether the outcome is cure or death. Palliative care can be provided alongside efforts to cure illness and/or prolong life, as appropriate and desired [5].

Older models depict curative and palliative care as being at opposite ends of the care continuum. However, newer recommendations encourage incorporating aspects of palliative care early, alongside more traditional aspects of care to accommodate varying goals and to maximize patients' quality of life (Fig. 24.1) [6].

Who Provides Palliative Care?

Every medical provider should practice palliative care to the extent of his/her abilities and comfort. *Primary palliative care* refers to basic skills and competencies required of all physicians and other healthcare professionals in areas such as pain management, guiding discussions regarding advance directives, and assisting in end-of-life decision-making.

Secondary palliative care refers to the specialist clinicians and organizations that provide consultation and specialty care. *Tertiary palliative care* refers to the academic medical centers where specialist knowledge for the most complex cases is practiced, researched, and taught.

Higher levels of palliative care are commonly accomplished through a multi- or trans-disciplinary palliative care team comprised of nurses, physicians, social workers, chaplains, counselors, child life specialists, and volunteers with the patient and family at its center (Fig. 24.2).

In general, referral to a specialist or center for palliative care should occur when the limit of the primary provider has been reached. Table 24.2 provides specific referral criteria.

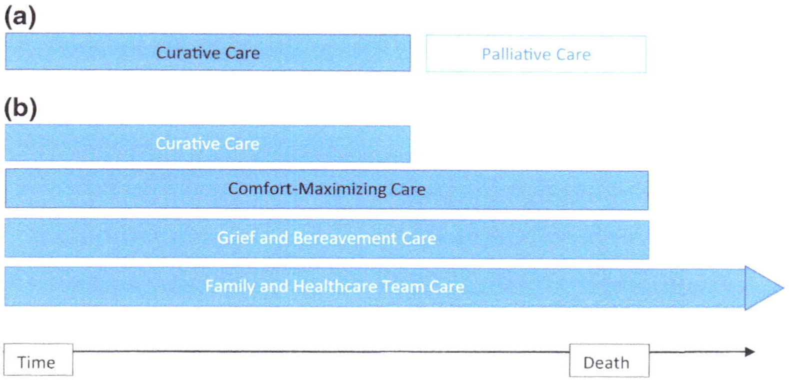

Fig. 24.1 Competing versus complementary domains of care. Adapted with permission from Carter B, Levetown M, Friebert S. Palliative Care for Infants, Children, and Adolescents. Baltimore, MD: The Johns Hopkins University Press 2011

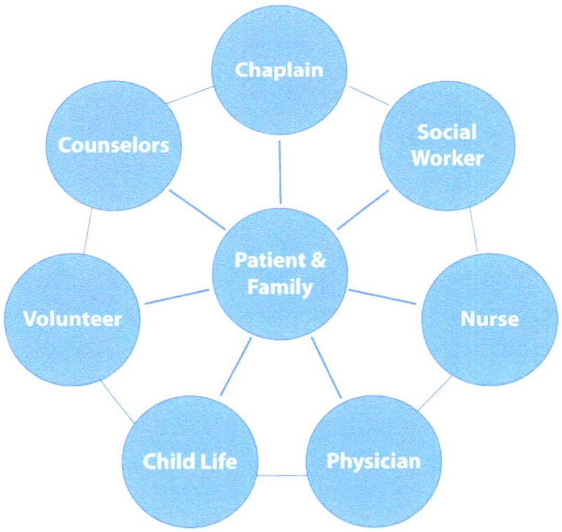

Fig. 24.2 Depiction of the trans-disciplinary palliative care team, where all disciplines work within and beyond the scope of their practice for the benefit of the patient unit at the center

Where Does Palliative Care Take Place?

Primary palliative care can take place in the context of every provider–patient relationship, regardless of place. Consultative palliative care can take place in the hospital setting, clinic setting, home setting, or in other post-acute facilities. A growing number of hospitals and institutions have multidisciplinary palliative care services that serve patients at various places along the care continuum.

Resources

To locate a palliative care provider or program near you, visit www.getpalliativecare.org.

Hospice

Definition

Palliative care and hospice are not synonyms. *Hospice is an expression of palliative care that is a collection of services provided at the end of life.*

Eligibility

In the United States, hospice is a benefit for individuals who are terminally ill and have a life expectancy of less than 6 months if their underlying disease runs its normal course; hospice is available to those who are eligible for Medicare Part A. Medicaid provides a hospice benefit to terminally ill patients in most states and territories, although the individual eligibility criteria and services provided vary by state. The

Table 24.2 Recommendations for referral to or consultation with secondary or tertiary palliative care specialists and teams

Palliative care referral criteria
• Advanced pain or other symptom management
• Functional decline; inability to complete activities of daily living
• Patient, family or physician uncertainty regarding goals of care
• Patient, family or physician uncertainty regarding prognosis
• Establishing or interpreting advance directives
• Complex medical decision-making (e.g., use of feeding tube in cognitively impaired or seriously ill patient)
• Assistance with end-of-life discussions
• Guidance in end-of-life care
• Assistance with hospice placement or other transitions in care
• Multiple or lengthy hospitalizations
• Multiple or lengthy intensive care unit (ICU) admissions
• Limited social supports in the setting of a serious illness
• Patient or family psychological or spiritual distress

Adapted from www.getpalliativecare.org

Department of Veterans Affairs, most private insurance plans, health maintenance organizations (HMOs), and other managed care organizations also provide a hospice benefit.

Patients who live beyond their expected 6-month prognosis may be recertified and continue hospice if their physician assesses them as having progressive clinical decline and ongoing hospice needs.

Services

Hospice beneficiaries are entitled to multiple services that can be provided at home, in a custodial care setting, or in a free-standing hospice unit. These services may include: nursing, physician, counseling, social work, chaplaincy, family support, short-term inpatient care, medical supplies and equipment, medications, home health aide, home-maker, physical therapy, occupational therapy, and speech-language pathology. Hospice continues to support the family for approximately 1 year after the patient has died.

When Hospice Is not Enough

Many patients and families have needs and desires that exceed what hospice can provide and require additional nursing, personal care services, therapy services, and familial support. These needs can be met through placing the hospice patient in custodial care or by acquiring additional services in the home setting via private duty nursing, home health care, or paid personal caregiver.

Concurrent Care

As part of the Patient Protection and Affordable Care Act of 2010, terminally ill individuals who are 21 years of age or younger and who are enrolled in a Medicaid or state Children's Health Insurance Plan (CHIP) may concurrently receive hospice care and curative care related to their terminal health condition [7].

The concurrent care model allows patients and families to continue therapeutic and supportive relationships with primary care and subspecialty providers with whom they have often had long-standing alliances.

Medicare beneficiaries can also receive concurrent care with primary and subspecialty providers while receiving hospice. However, the services must be separate and distinct in documentation and billing. The hospice physician and services bill for the terminal diagnosis and related symptoms under Medicare Part A, while the physician and services providing the concurrent care must address and treat non-hospice diagnoses and bill under Medicare Part B.

Resources

To find a hospice near you, visit http://www.nhpco.org/find-hospice.

Advance Care Planning

Definitions

Advance care planning is the process and documentation that clarifies an individual's wishes regarding their care in the event of illness or death. Advance care planning is important as it gives guidance to family members, friends, and healthcare providers in what can be a difficult time or situation. Additionally, it can provide patients with a sense of control and peace of mind regarding their future health care (Adapted from [8]).

The term "advance directives" is often used synonymously with "advance care planning" or used to refer to advance care planning documents.

Who Needs Advance Care Planning?

Advance care planning is not just for sick or dying people. All adults, emancipated minors, and children with chronic illnesses are encouraged to have conversations about and documentation of their wishes.

Some advance care planning, Out of Hospital DNR, and Physician Orders for Life Sustaining Treatment are for patients with serious illness or frailty.

Types of Advance Care Planning Documents

There are several types of advance care planning documents (Table 24.3), which vary by state. For example, most states recognize a Directive to Physicians as a legally binding document, but a few do not. Also, many states recognize a Physician Order for Life Sustaining Treatment while others only recognize an Out of Hospital DNR, with the former being a more inclusive directive than the latter for end-of-life treatment. Very few states recognize a Declaration for Mental Health. It is important to be aware of the advance directives specific to the state in which an individual lives or seeks care. Some patients have advance directives in multiple states.

How to Formalize Advance Care Plans

One does not need an attorney to obtain or complete advance care planning documents, but often lawyers or social workers can be helpful in the process. In most situations, advance care planning documents can be accessed and completed in the privacy of one's own home or in a physician's office. Physicians can play an important role in initiating and guiding the advance care planning process by making it a routine part of care for all patients, which is revisited regularly to explore any changes a patient may have in his or her wishes (Adapted from [8]).

The verification of advance care planning documentation also varies by state. Some states require two witnesses, some require notarization, and others require both witnesses and notarization.

Table 24.3 Types and descriptions of advance care planning documents

Directive to physicians ("Living Will")	Provides direction for inpatient care in the event of a sudden, severe illness and inability to participate in decision-making; typically differentiates between aggressive and comfort care; recommended for general population
Medical power of attorney	Designates surrogate or proxy for medical decision-making in the event of inability to participate in decision-making; recommended for general population
Out of hospital or pre-hospital do not resuscitate (OOH DNR)	Provides direction to emergency response teams for giving or withholding cardiopulmonary resuscitation; recommended for patients with serious illness or frailty, for whom a health care professional would not be surprised if they died within 1 year
Directive for mental health	Provides direction for inpatient treatment of mental health conditions regarding medications and restraints if unable to participate in decision-making; recommended for general population
Organ donation	Provides direction for organ and/or tissue donation; recommended for general population
Statutory durable power of attorney	Designates surrogate or proxy for financial and estate-related decision-making in the event of inability to participate in decision-making; recommended for general population
Physician orders for life sustaining treatment (POLST)	Provides direction to healthcare providers across the continuum of care for giving or withholding cardiopulmonary resuscitation as well as other treatments such as antibiotics or nutrition; recommended for patients with serious illness or frailty, for whom a health care professional would not be surprised if they died within 1 year

Resources

Social workers often have access to advance care planning forms. Useful Internet resources for obtaining state-specific advance care planning information and paperwork include www.caringinfo.org, and individual states' Departments of Aging and Disability. State-specific organ donor registries and forms can be accessed via http://donatelife.net.

Communication Regarding Advance Care Plans

Advance care plans should be talked about early and often, between patients and their families and patients and their healthcare teams. Copies should be made and given to physicians, put in the medical record, kept at home and given to family and friends, especially those serving as surrogates.

Palliative Care Issues Unique to Adults with Chronic Childhood Conditions

Due to the recent emergence of adults with chronic childhood conditions as a distinct patient population as well as the relative youth of palliative care as a distinct field, there is a paucity of research and literature specific to where these topics intersect. What literature exists does so mostly within the adolescent and young adult (AYA) oncology arena, but can be extrapolated to other populations that may be in need of palliative care, such as AYA with muscular dystrophy, congenital heart disease, and cystic fibrosis, as examples. Unique issues in the physical and psychosocial health of these patients, advance care planning, and systems-based issues have been identified.

Physical

Adults with chronic childhood illness may be small for their age and require pediatric or weight-based dosing of medications common in palliative care such as opioids or benzodiazepines. These patients may also require medical equipment that is more pediatric in nature due to its size, design, or function. For example, some AYA with chronic respiratory illnesses rely heavily on mechanisms more commonly used in children than in adults to maintain their comfort such as airway clearance devices or chest compression systems.

Psychosocial

Some of the AYA population may be developmentally delayed as a sequelae of their underlying disease process. However, even those AYA who are cognitively intact may have a more child-like mentality due to their protracted illness and physical dependence on proxy caregivers. Coping and decision-making skills may be at a developmental level that is far below the patient's chronological age. AYA patients with cancer seem to be more concerned with how they want to be treated and remembered than about decision-making [9].

Experimentation with risky behaviors, including substance abuse, is another psychosocial consideration in this population when considering palliative care [10]. One underutilized resource available to palliative care programs treating AYA patients is psychiatry [10].

Advance Care Planning

Voicing My Choices is an advance care planning guide designed for AYA patients to help them communicate their end-of-life preferences to family, caregivers, and friends [11]. Voicing My Choices is not a legal document but a legacy document developed through research with AYA with cancer and human immunodeficiency virus (HIV) infection [12].These guides can be found at agingwithdignity.org

Recommendations for advance care planning in AYA from this research include: that it be introduced by a trusted member of the healthcare team; that it be introduced when the patient's health is relatively stable and that the conversation evolve gradually over time, that the AYA's concerns be addressed throughout the advance care planning process, and that decisions regarding life support are best done witha healthcare professional [12].

Systems-Based Issues

Pediatric hospitals and palliative care programs are ill-equipped to care for AYAs with terminal conditions due to lack of provider education, staff training, and institutional policy [10]. Likewise, adult providers and institutions are similarly lacking in infrastructure and resources to adequately and effectively treat this population. Unique and novel forms of education are needed to equip healthcare providers to provide competent, confident, and compassionate palliative care to AYAs [13].

References

1. World Health Organization. WHO definition of palliative care. www.who.int/cancer/palliative/definition/en/.
2. Palliative Doctors. http://palliativedoctors.org/.
3. Temel JS, Greer JA, Muzikansky A, et al. Early palliative care for patients with metastatic non-small-cell lung cancer. N Engl J Med. 2010;363 (8):733–42.
4. Zimmermann C, Swami N, Krzyanowska M, et al. Early palliative care for patients with advanced cancer: a cluster-randomized controlled trial. Lancet. 2014;383(9930):1721–30.
5. American Academy of Pediatrics. Section on hospice and palliative medicine. June 2016. http://www2.aap.org/sections/palliative/.

6. Carter B, Levetown M, Friebert S. Palliative care for infants, children, and adolescents. Baltimore: The Johns Hopkins University Press. 2011.
7. Center for Medicaid, CHIP and Survey and Certification. Hospice Care for Children in Medicaid and CHIP. September 9, 2010. https://downloads.cms.gov/cmsgov/archived-downloads/SMDL/downloads/SMD10018.pdf.
8. American Medical Association. Opinion 2.191: advance care planning. June 2011. http://www.ama-assn.org/ama/pub/physician-resources/medical-ethics/code-medical-ethics/opinion2191.page.
9. Weiner L, Ballard E, Brennan T, et al. How I wish to be remembered: the use of an advance care planning document in adolescent and young adult populations. J Palliat Med. 2008;11(10):1309–13.
10. Humphrey L, Dell ML. Identifying unique aspects of adolescent and young adult palliative care: a case study to propel programmatic changes in pediatric hospitals. Semin Pediatr Neurol. 2015;22:166–71.
11. Voicing My Choices. www.agingwithdignity.org/voicing-my-choices.php.
12. Weiner L, Zadeh S, Battles H, et al. Allowing adolescents and young adults to plan their end-of-life care. Pediatrics. 2012;130:1–9.
13. Weiner L, Weaver M, Bell C, et al. Threading the cloak: palliative care education for care providers of adolescent and young adults with cancer. Clin Oncol Adolesc Young Adults. 2015;5:1–18.

Part V

Socio-Legal Aspects of Transition Care

25 Assessing and Enhancing Psychosocial Functioning

Daniel J. Coletti and Naomi S. Kane

Introduction

Development occurs through ongoing interactions with social networks that include family, peer groups, and larger systems such as community and culture. Positive social experiences are essential to patient health and wellbeing [1–3]. The primary care provider's office is an important social environment for an adolescent with special healthcare needs as physicians serve as both social agents as well as medical providers for these young people. Attaining the age of majority accelerates the transition to adult healthcare, and occurs at a time when social interactions are of paramount importance and among these patients' most salient preoccupations. The adult primary care provider (PCP) has a window into the social world of these patients. In light of evidence suggesting that young people with chronic conditions are at risk for problems in social competence and performance related to their illness [4, 5], the PCP has a unique opportunity to detect and address problems in social functioning. Through strategic communication and appropriate use of external resources, the PCP can promote healthy social engagement and positive social behaviors. The following chapter will (1) review the most relevant aspects of social development during the young adult period; (2) discuss ways to identify barriers to optimal social functioning; and (3) provide strategies for the PCP to facilitate this aspect of patient care.

Psychosocial Development and Young Adults with Chronic Health Conditions

Young Adults with Chronic Childhood Conditions (YACCC) face the same developmental milestones as unaffected peers, and the PCP assesses social development as part of comprehensive care [6]. Some social milestones have clear chronological markers, such as the age-related transfer of decisional capacity from guardian-to-patient at age 18, and dates of change in educational programming (starting college, aging out of special education services) and workforce entry. Most social milestones are processes that emerge over time, however, and are better defined by the *development* of peer and collegial social networks, *growth* toward independence from guardians and the family, and the *emergence* of sexual identity and an interest in intimate relationships. Adolescents with chronic

D.J. Coletti (✉)
Department of General Internal Medicine, Hofstra Northwell School of Medicine, 865 Northern Blvd, Suite 102, Great Neck, NY 11021, USA
e-mail: dcoletti@northwell.edu

N.S. Kane
Clinical Psychology Health Emphasis Program, Ferkauf Graduate School of Psychology, Yeshiva University, 1300 Morris Park Avenue, Rousso Building, Bronx, NY 10461, USA
e-mail: naomiskane@gmail.com

M. Pilapil et al. (eds.), *Care of Adults with Chronic Childhood Conditions*,
DOI 10.1007/978-3-319-43827-6_25

medical conditions also transition into young adulthood coping with the social effects (or late effects) of childhood disease and its treatment [7]. When treatment has required extended school absences, or when motor or communication deficits impair the quantity and quality of peer relationships, illness can *delay* the attainment of social skills and milestones. Conversely, illness can *accelerate* social development—either positively (e.g., when experience interacting with medical providers enhances a patient's ability to communicate with adults) or in a maladaptive way, when poor social adjustment and self-image fuels experimentation with risky health behaviors (such as substance use) [8]. Finally, social competence and support influence the ways young adults handle illness-related stressors. Social skills and well-developed social networks buffer the demands of managing a chronic medical condition, particularly when support from family and peers is perceived conjointly [9–11]. An extensive body of research has identified relations between social connectedness and enhanced psychological wellbeing [12, 13] that protects against premature mortality in adulthood [14, 15] and underscores the importance of attending to this aspect of patient functioning early for subsequent wellbeing across the lifespan.

Although social impairments in YACCC should not be assumed, it is important to consider the types of problems they are likely to experience. The increased caregiving supports YACCC required during childhood place them at heightened risk of developing dependency on caregivers in adulthood, as well as social exclusion [16]. YACCC may find that a disproportionate number of their interactions as children and adolescents were with adults rather than similarly aged peers, and less peer contact means fewer opportunities to develop social skills [17]. In addition, they were more likely to have faced bullying and ostracism from peer groups [18]. Although relations between severity and psychosocial functioning are complex and not always linear, the extent of social isolation may depend on illness severity [19]. For example, when mild illness severity has minimal impact on social development, and when individuals with severe illness are provided supports to help overcome social challenges, those patients with moderate levels of illness severity appear to be at greater risk of problems in social functioning [20]. The likelihood of developing social problems depends on the degree to which the condition is visibly recognizable [21] and if the condition involves the central nervous system and impacts motor development [22–25]. The association between the degree of motor impairment and psychosocial functioning is more equivocal [26]. In fact, some researchers identify a "disability paradox" or counterintuitive associations between *greater* impairment and *higher* levels of psychosocial satisfaction [27]. Therefore, chronic health conditions may foster resilience as well as insecurity.

Despite common perceptions that illness-related delays in social development might protect from experimentation with risky substances, YACCC may in fact be more likely than their peers to smoke cigarettes daily, endorse marijuana use, and perform antisocial behaviors (e.g., fighting, vandalism, fire-setting, etc.) [28]. For example, a study of young adults (ages 19–21) with congenital heart defects found that half endorsed alcohol consumption (including binge drinking) in the prior month [29]. Adolescents with chronic conditions are at least as likely as their peers to engage in sexual intercourse or risky sexual behaviors [30, 31]. Moreover, young people with chronic conditions may be more prone to adverse outcomes associated with experimentation [32]; for example, when patients with childhood-onset asthma smoke tobacco and increase their risk for adult respiratory dysfunction [33], when unplanned pregnancy creates risks for the young woman and to fetal health [34–36], and when young persons who are immunosuppressed engage in unprotected sex and are at an elevated risk of developing sexually transmitted infections (STIs) [37]. Finally, caution is urged in assuming that pediatric practitioners have adequately screened and addressed these social mediated risky health behaviors (e.g., smoking, alcohol use, sex education) in adolescence, as significant barriers to evaluation persist in pediatric practice [38].

Social problems are also more likely to occur in the presence of socioeconomic or environmental challenges. Patients must often handle a medical condition and its treatment with limited language proficiency [39], low healthcare related skills, inadequate housing, unemployment or low income, and in unsafe residential environments [16]. Strong associations between socioeconomic indicators and health status were identified across studies in a recent literature review of research in chronic kidney disease [40]. Finally, socioeconomic indicators such as parent level of education can influence the transition process when families lack knowledge and skills to assist their adolescent in preparing for adult-oriented medical care [41].

Perhaps the most significant negative impact on YACCCs social functioning occurs when integrated special education programming services end. Significant declines in social activity and perceived social wellbeing are often observed in young adults when support services end (typically at age 21). Young adults who require high levels of support can experience feelings of loneliness and greater social isolation when they leave school [42]. Forming a social network of peers with similar support needs or experience of illness can enhance social maturity and resiliency [18].

Potential accelerators of perceived social isolation are embedded in the healthcare transition process itself. YACCC often lack the skills to navigate a complex healthcare system with greater independence and less family involvement [43]. Young adult transition narratives have common themes of confusion about relationships with providers and feelings of alienation, with patients perceiving the adult healthcare environment to be significantly less engaging and person-centered than pediatric care [44, 45]. A successful healthcare transition augments self-efficacy, independence, responsibility, and self-sufficiency [46]. A person-centered approach during the transition process involves understanding the young patient's world by conveying interest in the patient's social functioning and observing the ways in which the patient interacts with others.

Assessment of Social Functioning in YACCC

The variable effects of chronic conditions on social functioning underscore the need for individualized assessment of each of the following: the patient's relationship to their illness, the type and severity of functional impairment, the impact of the illness on social adjustment, and the ways existing social supports facilitate or hinder wellbeing. To identify key areas for investigation, adolescent specialists have described a "Psychosocial Systems Review" where domains to assess correspond to the acronym HEEADSSS (Home environment, Education and employment, Eating, peer-related Activities, Drugs, Sexuality, Suicide/depression, and Safety from injury and violence) [47]. A fourth "S" might include "Social Media" involvement. Recent studies estimate that up to 83 % of young people aged 18–29 have an online presence [48]. Participation in social media sites can have enormous positive as well as negative effects on social wellbeing [49], and emerging evidence suggests that chronic illness-related social media interactions are increasing [50].

Optimal assessment integrates both formal (e.g., questionnaires, interviews, etc.) and informal (semi-structured questioning and observation) strategies to assess the social functioning of YACCC. Screening also facilitates improved communication about psychosocial functioning among providers, patients, and family [51]. Although screening for problems with psychological and behavioral functioning is now broadly implemented, identifying social impairments is rarely considered an active problem [52] or identified as a reason to refer for behavioral health services [53] despite its critical relationship to psychological health.

Screening and brief counseling for depression and alcohol misuse is a United States Preventive Services Task Force (USPSTF) recommendation in the general population [54, 55]. However, calls for comparable guidelines in young adults have yet to be articulated and evidence supporting universal screening for illicit substance use in adults or in adolescents has yet to be confirmed

[56, 57]. Given the overlap between social functioning, mood problems, and risky health behaviors, supplementing screening of these domains with a review of social competence, activities, and support can enhance broader psychosocial screening and provide context and solutions for identified difficulties.

Choosing appropriate standardized screening tools can be daunting. There are options for implementing universal screening strategies of substance and alcohol use, including the 4-item CAGE questionnaire [58] used for life-time drinking patterns, the 10-item Alcohol Use Disorders Identification Test (AUDIT) which focuses on current drinking problems [59], and subsets of the AUDIT designed to be rapid screenings (e.g., the reduced 3-item AUDIT-C used to screen based on consumption) [60, 61]. For illicit substance use disorders the Drug Abuse Screening Test (DAST) [62] is a 28-item survey (with a more commonly used 10-item version) [63] that assesses the impact of substance use on functioning. A single-item from the DAST—"How many times in the past year have you used an illegal drug or used a prescription medication for nonmedical reasons?"—was identified in a recent report as a highly sensitive (100 %) and specific (73.5 %) screen for drug use disorder in a large primary care trial [64].

Standardized assessment of social functioning is typically part of a more extensive psychosocial assessment. Questionnaire-based psychosocial assessments typically used in clinical research, such as the Medical Outcomes Study Health Survey [65], the Social Adjustment Scale [66], and the Social Adaptation Evaluation scale [67] were identified in one primary care study as strategies identified by patients as acceptable for real world self-report assessment [68]. However, each of these measures takes time, requires relatively high levels of patient literacy, and administration can impact patient workflow in busy practices. The broadly disseminated Patient Health Questionnaire (PHQ) [69] has items tapping social concomitants of depression (e.g., "little interest or pleasure in doing things"; "Feeling…as you have let your family down") and depression-related functional impairment, but is an inadequate screener for social functioning or distress.

For providers who collaborate with behavioral health professionals and implement comprehensive questionnaire assessment, the Adult Behavior Checklist (ABCL) [70] is a developmental extension of its widely used pediatric counterpart, the Child Behavior Checklist. The ABCL has both parent and Adult Self-Report forms and contains 137 items pertaining to youth problems, some of which tap social competence and functioning. Similarly, the Behavioral Assessment System for Children (2nd edition) [71] has normative data up to age 21 and includes parent-report data on constructs such as social skills and adaptive behavior. The Patient Reported Outcomes Measurement Information System (PROMIS) is a comprehensive set of larger "item banks" tapping a conceptually integrated "domain framework," with smaller breakout subscales tackling multiple areas of patient functioning. The PROMIS' Social Health and Social Function domains include subscales assessing patient satisfaction with "Participation in Social Roles" (work, household responsibilities, routines, etc.) and "Participation in Discretionary Activities (e.g., leisure activities, enjoyable activities with friends, etc.). Items are scored and compared with a normative database.

Many self-report questionnaires tend to skew toward assessing functioning within the normative ranges of social and behavioral development. For YACCC with known impairments in adaptive and intellectual functioning and/or with communication delays, parent/caregiver reports are paramount. An alternative assessment for social problems would be the Aberrant Behavior Checklist [72], a 58-item caregiver report of socially mediated behavioral problems such as lethargy/social withdrawal; stereotypic behaviors; hyperactivity, and inappropriate speech.

Screening for socially mediated problems (Table 25.1) should of course consider the social context of the screening itself [58, 59, 61, 63, 65–67, 70, 72]. For example, *when* the screening was completed (at home, in the office), *how* it was completed (on paper, via physician or medical assistant interview, alone at home on a

Table 25.1 Screening measures

Measure	Purpose	Description
Alcohol and substance use		
CAGE Questionnaire [58]	Life-time drinking patterns	4-Questions are asked to help provider diagnose problematic alcohol use: "Have you felt you should *cut down* on your drinking?" "Have people *annoyed* you by criticizing your drinking?" "Have you ever felt bad or *guilty* about your drinking?" "Have you ever had a drink first thing in the morning to steady your nerves or get rid of a hangover (*eye opener*)?"
Alcohol Use Disorder Identification Test (AUDIT) [59]	Problematic alcohol use screen	*10-item* self-report questionnaire that assesses problematic alcohol use across several domains: alcohol consumption, drinking-related behavior, and problems related to alcohol use. Scores range from 0 to 40, with scores of 8 or more indicative of problematic alcohol use. Also available as a brief screening instrument (AUDIT-C) [61].
Drug Abuse Screening Test (DAST) [63]	Influence of drug use on functioning	Clinician administered or self-report *28-item* questionnaire with yes/no responses that assesses the impact of drug use, excluding alcohol and tobacco, on health, withdrawal and family functioning. Also available as a briefer 10-item version (DAST-10) [63], with scores of 3 or greater requiring further assessment.
Quality of life and social functioning		
Medical Outcomes Study Health Survey (SF-36) [65]	General health status	Self-report *36-item* questionnaire measuring health functioning across 8 domains including limitations in social and physical functioning, pain, general wellbeing, and energy/fatigue level.
Social Adjustment Scale (SAS-SR) [66]	Social functioning	*42-item* self-report questionnaire evaluating an individual's level of satisfaction and role performance within social interactions in major domains of functioning including work/school, leisure and family. Also available as a screener and short form.
Social Adaptation Self-evaluation Scale (SASS) [67]	Social functioning in depression	*21-item* self-report measure assessing interest in initiating and maintaining social activities in patients with depression. Perceptions of social environment are sensitive to change with treatment for depression.
Behavioral functioning		
Adult Behavior Checklist (ABCL) and Adult Self-Report [70]	Social competence and behavioral functioning	Comprehensive measure of adaptive/social competence and behavioral functioning, parallel measures for self and parent/partner report.
Aberrant Behavior Checklist (ABC) [72]	Socially influenced behavioral problems for individuals with cognitive/adaptive impairments	*58-item* informant and/or caregiver report of socially mediated behavioral problems such as lethargy/social withdrawal; stereotypic behaviors; hyperactivity, and inappropriate speech among individuals 18–30.

tablet computer,) and *who* completed the assessment (patient, parent, case manager, etc.). These factors influence responses to social items more than other areas of functioning. Social desirability bias—the attempt to present oneself more favorably—should be considered when interpreting. Reviewing patient forms and questionnaires can be time consuming, though best practice for standardized screening suggests it is important to review the respondent's answers prior to or during the appointment—perhaps with a medical assistant, nurse, or extender flagging items above a threshold value. Pre-visit review can synthesize key findings, provide focus for further investigation, and engage the patient who appreciates that you are responding to his/her concerns. For example, noting a flagged response to an item on the ABCL assessing grades in school can be a jumping-off point to expand into a more in-depth review of health-related barriers in the classroom (e.g., insulin administration, use of PRN medication), future career goals, and social functioning in general outside the home.

In addition to questionnaire-based assessment, much can be learned by attending to patient verbal and nonverbal communication to detect problems in social functioning. The degree of apparent patient comfort within the medical encounter can hold clues to a patient's social functioning in other settings. Observing whether the patient can make and sustain eye contact, engage in reciprocal interactions, and respond to questions (particularly open-ended questions) may suggest social competence and/or difficulties in similarly structured environments. Young adults typically will involve their caregivers in some way during a visit, and noting the degree to which children expect parents to provide verbal reports to you may shed light on problems with independent functioning, social initiation, and family dynamics. For private conversations involving sexual activity and substance use, utilize questions that easily permit positive responses and that open the door to voluntary and authentic disclosure (e.g., "How many times have you tried smoking cigarettes?"; "Tell me about the drugs that you've tried…"). Ask patients about sensitive topics such as sexual matters in open-ended ways that allow a broad range of options including alternative identities, behaviors, and lifestyles—or lack of sexual activity, which can be equally uncomfortable to disclose ("Are you currently dating or are you having sex with anybody?"). Particularly with YACCC, variable development may make it necessary to assess multiple informants about social functioning. For example, YACCC may be more likely to present with uneven social development and more severe problems in one area than another. Therefore, obtaining a questionnaire from a vocational therapist in a special education program and then comparing it to a parent's report of the patient's social skills may identify areas of discrepancy across the home, work, and school environments. In addition, primary care providers should be mindful of the risk for diagnostic overshadowing [73]. This term was originally used to describe the tendency of physicians to misattribute the behavioral difficulties of people with intellectual disabilities to (more stable) cognitive deficits rather than to (potentially treatable) psychiatric conditions. More broadly defined and applied to the area of social functioning, providers should be cautious making assumptions about social competence, leisure interests, and supports based on initial presentation or on features of the illness. For example, diagnostic overshadowing might be at play if we were to assume that patients with intellectual disabilities fail to perceive subtle bullying, or struggle to communicate in a medical encounter because they lack communication skills (when they are actually socially anxious).

Ways Primary Care Providers Can Promote Young Patients' Social Functioning

Cross-validating sources and seeking additional information from a standardized screening or questionnaire with interview probes enhances the treatment validity of the assessment [74] by tying the content of the assessment to specific goals for interventions. Perhaps the most valuable thing a primary care provider can do to intervene in a young person's social development is to ask and assess—about their parents and family, their school and/or work life, and about their friends and partners. With regard to the illness, asking a patient "How do you explain your (illness, medical condition) to other people?" can open the door for more information about patients' social adaptation to their condition and whether they perceive support from their social environment. At the practice level, screening and assessment procedures are best integrated along the lines of the Screening, Brief Intervention, and Referral to Treatment (SBIRT) model for alcohol and substance use problems [75] in which universal screening identifies at-risk patients and subsequent assessment and treatment is triaged according to level of risk. SBIRT models have been shown to be effectively implemented in adult and adolescent primary care settings [76–78]. SBIRT processes rely on the therapeutic impact of brief interventions occurring in the medical setting, and provide clear criteria and mechanisms for referring within or outside the practice for behavioral health or substance abuse services.

Communicating with patients about their social world might incorporate the tenets of Motivational Interviewing (MI) [79], now widely used to negotiate behavior change and reduce high-risk patient behaviors. Although a complete primer on MI is beyond the scope of this chapter, interventions using this approach take a non-confrontative, person-centered stance to address patient ambivalence and resistance to making change or addressing problems. Key MI strategies include active listening techniques to elicit *patient-generated* motivations for making behavior change. Although proven effective in medical settings for a variety of patient behaviors [80], it has not been examined to promote social competence and support per se. One might speculate, however, that a therapeutic approach characterized by supportive but nondirective engagement, active listening, and support for positive change might effectively address social problems, and reduce gaps between patients' functional status and goals they have for themselves in areas such as school, home, friends, and the workplace. For example, one objective of a brief intervention using MI techniques might involve identifying "making more friends in my day program" as an important goal for a 20-year-old male patient with spina bifida and social anxiety. Active listening would identify specific people, behavioral settings, supportive adults, and potential barriers to attaining this goal as part of a behavioral plan, perhaps with family or day program personnel assistance.

Additional help for patients with problems involving social isolation or impaired social functioning would ideally be implemented in concert with behavioral health professionals integrated into your practice—through an integrative team, a co-located professional, or by collaborating with trusted community partners. Promising evidence exists for psychological interventions reinforcing social skills when these intervention teach effective communication techniques and are of adequate intensity and duration (>6 sessions over >3 months) [81]. In addition, effective group therapy has been developed targeting psychoeducation about illness [82], group training in coping skills with managing illness-related exchange of information, improving social competence, and learning positive self-talk [83]. Finally, an emerging body of literature supports the effectiveness of professionally moderated social support interventions provided over the Internet [84, 85].

In the absence of formalized treatment programs for YACCC in your community, an optimal referral to a Behavioral Health Professional (BHP) might best be seen as collaboratively engaging the BHP in recreating some of the best practices identified in laboratory settings. For example, providing information to the therapist about the young person's medical status—and what you have learned about his/her social adjustment—can help a BHP develop a treatment plan (Table 25.2) that fosters optimal physical functioning as well as psychological wellbeing [77, 79]. For example, to help a 22-year-old female with adolescent-onset Type 2 diabetes and social anxiety, sharing details about the patient's illness regimen with the therapist can help him/her develop a treatment

Table 25.2 Techniques to enhance the social functioning of YACCC

Strategy	Description	Rationale
Facilitated communicating about illness	"How do you explain your (illness, medical condition) to other people?" "How does it get in the way of what you want to do?"	Help patient articulate their relationship with their illness in the context of their social identity. Explore patient's perceptions of social support from peers, family, employers, etc.
Screening, Brief Intervention, and Referral to Treatment, (SBIRT) [77]	Universal screening, brief targeted interventions to address problem behavior; referral to community-based treatment for patients with clinical levels of misuse.	Provide education about the impact of alcohol and drug on physical functioning and illness status. Explore risks and benefits of continued drug use on condition. Develop patient goals for healthy behavior and assist obtaining behavioral health intervention if indicated.
Motivational interviewing [79]	Fostering social behavior change by providing information and support using an empathetic, non-confrontational approach.	Engages patient to create socially relevant goals (e.g., to participate in youth group/club, make friends with other YACCC, etc.). Help patient articulate and resolve ambivalence about change, focus conversation on areas according to patient priorities. Support and problem-solve practical changes the patient can make.
Collaborating with Behavioral Health Professionals (BHP)	Provide information about medical status to BHP; co-create behavioral goals that foster both social and physical functioning.	Help BHP integrate special healthcare needs into a treatment plan that is manageable within medical limitations; share in assessment of treatment outcomes, and maintain ongoing communication with the BHP.

based on both regimen-specific needs (e.g., understanding when diabetes tasks might interfere with social interactions) as evidenced-based psychological strategies. When evidence-based practices are unclear for optimizing social functioning, asking specific questions and making clear requests of the professional can improve the quality of the consultation as well as the intervention the patient receives. It might be particularly advantageous to identify behavioral health supports within school and day habilitation programs to work collaboratively in key environments where social processes unfold. Finally, becoming aware of the social activities sponsored by local disease-specific organizations, as well as local youth groups, sports clubs, theater and music associations, and church-based organizations can promote social functioning in clinically meaningful ways [86].

Conclusion

Primary care providers have a unique opportunity to keep YACCCs on track in all areas of functioning, and to help establish themselves in the world of interpersonal interactions and meaningful relationships. Consider ways to incorporate questions about social competence, activities, and perceived support into normative practice screening procedures. Evaluate features of the medical conditions most likely to impair social functioning such as central nervous system involvement, motor and communication impairments, facial anomalies, and severity of the condition. When problems in social functioning are pronounced, impairing, and might be amenable to intervention, engage behavioral health partners and community/social service agencies in collaborative care. Increasing comfort and expertise with engaging young patients around their social functioning can transform the healthcare transition process of a YACCC from one characterized by fear and alienation to an opportunity for you to promote mature adult interactions within the medical encounter and in the patient's social world.

References

1. Viner RM, Ozer EM, Denny S, Marmot M, Resnick M, Fatusi A, et al. Adolescence and the social determinants of health. Lancet. 2012;379 (9826):1641–52.
2. Rosendal M, Vedsted P, Christensen KS, Moth G. Psychological and social problems in primary care patients: general practitioners' assessment and classification. Scand J Prim Health Care. 2013;31(1):43–9.
3. Holt-Lunstad J, Smith TB, Layton JB. Social relationships and mortality risk: a meta-analytic review. PLoS Med. 2010;7(7):e1000316.
4. Pinquart M, Teubert D. Academic, physical, and social functioning of children and adolescents with chronic physical illness: a meta-analysis. J Pediatr Psychol. 2012;37(4):376–89.
5. Martinez W, Carter JS, Legato LJ. Social competence in children with chronic illness: a meta-analytic review. J Pediatr Psychol. 2011;36(8):878–90.
6. Geist R, Grdisa V, Otley A. Psychosocial issues in the child with chronic conditions. Best Pract Res Clin Gastroenterol. 2003;17(2):141–52.
7. Evan EE, Zeltzer LK. Psychosocial dimensions of cancer in adolescents and young adults. Cancer. 2006;107(7 Suppl):1663–71.
8. Zbikowski SM, Klesges RC, Robinson LA, Alfano CM. Risk factors for smoking among adolescents with asthma. J Adolesc Health. 2002;30(4):279–87.
9. Compas BE, Jaser SS, Dunn MJ, Rodriguez EM. Coping with chronic illness in childhood and adolescence. Annu Rev Clin Psychol. 2012;8:455.
10. Kyngäs H. Support network of adolescents with chronic disease: adolescents' perspective. Nurs Health Sci. 2004;6(4):287–93.
11. Oris L, Seiffge-Krenke I, Moons P, Goubert L, Rassart J, Goossens E, et al. Parental and peer support in adolescents with a chronic condition: a typological approach and developmental implications. J Behav Med. 2016;39(1):107–19.
12. Jose PE, Ryan N, Pryor J. Does social connectedness promote a greater sense of well-being in adolescence over time? J Res Adolesc. 2012;22(2):235–51.
13. Kearns A, Whitley E, Tannahill C, Ellaway A. Loneliness, social relations and health and well-being in deprived communities. Psychol Health Med. 2015;20(3):332–44.
14. Steptoe A, Shankar A, Demakakos P, Wardle J. Social isolation, loneliness, and all-cause mortality in older men and women. Proc Natl Acad Sci. 2013;110(15):5797–801.
15. Berkman LF, Syme SL. Social networks, host resistance, and mortality: a nine-year follow-up study of alameda county residents. Am J Epidemiol. 1979;109 (2):186–204.
16. Morris J. Social exclusion and young disabled people with high levels of support needs. Crit Soc Policy. 2001;21(2):161–83.
17. Reiter-Purtill J, Waller J, Noll R. Empirical and theoretical perspectives on the peer relationships of children with chronic conditions. In: Roberts M, Steele R, editors. Handbook of pediatric psychology. 4th ed. New York: The Guilford Press; 2009. p. 672–88.
18. Twyman KA, Saylor CF, Saia D, Macias MM, Taylor LA, Spratt E. Bullying and ostracism experiences in children with special health care needs. J Dev Behav Pediatr. 2010;31(1):1–8.
19. Vanhalst J, Rassart J, Luyckx K, Goossens E, Apers S, Goossens L, et al. Trajectories of loneliness in adolescents with congenital heart disease: associations with depressive symptoms and perceived health. J Adolesc Health. 2013;53(3):342–9.
20. Perrin JM, MacLean WE, Perrin EC. Parental perceptions of health status and psychologic adjustment of children with asthma. Pediatrics. 1989;83 (1):26–30.
21. Van Cleave J, Davis MM. Bullying and peer victimization among children with special health care needs. Pediatrics. 2006;118(4):e1212–9.
22. Nassau JH, Drotar D. Social competence among children with central nervous system-related chronic health conditions: a review. J Pediatr Psychol. 1997;22(6):771–93.
23. Rantanen K, Eriksson K, Nieminen P. Social competence in children with epilepsy: a review. Epilepsy Behav. 2012;24(3):295–303.
24. Gebauer-Bukurov K, Markovic J, Sekulic S, Bozic K. Social competence among well-functioning adolescents with epilepsy. Epilepsy Behav. 2015;42:54–60.
25. Yeates KO, Bigler ED, Gerhardt CA, Rubin KH, Stancin T, Taylor HG, et al. Theoretical approaches to understanding social function in childhood brain insults: toward the integration of social neuroscience and developmental psychology. In: Anderson V, Beauchamp M, editors. Developmental social neuroscience and childhood brain insult: theory and practice. New York: Guilford Press; 2012. p. 207–30.
26. Livingston MH, Rosenbaum PL, Russell DJ, Palisano RJ. Quality of life among adolescents with cerebral palsy: what does the literature tell us? Dev Med Child Neurol. 2007;49(3):225–31.
27. Albrecht GL, Devlieger PJ. The disability paradox: high quality of life against all odds. Soc Sci Med. 1999;48(8):977–88.

28. Suris J-C, Michaud P-A, Akre C, Sawyer SM. Health risk behaviors in adolescents with chronic conditions. Pediatrics. 2008;122(5):e1113–8.
29. Reid GJ, Irvine MJ, McCrindle BW, Sananes R, Ritvo PG, Siu SC, et al. Prevalence and correlates of successful transfer from pediatric to adult health care among a cohort of young adults with complex congenital heart defects. Pediatrics. 2004;113(3): e197–205.
30. Suris J-C, Parera N. Sex, drugs and chronic illness: health behaviours among chronically ill youth. Eur J Public Health. 2005;15(5):484–8.
31. Britto MT, Garrett JM, Dugliss MA, Daeschner C, Johnson CA, Leigh MW, et al. Risky behavior in teens with cystic fibrosis or sickle cell disease: a multicenter study. Pediatrics. 1998;101(2):250–6.
32. Sawyer SM, Drew S, Yeo MS, Britto MT. Adolescents with a chronic condition: challenges living, challenges treating. The Lancet. 2007;369 (9571):1481–9.
33. Aanerud M, Carsin A-E, Sunyer J, Dratva J, Gislason T, Jarvis D, et al. Interaction between asthma and smoking increases the risk of adult airway obstruction. Eur Respir J. 2015;45(3):635–43.
34. Hargrove A, Penny D, Sawyer S. Sexual and reproductive health in young people with congenital heart disease: a systematic review of the literature. Pediatr Cardiol. 2005;26(6):805–11.
35. Cardenas DD, Topolski TD, White CJ, McLaughlin JF, Walker WO. Sexual functioning in adolescents and young adults with spina bifida. Arch Phys Med Rehabil. 2008;89(1):31–5.
36. Kakleas K, Kandyla B, Karayianni C, Karavanaki K. Psychosocial problems in adolescents with type 1 diabetes mellitus. Diabetes Metab. 2009;35(5):339–50.
37. Orlicka K, Barnes E, Culver EL. Prevention of infection caused by immunosuppressive drugs in gastroenterology. Ther Adv Chronic Dis. 2013;2040622313485275.
38. Henry-Reid LM, O'Connor KG, Klein JD, Cooper E, Flynn P, Futterman DC. Current pediatrician practices in identifying high-risk behaviors of adolescents. Pediatrics. 2010;125(4):e741–7.
39. Eneriz-Wiemer M, Sanders LM, Barr DA, Mendoza FS. Parental limited english proficiency and health outcomes for children with special health care needs: a systematic review. Acad Pediatr. 2014;14 (2):128–36.
40. Vart P, Gansevoort RT, Joosten MM, Bultmann U, Reijneveld SA. Socioeconomic disparities in chronic kidney disease: a systematic review and meta-analysis. Am J Prev Med. 2015;48(5):580–92.
41. Knapp C, Huang IC, Hinojosa M, Baker K, Sloyer P. Assessing the congruence of transition preparedness as reported by parents and their adolescents with special health care needs. Matern Child Health J. 2013;17(2):352–8.
42. Ng S, Dinesh S, Tay S, Lee E. Decreased access to health care and social isolation among young adults with cerebral palsy after leaving school. J Orthop Surg. 2003;11(1):80.
43. Bonnie RJ, Stroud C, Breiner H. Investing in the health and well-being of young adults. Washington DC: 2015 by The National Academy of Sciences; 2015.
44. Fegran L, Hall EO, Uhrenfeldt L, Aagaard H, Ludvigsen MS. Adolescents' and young adults' transition experiences when transferring from paediatric to adult care: a qualitative metasynthesis. Int J Nurs Stud. 2014;51(1):123–35.
45. Reiss JG, Gibson RW, Walker LR. Health care transition: youth, family, and provider perspectives. Pediatrics. 2005;115(1):112–20.
46. Sawin KJ, Rauen K, Bartelt T, Wilson A, O'Connor RC, Waring WP III, et al. Transitioning adolescents and young adults with spina bifida to adult healthcare: initial findings from a model program. Rehabil Nurs. 2015;40(1):3–11.
47. Goldenring JM, Rosen DS. Getting into adolescent heads: an essential update. Contemp Pediatr. 2004;21 (1):64–92.
48. Duggan M, Brenner J. The demographics of social media users, 2012: Pew Research Center's Internet & American Life Project Washington, DC; 2013.
49. Best P, Manktelow R, Taylor B. Online communication, social media and adolescent wellbeing: a systematic narrative review. Child Youth Serv Rev. 2014;41:27–36.
50. Greene JA, Choudhry NK, Kilabuk E, Shrank WH. Online social networking by patients with diabetes: a qualitative evaluation of communication with facebook. J Gen Intern Med. 2011;26(3):287–92.
51. Hayutin LG, Reed-Knight B, Blount RL, Lewis J, McCormick ML. Increasing parent-pediatrician communication about children's psychosocial problems. J Pediatr Psychol. 2009;34(10):1155–64.
52. Rosendal M, Vedsted P, Christensen KS, Moth G. Psychological and social problems in primary care patients—general practitioners' assessment and classification. Scand J Prim Health Care. 2013;31(1): 43–9.
53. Linton JC. Psychological assessment in primary care. In: Hass LJ, editor. Handbook of primary care psychology. New York: Oxford University Press; 2004. p. 35–45.
54. Moyer VA. Screening and behavioral counseling interventions in primary care to reduce alcohol misuse: US preventive services task force recommendation statement. Ann Intern Med. 2013;159(3):210–8.
55. Siu AL, Bibbins-Domingo K, Grossman DC, Baumann LC, Davidson KW, Ebell M, et al. Screening for depression in adults: us preventive services task force recommendation statement. JAMA. 2016;315 (4):380–7.
56. Saitz R, Palfai TP, Cheng DM, Alford DP, Bernstein JA, Lloyd-Travaglini CA, et al. Screening and brief intervention for drug use in primary care: the

aspire randomized clinical trial. JAMA. 2014;312 (5):502–13.
57. Moyer VA. Primary care behavioral interventions to reduce illicit drug and nonmedical pharmaceutical use in children and adolescents: US preventive services task force recommendation statementinterventions to reduce drug use in children and adolescents. Ann Intern Med. 2014;160(9):634–9.
58. Ewing JA. Detecting alcoholism: the cage questionnaire. JAMA. 1984;252(14):1905–7.
59. Saunders JB, Aasland OG, Babor TF, De la Fuente JR, Grant M. Development of the alcohol use disorders identification test (audit): who collaborative project on early detection of persons with harmful alcohol consumption-ii. Addiction. 1993;88 (6):791–804.
60. Gomez A, Conde A, Santana J, Jorrin A. Diagnostic usefulness of brief versions of alcohol use disorders identification test (audit) for detecting hazardous drinkers in primary care settings. J Stud Alcohol. 2005;66(2):305–8.
61. Bush K, Kivlahan DR, McDonell MB, Fihn SD, Bradley KA. The audit alcohol consumption questions (audit-c): an effective brief screening test for problem drinking. Ambulatory care quality improvement project (acquip). Alcohol use disorders identification test. Arch Intern Med. 1998;158(16):1789–95.
62. Yudko E, Lozhkina O, Fouts A. A comprehensive review of the psychometric properties of the drug abuse screening test. J Subst Abuse Treat. 2007;32 (2):189–98.
63. Bohn M, Babor T, Kranzler H. Validity of the drug abuse screening test (dast-10) in inpatient substance abusers. Probl Drug Depend. 1991;119:233–5.
64. Smith PC, Schmidt SM, Allensworth-Davies D, Saitz R. A single-question screening test for drug use in primary care. Arch Intern Med. 2010;170 (13):1155–60.
65. Ware JE Jr, Sherbourne CD. The mos 36-item short-form health survey (sf-36). I. Conceptual framework and item selection. Med Care. 1992;30(6):473–83.
66. Weissman MM, Bothwell S. Assessment of social adjustment by patient self-report. Arch Gen Psychiatry. 1976;33(9):1111.
67. Bosc M. Assessment of social functioning in depression. Compr Psychiatry. 2000;41(1):63–9.
68. Weissman MM, Olfson M, Gameroff MJ, Feder A, Fuentes M. A comparison of three scales for assessing social functioning in primary care. Am J Psychiatry. 2001;158(3):460–6.
69. Kroenke K, Spitzer RL, Williams JB. The phq-9. J Gen Intern Med. 2001;16(9):606–13.
70. Achenbach T, Rescorla LA. Manual for the aseba adult forms and profiles. Burlington: Research Center for Children and Families, University of Vermont; 2003.
71. Reynolds CR, Kamphaus RW. Basc-2 behavioral assessment system for children manual. Circle Pines: AGS Publishing; 2004.
72. Aman MG, Singh NN, Stewart AW, Field CJ. The aberrant behavior checklist: a behavior rating scale for the assessment of treatment effects. Am J Ment Defic. 1985;89(5):485–91.
73. Reiss S, Levitan GW, Szyszko J. Emotional disturbance and mental retardation: Diagnostic overshadowing. Am J Ment Defic. 1982;86(6):567–74.
74. Hayes SC, Nelson RO, Jarrett RB. The treatment utility of assessment: a functional approach to evaluating assessment quality. Am Psychol. 1987;42 (11):963.
75. Muench J, Jarvis K, Gray M, Hayes M, Vandersloot D, Hardman J, et al. Implementing a team-based sbirt model in primary care clinics. J Subst Use. 2015;20(2):106–12.
76. Kaner E, Beyer F, Dickinson H, Pienaar E, Campbell F, Schlesinger C, et al. Effectiveness of brief alcohol interventions in primary care populations. Cochrane Database Syst Rev. 2007;2.
77. Gryczynski J, Mitchell SG, Peterson TR, Gonzales A, Moseley A, Schwartz RP. The relationship between services delivered and substance use outcomes in new mexico's screening, brief intervention, referral and treatment (sbirt) initiative. Drug Alcohol Depend. 2011;118(2):152–7.
78. Ozechowski TJ, Becker SJ, Hogue A. Sbirt-a: adapting sbirt to maximize developmental fit for adolescents in primary care. J Subst Abuse Treat. 2016;62:28–37.
79. Miller WR, Rollnick S. Motivational interviewing: helping people change. New York: Guilford Press. 2012.
80. Lundahl B, Moleni T, Burke BL, Butters R, Tollefson D, Butler C, et al. Motivational interviewing in medical care settings: a systematic review and meta-analysis of randomized controlled trials. Patient Educ Couns. 2013;93(2):157–68.
81. Sansom-Daly UM, Peate M, Wakefield CE, Bryant RA, Cohn RJ. A systematic review of psychological interventions for adolescents and young adults living with chronic illness. Health Psychol. 2012;31(3):380–93.
82. Roberts CS, Piper L, Denny J, Cuddeback G. A support group intervention to facilitate young adults' adjustment to cancer. Health Soc Work. 1997;22 (2):133–41.
83. Scholten L, Willemen AM, Last BF, Maurice-Stam H, van Dijk EM, Ensink E, et al. Efficacy of psychosocial group intervention for children with chronic illness and their parents. Pediatrics. 2013;131 (4):e1196–203.
84. Stewart M, Letourneau N, Masuda JR, Anderson S, McGhan S. Impacts of online peer support for

children with asthma and allergies: "It just helps you every time you can't breathe well". J Pediatr Nurs. 2013;28(5):439–52.
85. Maurice-Stam H, Scholten L, de Gee EA, van der Zanden RA, Conijn B, Last BF, et al. Feasibility of an online cognitive behavioral-based group intervention for adolescents treated for cancer: a pilot study. J Psychosoc Oncol. 2014;32(3):310–21.
86. Suris J-C, Michaud P-A, Viner R. The adolescent with a chronic condition. Part I: developmental issues. Arch Dis Child. 2004;89(10):938–42.

Adherence and Self-Management 26

Gregory S. Sawicki

Overview

Advances in medical care have led to an increasing number of adolescents and young adults (AYA) surviving into adulthood with childhood onset chronic health conditions. Examples of such conditions include asthma, cystic fibrosis, diabetes, human immunodeficiency virus (HIV), inflammatory bowel disease, sickle cell disease, chronic renal disease, and cerebral palsy. As AYA with a range of diagnoses transition from pediatric to adult-focused healthcare systems, developing strategies to maintain health outcomes during this period is critical [1]. A key driver for maintaining optimal outcomes is adherence to recommended care therapies and condition-specific management plans. However, for AYA, particularly those with complex chronic health conditions, adherence to a daily regimen is a challenge. Therapeutic regimens are often complex, multifaceted, and time consuming to administer. Chronic health conditions often progress during adolescence and early adulthood, so the need to maintain prescribed regimens increases at a very time of life when youth are vulnerable from a physiologic perspective. Additionally, normal adolescent development, including a desire for independence from caregivers, can hinder appropriate adherence behaviors and disease self-management. Illness perceptions and beliefs are being established during this period, and struggles with parents and caregivers over roles and responsibilities can negatively influence adherence behaviors. Therefore, improving adherence is a key part of transitional care. This chapter reviews the clinical approach to adherence for AYA with chronic health conditions, including the recognition of distinct patterns of adherence behaviors, outlines barriers to optimal adherence, and suggests strategies to improve adherence in this high-risk population.

Defining Adherence Behaviors

Broadly defined, adherence to medical therapies is the extent to which an individual completes a mutually agreed upon treatment plan. "Adherence" and "disease self-management" are sometimes used as interchangeable terms to describe an individual patient's behavior related to maintaining a chronic therapeutic regimen [2]. Unlike the term "compliance," which indicates a unidirectional directive in which an individual receives a treatment plan or prescription from a healthcare provider, the term "adherence" encompasses a shared decision-making approach to therapies in which both the individual and their healthcare provider have provided input

G.S. Sawicki (✉)
Division of Respiratory Diseases, Boston Children's Hospital, Harvard Medical School, 300 Longwood Avenue, Boston, MA 02115, USA
e-mail: Gregory.sawicki@childrens.harvard.edu

M. Pilapil et al. (eds.), *Care of Adults with Chronic Childhood Conditions*,
DOI 10.1007/978-3-319-43827-6_26

into the therapeutic regimen. Therefore, labeling health behavior as "non-compliance" suggests that the individual is solely responsible for the failure to complete a therapeutic plan, whereas "non-adherence" implicates challenges for an individual, their support network, and their healthcare providers and system.

Although non-adherence is a common occurrence among AYA with chronic health conditions, an understanding of the type of non-adherence behaviors is important to develop appropriate individualized interventions. An individual may exhibit *unwitting* non-adherence in which they do not realize that they are failing at maintaining a prescribed treatment plan. An example of unwitting non-adherence is an adolescent with asthma who uses their controller medication once daily instead of twice daily as prescribed. They may not understand the prescription directions, or may have been misinformed, but they do not realize that they are not following a prescribed plan. A second type of non-adherence behavior is *erratic*, in which an individual has periods of good adherence interspersed with periods of non-adherence. Such an individual likely understands and agrees with therapy but has difficulty consistently maintaining their regimen. An example of erratic non-adherence is a young adult with cystic fibrosis who is able to complete all recommended therapies during the week, but on weekends often neglects his therapies as his schedule differs during those days. Similarly, a transplant patient may not consistently take oral anti-rejection medication on a daily schedule. Erratic non-adherence generally results from lack of structure, forgetfulness, or competing priorities, which may be variable. A third type of non-adherence is *intentional*, in which an individual understands their treatment plan but chooses not to follow it. For instance, an adolescent with diabetes may not use insulin during every meal or snack or a young adult with inflammatory bowel disease may avoid her anti-inflammatories on a regular basis. Such intentional non-adherence often results from anger at a health condition, health system, or caregivers, or may be due to underlying depression or other mental health comorbidities common with chronic illness. Similarly, such behaviors may be due to the avoidance of side effects or a desire to remain "normal" in the eyes of peers by not disclosing an illness. Finally, *rationalized* non-adherence, occurs when an individual deliberately alters or discontinues therapy, often without consulting with their healthcare team. This type of behavior may result if an individual does not believe that they need a particular therapy or they feel no immediate benefit from a therapy. For instance, an individual with epilepsy may perceive no immediate benefit symptomatically from a daily medication, or a person with asthma may not notice any difference after several weeks of not taking a daily inhaler. For AYA, such rationalized behavior is quite common, and may indicate a desire for risk taking, or, similar to intentional non-adherence, be a manifestation of anger, depression, or misinformation.

When approaching non-adherence, therefore, a clinician needs to evaluate the type of behavior that each individual is exhibiting and use that information and assessment to guide intervention plans.

Assessing Adherence: Measurement Tools

It is important for clinicians to obtain measurement data to help assess adherence among their patients. Biomarkers, such as serum drug levels, would appear to be the best measure of adherence, but are only routinely available for certain classes of medications. For most therapies, there is no "gold standard" for adherence measurement, and types of measures vary depending on therapies prescribed. It is clear, however, that self-report and caregiver report of adherence is inadequate. Multiple studies have shown that self-report is subjective and overestimates true adherence behaviors when compared to direct observation, monitoring, or other measurement methods [3]. This does not mean that clinicians should not ask subjectively about non-adherence during routine clinical care; rather, they should carefully phrase questions about adherence to allow an individual to report their challenges. Asking "do you take medication X?" sets up a response that will lead to overreporting, whereas framing a question "over the past week, how often did you miss taking medication X?" may elicit more accurate self-report.

Ideally, a clinician has access to additional objective measures of adherence. Various measurement tools exist, including data from prescription refills and electronic monitors [4]. Each of these tools has advantages and disadvantages as outlined in Table 26.1. Access to such measurements may be limited to research studies, but increasingly, electronic medical records have improved capabilities for such data to be captured in the context of routine chronic disease case management. With such data becoming more available, clinician training on how to communicate adherence data to individuals is also critical. Accurate, yet practical measures of adherence that provide real-time data are essential to provide patients, families, and their care team useful information to guide interventions if needed, and these measures need to be aligned with efficacious adherence interventions. Several monitoring devices are on the market or in development and are increasingly acceptable in our society as we become more "quantified," yet there is little evidence that this big data approach has improved health [5]. Online data platforms in which individuals with a chronic illness interact with the healthcare system present a viable opportunity for both adherence measurement and intervention designs. There is also an increasing desire for cell phone applications to be tailored to the chronic illness experience, include multiple functions, and facilitate coordination and communication, yet be low burden and customizable [6]. Currently, there is still a need for technology-based systems that integrate adherence and clinical data with decision support and also provide a platform for coordinating and executing effective adherence promotion interventions. Such technology also needs to be created in a practical and feasible manner to enable wider spread dissemination.

Barriers and Facilitators of Adherence

Adherence behaviors are affected by multiple factors stemming from (1) individuals, (2) fami-

Table 26.1 Measuring adherence

Measurement tool	Example	Advantages	Disadvantages
Prescription refill history	Medication possession ratio (MPR) Number of refills Proportion of days covered (PDC)	Identify what medications an individual has obtained as opposed to what is prescribed Allows for evaluation of adherence over a longer time period without need for individual input/recall	Only measures dispensing of medication Not always clear exactly what has been prescribed Does not account for "overfilling" of a prescription May not correlate with written treatment plans May not account for changing treatments over time
Electronic monitors	Metered-dose inhaler counters Continuous glucose monitors CPAP monitors	Continuous, long-term, real-time measures More objective than diaries or self-report Can identify a spectrum of issues Underdosing Delayed dosing Drug "holidays" "White-coat" adherence	Device malfunction/Technology failure Recording events that did not occur or failure to record events that did occur Cost Privacy concerns

CPAP continuous positive airway pressure

lies, (3) health systems, and (4) communities [2]. For many chronic health conditions, treatment complexity is an important barrier to adherence, and the degree of complexity may be associated with differing rates of adherence. In cystic fibrosis, for example, adherence rates vary between types of treatments, with higher rates of adherence with oral medications, lower rates with nebulized therapy, exercise and physiotherapy, and nutritional care [7]. Broadly, treatment complexity can lead to time tradeoffs based on other competing priorities, particularly those that allow a youth to engage in "normal" developmentally appropriate activities with their peers. Other key barriers include immediate time pressures, lack of time to complete therapies, uncertain schedules, and forgetfulness, either accidental or purposeful. Many youth may avoid therapies in favor of other activities and may skip therapies in order to be "normal." Finally, for many youth a barrier to adherence is a lack of perceived consequences, specifically not seeing an impact on one's health right away after skipping treatments or medications.

Conversely, key motivators for adherence behaviors for AYA include developing trusting relationships with clinicians, being treated as an adult, and early and repeated practice and skill building. Therefore, effective health care for AYA needs to address the developmental progression from adolescence to young adulthood. While in childhood, self-management of a chronic disease generally rests in the hands of the parents. At school age, optimally there should be an initiation of the transition to a shared model based on partial self-management, and in adolescence, there should be an increasing assertion of independence on the part of the teenager. The gradual immersion into independent self-management needs to be tracked by clinicians throughout adolescence, and parental support needs to be augmented. Encouragement of this progression into adulthood should be the cornerstone for programs to enhance adolescent disease knowledge, skills, and self-management. Additional facilitators such as improved communication and engagement of social support have been identified in multiple studies of adherence interventions [8].

Strategies to Improve Adherence

Interventions to improve adherence often are multicomponent, and may be costly, labor-intensive, and complex [9, 10]. However, there are relatively straightforward interventions that clinicians in practice can use to address non-adherence among individuals. One mnemonic that has been developed is "SIMPLE": Simplifying regimen characteristics; Imparting knowledge; Modifying patient beliefs; Patient communication; Leaving the bias; and Evaluating adherence [11]. Examples of behavioral intervention strategies aligned with these strategies are shown in Table 26.2 [11].

Adherence interventions can also be embedded into the Chronic Care Model (CCM), a framework with documented success for improving chronic illness care that can be used to incorporate the patient, caregiver, and healthcare system in designing interventions [12]. In this model, focusing on self-management support, delivery system design, decision support, and clinical information systems is proposed to facilitate the development of systems in which informed, activated patients work collaboratively with prepared, proactive care teams. In a review of the evidence for the CCM, 32 of 39 studies examined found that interventions based on the CCM components improved at least 1 process or outcome measure when utilized for patients with diabetes [13]. Application of the CCM has demonstrated improvements in adherence in individuals with either diabetes or asthma [14, 15].

A clinician needs to evaluate the multiple factors affecting adherence for an individual patient. In this way, addressing non-adherence is a part of routine personalized medical care. Identifying the type of non-adherence for an individual, including a recognition and understanding of individual barriers, can guide an appropriate intervention strategy. As an example,

Table 26.2 Strategies to improve adherence

"SIMPLE" strategies	Behavioral approaches
Simplifying the regimen	Creating reminders Promoting self-monitoring Tailoring the regimen Developing contingencies and rewards
Imparting knowledge	Improving health education Assessing health literacy
Modifying beliefs	Health and behavioral feedback/coaching Cognitive behavioral therapy Motivational Interviewing
Patient communication	Problem solving Family therapy Social support
Leaving the bias	Addressing mental health Assessing individual barriers Assessing type of adherence behavior
Evaluating adherence	Asking open-ended questions Electronic monitors Pharmacy refill data

Adapted from [11]

for those with unwitting non-adherence, efforts to improve knowledge of the condition and its treatments could be the cornerstone for adherence interventions. An adolescent that only uses their asthma controller medication when they are feeling unwell could be educated about the chronicity of airway inflammation even in the absence of symptoms. In this type of case, the lack of immediate perceived benefits to chronic therapies also needs to be discussed as part of an adherence intervention approach. Similarly, reminder systems may provide a structure for those with unwitting non-adherence. Automated reminders such as mobile text messages align with the self-management support component of the CCM, and have led to improvements in adherence behaviors in varied populations, including individuals with asthma, diabetes, and HIV [16–18]. Messaging interventions can be designed as one-way or two-way, enabling communication between an individual and the healthcare system. Small studies of adolescents with asthma showed high satisfaction with tailored, individual messaging reminders targeting self-management [19]. However, these interventions alone, particularly in a complex therapeutic regimen for a youth with a chronic health condition, likely would not lead to dramatic changes if not accompanied by a greater understanding of the global context of an individual's day-to-day needs. For those with rationalized non-adherence, particularly those who identify time as a key barrier, reminders likely would not help as much. Interventions to address time pressures and competing priorities would be an appropriate strategy. Interventions would require more than simply reducing the number of prescribed therapies or shortening the actual administration of medications. Discussions would need to identify the reason that time is an issue and likely address the overall place of therapies in the context of an individual's other daily routines. Examining family relationships, focusing on problem-solving skills, are robust targets for adherence interventions. Such interventions might best be implemented using techniques such as motivational interviewing [20].

Across all types of adherence interventions, developing a strong relationship with the clinical care team, particularly with respect to communication and respect, is a key driver of improved adherence. Recent opportunities for improving such interactions have entered the realm of health information technology. For example, a cell phone support program for teenagers and young adults with CF was designed to provide CF information and social support [21]. Such technologies are likely to enhance existing care models and allow for innovative adherence interventions outside routine clinical visits. However, such programs would still need to promote structured knowledge, support, and shared decision-making while enabling youth to develop effective communication with their treating clinicians.

Since poor communication with clinicians has been associated with lower levels of adherence [8], enhancing communication efforts may lead to adherence improvements. One way to support communication is providing feedback on adherence data to clinical care teams. Such feedback can enhance patient-provider communication, alert clinicians to lapses in adherence in periods between routine clinical visits, and therefore aligns with the decision support and clinical information system components of the CCM. Feedback of adherence data to patients combined with counseling to overcome adherence barriers is increasingly being evaluated in other chronic health conditions (e.g., asthma, transplant, heart failure, hypertension, sickle cell disease) and has been shown to be superior to usual care or counseling alone in improving medication adherence [22–26]. Offering objective feedback of behaviors can be eye-opening for patients and, if provided in a supportive, patient-centered conversation, can encourage patients to play a more informed and activated role in their care.

Conclusion

In summary, youth transitioning from pediatric to adult-focused care, particularly those with chronic health conditions, may struggle with adherence to recommended therapies and care plans. Clinicians need to be able to identify non-adherence and differentiate the type of non-adherence behaviors that an individual patient may exhibit. They should also work with patients to identify their unique barriers and possible strategies to improve adherence. Interventions to improve adherence need to be multifaceted, incorporating an understanding of barriers and behaviors. Technology, including monitoring and reminders, clearly has a role in adherence promotion, but needs to ultimately be coupled with personalized approaches tailored to the challenges facing each individual patient.

References

1. American Academy of Pediatrics, American Academy of Family Physicians, American College of Physicians, Transitions Clinical Report Authoring Group, Cooley WC, Sagerman PJ. Supporting the health care transition from adolescence to adulthood in the medical home. Pediatrics. 2011;128(1):182–200.
2. Modi AC, Pai AL, Hommel KA, Hood KK, Cortina S, Hilliard ME, Guilfoyle SM, Gray WN, Drotar D. Pediatric self-management: a framework for research, practice, and policy. Pediatrics. 2012;129(2):e473–85.
3. Stirratt MJ, Dunbar-Jacob J, Crane HM, Simoni JM, Czajkowski S, Hilliard ME, et al. Self-report measures of medication adherence behavior: recommendations on optimal use. Transl Behav Med. 2015;5(4):470–82.
4. Ingerski LM, Hente EA, Modi AC, Hommel KA. Electronic measurement of medication adherence in pediatric chronic illness: a review of measures. J Pediatr. 2011;159(4):528–34.
5. Almalki M, Gray K, Sanchez FM. The use of self-quantification systems for personal health information: big data management activities and prospects. Health Inf Sci Syst. 2015;3(Suppl 1):S1.
6. Hilliard ME, Hahn A, Ridge AK, Eakin MN, Riekert KA. User preferences and design recommendations for an mHealth app to promote cystic fibrosis self-management. JMIR Mhealth Uhealth. 2014;2(4):e44.
7. Zindani GN, Streetman DD, Streetman DS, Nasr SZ. Adherence to treatment in children and adolescent patients with cystic fibrosis. J Adolesc Health. 2006;38(1):13–7.
8. Ratanawongsa N, Karter AJ, Parker MM, Lyles CR, Heisler M, Moffet HH, et al. Communication and medication refill adherence: the Diabetes Study of Northern California. JAMA Intern Med. 2013;173(3):210–8.
9. Nieuwlaat R, Wilczynski N, Navarro T, Hobson N, Jeffery R, Keepanasseril A, et al. Interventions for enhancing medication adherence. Cochrane Database Syst Rev. 2014;20(11):CD000011.
10. Kahana S, Drotar D, Frazier T. Meta-analysis of psychological interventions to promote adherence to treatment in pediatric chronic health conditions. J Pediatr Psychol. 2008;33(6):590–611.

11. Atreja A, Bellam N, Levy SR. Strategies to enhance patient adherence: making it simple. MedGenMed. 2005;7(1):4.
12. Coleman K, Austin BT, Brach C, Wagner EH. Evidence on the chronic care model in the new millennium. Health Aff (Millwood). 2009;28(1):75–85.
13. Bodenheimer T, Wagner EH, Grumbach K. Improving primary care for patients with chronic illness: the chronic care model, part 2. JAMA. 2002;288 (15):1909–14.
14. Mackey K, Parchman ML, Leykum LK, Lanham HJ, Noel PH, Zeber JE. Impact of the Chronic Care Model on medication adherence when patients perceive cost as a barrier. Prim Care Diabetes. 2012;6 (2):137–42.
15. Moullec G, Gour-Provencal G, Bacon SL, Campbell TS, Lavoie KL. Efficacy of interventions to improve adherence to inhaled corticosteroids in adult asthmatics: impact of using components of the chronic care model. Respir Med. 2012;106(9):1211–25.
16. Hamine S, Gerth-Guyette E, Faulx D, Green BB, Ginsburg AS. Impact of mHealth chronic disease management on treatment adherence and patient outcomes: a systematic review. J Med Internet Res. 2015;17(2):e52.
17. Fischer HH, Moore SL, Ginosar D, Davidson AJ, Rice-Peterson CM, Durfee MJ, et al. Care by cell phone: text messaging for chronic disease management. Am J Manag Care. 2012;18(2):e42–7.
18. de Jongh T, Gurol-Urganci I, Vodopivec-Jamsek V, Car J, Atun R. Mobile phone messaging for facilitating self-management of long-term illnesses. Cochrane Database Syst Rev. 2012;12:CD007459.
19. Britto MT, Munafo JK, Schoettker PJ, Vockell AL, Wimberg JA, Yi MS. Pilot and feasibility test of adolescent-controlled text messaging reminders. Clin Pediatr (Phila). 2012;51(2):114–21.
20. Spoelstra SL, Schueller M, Hilton M, Ridenour K. Interventions combining motivational interviewing and cognitive behaviour to promote medication adherence: a literature review. J Clin Nurs. 2015;24 (9–10):1163–73.
21. Marciel KK, Saiman L, Quittell LM, Dawkins K, Quittner AL. Cell phone intervention to improve adherence: cystic fibrosis care team, patient, and parent perspectives. Pediatr Pulmonol. 2010;45 (2):157–64.
22. Creary SE, Gladwin MT, Byrne M, Hildesheim M, Krishnamurti L. A pilot study of electronic directly observed therapy to improve hydroxyurea adherence in pediatric patients with sickle-cell disease. Pediatr Blood Cancer. 2014;61(6):1068–73.
23. Foster JM, Usherwood T, Smith L, Sawyer SM, Xuan W, Rand CS, et al. Inhaler reminders improve adherence with controller treatment in primary care patients with asthma. J Allergy Clin Immunol. 2014;134(6):1260–8.
24. Wu JR, Corley DJ, Lennie TA, Moser DK. Effect of a medication-taking behavior feedback theory-based intervention on outcomes in patients with heart failure. J Card Fail. 2012;18(1):1–9.
25. Russell C, Conn V, Ashbaugh C, Madsen R, Wakefield M, Webb A, et al. Taking immunosuppressive medications effectively (TIMELink): a pilot randomized controlled trial in adult kidney transplant recipients. Clin Transplant. 2011;25(6):864–70.
26. Ruppar TM. Randomized pilot study of a behavioral feedback intervention to improve medication adherence in older adults with hypertension. J Cardiovasc Nurs. 2010;25(6):470–9.

Education

27

Kitty O'Hare and Alice A. Kuo

Introduction

Americans who obtain more education after high school have a higher likelihood of earning more, leading healthier lives, and living longer. In general, about 75 % of high school graduates go on to obtain some form of post-secondary education, and 66 % enroll in college. However, for graduates with a chronic childhood condition, the rates are lower. For example, for students on the autism spectrum, only 36 % attended any type of post-secondary education [1].

Post-secondary education can include 2-year college, 4-year college, or vocational, business, or technical school. For some, 2-year college is their sole post-secondary experience; for others, attending 2-year college first before transferring to a 4-year college to graduate offers the opportunity to save some money or obtain general education units in a less competitive environment.

Vocational education is education that prepares people to work in a trade, in a craft, as a technician, or in support roles in professions such as engineering, accountancy, nursing, medicine, architecture, or law. Craft vocations are usually based on manual or practical activities and are traditionally nonacademic but related to a specific trade or occupation, such as culinary arts, hospitality management, or fire science. Vocational education is sometimes referred to as career education or technical education.

More and more young adults with chronic childhood conditions (YACCC) and youth with intellectual disabilities/developmental disabilities (ID/DD) are pursuing post-secondary educational opportunities. As a result, internists as well as pediatricians are likely to encounter concerns about educational attainment. YACCCs have lower rates of educational attainment than do their peers without chronic medical conditions. Having a coexisting mental health condition, as well as a physical condition, has particular effects on educational success. YACCCs who do not graduate from high school are less likely to be employed and more likely to receive financial assistance.

Beginning with the Rehabilitation Act of 1973 [2], and then with the Individuals with Disabilities Education Act of 1975 [3] and the Americans with Disabilities Act of 1990, [4] educational opportunities for youth with chronic medical conditions and disabilities have expanded rapidly

K. O'Hare (✉)
Department of Medicine, Boston Children's Hospital, Boston, MA, USA
e-mail: frances.ohare@childrens.harvard.edu

A.A. Kuo
Departments of Medicine and Pediatrics, Health Care Transitions Research Network, University of California, Los Angeles, CA, USA
e-mail: AKuo@mednet.ucla.edu

K. O'Hare
Department of Medicine, Brigham and Women's Hospital, Boston, MA, USA

K. O'Hare
Harvard Medical School, Boston, MA, USA

M. Pilapil et al. (eds.), *Care of Adults with Chronic Childhood Conditions*,
DOI 10.1007/978-3-319-43827-6_27

Table 27.1 Definitions

Rehabilitation Act (Rehab Act)	Prohibits discrimination on the basis of disability in programs run by federal agencies; programs that receive federal financial assistance; in federal employment; and in the employment practices of federal contractors.
504 Plan	Ensures that students with a disability receive reasonable accommodations in their primary or secondary education. Used for students who need accommodations for equal access to their learning environment, but who do not require the specialized instruction stipulated by an individualized education plan (IEP).
Individuals with Disabilities Education Act (IDEA)	Stipulates that children and youth with disabilities must be provided with a free, appropriate public education in the least restrictive environment. The law allows for early intervention services for children ages 0–2 years, and special education services for children and youth ages 3–21 years.
Individualized Education Plan (IEP)	A plan or program that ensures that students with a disability receive specialized instruction in their primary or secondary education.
Transition Plan	Under the IDEA, students with an IEP must have a personalized transition plan by age 16 years. Must incorporate the student's strengths, preferences, and interests. Geared toward developing functional skills for work and for community life.
Americans with Disabilities Act (ADA)	Stipulates that public accommodations, including private schools, may not discriminate on the basis of disability. Certain physical modifications are necessary to make buildings and public spaces accessible. Services must also be provided to individuals with visual or hearing impairments.
Accommodations	Modifications that allow a student to learn and demonstrate learning without the interference of their disability.
Family Educational Rights and Privacy Act (FERPA)	Protects the privacy of student records. At the level of primary and secondary education, FERPA (rather than HIPAA) applies to immunization records, school nurse records, and special education records.
Higher Education Opportunity Act	Provides some federal financial aid for some students with ID/DD pursuing post-secondary education. Creates and expands college level programs for students with ID/DD.

HIPAA health insurance portability and accountability act, *ID/DD* intellectual disabilities/developmental disabilities

(Table 27.1). Now all primary and secondary students are entitled to supports that optimize their educational experiences when compared with their nondisabled peers. These supports can include testing accommodations, human aides, assignment accommodations, materials/technical adaptations, and physical adaptations.

Preparing for Post-Secondary Education

While college students are afforded some legal protections, they do not have the same entitlements as primary and secondary (K-12) students; special education plans do not extend beyond high school. The burden is on the student to identify themselves to the college as needing accommodation, and to work with the college to determine whether the college can provide reasonable accommodations. Added to the challenge is that, in most states, students ages 18 or older are legal adults; they must advocate for themselves without the direct intervention of parents or other family members. Nevertheless, colleges can provide a number of accommodations, from note-taking services to extended time for tests. Responsibility for providing accommodations may be divided among multiple college offices. Most colleges do not have a systematic way to identify YACCCs on their

Table 27.2 College resources for students with disabilities

Student health
This office varies in scope from school to school. Some larger institutions have a health service that is staffed 24/7 by physicians and nurses, with some primary and specialty care available. Other institutions may have a physician or nurse practitioner available for urgent care needs. Some student health services are staffed only by a nurse for limited hours. It is important for YACCCs to ask about the scope of the student health service prior to enrolling in college.
Disability services
This is the office that manages accommodations, ranging from physical access, to low vision and hard-of-hearing services, to learning disabilities. If a student will require accommodation for any reason then they must notify the disability services office at the time of enrollment.
Dean of students
This is the office that is often involved if a student withdraws due to medical concerns, either temporarily or permanently. YACCCs should inquire about school policies regarding withdrawals prior to enrollment.
Student life
This is the office that, in many schools, trains resident advisors and manages student housing. YACCCs may interact with this office if their condition is disclosed to their resident advisor or if their condition will impact their housing services.

campuses. Students typically must initiate the disclosure of a chronic condition and advocate for their needs. Although the federal government does not mandate accommodating students with disabilities on college campuses, most institutions of higher learning have Offices for Students with Disabilities (Table 27.2), which can coordinate services and provide accommodations such as longer time on tests or a quieter location in to take tests; note-taking services; transportation; audio-visual (AV) equipment for the visually or hearing impaired; or arrangements for testing accommodations for major standardized tests. These services are completely voluntary and require the student to self-identify and seek them out.

Chronic Disease Management in the College Setting

Healthcare Access

As YACCCs begin to consider different options for post-secondary education, a discussion with their healthcare provider could be useful. In particular, health insurance status is an important consideration. The Affordable Care Act (ACA) [5] allows for children to stay on their parents' health insurance until age 26-years, provided that parents have health insurance in the first place. However, for parents who are self-employed, uninsured, or have insurance in which the premiums to add dependents are too costly to afford, YACCCs may lose their health insurance upon reaching adulthood. If these YACCCs are considering post-secondary education, then a 4-year college may be the best option, given that most universities provide relatively affordable student health insurance. YACCCs opting to attend vocational school or 2-year college may end up uninsured, which for those with chronic medical conditions may be a challenging situation. YACCCs and their families should be counseled on the importance of maintaining health insurance through the college years. Students do need to compare what is offered through their college versus the benefits on their parents' insurance plan. If the student is attending an out-of-state school then they should be especially vigilant about what services are covered near their school.

The ACA expands Medicaid eligibility for individuals with disabilities in states that chose to implement the Medicaid expansion. Because some people may be reluctant to self-identify as having a disability, it is important for YACCCs seeking insurance coverage with Medicaid to understand that answering the disability screening questions can affect the contents of their benefits package. States must provide information to applicants and beneficiaries about the different Medicaid coverage groups and associated benefits packages so that people can make an informed decision about whether to seek coverage in a disability-related group with a benefits package that may better meet their needs. The online version of the single streamlined application contains two questions designed to identify people with disabilities: applicants are asked whether they have a physical disability or mental health condition that limits their ability to work, attend school, or take care of their daily needs; and whether they need help with activities of daily living (such as bathing, dressing, and using the bathroom) or live in a medical facility or nursing home. For YACCCs seeking Medicaid coverage with the intention of attending post-secondary education, accommodations for the health condition or disability should qualify them under the first question.

States generally must provide Medicaid to people who receive Supplemental Security Income (SSI) benefits [6]. To be eligible for SSI, beneficiaries must have low incomes, limited assets, and a significant disability that impairs their ability to work at a substantial gainful level. States also have the option to provide Medicaid to certain other related groups, including people with disabilities whose income exceeds the SSI limits but is still below the federal poverty level (FPL, $11,670 per year for an individual in 2014) [7]. In some situations, making parents aware of these benefits and guidelines can help them determine how to structure their family's financial assets so that the YACCC can qualify and obtain health insurance and financial assistance in the long term.

General Healthcare

During the college exploration and admission process, YACCCs can explore the health services available at the schools they are considering. Based on the availability of care at the school, YACCCs and their healthcare teams can negotiate how care will be provided during the college years. One area of anxiety for many YACCCs is how to reach their provider with questions or urgent care needs. Providers can share the options available through their practice, whether an online patient portal, email, text messaging, or even virtual consultations. Providers should discuss their expectations regarding visit frequency, particularly in regard to medication refills. Most YACCCs prefer to coordinate appointments during school vacations. Assessment of a YACCCs ability to describe their health conditions, name their allergies, name their medications, fill a prescription, and name the common side effects of their medication should be a routine part of office visits.

Every pediatric practice has its own transfer policy. Some practices continue to see their YACCCs until they graduate college; others encourage their patients to transfer to adult providers at age 18 years. It is important for practices to be transparent about their policies and to notify patients, in advance, when they will need to transfer care, especially if a care transfer is expected before or during the college experience. If the practice is not transparent, then parents or the YACCC should ask what the transfer policy is. The transfer policy should be posted where all patients can see it, including the office Website and waiting area. Frontline staff should be trained in the specifics of the policy. Pediatric providers should give specific recommendations for finding an adult healthcare team.

Mental Health

Mental health concerns are very common among college students, from attention deficit/hyperactivity disorder (ADHD) to depression and anxiety. Some students enter college with a preexisting mental health concern, while others will develop a mental health problem after starting post-secondary school. Just as with physical health services, mental health services vary from college to college. Students should be encouraged to explore the options for services at their school, particularly counseling/psychotherapy versus medication management. Prescribers of mental health related medications need to assess the student's understanding of its side effects and its potential impact on college habits, including alcohol use. Prescribers should be clear about their expectations regarding frequency of office visits and management of refills. Diversion of mental health medications is unfortunately common on college campuses; prescribers should be very clear about the consequences of improper medication use. In many cases, routine drug testing is carried out for young adults with ADHD on stimulant medications with each set of refills because of the high diversion potential of these medications.

Confidentiality

YACCCs may be nervous about sharing their health information. However, selective sharing is an important part of safety planning. Selective sharing of information is particularly valuable for YACCCs who are living on campus. While Student Health or Disability Services may be aware of students' medical needs, these offices generally are not available during off hours or weekends/holidays. YACCCs should be encouraged to disclose their condition to someone in proximity to their residential environment, such as the dorm resident advisor, or a roommate. In the classroom, some selective sharing is necessary to ensure that students get appropriate accommodations. For example, professors need to be aware of accommodations needed for visual impairment or hearing impairment. However, professors do not need to know extensive details of a student's health history. Students should know that the Family Educational Rights and Privacy Act (FERPA) [8] prevents colleges from disclosing educational records, including student health information, to third parties.

Routine office visits provide an opportunity for YACCCs to practice selective sharing. YACCCs should have the opportunity to spend a portion of each office visit alone with their provider, to develop some trust in sharing confidential information. YACCCs can sign a release for the practice to share health information with student health services, or vice versa. The provider and the youth can discuss which information is most important for the college to have.

Emergency Planning

Many YACCCs will experience a medical emergency while on campus. With advanced preparation, emergency management can proceed much more smoothly. Prior to coming to campus, YACCCs and their families should decide who the best emergency contact is. YACCCs should also identity a healthcare proxy (HCP) who is authorized to make health decisions if the student becomes incapacitated. No-cost state-specific HCP forms are available online. There is some provision in FERPA to allow notification of a student's family in case of emergency, even if the student has not identified a specific HCP.

A portable healthcare summary is a useful tool for communicating with hospitals and emergency responders. These allow first responders to triage appropriately and in a timely fashion based on the YACCCs situation. Examples of portable healthcare summaries are available online through the American Academy of Pediatrics and the Center for Health Care Transition Improvement (Got Transition; www.gottransition.org). If saved as a portable document file (PDF), then the summary can be easily available via a cell phone, tablet, or encrypted portable flash drive. Given the sensitive nature of the information, ensuring that a cell phone or tablet is properly encrypted could be an important consideration.

Medical alert bracelets or similar identifiers are helpful for first responders. YACCCs can find a variety of styles online. Healthcare providers can encourage YACCCs to introduce themselves to student health when they arrive on campus. Even if the student does not plan to utilize student health services on a regular basis, the student health service should still be aware of how to respond if the student experiences a medical emergency. In particular, student health should know how to contact the YACCCs primary care physician and specialists.

Wellness

Like all college students, YACCCs need to learn how to incorporate wellness into their daily routine. Regular exercise is important for all college students; healthcare providers can stress the benefits of exercise for specific chronic conditions. Guidance on nutrition is also essential, given the variety of options available on most college campuses. Adequate sleep is being appreciated more and more as an important component of overall wellness. YACCCs can be counseled on the effects of sleep deprivation on their specific condition. Finally, stress management is an essential component of wellness and most college campuses offer some stress management services through psychological counseling or the Office of Student Life.

Social Life

College is often a time of exploration and of testing limits. Most YACCCs report that their provider did not discuss the impact of cigarettes, alcohol, and drugs on their health. It is important for healthcare providers to demonstrate their openness to discussing challenging topics such as substance use. Healthcare providers can counsel YACCCs on how tobacco, alcohol, marijuana, and other drugs can impact their particular chronic condition. Medication interactions with substances are a common concern. Complete abstinence from tobacco products (including cigarettes, e-cigarettes, chewing tobacco, and hookah) is the best approach, though providers should also offer cessation materials when needed.

Many female YACCCs have not been counseled about the impact of pregnancy or of hormonal birth control on their health condition. Young women may be unaware of the impact that pregnancy can have on their health. Healthcare providers should demonstrate openness to questions about contraception and pregnancy. While many college campuses offer contraception, emergency contraception, and testing for sexually transmitted infections, these supports are not universal. YACCCs may need assistance in identifying sexual health services. Long-acting reversible contraception (LARC) is a reasonable choice for female YACCCs during their post-secondary education period.

Post-Secondary Education for People with Intellectual Disabilities/Developmental Disabilities

Students with ID/DD also benefit from post-secondary educational experiences. According to national surveys, youth with ID/DD value their college experiences as opportunities to interact with same-age peers, as well as to develop independent living skills. Youth with ID/DD who receive post-secondary educational services are more likely to sustain paid employment. This can lead to improved quality of life. Post-secondary education is a time for youth to explore their self-identity. Some students may have strong feelings about the labels applied to them as they enroll in services.

Whether or not young adults with ID/DD are able to attend some post-secondary education is often dependent on their adaptive skills (i.e., practical, everyday skills needed to function and meet the demands of one's environment, including the skills necessary to effectively and independently take care of oneself and to interact with other people). If young adults with ID/DD are planning to go away to college, a discussion about the ability to function independently could be valuable for the young adult and his/her parents. Often, it is not the academic work that proves to be challenging for the young adult with ID/DD but navigating adult social situations that can ultimately lead to the young adult leaving school and moving back home. Parents should be aware of this possibility and be prepared to consider post-secondary opportunities closer to home, with the ability for the young adult to be with trusted friends and family members more frequently.

A variety of post-secondary education options are available to youth with ID/DD. Vocational or working-training programs can offer young adults with ID/DD practical education while preparing them to enter the workforce in a supported environment. Often times, programs such as these offer a wide variety of job opportunities that can be tailored to the interests of the young adult. The young adult works part time and still receives some training or education for new jobs, with coaching or mentoring included. A recent movement has been to shift from a readiness model (train and place) to a support model (place and train) so that the YACCC with an ID/DD can have work that is customized and yet still meets the needs of an employer.

Conclusion

Post-secondary education should be encouraged in YACCCs with or without ID/DD. A primary care provider can counsel on appropriate placement and health insurance considerations ("Appendix"). In addition, emergency plans, healthcare proxies, and confidentiality are issues that should be discussed and planned appropriately with the help of a primary care provider.

Appendix

Resources

- Disability.gov: www.disability.gov.
- Champaloux SW, Young DR. Childhood chronic health conditions and educational attainment: a social ecological approach. J Adol Health. 2015;(56):98–105.
- Maslow GR, Haydon A, Ford CA, Halpern CT. Young adult outcomes of children growing up with chronic illness: an analysis of the National Longitudinal Study of Adolescent Health. Arch Pediatr Adolesc Med. 2011;(165):256–61.
- HEATH Resource Center at the National Youth Transitions Center, Graduate School of Education and Human Development, The George Washington University. http://heath.gwu.edu/transitioning-high-school-college-spotlight-section-504.
- Got Transition: www.gottransition.org.
- Lemly DC, Lawlor K, Scherer EA, Kelemen S, Weitzman ER. College health service capacity to support youth with chronic medical conditions. Pediatrics. 2014;134(5):885–91.
- Massachusetts Child Health Quality Coalition. Communication matters: a guide for sharing information about a child's care. 2014. http://www.masschildhealthquality.org/wp-content/uploads/2014/06/Communication_Matters1.pdf.
- Think College: www.thinkcollege.net.
- American Academy of Pediatrics Emergency Information Form. http://www2.aap.org/advocacy/blankform.pdf.

References

1. Roux AM, Shattuck PT, Rast JE, Rava JA, Anderson KA. National autism indicators report: transition into young adulthood. Philadelphia, PA: Life Course Outcomes Research Program, A.J. Drexel Autism Institute, Drexel University; 2015. http://drexel.edu/autisminstitute/research-projects/research/ResearchPrograminLifeCourseOutcomes/IndicatorsReport/. Accessed 25 Jan 2016.
2. Disability.gov. Rehabilitation Act of 1973. https://www.disability.gov/rehabilitation-act-1973/. Accessed 17 June 2016.
3. Disability.gov. Individuals with Disabilities Education Act (IDEA). https://www.disability.gov/individuals-disabilities-education-act-idea/. Accessed 17 June 2016.
4. Disability.gov. https://www.disability.gov/americans-disabilities-act/. Accessed 17 June 2016.
5. US Department of Health and Human Services. Affordable Care Act. http://www.hhs.gov/healthcare/about-the-law/read-the-law/. Accessed 17 June 2016.
6. Social Security Administration. Supplemental Security Income (SSI) Benefits. https://www.ssa.gov/disabilityssi/ssi.html. Accessed 17 June 2016.
7. US Department of Health and Human Services, Office of the Assistant Secretary for Planning and Evaluation (ASPE). 2014 Poverty Guidelines. December 1, 2014. https://aspe.hhs.gov/2014-poverty-guidelines. Accessed 17 June 2016.
8. US Department of Education. Family Educational Rights and Privacy Act (FERPA). http://www2.ed.gov/policy/gen/guid/fpco/ferpa/index.html. Accessed 17 June 2016.

Employment

28

Alice A. Kuo and Cory Ellen Nourie

Introduction

Employment for adults fulfills many needs. The first and foremost is a paycheck—an ability to have some financial independence, whether it be for pocket money or complete living expenses. However, having a job also anchors one's identity and can influence quality of life. Being successfully employed can give purpose and build self-esteem in one's life. More practically, paying into the US Social Security system for 40 quarters (10 years) makes an adult eligible to draw upon the Social Security system as a senior citizen and also be eligible for Medicare.

For young adults with chronic childhood conditions (YACCC) with intellectual disabilities/developmental disabilities (ID/DD), the road to employment can be arduous, depending on the level of cognitive impairment. Many young adult students with disabilities have the option to remain public school students until the year they turn 21. These extra years of schooling can focus on academic supports or vocational training. Every high school year, during their Individualized Education Plan (IEP) meeting, some level of transition planning should have occurred, focusing on what the student was going to do once he finished his school experience. Typically, options range from going on to college, into a job training program, to a vocational support environment, or to an adult day program focused on recreation.

For those young adults who are interested in obtaining employment, whether full or part time, it is essential that they connect with their local vocational rehabilitation (VR) program. VR services are offered to people who have "barriers to employment." Those barriers can be anything from a physical disability to an intellectual/developmental disability, visual impairment, or psychiatric condition. VR programs are funded by both federal and state governments and administered by states to help people with disabilities obtain gainful employment. VR programs have their origins in the rehabilitation for disabled World War I veterans. The Rehabilitation Act of 1973 (the "Rehab Act") is the legal basis for today's VR system and shifted the focus in vocational services for people with ID/DD through its emphasis on services and individualized plans for employment [1]. In addition, Employment First is a national movement that promotes integrated employment as the primary and preferred outcome for people with ID/DD and establishes that the default setting of services should be a presumption of ability [2].

A.A. Kuo (✉)
Departments of Medicine and Pediatrics, Health Care Transitions Research Network, University of California, Los Angeles, CA, USA
e-mail: AKuo@mednet.ucla.edu

C.E. Nourie
Division of Transition of Care, Nemours Alfred I. duPont Hospital for Children, 1600 Rockland Road, Wilmington, DE 19803, USA
e-mail: cory.nourie@nemours.org

M. Pilapil et al. (eds.), *Care of Adults with Chronic Childhood Conditions*,
DOI 10.1007/978-3-319-43827-6_28

VR services can provide a bridge as high school students prepare to leave school and enter the workforce; however, the involvement of VR during the special education transition process has been rare. Although VR primarily provides services for working age adults, due to recent shifts in federal funding toward transition-age services, VR should be increasingly involved with younger adults just entering the workforce for the first time.

Transition from Education to Employment

High school students with a disability can receive supports through special education, as mandated by the Individuals with Disabilities Education Act (IDEA) [3]. When a high school student is 16 or older, a transition plan should be developed that specifies the supports needed to get a job, continue postsecondary education and/or live independently. If the immediate goal after high school is to get a job, then special education services could include vocational education (including part-time employment during high school), career counseling, life skills, and transportation training.

The challenge for many young adults with a disability is that there is no entitlement for services in adulthood. After exiting the public K-12 school system, young adults and their families must apply for services from a myriad of adult-serving public systems. Young adults with a documented intellectual disability may have an easier time qualifying for these services; however, many young adults with a developmental disability without an intellectual disability (such as autism) may need significant support in order to function in the workplace.

Eligibility for Vocational Rehabilitation Services

All individuals with disabilities are eligible for VR services. Specifically, this includes a person:

1. who has a physical or mental impairment;
2. whose impairment substantially interferes with the ability to get a job;
3. whose impairment requires VR services to prepare for, secure, retain, or regain employment; and
4. who intends to achieve an employment outcome.

The federal Rehabilitation Act specifies that VR should operate with the presumption that the person can achieve an employment outcome through VR services [1]. If it is decided that a person cannot benefit from VR services, there must be clear and convincing evidence as to why. Additionally, a person who is eligible for Social Security Income (SSI) benefits is also automatically presumed eligible for VR services [4].

In regard to VR services for transition-age youth, the Rehabilitation Services Administration clarified that since all individuals with disabilities are eligible for VR services, "...all students with disabilities, including those with significant and the most significant disabilities, are presumed to be eligible for VR services, unless the VR agency concludes, based on clear and convincing evidence, that the individual cannot benefit from the VR program through the achievement of an employment outcome (i.e., integrated employment) because he or she is too severely disabled" [5].

Vocational Rehabilitation Services

VR services can assist clients with resume writing, interview skills, job trials, volunteer opportunities, job coaching, and job placement. They can also pay for job-required training, including certifications or college degrees. In some cases, if someone has a physical disability that requires an accessible vehicle to get to and from work, VR services may pay for modifications to a vehicle, already owned by the client, to make it accessible. A more complete list of VR service categories is provided in Table 28.1 [6].

VR services also have Benefits Counselors who can guide young adults through the confusing maze of eligibility for government benefits, such as Supplemental Security Income

Table 28.1 Vocational rehabilitation service categories and definitions

Assessment

Assessment means services and activities used to determine an individual's eligibility for VR services, to prioritize level of employment needs, and/or to determine the nature and scope of VR services to be included in the IPE. Assessment services might include:

- Trial work experiences and extended evaluation
- Psychological assessments
- Dental and medical exams
- Assessments of personality, interests, interpersonal skills, intelligence and related functional capacities, educational achievements, work experience, vocational aptitudes, personal and social adjustments, and employment opportunities of the individual

VR Counseling and Guidance

VR counseling and guidance provides information and support services to assist people in making informed choices about employment.

Job Placement Services

Job placement assistance is a referral to a specific job resulting in an interview, whether or not the individual obtained the job.

Job Search Assistance

Job search activities support and assist an individual in searching for an appropriate job. Job search assistance may include help in resume preparation, identifying appropriate job opportunities, developing interview skills, and contacting businesses.

Information and Referral

Information and referrals to other agencies are provided for services that are not available through the VR program.

On-the-Job Supports (Supported Employment)

On-going support services and other appropriate services needed to support and maintain an individual with a most significant disability in supported employment for a period of time generally not to exceed 18 months. Such services, such as job coaching, are for individuals who have supported employment and long-term supports identified on their IPE. For example, an employee may need support in understanding job tasks or workplace rules, or learning how to navigate to/from work or within the workplace.

Job Readiness Training

Training provided to prepare an individual for the world of work (e.g., appropriate work behaviors, getting to work on time, appropriate dress and grooming, increasing productivity).

Diagnosis and Treatment of Impairments

VR services will pay for diagnosis and treatment of the listed physical and mental impairments, *if and only if* other sources of funding (i.e., grant funding) cannot be secured, and if the physical or mental impairment negatively affects ability to work. Services include, but are not limited to:

- Diagnosis and treatment for mental and emotional disorders by licensed providers
- Nursing services
- Prescription of eyeglasses and visual services
- Physical, occupational, and speech or hearing therapy
- Mental health services
- Other medical or medically related rehabilitation services

On-the-Job Supports, Short Term

Services provided to support a person in maintaining their job once he or she is employed. Such services include short-term job coaching for persons who do not have a supported employment goal in their IPE.

Reprinted with permission from Roux AM, Rast JE, Anderson KA, Shattuck PT. National Autism Indicators Report: Vocational Rehabilitation. Philadelphia, PA: Life Course Outcomes Research Program, A.J. Drexel Autism Institute, Drexel University; 2016

VR vocational rehabilitation, *IPE* individual plan for employment

(SSI) and Medicaid, while earning a paycheck. These professionals can explain about programs that will allow them to save their income while not losing their benefits (called a Plan to Achieving Self-Support or PASS) [7].

Another service VR can help with is for legal rights of employees with disabilities. Many adults are unsure of their legal rights under the Americans with Disabilities Act (ADA) [8]. Prospective employers are not allowed to ask an applicant if she has any disabilities or medical conditions. They are allowed to ask, "With proper accommodations, are you able to fulfill the duties of this job?" VR can direct applicants how to answer interview questions and protect themselves from discrimination.

Vocational Rehabilitation Service Use and Outcomes

Few studies have been published in the traditional research literature about use of VR services and outcomes. However, the 2016 National Autism Indicators Report produced by researchers at Drexel University focused on VR and examined service use and outcomes using administrative data from the Rehabilitation Services Administration for federal fiscal year 2014 [6]. Their key findings included the following:

- Overall, 80 % of those who got a job were employed part time with median weekly earnings of $160. Earnings were slightly higher for those who were employed without supports and lower for those in supported employment.
- The most common job type was office and administrative support. About 1 in 4 people worked in an office job.
- The employment rates following VR services were comparable for those with autism (60 %), intellectual disability (55 %), and other disabilities (56 %). A lower percentage with autism had supported employment compared to those with ID.
- The rate of working part time was the same for those with autism and those with ID: nearly 90 %.
- Those with autism were more likely to work in office jobs compared to their peers who received VR services. Working in food service or cleaning jobs was less likely compared to those with ID.

Individuals who receive job placement services with VR are more likely to exit VR with employment [9–13]. Job placement services are the most predictive of a positive employment outcome in VR.

Job Training or Placement

Besides VR, individual agencies may provide job training or job placement services. Companies like Goodwill Industries and Salvation Army are some of the larger, more established organizations in the country, but each state has many options. Young adults can find a list of providers through their state agency on disability, either for intellectual/developmental disabilities or the department of aging and physical disabilities.

Two models of job training/placement are worth mentioning, especially as programs are moving toward a Support Model (place then train) as opposed to a Readiness Model (train then place).

Project SEARCH

Project SEARCH was developed at Cincinnati Children's Hospital [14] and has been disseminated internationally with strong program fidelity to replicate impressive outcomes. More information about Project SEARCH and its model is available at: www.projectsearch.us.

TEACCH Autism Program

A second model of supported employment was developed in 1972 at the University of North Carolina, called the TEACCH Autism Program [15]. In an effort to provide each individual with ASD the greatest chance of obtaining and maintaining successful, competitive employment, the

TEACCH® Supported Employment Program has developed 4 models of support: One-to-One Placement, Mobile Crew, Group Shared Support Site, and Standard Placement. More information about the TEACCH model is available at: www.teacch.com/clinical-services/supported-employment-1

Family Medical Leave

As adults with chronic disease or disabilities enter the workforce, it is important for them to know about and understand the Family Medical Leave Act (FMLA) [16]. FMLA is federal protection against termination from employment for missing work due to a disclosed medical condition. Once an adult has accepted employment, it is suggested he talk with his Human Resources department about completing FMLA paperwork. This entails his physician attesting to the diagnosis and giving an estimate of the amount of time the employee may need to miss work over the course of the year. FMLA protection is effective for up to 12 weeks per year. There are some exclusion to FMLA protections, particularly around the length of employment and the size of the business. It is advised to learn more about FMLA at the Department of Labor Website at http://www.dol.gov/whd/fmla/fmla-faqs.htm.

References

1. Disability.gov. Rehabilitation Act of 1973. https://www.disability.gov/rehabilitation-act-1973/. Accessed 17 June 2016.
2. US Department of Labor Office of Disability Employment Policy. Employment First. https://www.dol.gov/odep/topics/employmentfirst.htm. Accessed 17 June 2016.
3. Disability.gov. Individuals with Disabilities Education Act (IDEA). https://www.disability.gov/individuals-disabilities-education-act-idea/. Accessed 17 June 2016.
4. Assessment for Determining Eligibility and Priority for Services [Internet]. United States Code of Federal Regulations, Title 34 Ch. III § 361.42 Jul 1, 2006. http://edocket.access.gpo.gov/cfr_2006/julqtr/pdf/34cfr361.42.pdf.
5. Transition Planning and Services Provided through the State Vocational Rehabilitation Services Program. Washington, DC: U.S. Department of Education Office of Special Education and Rehabilitative Services, Rehabilitation Services Administration; 2014 May p. 4. (Technical Assistance Circular). Report No.: RSA-TAC-14-03. https://www2.ed.gov/policy/speced/guid/rsa/tac/2014/tac-14-03.pdf. Accessed 25 Jan 2016.
6. Roux AM, Rast JE, Anderson KA, Shattuck PT. National Autism Indicators Report: Vocational Rehabilitation. Philadelphia, PA: Life Course Outcomes Research Program, A.J. Drexel Autism Institute, Drexel University; 2016. http://drexel.edu/~/media/Files/autismoutcomes/publications/2016%20National%20Autism%20Indicators%20Report%20-%20Vocational%20Rehabilitation%20Autism.ashx. Accessed 25 Jan 2016.
7. Social Security Administration. Plan to Achieve Self-Support (PASS). https://www.ssa.gov/disabilityresearch/wi/pass.htm Accessed June 17, 2016.
8. Disability.gov. https://www.disability.gov/americans-disabilities-act/. Accessed 17 June 2016.
9. Chen JL, Sung C, Pi S. Vocational rehabilitation service patterns and outcomes for individuals with autism of different ages. J Autism Dev Disord. 2015;45(9):3015–29.
10. Schaller J, Yang NK. Competitive employment for people with autism correlates of successful closure in competitive and Supported Employment. Rehabil Couns Bull. 2005;49(1):4–16.
11. Lawer L, Brusilovskiy E, Salzer MS, Mandell DS. Use of vocational rehabilitative services among adults with autism. J Autism Dev Disord. 2009;39(3):487–94.
12. Butterworth J, Migliore A, Timmons J. Services and outcomes for transition age young adults with autism spectrum disorders: secondary analysis of the NLTS2 and RSA 911. November 2010. Boston, MA: Institute for Community Inclusion, University of Massachusetts Boston. http://media.mchtraining.net/research/documents/finalreports/butterworth_r40_mc_16396_final_report_updated.pdf. Accessed 25 Jan 2016.
13. Alsaman MA, Lee C-L. Employment outcomes of youth with disabilities in vocational rehabilitation. A multilevel analysis of RSA-911 Data. Rehabil Couns Bull. 2016. doi:10.1177/0034355216632363 Epub ahead of print. Accessed 12 August 2016.

14. Cincinnati Children's Hospital Medical Center. Project SEARCH. Educating people with disabilities. http://www.projectsearch.us/OurPROGRAM/ProgramModel.aspx. Accessed 17 June 2016.
15. University of North Carolina. TEACCH Autism Program. TEACCH® Supported Employment Program. http://teacch.com/clinical-services/supported-employment-1/introduction-to-models-of-support. Accessed 17 June 2016.
16. US Department of Labor. Wage and Hour Division. Family and Medical Leave Act. https://www.dol.gov/whd/fmla/ Accessed 17 June 2016.

Independent Living

29

David E. DeLaet and Cory Ellen Nourie

Introduction

This chapter will focus on challenges faced by young adults from vulnerable populations as they attempt to transition to an independent living environment as well as existing programs and legislation that can help young adults address these obstacles. Vulnerable populations to be considered include young adults with chronic childhood conditions (YACCC), those with learning and developmental disabilities, individuals with mental health conditions, and those emerging from the foster care system.

Vulnerable Populations and Scope of the Problem

As has been highlighted throughout this text, advances in medicine over the last several decades have resulted in a significant increase in the population of YACCC. For example, whereas the median age of survival among individuals with sickle cell disease was estimated to be 14.3 years in 1973 [1], more recent data indicates that the average life expectancy of those diagnosed with sickle cell anemia was 42 years for males and 48 years for females [2]. Likewise, the median predicted age of survival for patients with cystic fibrosis has risen from approximately 25 years of age in 1985 to 37.4 years in 2007 [3]. Similar trends of improved survival have been seen for pediatric and adolescent patients diagnosed with malignancies and congenital heart disease [4, 5]. This diverse and growing population of YACCC represents a group of patients for whom the transition period from adolescence to young adulthood can be particularly difficult.

Another population for whom this transition can be challenging is those patients with intellectual disability, developmental delay, or mental health illness. Recent estimates suggest that the prevalence of intellectual disability in the non-institutionalized population of the United States is about 7.8 people per thousand and of developmental disabilities to be about 11.3 people per thousand; it would be expected that as many as 1 million individuals with intellectual and developmental disabilities would likely transition into adulthood over a period of 5 years [6]. Additionally, the estimated prevalence of serious mental illness among noninstitutionalized adults age 18–26 years is 4.8% [7].

Lastly, those young adults transitioning from foster care are also susceptible to the obstacles

D.E. DeLaet (✉)
Departments of Medicine and Pediatrics, Icahn School of Medicine at Mount Sinai, New York, NY 10029, USA
e-mail: David.delaet@mountsinai.org; david.delaet@mssm.edu

C.E. Nourie
Division of Transition of Care, Nemours Alfred I. duPont Hospital for Children, 1600 Rockland Road, Wilmington, DE 19803, USA
e-mail: cory.nourie@nemours.org

M. Pilapil et al. (eds.), *Care of Adults with Chronic Childhood Conditions*,
DOI 10.1007/978-3-319-43827-6_29

inherent to this period of transition. According to the most recently available data from the Adoption and Foster Care Analysis and Reporting System (AFCARS), there were an estimated 415,129 children in foster care on September 30, 2014. Of those, 103,916 were between the ages of 14 and 18 years and an additional 5631 ages 19 and 20 years [8]. Though a few states define the legal age of majority as 19 or even 21 years of age, most states recognize 18 years as the age of majority. It is this legal definition by states that largely dictates when a young adult will age out of the foster care system. During fiscal year (FY) 2014, an estimated 22,392 young adults in the United States were so emancipated [8].

Transition to Independent Living Among Young Adults

Multiple studies have demonstrated that the transition to independent living can be difficult for many young adults. The 1999 National Survey of Families and Households, a survey of a representative sample of 13,009 adults, revealed that the proportion of young adults who leave home only to subsequently return increased dramatically over the last century such that nearly 50 % do so for at least some period of time [9]. Other studies have demonstrated that many young adults continue to receive financial support from their parents as they transition to independence [10]. Further, young adults also continue to rely on their parents for emotional support and guidance, with degree of dependence perhaps influenced by race and ethnicity. A 2001 survey of 300 subjects 18–22 years of age suggested that African American and Hispanic young adults were more reliant on caregivers for direction and nurturing than white counterparts [11]. While this period of transition appears to be difficult for many young adults, it would be anticipated to be even more challenging for the susceptible populations previously described.

Independent Living Issues for Young Adults with Chronic Medical and Mental Health Conditions and Disabilities

Adolescents and young adults with chronic medical conditions and disabilities, intellectual disabilities, developmental disabilities, and mental health disease are likely to face many obstacles as they attempt to transition to independent living. Similar to their peers in the general population, adolescents and young adults with disabilities rely on their parents for financial support during this period of transition. In fact, many of these young adults are more likely than their peers to remain in the family home as they complete secondary education or vocational training [12]. However, families with children with disabilities are significantly more likely to suffer financial hardship [13], and this may limit available resources for continued support. Such financial hardship is further aggravated by limited employment opportunities for these young adults: 35% of people with disabilities as compared to 78% of those who do not have disabilities are working [14]. The majority of these unemployed disabled individuals would like to be working [14, 15]. The independence of many disabled adults is also limited by inadequate transportation [14]. These obstacles may lead to increased emotional stressors on these individuals. As compared with their peers in the general population, individuals with disabilities are twice as likely to be worried about not being able to care for themselves or being a burden to their families [14].

The successful transition to a minimally restrictive living environment may be particularly problematic for those individuals with intellectual disabilities and mental health diseases. The Community Mental Health Centers Act of 1963 initiated the era of community mental health and deinstitutionalization practices in the United States [16]. Over the subsequent decades, the result was a dramatic decrease in the number of individuals with mental illness who were institutionalized in state mental hospitals [17]. Legislative efforts have been made to assure adequate housing opportunities for the mentally disabled such as the Fair Housing Act of 1968, which prohibits discrimination in the sale, rental, and financing of dwellings, and in other housing-related transactions, based on race, color, national origin, religion, sex, familial status, and disability [18]. Despite such legislation, access to adequate community alternatives to hospitalization has not kept pace with such deinstitutionalization [19]. For example, options for out-of-home placement, such as small group homes, for disabled individuals are limited [12]. As a likely consequence of these policy changes, recent estimates have suggested that while 11 % of adults with intellectual or developmental disabilities live in publicly funded residential homes and an additional 28 % in their own household, 61 % of these disabled adults live at home with their parents [20].

As another example of inadequate access to mental health resources, which negatively impacts transitioning youth, research has demonstrated that the majority of youth who receive publicly funded mental health services do not continue to receive such services as young adults [21, 22]. This lack of service support is underscored by the high rate of unemployment, poverty, substance abuse, criminal activity, and homelessness these young adults with mental health conditions exhibit [22, 23].

Given these difficulties with transition, it is important for young adults from susceptible populations and their families to be aware of available resources that might assure a better transition experience. From the standpoint of financial assistance, patients and their families should inquire about eligibility for Supplemental Security Income (SSI) and Social Security Disability Insurance (SSDI) through the United States Social Security Administration [24]. Though many patients may have already been receiving benefits through SSI prior to the age of 18 years, eligibility standards for adults are not identical to those for individuals less than 18 years of age; as such, patients may no longer qualify for assistance [24]. For planning purposes, it is therefore critical to clarify eligibility well in advance of reaching the age of majority. Additionally, some states provide additional cash subsidies to children and adults with intellectual and developmental disabilities living in the family home, though this support varies greatly from state to state [25].

For the large majority of unemployed individuals with disabilities who want to work, it is important that they be familiar with programs and legislation that support this goal. Historically, SSI has had employment and income restrictions, which served as disincentives to becoming self-supportive through work [26]. The Center for Medicare & Medicaid Services "Ticket to Work and Work Incentives Improvement Act of 1999" was enacted to allow patients to work while continuing to receive SSI and the associated Medicaid benefits [27]. Despite such initiatives, a large percentage of individuals receiving SSI remain unemployed [6]. It is essential then that these individuals understand their protected rights for employment under the 1990 Americans with Disabilities Act (ADA), which states that "no covered entity shall discriminate against a qualified individual on the basis of disability in regard to job application procedures, the hiring, advancement, or discharge of employees, employee compensation, job training, and other terms, conditions, and privileges of employment" [28]. It would also be beneficial that these young adults are aware of the federally supported state vocational rehabilitation programs that can assist youth with disabilities in vocational education and supported employment services and that such education begin before 18 years of age [29]. Benefits counselors at these vocational rehabilitation programs can additionally help guide young adults regarding their eligibility for the aforementioned SSI and SSDI benefits and the related "Ticket to Work" program as well as assist with issues pertaining to legal rights of employees with disabilities.

Patients with physical or developmental disabilities should be familiar with provisions of the

ADA in terms of being able to secure independent housing. The law allows individuals, at their own cost, "to make reasonable structural modifications to units and public/common areas in a dwelling when those modifications may be necessary for a person with a disability to have full enjoyment of a dwelling" [30]. They should also explore with a social worker or other support providers in the local community the availability of family support services such as respite services for families, home health attendant or homemaker services, assistive technology and environmental modification, adaptive medical equipment, transportation services, as well as respite services and counseling services for caretakers [25].

Additionally, young adults with physical, mental, or developmental disabilities might benefit from involvement with one or more of several available community resources in addressing concerns about independence. Examples of such community resources include, but are not limited to, the vocational rehabilitation programs previously discussed as well as Centers for Independent Living, Aging and Disability Resource Centers, Assistive Technology Resource Centers, and state agencies for individuals with intellectual or developmental disabilities.

Centers for Independent Living are consumer-controlled, community-based, cross-disability, nonresidential, private, nonprofit agencies that are designed and operated within local communities by individuals with disabilities and that provide an array of independent living services, including the core services of information and referral, independent living skills training, peer support, and individual and systems advocacy [31]. Similarly, patients with mental health disorders should be, where available, referred to community-based transition programs. There are several examples of the success of such programs, which provide patients with such services as individualized counseling, vocational training, and educational support [32, 33].

Young adults with chronic physical conditions or disabilities should register with their state's office of aging and/or physical disabilities (the name of the agency will vary from state to state). Every state has an Aging and Disability Resource Center run by this agency. By connecting with an Aging and Disability Resource Center, clients can talk with an Options Counselor to discuss their specific needs for supports to live independently. Depending on funding, waivers and insurance, some people are eligible for home healthcare attendants, nurses, aides, or funding to pay a private caregiver of her choice [34].

Living on one's own may be full of challenges for the adult with physical or intellectual disabilities. Oftentimes the young adult and his or her family may worry about physical accessibility, safety, and the ability to handle functional needs. Every state has Assistive Technology Resource Centers, where residents can meet with an assistive technology (AT) specialist to discuss needs and then be given a device to take home for a free trial, typically for 2 weeks. Once an individual knows if a device meets his or her needs, the AT specialist can recommend places to purchase the item. The assistive technology options can range from simple items, such as a doorknob lever, to more complex items, such as a communication device. Access to such devices often affords an individual with a disability greater ability to live in a more independent, less restrictive environment.

Those young adults with intellectual or developmental disabilities should register with their state agency for individuals with intellectual or developmental disabilities (the name of the agency will vary from state to state), found through their Department of Health and Human Services. Types of residential supports vary amongst states, but the state agency provides funds to the individual service providers. Adults can live in a variety of settings, from totally independent with no care giving needs to a community group home with staff members who assist with activities of daily living to an institutional facility or nursing home with around-the-clock care. As there are substantial waitlists/registries for access to residential programs in every state, adults with disabilities and their caregivers should register as soon as possible.

Independent Living Issues for Young Adults Emerging from the Foster Care System

Young adults who are "aging out" of the foster care system may find this period of transition particularly daunting. As compared to peers among the general population, youths in the foster care system tend to have a higher incidence of physical, developmental, and mental health illness and disabilities as well as higher rates of alcohol and drug abuse [35–38]. Further, given the instability of their social and family relationships, youth emerging from foster care are less likely to have available to them a sustained support network [39, 40]. As previously described, minorities may be even more susceptible to the absence of ongoing family support systems as they transition to adulthood, and minorities tend to be relatively overrepresented among youths in the foster care system, with the 2014 AFCARS data revealing that 42 % were non-Hispanic whites as compared to 24 % African American and 22 % Hispanic [8].

Existing data confirm that young adults who have recently emancipated from the foster care system are a vulnerable population with poor social status. A recent survey of 100 young adults who had been out of the foster care system for at least 6 months yielded many concerning findings. Of those surveyed, 26 % reported not having steady employment since leaving care, and 41 % indicated that they did not have enough money to cover living expenses; 24 % had dealt drugs and 11 % had exchanged sex for money. Additionally, 41 % admitted to having legal issues and 7 % reported having been incarcerated, while 2 % admitted to being homeless at some point since emancipation [40].

There are many barriers to a successful transition for young adults leaving foster care. Importantly, many young adults leaving foster care cite that, while they had received independent living services training, very few actually receive concrete assistance for independence. For example, it has been demonstrated that less than 70 % of individuals identified having a place to live and 50 % noted having less than $250 at time of discharge from foster care [40]. This situation might be aggravated by the fact that very few emancipating young adults had regular, if any, contact with their case worker in their final year in the system [40]. Additionally, as discussed previously, the failure of many of these young adults to establish reliable family and social relationships contributes to difficulty with the transition period. Difficulty placing older children in permanent homes from the foster care system contributes to this problem. During FY2014, the mean age of adoption was 6.2 years of age, with only 7.2 % of the 50,643 adopted age 14 years or older [8]. Many surveyed foster system case workers, in fact, have the perception that older youth are unlikely to be placed [41].

In an effort to diminish these problems in transition, federal legislation has been enacted over the years to fund independent living programs. The first such piece of legislation was the 1986 Independent Living Initiative, which amended the Title IV-E Social Security Act in order to establish the distribution of federal funding to states for independent living programs. The focus of these programs was on education and employment assistance, training in daily living skills, individual and group counseling, integration and coordination of services, and a transitional independent living plan for each participant [42]. Given the continued hardships of many emancipated young adults, the Foster Care Independence Act of 1999 was passed and so created the John Chafee Foster Care Independence Program, which not only doubled federal funding for state independent living programs but, in part, also allowed for funds to be used for housing and allowed for vouchers for postsecondary education and training [43]. In some states, such as California and Illinois, there has been an increased emphasis by the courts that foster care agencies and minors preparing for emancipation demonstrate that they have met specific requirements and developed plans for independent living that would increase the success of transitioning out of the foster care system [44]. As an important part of this process, as early as age 14 and continuing through the age of 21 years, foster youth should establish regular contact with the Independent Living Coordinator for their state.

There are data to support the effectiveness of such legislation. One survey of 100 subjects revealed that young adults who had received more independent living training and services prior to discharge were less likely to report legal trouble, felt better prepared to live on their own, and were more satisfied with their current living arrangements [40]. An additional survey of 479 young adults formerly in the foster care system demonstrated that those who had received better independent living preparation had a decreased risk for drug dependency [45].

While such programs have improved outcomes, there has been more recent emphasis on the continued importance of improving social support for these young adults, suggesting the ideal scenario would be concurrent efforts to establish stable relationships with at least one adult while providing independent living services and training [44]. An obvious opportunity for providing such a relationship would be through legal adoption. Though this has long been considered an unlikely option for older youths, recent data have suggested more significant success in finding permanent families for these adolescents, often through existing relationships [46]. In cases where this is not possible, emphasizing the benefit of having a non-kin mentor is critical. One recent survey of 339 foster youths approaching 18 years of age revealed that 62% revealed the presence of a non-kin mentor relationship, many of which were established through formal care systems, including adults that work in child welfare, education, and mental health systems. Of note, minorities were less likely than whites to identify the presence of a mentor [47], making this perhaps an even greater challenge among these subpopulations. There are examples of successful programs in several cities and states that have focused on the development of such relationships, with an important component being the involvement of the youth in the process of identifying such mentors [44].

Conclusion

Young adults with chronic childhood conditions, learning and developmental disabilities, mental health conditions, and those emerging from the foster care system comprise a diverse population that faces numerous barriers to a successful transition to independent living. However, there are a large number of existing programs, legislation, and community resources that can aid these vulnerable young adults in overcoming these barriers ("Appendix"). Adult medical providers should be familiar with these resources to assure that their young adult patients achieve their maximum level of independent functioning and are able to live in as minimally restrictive of a living environment as possible.

Appendix

Resources

- Titles I and V of the Americans with Disabilities (ADA) Act of 1990: https://www.eeoc.gov/laws/statutes/ada.cfm
- Independent Living Research Utilization Directory of Centers for Independent Living: http://www.ilru.org/projects/cil-net/cil-center-and-association-directory
- Find a Local Aging and Disability Resource Center: https://www.adrc-tae.acl.gov/tiki-index.php?page=ADRCLocator
- John H. Chafee Foster Care Independence Program: http://www.acf.hhs.gov/programs/cb/resource/chafee-foster-care-program

References

1. Diggs LM. Anatomic lesions in sickle cell disease. In: Abramson H, Bertles JF, Wethers DL, editors. Sickle cell disease: diagnosis, management, education, and research. St. Louis, LA: C.V. Mosby; 1973.
2. Platt OS, Brambilla DJ, Rosse WF, Milner PF, Castro O, Steinberg MH, et al. Mortality in sickle cell disease—life expectancy and risk factors for early death. NEJM. 1994;330(23):1639–44.

3. Cystic Fibrosis Foundation Patient Registry. 2015 annual data report. Bethesda, MA. © 2008 Cystic Fibrosis Foundation. https://www.cff.org/About-Us/Assets/2015-Annual-Report.pdf Accessed 26 May 2016.
4. Horner MJ, Ries LAG, Krapcho M, Neyman N, Aminou R, Howlader N, et al editors. SEER cancer statistics review, 1975–2006. Bethesda, MD: National Cancer Institute; 2008. http://seer.cancer.gov/csr/1975_2006. Accessed 26 May 2016.
5. Moller JH, Taubert KA, Allen HD, Clark EB, Lauer RM, a Special Writing Group from the Task Force on Children and Youth, American Heart Association. Cardiovascular health and disease in children: current status. Circulation. 1994;89(2):923–30.
6. Larson SA, Lakin KC, Anderson L, Kwak L, Nohoon L, Jeoung H, Anderson D. Prevalence of mental retardation and developmental disabilities: estimates from the 1994/1995 National Health Interview Survey Disability Supplements. Am J Ment Retard. 2001;106(3):231–52.
7. National Institute of Mental Health. Serious mental illness (SMI) among U.S. adults. Washington, DC: United States Department of Health and Human Services, National Institute of Mental Health; 2014. http://www.nimh.nih.gov/health/statistics/prevalence/serious-mental-illness-smi-among-us-adults.shtml. Accessed 26 May 2016.
8. U.S. Department of Health and Human Services. The AFCARS report: preliminary FY 20014 estimates as of July 2015. Washington, DC: DHHS; 2015. http://www.acf.hhs.gov/sites/default/files/cb/afcarsreport22.pdf. Accessed 26 May 2016.
9. Goldscheider F, Goldscheider C, St. Clair P, Hodges J. Changes in returning home in the United States, 1925–1985. Soc Forces. 1999;78(2):695–728.
10. Schoeni R, Ross K. Material assistance received from families during the transition to adulthood. In: Setterson Jr R, Furstenberg Jr F, Rumbaut R, editors. On the frontier of adulthood: theory, research, and public policy. Chicago, IL: University of Chicago Press; 2004.
11. Gnaulati E, Heine BJ. Separation-individuation in late adolescence: an investigation of gender and ethnic differences. J Psychol. 2001;135(1):59–70.
12. Hallum A. Disability and the transition to adulthood: Issues for the disabled child, the family, and the pediatrician. Curr Prob Pediatr. 1995;25(1):12–50.
13. Parish SL, Rose RA, Grinstein-Weiss M, Richman EL, Andrews ME. Material hardship in U.S. families raising children with disabilities. Except Child. 2008;75(1):71–92.
14. National Organization on Disability. Harris Survey of Americans with disabilities. Washington, DC: National Organization on Disability; 2004. http://205.186.160.39/research_publications/surveys_research//survey_americans_disabilities_2004. Accessed 26 May 2016.
15. Blomquist KB. Health, education, work, and independence of young adults with disabilities. Orthop Nurs. 2006;25(3):168–86.
16. Rochefort DA. Origins of the "Third Psychiatric Revolution": the community mental health centers act of 1963. J Health Polit Policy Law. 1984;9(1):1–30.
17. Lamb HR, Bachrach LL. Some perspectives on deinstitutionalization. Psychiat Serv. 2001;52(8):1039–45.
18. U.S. Department of Housing and Urban Development. Fair housing laws and presidential executive orders: fair housing act. Washington, DC: U.S. Department of Housing and Urban Development. http://www.fhasecure.gov. Accessed 26 May 2016.
19. The past and future of mental health services: an interview with Leona Bachrach. Psychiat Serv. 2000; 51(12):1511–1512.
20. Fujiura GT. Demography of family households. Am J Ment Retard. 1998;103(3):225–35.
21. Davis M, Sondheimer DL. State child mental health efforts to support youth in transition to adulthood. J Behav Health Serv Res. 2005;32(1):27–42.
22. Davis M, Vander Stoep A. The transition to adulthood for youth who have serious emotional disturbance: developmental transition and young adult outcomes. J Ment Health Adm. 1997;24(4):400–27.
23. Vander Stoep A, Beresford S, Weiss NS, McKnight B, Cauce AM, Cohen P. Community-based study of the transition to adulthood for adolescents with psychiatric disorder. Am J Epidemiol. 2000;152(4):352–62.
24. U.S. Social Security Administration. Red book: overview of our disability programs. Washington, DC: U.S. Social Security Administration; 2016. http://www.ssa.gov/redbook/eng/overview-disability.htm. Accessed 26 May 2016.
25. Rizzolo MC, Hemp R, Braddock D, Schindler A. Family support services for persons with intellectual and developmental disabilities: recent national trends. Intellect Dev Disabil. 2009;47(2):152–5.
26. Parsons DO. The decline in male labor force participation. J Pol Econ. 1980;88(1):117–34.
27. U.S. Department of Health and Human Services. HHS historical highlights. Washington, DC: U.S. DHHS. http://www.hhs.gov/about/historical-highlights/index.html. Accessed 26 May 2016.
28. U.S. Equal Employment Opportunity Commission. Titles I and V of the Americans with Disabilities Act of 1990 (ADA). Washington, DC: The U.S. Equal Employment Opportunity Commission. https://www.eeoc.gov/laws/statutes/ada.cfm. Accessed 26 May 2016.
29. American Academy of Pediatrics. Committee on children with disabilities and committee on adolescence. Transition of care provided for adolescents

with special health care needs. Pediatrics. 1996;98 (6):1203–6.
30. U.S. Department of Justice and the U.S. Department of Housing and Urban Development. Joint Statement on the Department of Housing and Urban Development and the Department of Justice: Reasonable Accommodations Under the Fair Housing Act. Washington, DC: The U.S. Department of Justice and the U.S. Department of Housing and Urban Development. 2004. http://www.hud.gov/offices/fheo/library/huddojstatement.pdf. Accessed 26 May 2016.
31. National Council on Independent Living. About independent living. Washington, DC: National Council on Independent Living; 2016. http://www.ncil.org/about/aboutil. Accessed 26 May 2016.
32. Bullis M, Moran T, Benz MR, Todis B, Johnson MD. Description and Evaluation of the Aries Project: achieving rehabilitation, individualized education, and employment success for adolescents with emotional disturbance. Career Dev Except Individ. 2002;25(1):41–58.
33. Baker AJL, Olsen D, Mincer C. The WAY to Work: an independent living/aftercare program for high risk youth. Washington, DC: Child Welfare of American League Press; 2000.
34. U.S. Department of Health and Human Services, Administration for Community Living. No wrong door system. Washington, DC: US DHHS, Administration for Community Living; 2013. https://www.adrc-tae.acl.gov/tiki-index.php?page=ADRCLocator. Accessed 26 May 2016.
35. Schor EL. The foster care system and health status of foster children. Pediatrics. 1982;69(5):521–8.
36. Chernoff R, Coombs-Orme T, Risley-Curtiss C, Heisler A. Assessing the health status of children entering foster care. Pediatrics. 1994;93(4):594–601.
37. Pilowsky D. Psychopathology among children placed in family foster care. Psychiatr Serv. 1995;46(9):906–10.
38. Pilowsky DJ, Wu L-T. Psychiatric symptoms and substance use disorders in a nationally representative sample of American adolescents involved with foster care. J Adolesc Health. 2006;38(4):351–8.
39. Courtney ME, Piliavin I, Grogan-Kaylor A. Foster youth transition to adulthood: a longitudinal view of youth leaving care. Child Welf. 2001;80(6):685.
40. Reilly T. Transition from care: status and outcomes of youth who age out of foster care. Child Welf. 2003;82 (6):727–46.
41. Avery RJ. Perceptions and practice: agency efforts for the hardest-to-place children. Child Youth Serv Rev. 2000;22(6):399–420.
42. Collins ME. Transition to adulthood for vulnerable youths. Soc Serv Rev. 2001;75(2):271–91.
43. Fernandes AL. CRS report for congress. Child Welfare: the Chafee Foster care Independence Program (CFCIP). Washington, DC: Congressional Research Service, Library of Congress. Order Code RS22501; 2006. http://www.nilausa.org/membersonly/Chafee%20Report%20RS22501.pdf. Accessed 26 May 2016.
44. Bussiere A. Adoption and foster care: permanence for older foster youth. Fam Court Rev. 2006;44(2):231–43.
45. White CR, O'Brien K, White J, Pecora PJ, Phillips CM. Alcohol and drug use among alumni of foster care: decreasing dependency through improvement of foster care experiences. J Beh Health Serv Res. 2007;35(4):419–34.
46. Avery RJ. An examination of theory and promising practice for achieving permanency for teens before they age out of foster care. Child Youth Serv Rev. 2009;32(3):399–408.
47. Munson MR, McMillen JC. Nonkin natural mentors in the lives of older youths in foster care. J Beh Health Serv Res. 2008;35(4):454–68.

30 Decision-Making and Guardianship

Jennifer H. Chuang and Jane Subak Kennedy

The Healthcare Provider's Role in Assessing Medical Decision-Making

Healthcare providers at times find themselves needing to assess whether the patient has the capacity to make medical decisions. The terms competency and capacity are often used interchangeably, though competency refers to a legal decision whereas capacity refers to a clinical assessment. The person consenting to medical care must be competent to do so. In this regard, the competent person should be able to: (1) understand the potential benefits, risks, and alternatives involved in a specific treatment or procedure; (2) make the healthcare decision on his/her own behalf; and (3) communicate that healthcare decision to any other person. A person may be competent to make some healthcare decisions but not others. Given that capacity refers to a clinical assessment, it may be transient due to conditions related to altered level of consciousness, hypoglycemia, hyperglycemia, medication toxicity, or mental health concerns.

In some instances the parent and provider may determine early on that some patients with long-term cognitive disabilities will not have the capacity to make medical decisions. At other times the assessment as to whether the patient has the capacity to make informed consent may be more urgent, such as during an acute psychiatric crisis or if the patient is experiencing dementia or delirium. Capacity is also a fluid process and an assessment made the previous day may not apply to the present day.

The provider should consider the following four legally relevant areas in the assessment: (1) the ability to communicate a choice; (2) the ability to understand relevant information about their condition and treatment; (3) the ability to appreciate how that information applies to their own situation and the consequences of treatment options (including no treatment); and (4) the ability to reason with that information [1–3].

Although the healthcare provider may be in the position to determine medical decision-making capacity, there are currently no formal guidelines from professional societies to assess a patient's capacity. Resources and tools are available to assist providers to assess their patients' capacity [1–3]. Examples of the following questions may be used:

1. To assess the ability to communicate a choice:
   - We have discussed a lot of information about your condition. Have you decided

J.H. Chuang (✉)
Craig-Dalsimer Division of Adolescent Medicine, Children's Hospital of Philadelphia, 3401 Civic Center Boulevard, Philadelphia, PA 19104, USA
e-mail: chuangj@email.chop.edu

J.S. Kennedy
Department of Social Work and Family Services, Children's Hospital of Philadelphia, 3401 Civic Center Boulevard, Philadelphia, PA 19104, USA
e-mail: kennedyj@email.chop.edu

M. Pilapil et al. (eds.), *Care of Adults with Chronic Childhood Conditions*,
DOI 10.1007/978-3-319-43827-6_30

which medical option is best for you right now?

2. To assess the ability to understand relevant information about their condition and treatment:
   - What is your understanding of your condition? What are the options for your condition? What are the risks and benefits of the treatment options? What are the risks and benefits if nothing is done?
3. To assess the ability to appreciate how that information applies to their own situation and the consequences of treatment options:
   - Why do you think your doctor has recommended this specific test or treatment for you? Do you think that treatment is the best treatment for you? Why or Why not? What do you think will happen if you accept this treatment? What do you think will happen if you do not accept this treatment?
4. To assess the ability to reason with the information regarding the patient's condition, situation, and treatment options:
   - What factors are most important to you in deciding about your options? How are you balancing the pluses and minuses of the treatments? What do you think will happen to you now? How did you decide to accept or reject the recommended treatment? What makes one option better than another option?

The practitioner should keep in mind that decision-making capacity is not equivalent to agreeing with the practitioner's recommendation. The patient may make a decision that will result in greater harm or potentially death, but the patient may still have capacity to make the decision if the above four criteria were met.

In the event that the healthcare provider determines that the patient lacks the capacity for medical decision-making, then a substitute decision-maker will be necessary. If a surrogate has not been appointed in an advanced directive, living will, healthcare proxy, or durable power of attorney, then the usual recourse is to contact family members. There is variation between states in terms of the priority order in which the family members are approached. In emergency cases in which no surrogate is available, physicians can provide treatment under the premise that a reasonable person would have consented to the given care.

In the case of an acute psychiatric emergency, the patient may not have the capacity to refuse the recommended treatment. If the patient is 18-years or older, then one may petition for emergency psychiatric hospitalization for the patient. After the initial emergency psychiatric hold, a judge may determine whether the patient meets civil commitment to be held in a hospital beyond the emergency period. Some states allow a commitment for assisted outpatient treatment. The details of involuntary commitment for psychiatric emergencies vary from state to state [4, 5].

Decisions regarding guardianship and medical decision-making capacity can be lengthy and emotional. The healthcare provider is in a key role to facilitate discussions with the patient and family regarding these decisions in a proactive and thoughtful manner well before the patient turns 18-years-old. Allowing the patient and family the time and space to process these important decisions in advance may ease concerns that may arise in the event of an emergency.

Shared Decision-Making

To every extent possible, the adult-aged patient, including those with disabilities, is entitled to exercise their legal capacity on an equal basis with others in all areas of life. Article 12 of the United Nations Convention on the Rights of Persons of Disabilities provides that persons with disabilities have equal rights as others and that parties should take appropriate measures to provide that person with the support they need to exercise their legal capacity [6]. Rather than obtaining guardianship or conservatorship (described later), a shared decision-making role between the adult-aged patient and persons that they choose allow the patient to make their own choices about their life. Supported decision-making allows the adult-aged patient with disabilities to retain their decision-making capacity by choosing supporters to help them make choices. Examples of important choices that may be included in supported decision-making include how to manage money, make healthcare decisions, decide where to live and with whom, and activities to partake in during the day.

Laws regarding supported or shared decision-making vary state by state [7, 8]. Recently, Supported Decision-Making has been formally recognized in the state of Texas under the "Supported Decision-Making Agreement Act" passed in 2015 [7]. It allows a "process of supporting and accommodating an adult with a disability to enable the adult to make life decisions, including decisions related to where the adult wants to live, the services, supports, and medical care the adult wants to receive, whom the adult wants to live with, and where the adult wants to work, without impeding the self-determination of the adult" [7]. Further information about supported decision-making for patients and families can be found at the American Civil Liberties Union (ACLU) Disability Rights Program (www.aclu.org/disability) [9], the National Resource Center for Supported Decision-Making (supporteddecisionmaking.org) [10], or Quality Trust for Individuals with Disabilities (dcqualitytrust.org) [11].

Guardianship/Conservatorship

Conservatorship Versus Adult Guardianship

In some states, conservatorships are called adult guardianships, but the terms mean roughly the same thing. For the rest of this article, we will use the term "guardianship" to refer to adult guardianships and conservatorships.

If a court appoints someone to take care of financial matters, that person is usually called a "conservator of the estate," while a person in charge of medical and personal decisions is a "conservator of the person." An incapacitated person may need just one type of representative, or both. The same person can be appointed to take both the roles. Both types of conservators are supervised by and held accountable to a court.

When the individual turns 18, the parent or previous legal guardian will no longer be the guardian without a court-approved process. Many young adults with medical conditions, including mental health illnesses, are able to assume legal responsibility regarding their healthcare and financial decision-making. If there is concern that the patient is incapable of handling medical and financial manners, then the parent or previous legal guardian may wish to consider petitioning for guardianship.

Guardianship is a legal process whereby the court appoints a guardian to make legal decisions about the individual's person and property, including medical decision-making [12]. It is utilized in situations where the individual is unable to make decisions about person, property, or is susceptible to fraud or undue influence. The guardian who is appointed should take into account the wishes and desires of the individual regarding decisions about medical treatment, living arrangements, finances, and end-of-life care. Other areas that guardianship may affect include the ability to possess a driver's license, own or possess a firearm, marry, vote, file lawsuits, and property management (including buying and selling). The guardian may be a parent, other family member, a friend, or a court-appointed public or private entity.

The process of applying for guardianship varies from state to state (Table 30.1). The procedure includes a court petition filed by the potential guardian. The petition usually includes a description of the physical and mental condition of the patient as well as any functional limitations. The healthcare provider may be asked to provide an evaluation of the patient's capabilities and limitations [12, 13]. An annual court review and assessment will monitor the need to continue the guardianship, as the

Table 30.1 Steps on establishing guardianship (details vary state by state)

Establishing adult guardianship
1. The guardian applicant determines that the adult-aged patient may not have the capacity to fully make his or her own decisions
2. The guardian applicant should fill out a court petition or application for legal guardianship of the adult-aged patient
3. The adult-aged patient should have a medical and psychological evaluation to determine his or her capabilities and limitations
4. The guardian applicant is required to give notice of the application to the adult-aged patient and attend a hearing before a judge
5. Consultation with a lawyer by the guardian applicant may be helpful to coordinate the guardianship process

individual's rights may be reinstated if the patient's capacity is restored.

Circumstances may arise where the consent is needed from the guardian, and assent is needed from the patient to participate in the activity. These situations may include research studies, medication administration, or surgical procedures. Consent may only be given by the individuals who are legally authorized to give consent for the patient, whether that be the adult-aged patient with decision-making capacity, the emancipated minor, or the legal guardian. Assent is the agreement of the patient if they are not able to legally consent to participate in the activity. Information should be given to the patient in an easily understood manner by the participant so they can assent in an affirmative manner.

Variations or Alternatives to Guardianship

There do exist variations or alternatives to guardianship which vary state to state. The least intrusive measures on the patient's autonomy should be sought when considering guardianship (see earlier section on Shared Decision-Making). Options include the following:

- A guardian of the estate—a person who is responsible for the individual's finances.
- Limited guardianship—limits decision-making to certain discrete areas, such as medical decision-making.
- Temporary guardianship—limits decision-making to a guardian for a defined period of time.
- Joint bank accounts—a joint account may allow the guardian to monitor spending activity on the account, or the guardian and adult-aged patient may choose to have a joint account where both signatures are needed for transaction activity.
- Living Will—a document that states a patient's wishes for end-of-life medical care in the circumstance that they become unable to communicate their decisions.
- Representative payee—a person who manages funds received by government agencies, such as Social Security.
- Durable powers of attorney for property and for healthcare—grants a person legal authority to make decisions on another's behalf in the event that the patient is unable to do so. When appointing a Durable Power of Attorney, that person may carry out the patient's wishes of whether to remain on machines to keep the patient alive, whether to be hooked up to feeding tubes that provide nutrition and hydration, how the patient's body should be disposed of in the event of the patient's death, and whether the patient's organs should be used for donation.
- Advanced Directives and Healthcare Proxies—allows the patient to designate ahead of time a healthcare agent who is allowed to make healthcare decisions if the patient is unable to make them. The patient must be competent to make healthcare decisions at the time of appointment.
- Appointment of a Community Advocate—allows an agent to advocate on the

individual's behalf with administrative and government agencies.

- A Trust—to place funds and other assets in the control of a trustee. Access to these funds by the patient would need to be coordinated with the trustee.

Planning for Guardianship of the Child in the Event of a Parent's Death

Planning for care of a disabled or well child should begin well before the age of 18 (Appendix). In the event of a parent or guardian's death, it can be a lengthy process through the courts to determine who would have clear legal authority of the child. The parent or guardian should consider the long-term care of their child in their estate planning. Without legal documentation, the child may be placed with Child Protective Services or the court may appoint a family member as a guardian, though that may or may not have been the intent of the deceased parent or guardian. Legal processes may also become lengthy and emotional for families if the deceased parent or guardian's expressed wishes were not clearly documented in writing. In addition to appointing legal authority to a guardian, estate planning should include distribution of financial assets—even if the sum is modest—in order to avoid lengthy proceedings for banks to release funds. The parent may wish to consider putting the potential inheritance in a trust until the child reaches an age or maturity that is deemed appropriate.

Appendix

Resources

- American Civil Liberties Union: ACLU Supported Decision-Making Resource Library. www.aclu.org/supported-decision-making-resource-library.
- The Arc: for people with intellectual and developmental disabilities. www.thearc.org.
- Department of Developmental Services: offices available in each state
- National Center for Medical-Legal Partnership. medical-legalpartnership.org.
- National Guardianship Association. www.guardianship.org.
- "What happens when my child turns 18?" published by Boston Children's Hospital.

References

1. Tunzi M. Can the patient decide? Evaluating patient capacity in practice. Am Fam Physician. 2001;64:299–306.
2. Grisso T, Appelbaum PS. Assessing competence to consent to treatment: a guide for physicians and other health professionals. New York: Oxford University Press; 1998.
3. Appelbaum PS. Assessment of patients' competence to consent to treatment. N Engl J Med. 2007;357:1834–40.
4. American Bar Association. Guardianship Law and Practice. http://www.americanbar.org/groups/law_aging/resources/guardianship_law_practice.html. Accessed 1 Dec 2015.
5. National Alliance on Mental Illness. https://www.nami.org/. Accessed 1 Dec 2015.
6. United Nations Convention on the Rights of Persons with Disabilities. http://www.un.org/disabilities/convention/conventionfull.shtml. Accessed 17 June 2016.
7. Texas Council for Developmental Disabilities. Supported Decision-Making Agreement Act. http://www.tcdd.texas.gov/resources/guardianship-alternatives/supported-decision-making/. Accessed 17 June 2016.
8. "Guardianship in Pennsylvania" Prepared by Disability Rights Network of Pennsylvania. www.drnpa.org. Accessed 4 Dec 2015.
9. American Civil Liberties Union (ACLU) Disability Rights Program. www.aclu.org/disability. Accessed 17 June 2016.
10. National Resource Center for Supported Decision-Making. supporteddecisionmaking.org. Accessed 17 June 2016.
11. Quality Trust for Individuals with Disabilities. dcqualitytrust.org. Accessed 17 June 2016.
12. National Guardianship Association. http://www.guardianship.org/. Accessed 17 June 2016.
13. National Disability Rights Network. http://www.ndrn.org/. Accessed 4 Dec 2015.

31 Access to Health Insurance

Beth Sufian, James Passamano and Amy Sopchak

Introduction

Adults with chronic illness must have some form of insurance coverage to help pay for medical care and the medications needed to treat their disease. Often when young adults transition to adult care there is a change in their ability to access insurance coverage, which affects their ability to access medical care and treatment. Transitioning adults may find they have less options when it comes to accessing health insurance than in childhood.

This chapter will provide an overview of the laws and programs that may provide health insurance options for young adults with chronic illness who are transitioning to adult care.

Disclaimer The information in this chapter is general in nature and is not meant to be legal advice regarding a specific situation. Nothing in this chapter should be considered as legal advice regarding a specific individual's situation. There is no guarantee that the information in this chapter has not changed between the time it was drafted and the time the chapter was published. Please consult with an attorney for specific advice regarding your situation.

B. Sufian (✉) · J. Passamano · A. Sopchak
Sufian & Passamano, LLC, 712 Main Street, Suite 2130, Houston, TX 77002, USA
e-mail: bsufian@sufianpassamano.com; cflegal@sufianpassamano.com

J. Passamano
e-mail: jpassamano@sufianpassamano.com

A. Sopchak
e-mail: asopchak@sufianpassamano.com

M. Pilapil et al. (eds.), *Care of Adults with Chronic Childhood Conditions*,
DOI 10.1007/978-3-319-43827-6_31

Some options include eligibility for Social Security benefits that will result in Medicaid or Medicare eligibility, coverage offered by certain state government programs, group health insurance policies offered by an employer or a health insurance plan that can be purchased on the Healthcare Exchange operated by the federal government or a state run Healthcare Exchange. In addition, this chapter will explain situations that will allow health insurance coverage to be extended to a disabled dependent child.

Social Security Benefits

Overview

The Social Security Administration (SSA) administers two programs that also provide health insurance coverage to an individual who is eligible for the Social Security program. It is easy to confuse the two programs but important to understand the differences.

Social Security Disability Insurance (SSDI) is a program that provides a monthly benefit and Medicare coverage. Medicare coverage begins after receipt of the actual SSDI benefit for 24 months. A person must meet work and medical requirements in order to receive SSDI benefits. A person who has never worked will not be eligible for SSDI benefits.

Supplemental Security Income (SSI) is a program that provides a monthly benefit and Medicaid coverage. Eligibility for Medicaid coverage begins after SSI benefit approval in 39 states. In 11 states, Medicaid eligibility begins after a separate application for Medicaid is approved. A person must meet certain low income and medical requirements in order to receive SSI benefits.

Social Security Administration Medical Criteria

A diagnosis of a chronic illness alone does not make a person eligible for Social Security benefits. A person applying for SSDI or SSI benefits must meet certain medical criteria. Both SSI and SSDI use the same medical criteria for eligibility. Social Security often calls the medical criteria "The Social Security Listing."

Children and adults with chronic illness can determine if they meet a Social Security Medical Listing by going to www.ssa.gov and looking for the SSA Blue Book. The blue book will list a number of medical conditions and the criteria a person must show in order to prove the person meets the SSA medical eligibility criteria. The SSA Medical Listing for children is often different from the SSA Medical Listing for an adult with the same medical condition. This means that when a child transitions to adulthood the medical eligibility criteria for Social Security benefits may change.

A person who receives SSI benefits as a child will have their benefit eligibility reviewed by Social Security when the person reaches his 18th birthday. Social Security reviews the person's eligibility for benefits using the SSA Adult Medical Listing. At the end of the review, an SSI recipient may become ineligible for the SSI benefits he has received throughout childhood. An adult who does not meet one of the Social Security Medical Listing eligibility criteria will have to show that her condition is as severe as one of the listed criteria.

Medical Records

SSA will base its decision about medical eligibility on the medical records it receives to support a finding the person meets the Social Medical Listing for their condition or that their medical condition is as severe as a listed medical criteria.

- Typically Social Security will consider medical records from the year prior to the application date because Social Security will consider the applicant's medical condition in the year prior to the application date. However, there are certain circumstances that will result in Social Security needing additional medical records for a longer period of time, such as when a person must prove he met the eligibility criteria more than 1 year prior to applying for benefits.
- Social Security must have medical records that will support a finding that the applicant meets the Social Security medical eligibility requirements. Social Security will request medical records from medical providers but often the records are lost or never sent by the medical provider. Many advocates suggest the applicant provide medical records to Social Security. Keeping a copy of the medical records is a good idea.
- A letter from the treating physician can help Social Security understand how the applicant meets the medical criteria. The letter can be submitted with the SSA application.

Social Security Disability Insurance (SSDI)

Who Is Eligible for SSDI Benefits

Social Security Disability Insurance (SSDI) is a program that provides a monthly benefit and Medicare coverage [1]. Medicare coverage begins after 29 months of SSDI benefit eligibility.

- A person who has never worked will not be eligible for SSDI benefits. Often parents of transitioning young adults mistakenly believe their child can apply for SSDI benefits. If the child has never worked then the child is not eligible for SSDI benefits even if the child meets the medical eligibly criteria for benefits.

- Adults with chronic illness who must stop work due to an increase in the time needed to deal with health issues may be eligible for SSDI.
- In order to be eligible for SSDI benefits a person must meet one of the Social Security medical requirements and must have worked for a certain period of time before applying for benefits.
- In addition, the person cannot be engaged in substantial work activity at the time the application for SSA benefits is filed. In 2016, an applicant for SSDI benefits cannot be making more than $1130 from part-time work. This dollar amount changes each year. This monthly dollar amount only applies to those who are applying for SSDI.

If the person is working more than part-time or working making more than $1130 a month, the person will be considered to be engaged in substantial gainful activity. A person who is engaged in substantial gainful activity is not eligible for SSDI benefits.

- A person who is self-employed has a different earnings cutoff he must stay within in order to be eligible for SSDI benefits. A person must contact Social Security for more information on work limits for a person who is self-employed.
- A monthly SSDI benefit will be based on the applicant's work history. Benefit checks do not start until 5 full months after the person becomes unable to work full time. Therefore, it is important to start the application process when a person becomes unable to work due to his health. Saving money that can be used to pay living expenses during the 5-month waiting period is helpful.

Appealing a Denial of Benefits

If the applicant meets both the medical and work requirements but his initial application is denied he can file an appeal. Filing an appeal allows the applicant to accrue benefits while the appeal is pending.

For example, Jack's application for SSDI benefits is denied. Jack has 60 days to appeal the denial. Jack's appeal results in an approval for benefits 10 months after he filed his application. Jack will receive 5 months of back benefits. Jack will never receive benefits for the first 5 months he was unable to engage in full-time work.

Insurance: SSDI Benefits and Medicare Eligibility

A person will become eligible for Medicare coverage after he has been receiving SSDI benefits for 24 full months. SSDI benefits begin after a 5-month waiting period has been satisfied. Therefore, the person will actually become eligible for Medicare 29 full months after he became unable to work. To prevent a lapse of coverage, the individual can COBRA his employer-based insurance for 29 months until Medicare starts. (See COBRA section below.) A person may also choose to purchase an insurance policy on either the federal Healthcare Exchange or a state Healthcare Exchange offered to residents of his state.

Supplemental Security Income (SSI)

Who Is Eligible for SSI Benefits

There are 3 groups of individuals who may be eligible for SSI benefits [2]:

- A child under the age of 18 who meets medical criteria and whose parents meet the income guidelines,

- An adult who meets the medical criteria but has not worked enough to receive SSDI benefits.
- An adult who meets the medical criteria and who receives an SSDI benefit, that is, less than the SSI benefit amount in their state.

Benefit Review at Age 18

A child who receives SSI will have a benefit review once he reaches the age of 18. The child will have to show that he still meets the SSA medical criteria, income, and asset requirements at that time. If Social Security determines the 18-year-old is no longer eligible for SSI benefits he has 10 days to appeal.

Filing the appeal within 10 days allows the SSI and Medicaid benefits to continue while the appeal is processed by Social Security. Otherwise, the young adult has 60 days to file an appeal from the date of the denial of benefits.

SSI Issues Specific to Transitioning Adult

An adult applying for SSI benefits must meet the medical, income, and asset criteria. During the application process the adult cannot be engaged in work activity that results in earnings that would result in making the SSI benefit to zero.

An adult age 18 or older will not have his parent's income and assets counted when SSA determines if the applicant meets the SSA income and asset criteria. Therefore, a child who was not eligible for SSI prior to age 18 may be eligible for SSI when he turns 18 if his own income and assets meet the Social Security eligibility guidelines. Identifying potential eligibility for SSI by an adult with chronic illness who is transitioning to adult care is helpful.

In a situation where the transitioning young adult with chronic illness lives with her parents, the amount of money the parents are contributing to the support of the adult will be counted by Social Security as income to the adult. Without an agreement to pay her portion of household expenses, the SSI benefit will be reduced to account for support provided by the parent.

However, if the adult who is applying for SSI benefits has a valid written agreement to pay her share of household expenses, there should not be a reduction in the SSI benefit amount. The written agreement is submitted to Social Security when the application for benefits is submitted. The written agreement must contain specific language in order for the agreement to be valid. An applicant for benefits can discuss the elements of a valid loan agreement with a Social Security representative.

Eligible for Both SSDI and SSI

Some young adults with chronic illness may have worked a short amount of time before becoming unable to work. These young adults may be eligible for a small SSDI benefit and a SSI benefit that subtracts any amount received from SSI. These individuals are often called "Dual Eligibles." The SSI benefit will be reduced by the SSDI benefit amount received. For example, if Isabella is eligible to receive an SSDI benefit of $200, her SSI benefit would be $530. The 2016 SSI basic benefit amount is $730. Some states supplement the basic SSI amount with state funds so the monthly SSI amount is higher.

If the SSI amount in the state is $730 then a person who receives an SSDI benefit amount will receive an SSI benefit check in the amount of $530 a month. Dual Eligibles will be eligible for Medicaid and Medicare after meeting the eligibility requirements for SSI and SSDI.

Insurance: SSI Benefits and Medicaid Coverage

In 39 states, SSI benefit approval automatically qualifies a child or adult for Medicaid coverage. In 11 states, once the SSI application has been approved, a separate application for Medicaid must be filed. The 11 states that require a separate application are: Connecticut, Hawaii, Illinois, Indiana, Minnesota, Missouri, New

Hampshire, North Dakota, Ohio, Oklahoma, and Virginia. Notice of SSI approval in these 11 states will instruct the SSI recipient on where to file the Medicaid application.

In most states, children under the age of 18 who live in a household that meets certain low-income guidelines may be eligible for Medicaid even if the child is not eligible for SSI.

The Affordable Care Act expanded Medicaid benefits to low-income adults who met certain low income and asset criteria. The United States Supreme Court held that the federal government could not mandate that states expand their Medicaid programs to nondisabled low-income adults. The Supreme Court held that such expansion of Medicaid must be voluntary not mandatory. As a result, 32 states (including the District of Columbia) have expanded Medicaid to low-income citizens in their states. A transitioning young adult who lives in 1 of the 32 states that has expanded Medicaid to low-income adults can apply for Medicaid coverage even if the person is not eligible for SSI benefits.

However, in the 19 states that have not expanded Medicaid, the only way for an adult to receive Medicaid is if the adult is also receiving SSI benefits. There are limited programs in some states that allow an adult to obtain Medicaid benefits, but these types of Medicaid waiver programs are disappearing quickly.

State Programs

Children with Special Healthcare Needs (CSHCN)

- Children with Special Healthcare Needs (CSHCN) state programs [3] offer health insurance to children that have certain medical conditions.
- CSHCN has higher income guidelines than Medicaid.
- States differ on age limits for the CSHCN program. In some states CSHCN may provide insurance coverage to some transitioning young adults with chronic illness.

State Children's Health Insurance Program (SCHIP)

The State Children's Health Insurance Program (SCHIP) [4] provides Medicaid coverage to children whose household income exceeds the Medicaid guidelines.

- Coverage under SCHIP is limited to children under the age of 18 (or in some states under the age of 19).
- Young adults with chronic illness should plan ahead and understand what type of health insurance coverage will be available to them in their state before SCHIP coverage ends.

The Affordable Care Act

Preexisting Condition Clauses

Prior to the Affordable Care Act's effective date, preexisting condition clauses [5] were typically used to deny coverage for an individual health insurance policy if the applicant for insurance had expenses related to a health condition that was treated or diagnosed within 6 months prior to enrollment on the policy. The Affordable Care Act abolished preexisting condition clauses in health insurance policies sold in the United States. A person can no longer be denied the ability to purchase a health insurance policy due to a preexisting condition.

Limiting Age of 26

The Affordable Care Act provides that all dependents must be allowed to stay on their parent's health insurance policy until the dependent reaches the age of 26 years old. This section of the Affordable Care Act went into effect in September 2010. The dependent can be married and still continue on their parent's health insurance policy. The dependent child can be employed and still continue on their parent's health insurance policy. Age is the governing factor. A dependent child does not need to be a full-time student in order to continue coverage until age 26. There is no requirement that the dependent be receiving Social Security benefits in order to continue as a covered dependent on their parent's health insurance policy until he is 26-years-old.

Caps on Coverage

The Affordable Care Act prohibits individual and group health plans from placing a lifetime limit on the aggregate dollar value of coverage that will be provided to a policyholder. Beginning in January 2014, insurers are prohibited from placing annual limits on overall plan coverage. There are 45 services that must be covered as essential services under the Affordable Care Act and these services cannot be limited or excluded under a health insurance plan. However, insurers can still exclude certain services from coverage or place a limit on the amount of services the insurer will pay for a certain service.

Health Insurance Exchanges

A Health Insurance Exchange is a government-operated Internet site that offers eligible health insurance plans in the state where the citizen resides. Each health insurance plan is operated by a private insurance company. The government does not operate the health insurance plan. A Health Insurance Exchange can also offer health insurance plans to small businesses for purchase. The federal Health Insurance Exchange can be found at www.healthcare.gov. A few states operate their own State Healthcare Exchange.

A person is not required to purchase a health insurance plan through either a federal or state Healthcare Exchange. However, if the person wants to obtain a subsidy from the government to help pay for a portion of their health insurance premium the person must purchase the policy through a Healthcare Exchange. The Healthcare Exchange will have an income and family size calculator that will determine the amount of premium subsidy a specific person will receive if the person purchases a health insurance policy on the Healthcare Exchange.

Special Enrollment Period

A person can only enroll in a health insurance plan outside of the open enrollment period if the person had health insurance coverage during the Healthcare Exchange open enrollment period but has had a change in circumstance after the close of the open enrollment period. Typical changes in circumstances that will allow a person a special enrollment period and the opportunity to purchase a health insurance policy on a Healthcare Exchange are:

- A move to another state
- A change in income
- A loss of health insurance coverage
- A change in family size

State Insurance Law: Continued Coverage if Child Is Incapable of Self-Support

Private insurance policies only have to provide coverage for dependent children up to their 26th birthday. A few states have state laws that extend dependent coverage after the dependent's 26th birthday.

Young adults with chronic illness who reach the age of 26 may qualify for an extension of benefits under a state law that provides for a continuation of coverage if the dependent child is incapable of self-support due to a mental or physical condition. The health insurance coverage is extended until the dependent is able to self-support.

If the employer is contributing to premium payments the employer will typically be required to continue to do so.

For example, Amy is covered under her mother's employer-based policy. The mother contributes $100 toward the premium and her employer pays the other $400. Amy reaches the limiting age on the policy. Amy's treating physician certifies in writing that Amy is incapable of self-support due to her medical condition. The employer continues to pay the $400 portion of the premium.

The following steps typically have to be taken in order to apply for an extension of benefits under a state law that extends health insurance coverage to a dependent child if the child is incapable of self-support due to a mental or physical condition:

- Obtain a form from the heath insurance company prior to the young adult reaching the limiting age on the policy.
- The treating physician must certify in writing that the young adult is incapable of self-support due to their medical condition.
- The insurance company can request information about income the young adult has earned from work activity.
- The young adult who has made enough money to support himself will not be able to extend coverage under his parent's health insurance policy.
- Some state laws allow an insurance company to determine the amount a person can make that will be considered self-support based on cost of living in the state. Most state laws do not have dollar limits on the amount of money a child can make from work activity and still be considered incapable of self-support.
- The insurance company can require annual recertification by the treating physician certifying that the child continues to be unable to self-support due to medical condition and has not made enough money in the prior year to self-support.
- The young adult must be unmarried.
- The following states do not have a state law that extends coverage to young adults incapable of self-support: Alabama, Alaska, Kansas, Maine, Oklahoma, and Oregon.
- A young adult who is not eligible for an extension of coverage based on his inability to self-support can extend coverage under COBRA for 36 months. Under COBRA, the policyholder must pay the full premium amount. See following section on COBRA.

COBRA Extension of Benefits

COBRA Overview

For employers with 20 or more employees, the Consolidated Omnibus Budget Reconciliation Act of 1985 (COBRA) [6] provides a continuation of health insurance coverage if a qualifying event takes place. The coverage under the policy remains the same. An employee is eligible for an extension of coverage under COBRA if a "qualifying event" takes place. The COBRA extension period varies depending on the qualifying event (Table 31.1).

Under COBRA the employee pays the full premium. Often employers pay part of the health insurance premiums for employees. Some employees do not know the actual full cost of the health insurance policy. It is important to know the full premium amount for any employer-provided health insurance coverage.

In the event coverage must be extended under COBRA, it is important to have the funds to pay the full COBRA premium. Saving money in advance will ensure the employee has the funds

Table 31.1 COBRA qualifying events and related extension periods

COBRA qualifying event	Extension period (months)
Termination, resignation, or layoff	18
Death of policyholder	36
Divorce or separation from policyholder	36
Adult becomes eligible for SSDI benefits	29
Child reaches a limiting age under the policy	36

SSDI Social Security Disability Insurance

to pay for COBRA coverage. A late premium payment will result in loss of coverage.

COBRA Time Table

The following time tables are important under COBRA:

- The employer has up to 14 days after the employee notifies employer of a qualifying event to provide a COBRA election notice.
- The employee then has 60 days to decide whether to elect COBRA continuation coverage.
- The employee has 45 days after the day the COBRA coverage is elected to pay the initial premium.
- Failure to pay the COBRA premium will result in cancellation of the policy.

Conclusion

Transitioning young adults have a variety of options for health insurance coverage (Appendix). Understanding those options is important to accessing the care needed to treat their chronic conditions.

Appendix

Resources

- To obtain each state's Department of Insurance contact information go to: www.naic.org/state_web_map.htm.
- The Social Security Administration's Website has information on the different SSA programs and application procedures at: www.ssa.gov.
- To apply for Social Security benefits call SSA at 1-800-772-1213. An application may also be completed on line at www.ssa.gov or at a local Social Security office but only for those applying for Social Security Disability Insurance benefits.
- A list of the SSA medical criteria can be found at: www.ssa.gov/disability/professionals/bluebook.
- For a list of Medicaid eligibility income guidelines by state visit: http://www.statehealthfacts.org/comparetable.jsp?ind=203&cat=4.
- For more information about each state's SCHIP program please visit: http://www.insurekidsnow.gov.
- The Department of Labor has information on COBRA at: www.dol.gov/ebsa/faqs/faq_consumer_cobra.html.

References

1. USC 1382. Eligibility for benefits. US Government Publishing Office. https://www.gpo.gov/fdsys/pkg/USCODE-2010-title42/html/USCODE-2010-title42-chap7-subchapXVI-partA-sec1382.htm. Accessed 6 June 2016.
2. USC 701(a)(1)(D). Authorization of appropriations; purposes; definitions. US Government Publishing Office. https://www.gpo.gov/fdsys/pkg/USCODE-2010-title42/html/USCODE-2010-title42-chap7-subchapV-sec701.htm. Accessed 6 June 2016.
3. USC 1397bb. General contents of State child health plan; eligibility; outreach. US Government Publishing Office. https://www.gpo.gov/fdsys/pkg/USCODE-2010-title42/html/USCODE-2010-title42-chap7-subchapXXI-sec1397bb.htm. Accessed 6 June 2016.
4. USC 1181. Increased portability through limitation on preexisting condition exclusions. US Government Publishing Office. https://www.gpo.gov/fdsys/pkg/USCODE-2010-title29/html/USCODE-2010-title29-chap18-subchapI-subtitleB-part7-subpartA-sec1181.htm. Accessed 6 June 2016.
5. CFR 54.4980H-1. Definitions. US Government Publishing Office. https://www.gpo.gov/fdsys/pkg/CFR-2014-title26-vol17/xml/CFR-2014-title26-vol17-sec54-4980H-1.xml. Accessed 6 June 2016.
6. US Department of Labor. Health Plans & Benefits: Continuation of Health Coverage – COBRA. https://www.dol.gov/general/topic/health-plans/cobra. Accessed 17 June 2016.

Index

Note: Page numbers followed by *b*, *f*, and *t* indicate boxes, figures, and tables, respectively

M. Pilapil et al. (eds.), *Care of Adults with Chronic Childhood Conditions*,
DOI 10.1007/978-3-319-43827-6

D

N

Printed by Printforce, the Netherlands